Bioactive Phytochemicals

Perspectives for Modern Medicine

— Volume 1 —

Bioactive Phytochemicals

Perspectives for Modern Medicine

— *Volume 1* —

Editor
V.K. Gupta
Sr. Principal Scientist & Head,
Central Animal Facility
Indian Institute of Integrative Medicine (CSIR),
Canal Road, Jammu – 180 001,
India

2012
DAYA PUBLISHING HOUSE®
New Delhi - 110 002

ISBN 978-81-7035-778-0 (Series)
ISBN 978-81-7035-779-7 (Volume 1)

Published by : **Daya Publishing House®**
4760-61/23, Ansari Road, Darya Ganj,
New Delhi - 110 002
Phone: 23245578, 23244987
Fax: (011) 23260116
e-mail : dayabooks@vsnl.com
website : www.dayabooks.com

Laser Typesetting : **Classic Computer Services**
Delhi - 110 035

Printed at : **Salasar Imaging Systems**
Delhi - 110 035

PRINTED IN INDIA

DEDICATION

**This book is dedicate to my wife.
without her patience, understanding,
support, and most of all love, the
completion of this work would
not have been possible**

Nagasaki
International University

Nagasaki International University

2825-7 Huis Ten Bosch, Sasebo,
Nagasaki 859-3298 Japan

Tel +81-956-2020

Fax +81-956-39-311

URL http://www.niu.ac.jp

Foreword

"Bioactive Phytochemicals: Perspectivs for Modern Medicine" has been born from the editor's hope that the readers will be able to obtain the different kinds of knowledge from many contributors. Therefore, the authors were invited from wide fields, like isolation, structure elucidation and pharmacological activity related to plants and marine products. The authors in this thematic issue provide a comprehensive summary of latest knowledge and references on the field of bioactive phytochemicals. Phytochemicals have supplied a huge resource of organic substances having different structural features¡¡and different biological activities. For example at least 470 different compounds have been determined to be in the licorice root. It is well known that the accumulated data in bioactive phytochemicals did bring not only a large amount of lead compound for drugs, but also the discovery and development of drugs. In this issue of "Bioactive phytochemicals: Perspectives for modern medicine", fifteen reviews have been incorporated and highlighted their detail related to phytochemicals. It might be evaluated that these evidences reviewed in this issue can be applied widely in the field of drug discovery. Moreover, the more than 1223 references found at the end of the individual reviews, will make this thematic issue useful for not only phytochemical researchers but also many scientists working in the numerous fields of natural products emphasizing the high scientific standing of the issue.

Much energies have been accumulated to share current information by the contributors. Without their efforts and input this term issue has not been published. The editor sincerely appreciate the time spent and the wisdom shared in bringing this term book to fruition.

Yukihiro Shoyama
Faculty of Pharmaceutical Science

Preface

Biologically active compounds from plant sources have always been of great interest to scientists throughout the world and are getting much attention now-a-days for treating various diseases. Primitive man, through trial and error, gained knowledge of herbals and passed it on to their progeny. It appears that for thousands of years herbs were perhaps used for both their magical powers as well as medicinal values. Ancient civilization flourished in 3000 BC onward in Egypt, Middle East, India and China, with a parallel growth in the refinement of herbal medicine. The Egyptian *Ebers Papyrus* (1500 BC) is one of the earliest records providing information on herbs. In India, *circa* 1500 BC, *Vedas* included the *Ayurveda* system of medicine along with its vastly sophisticated information-base on herbs, with about 350 herbals cited in this compilation. Chinese traditional pharmacopoeia lists over 5700 traditional medicines which are mostly of herbal origin. Over the last 10 years Europe has witnessed a growth in the practice of Herbal Medicine.

In spite of the great advances in synthetic and combinatorial chemistry, medicinal plants still make an important contribution in pharmaceutical innovation. According to the World Health Organization (WHO), about 65-80% of the world's population living in developing countries, still depends essentially on plants for primary health care because of poverty and lack of access to modern medicine. Some Western countries such as Germany, France, Italy and the United States have developed appropriate guidelines for registration of herbal medicines. Discovery of the blockbuster anticancer drug paclitaxel (Taxol) from the yew tree (*Taxus brevifolia*) once again helped to revive the interest towards herbal medicine both among the academia as well as in pharmaceutical companies. There are around 250,000 species of higher plants that exist on earth, but merely only 5 to 10 per cent of these have been investigated so far. In USA, the botanical market, including herbs and medicinal plants is estimated around US$1.6 billion per annum. The dominating countries are China with exports of over 120,000 tonnes annually and India with some 32,000 tonnes annually. It is estimated that Europe imports medicinal plant from Asia and Africa is about 400,000 tonnes annually which cost approximately US$ 1 billion. With the growing awareness about this new commodity towards the foreign-exchange reserves, a number of national economies are beginning to emerge. Surveys are being conducted to unearth new plant sources of herbal remedies and medicines to satisfy this growing demands.

The development of organic chemistry has shown that the ability of herbal medicine to treat the body depended upon its chemical constituents. Chemists first began extracting and isolating chemicals from plants in the 18th century. A number of medicinal plants have been subjected to detailed chemical investigations and this has lead to the isolation of pure bioactive molecules which have been pharmacologically evaluated. This has led to the discovery of new drugs along with new applications. These bioactive molecules are used as therapeutic agents, starting materials and new reagents for molecular biology research. At present there are 125 clinically useful drugs of known constitution which have been isolated from about 100 species of higher plants. It has been estimated that about 5000 plant species have been studied in detail as possible sources of new drugs. The bulk production of plant based drugs is one of the most important tasks for the pharmaceutical industry. At least 25% of the prescription drugs issued in the USA and Canada contain bioactive compounds that are derived from or modeled after plant natural products. Medicinal plants would be the best source to obtain a variety of drugs and therefore such plants should be investigated to understand better about their properties, safety and efficacy.

Encouraging results accelerated their enterprise and natural product chemists have given to the world some of its most useful drugs such as morphine, digoxin, d-tubocurarine, ephedrine, quinine, vincristine, paclitaxel etc.

The present book "*Bioactive Phytochemicals: Perspectives for Modern Medicine Vol. 1*" comprises the vast body of research on the subject and includes fifteen review chapters written by eminent scientists and researchers from India, Brazil, China, Japan, México, Singapore and South Africa. The editor express his gratefulness to the contributors who have shared valuable thoughts through their scholarly contributions and timely submission of manuscripts for the present volume and also thanks to the publisher, *M/s Daya Publishing House, New Delhi* and their staff for timely and expeditious job rendering the manuscript press-ready.

V.K. Gupta

Contents

	Foreword	*vii*
	Preface	*ix*
1.	**Bioactive Pregnanes and Cardenolides from *Nerium oleander*** *Liming Bai, Ming Zhao, Yuhua Bai, Asami Toki, Ryo Hasegawa, Junichi Sakai, Toshiaki Hasegawa, Mariko Ando, Tomokazu Mitsui, Hirotsugu Ogura, Takao Kataoka, Katsutoshi Hirose and Masayoshi Ando* **(Japan, China)**	1
2.	**Flavonoids and their Anti-Diabetic Potentials** *A.O. Ayeleso, O.O. Oguntibeju and N. Brooks* **(South Africa)**	79
3.	**Limonene: A Systematic Overview for its Chemistry and Bioactivity** *P. Koul, G. D. Singh, R. Sharma, V. K. Gupta and S. Singh* **(India)**	107
4.	**Phytochemicals Against Liver Disease I: Recent Progress in the Treatment of NAFLD and AFLD by Natural Drug Products and their Active Chemical Entities, in China and other Countries** *Fang Peng, Shawn Spencer, Xiumei Wu, Yan Xu, Su Zeng, Guangming Liu, Chenggui Zhang, Pengfei Gao, Yu Zhao and Xiaojiang Hao* **(China)**	127
5.	**Phytochemicals Against Liver Disease II: Recent Progress in the Treatment of Liver Fibrosis by Natural Drug Products and their Active Chemical Entities, in China and Other Countries** *Pengfei Gao, Lu Xu, Mengxi Xu, Xiumei Wu, Hui Li, Yan Xu, Guangming Liu, Guoping Yang, Xiaoman Lv, Ping Gan, Li Lu, Shawn Spencer, Yu Zhao, and Xiaojiang Hao* **(China)**	177
6.	**Anti-Allergic Leads from Indian Medicinal Plant** *Pulok K. Mukherjee and P. Venkatesh* **(India)**	215

7. **Essential Oils from Brazilian Amazonia** **255**

Valdir F. Veiga Junior, Ana P. M. Rodrigues-Bastos, André L. Rüdiger, Iuri B. Barros, Joelma M. Alcântara, Klenicy K.L. Yamaguchi, Lidiam M. Leandro, Priscilla A. Oliveira And Roosevelt H. Leal ***(Brazil)***

8. **Phytochemical and Pharmacological Profile of Plants belonging to *Strychnos* Genus: A Review** **277**

P. Rajesh, V. Rajesh Kannan, S. Latha and P. Selvamani ***(India)***

9. **Phytochemicals as Natural Antimicrobials: Prospects and Challenges** **331**

Sujogya K. Panda and Chandi C. Rath ***(India)***

10. **Biomedical Potentials of Filamentous Marine Cyanobacterial Natural Products** **381**

Lik Tong Tan and Ashootosh Tripathi ***(Singapore)***

11. **Natural Bioactive Compound from Marine Plants with Anticancer Potential: A Review** **395**

S. Arif Nisha, R. Sakthivel, S. Karutha Pandian and K. Pandima Devi ***(India)***

12. **The Lauraceae Alkaloids** **413**

Dayana L. Custódio, Diego C. Squinello and Valdir F. Veiga Junior ***(Brazil)***

13. **Phytochemical and Pharmacological Profile of *Lepidium sativum* Linn.** **437**

Alok Shukla, C.S. Singh and Papiya Bigoniya ***(India)***

14. **Chemistry and Pharmacology of Selected Asian and American Medicinal Species of *Justicia*** **457**

Juan Carlos Gomez-Verjan, Ricardo Reyes-Chilpa and María Isabel Aguilar ***(Mexico)***

15. **Biological Activities of *Anoectochilus formosanus* Hayat and its Active Component** **477**

Xiao-Ming Du and Yukihiro Shoyama ***(China, Japan)***

Index **495**

Bioactive Phytochemicals: Perspectives for Modern Medicine Vol. 1 (2012) *Pages* **1–77**
Editor: **V.K. Gupta**
Published by: **DAYA PUBLISHING HOUSE, NEW DELHI**

1

Bioactive Pregnanes and Cardenolides from *Nerium oleander*

Liming Bai[1,3], Ming Zhao[1,3], Yuhua Bai[7], Asami Toki[1], Ryo Hasegawa[1], Junichi Sakai[2], Toshiaki Hasegawa[1,5], Mariko Ando[6], Tomokazu Mitsui[4], Hirotsugu Ogura[4], Takao Kataoka[4], Katsutoshi Hirose[8] and Masayoshi Ando[2,*]

ABSTRACT

*Four new pregnanes, 21-hydroxypregna-4,6-diene-3,12,20-trione (**1**), 20R-hydroxypregna-4,6-diene-3,12-dione (**2**), 16β,17β-epoxy-12β-hydroxypregna-4,6-diene-3,20-dione (**3**) 20S,21-dihydroxypregn-4-en-3,12-dione (**6**) were isolated from Nerium*

1 Graduate School of Science and Technology, Niigata University, Ikarashi, 2-8050, Niigata, 950-2181, Japan.

2 Department of Chemistry and Chemical Engineering, Faculty of Engineering Niigata University, Ikarashi, 2-8050, Niigata, 950-2181, Japan.

3 College of Chemistry and Chemistry Engineering, Qiqihar University, Wenhuadajie, Qiqihar, Heilongjiang Province,161006, People's Republic of China.

4 Center for Biological Resources and Informatics, Tokyo Institute of Technology, 4259 Nagatsuta-cho, Midori-ku, Yokohama 226-8501, Japan

5 Mitsubishi Gas Chemical Company Inc., Niigata Research Laboboratory, 182, Shinwari, Tayuhama, Niigata 950-3112, Japan.

6 Technical Division, School of Engineering, Tohoku University, 6-6 Aramaki-aza- Aoba, Aoba-ku, Sendai 980-8579, Japan

7 Department of Medicinal Chemistry, Pharmaceutical Department, Daqing Campus of Harbin Medical University, Xinyang Road, Hi-Tech Zone, Daquig, Heilongjiang Province, 163319, People's Republic of China.

8 KNC Laboratories Co. Ltd. 3-2-34 Takatsukadai, Nishi-ku, Kobe, Hyogo 651-2271, Japan.

* *Corresponding author*: E-mail: andomasa@kdp.biglobe.ne.jp;Tel and Fax: +81-22-229-2916

Present address: 22-20 Keiwa-machi, Taihaku-ku, Sendai, 982-0823, Japan.

*oleander, together with four known compounds, 12β-hydroxypregna-4,6,16-triene-3,20-dione (neridienone A, **4**), 20S,21-dihydroxypregna-4,6-diene-3,12-dione (neridienone B, **5**), 21-O-(β-glucopyranosyl)-4-ene-3,20-dione (**7**), and 3β-O-{β-D-glucopyranosyl-(1→2)-[β-D-glucopyranosyl-(1→4)]-β-D-glucopyranosyl}-17α-pregn-5-en-20-one (**8**). The structures of compounds **1–3** and **6** were established on the basis of their spectroscopic data. The anti-inflammatory activity in vitro of compounds **1–8** was examined based on inhibitory activity against the induction of intercellular adhesion molecule-1 (ICAM-1), and compound **4** was active. The cytotoxic activity of compounds **1–8** was evaluated against three human cell lines, normal human fibroblast cells (WI-38), malignant tumor cells induced from WI-38 (VA-13), human liver tumor cells (HepG2). Compound **4** showed significant cell growth inhibition of VA-13 and HepG2 cells. The MDR-reversal activity of compounds **1–8** was evaluated based on the amount of calcein accumulated in MDR human ovarian cancer 2780AD cells in the presence of each compound. Compounds **1**, **2**, and **5** showed significant effects on calcein accumulation.*

*Four new cardenolide monoglycosides, named cardenolides N-1 (**9**), N-2 (**10**), N-3 (**11**), and N-4 (**12**) were isolated from the less polar fraction of ethyl acetate extracts of N. oleander, together with two known cardenolides **13** and **20**, and seven cardenolide monoglycosides **14–19** and **21**. The structures of compounds **9–12** were established on the basis of their spectroscopic data. The anti-inflammatory activity in vitro of compounds **9–21** was examined on the basis of inhibitory activity against ICAM-1, and compounds **9**, **13**, **14** and **19–21** were active at an IC_{50} value of less than 1 μM. The cytotoxic activity of the isolated thirteen compounds **9–21** was evaluated against WI-38, VA-13, and HepG2 cells. Compounds **9**, **14**, and **19–21** were active toward VA-13 cells and compounds **9**, **19**, and **2 0** were active toward HepG2 cells at IC_{50} values of less than 1 μM. Compounds **12**, **13**, **18**, and **20** showed selective cell growth inhibitory activity toward VA-13 cells compared with that of parental normal WI-38 cells. The MDR-reversal activity of compounds **9–21** was evaluated and compounds **12**, **17**, and **18** showed significant effects on calcein accumulation.*

*Twelve polar cardenolide monoglycosides, **22**, **23**, **25–34** and oleagenin (**24**) were isolated from the more polar fraction of ethyl acetate extracts of stems and twigs of N. oleander. The structures of two new cardenolide monoglycosides, cardenolides B-1 (**22**) and B-2 (**23**) were established on the basis of their spectroscopic data. The in vitro anti-inflammatory activity of compounds **22–34** was examined on the basis of inhibitory activity against ICAM-1. Compounds **25–28** were active at an IC_{50} value of less than 0.4 mM. The cytotoxic activity of compounds **22–34** was evaluated against WI-38, VA-13, and HepG2. Compounds **25**, **27**, and **28** were active toward these three cell lines at IC_{50} values of less than 0.7 mM and compounds **26** and **29** were active toward them at IC_{50} values of less than 1.5 μM. The MDR cancer-reversal activity of compounds **22–34** was evaluated on the basis of the amount of calcein accumulated in MDR human ovarian cancer 2780AD cells in the presence of each compound. Compound **22** and **33** showed significant effects on calcein accumulation.*

*One new cardenolide diglycosides **35** was isolated from N. oleander, together with ten known cardenolide diglycosides **36–45**. The structure of compound **35** was established to be 3β-O-[β-D-glucopyranosyl-(1→4)-β-D-diginopyranosyl]-14α-hydroxy-8-oxo-8,14-seco-5β-card-20(22)-enolide on the basis of their spectroscopic data. The anti-inflammatory activity in vitro of compounds **35–45** was examined on the basis of inhibitory activity against the induction of ICAM-1, and compounds **35– 39** were active at an IC_{50} value of less than 1 μM.*

The cytotoxic activity of compounds **36–45** *was evaluated against WI-38, VA-13, and HepG2 cells. Compounds* **36–39** *were active toward WI-38 cells, and compounds* **36**, **37**, *and* **39** *were active toward HepG2 cells at IC_{50} values of less than 1 µM. The MDR-reversal activity of compounds* **35–45** *was evaluated and compounds* **35** *and* **42** *showed significant effects on calcein accumulation.*

Sixteen cardenolide triglycosides **46–61** *were isolated from stems and twigs, and leaves of N. oleander. Among them, 3β-O-(4-O-gentiobiosyl-D-diginosyl)-7β,8-epoxy-14-hydroxy-5β,14β-card-20(22)-enolide named cardenolide B-3 (***61***) was isolated first from natural sources by us and the structure was determined by spectroscopic analyses. The in vitro anti-inflammatory activity of compounds* **46–61** *was examined on the basis of inhibitory activity against ICAM-1. Compounds* **46–50** *were active at an IC_{50} value of less than 7µM. The cytotoxic activity of isolated compounds was evaluated against WI-38, VA-13, HepG2. Compounds* **46–50** *were active toward WI-38 cells, compounds* **46** *and* **50** *were active toward V-13 cells, and compounds* **46–50** *were active toward HepG2 cells at an IC_{50} value of less than 10 µM. The MDR cancer-reversal activity of compounds* **46–61** *was evaluated on the basis of the amount of calcein accumulated in MDR human ovarian cancer 2780AD cells in the presence of each compound. Compounds* **58** *and* **59** *showed significant effects on calcein accumulation.*

Keywords: *Nerium oleander, Pregnane, Cardenolide monoglycoside, Cardenolide* diglycoside, Cardenolide triglycoside, Anti-inflammatory activity *in vitro*, Cytotoxic activity, MDR reversal activity.

Introduction

Nerium oleander L. (synonyms: *Nerium indicum; Nerium odorum*) (Apocyaceae) is a medium-sized evergreen flowering tree of 2–5 m in height and is planted throughout Japan as a garden and roadside trees. This species was distributed originally in the Mediterranean region, sub-tropical Asia, and the Indo-Pakistan subcontinent, and has been used as a traditional medicine because of its antibacterial, anticancer, antidote, antileprotic, and cardiotonic properties (Chopla *et al.*, 1956). Abe and Yamauchi reported the isolation of five pregnanes from the root bark of this plant (Abe and Yamauchi, 1976). Recently, we reported the results of the examination of the triterpenoid constituents from the leaves of *N. oleander* (Fu *et al.*, 2005; Chao *et al.*, 2006). In this chapter, we report the results of a phytochemical and biological investigation of pregnanes and cardenolides from leaves, stems, and twigs of this plant. Cardenolides in the leaves (Abe and Yamauchi, 1978; Yamauchi and Abe, 1978; Abe and Yamauchi, 1979; Yamauchi and Abe, 1983; Abe and Yamauchi, 1992; Abe and Yamauchi, 1996; Siddiiqui *et al.*, 1997; Begum *et al.*, 1999) roots and root bark (Yamauchi *et al.*, 1976; Hanada *et al.*, 1992; Huq *et al.*, 1999) have been investigated because of interest in their biological activity (Fieser and Fieser, 1959). The cardiac glycosides, digitoxin and digoxin, have been used in the treatment of cardiac diseases for many years (Fieser and Fieser, 1959; Hong *et al.*, 2006), but they have a narrow therapeutic window because of arrhythmia and disturbance of atrio-ventricular contraction. Anticancer utilization of digitoxin, digoxin, and related cardenolides has been also investigated (López-Lázaro *et al.*, 2005; Roy *et al.*, 2005). These reports prompted us to reinvestigate cardenolides in*N. oleander* and their biological activities.

Materials and Methods

General Experimental Procedures

Melting points are uncorrected. Optical rotation values were measured using a Horiba Sepa-200 polarimeter. IR spectra were recorded on a Shimadzu FTIR-4200 infrared spectrometer. UV spectra were measured using a JASCO V-530 UV/vis spectrometer. ^1H and ^{13}C NMR spectra were measured with a Varian Unity-plus instrument at 500 and 125 MHz. ^1H NMR assignments were determined by ^1H–^1H COSY experiments. ^{13}C NMR assignments were determined using DEPT, HMQC, and HMBC experiments. HRFABMS were recorded on a JEOL JMS-HX110 instrument and HREIMS were recorded on a JEOL GC mate-BU20 and JEOL JMS-HX110 instruments. Silica gel (70–230 mesh) was employed for column chromatography and silica gel (230–400 mesh) for flash column chromatography. HPLC separations were performed on a Hitachi L-6200 HPLC instrument with an Inertsil Prep-sil GL 10 × 250 mm stainless steel column and an Inertsil Prep-ODS GL 10 × 250 mm stainless steel column and monitored by a Hitachi L-7400 UV detector and a Shodex SE-61 RI detector.

Plant Material

The leaves, stems, and twigs of *Nerium oleander* were collected in Niigata City, Niigata Province, Japan, in November 2001. The plant was identified by Dr. K. Yonekura, Department of Biology, Faculty of Science, Tohoku University, Sendai, Japan. A voucher specimen (2001-11-10) was deposited at the Department of Chemistry and Chemical Engineering, Niigata University.

Extraction, Isolation, and Identification of Pregnanes 1–6 and Pregnane Glycosides 7 and 8

The air-dried bark and twigs (19.5 kg) were combined and extracted with MeOH (85 l) for 20 days. The MeOH extract was concentrated to 4 l and extracted with hexane (8 × 1.0 l). Water (1.3 l) was added to the MeOH layer, extracted with EtOAc (3 × 3.0 l), dried (Na_2SO_4), and concentrated to give an oily material (96.5 g). This was separated by column chromatography [silica gel (1.1 kg), gradient mixture of hexane, EtOAc, and MeOH] into five fractions, A–E. Fraction B [hexane–EtOAc (1:1), EtOAc], fraction C (EtOAc), and fraction D [EtOAc–MeOH (1:1)] gave on drying viscous oils, weighing 29.58 g, 23.33 g, and 32.14 g, respectively. Fraction B was dissolved in EtOAc (110 ml), stirred for 1 h, filtered, and concentrated to give a viscous oil (30 g). This was separated into nine fractions (B1–B9) by column chromatography [silica gel (1.5 kg), gradient mixture of hexane, EtOAc, and MeOH]. Fraction B5 [hexane–EtOAc (4:6)] gave on drying a viscous oil (0.670 g). Fractions B6 and B7 [EtOAc (100 per cent)] gave on drying additional viscous oils (B6; 13.39 g, B7; 2.61 g). Fraction B5 afforded compound **3** (34.2 mg, 0.00018 per cent) by separation using HPLC [silica gel, hexane–EtOAc (4:6)] and further separation of the second fraction obtained (404 mg) by HPLC [ODS, MeOH–MeCN–H_2O (1:9:10)]. Fraction B6 was subjected to silica gel column chromatography [silica gel (700 g), gradient of hexane, EtOAc, and MeOH] to give seven fractions, B61–B67 [hexane–EtOAc (1:1), B64 (11.5 g)], and B64 was separated using HPLC [ODS, MeOH–MeCN–H_2O (1:6:9)] to give sub-fraction B642 (827 mg). This sub-fraction was further separated by HPLC [ODS, MeOH–MeCN–H_2O (1:9:10)] to give B6422 (283 mg), which in turn, was purified by HPLC [ODS, MeOH–MeCN–H_2O (1:6:9.3)] to give B64222 (180 mg), and then by additional HPLC [ODS, MeOH–MeCN–H_2O (1:9:10)] to give **4** (131.4 mg, 0.00067 per cent). Fraction C was separated by HPLC [silica gel, hexane-EtOAc (1:59)] into six fractions, C1– C6, and C3 (9.32 g) was separated by HPLC [silica gel, hexane-EtOAc (3:7)] into four further fractions, C31–C34. Fraction C33 (4.10 g) was separated by HPLC [ODS, MeOH–MeCN–H_2O (1:6:9)] to give thirteen fractions (C33-1– C33-13), with **1** (55.9 mg, 0.00029 per cent) obtained from C33-4 without further purification. Fraction C33-9 (950 mg) was further separated by HPLC [ODS, MeOH–MeCN–H_2O (4:4:9)] to give **2** (43.0 mg, 0.00022 per cent). Fraction D (30.66 g) was dissolved in EtOAc (75 mL) and filtered. The filtrate gave on dryness a viscous oil (17.06 g), which was separated by column chromatography [silica gel, 620 g; gradient of $CHCl_3$ and MeOH; $CHCl_3$–MeOH (98:2)–MeOH(100 per cent)] to give twelve fractions (D1–D12). Fraction D4 [$CHCl_3$–MeOH (98:2), 1.66 g] was further separated by HPLC [silica gel, EtOAc (100 per cent)] to give six fractions (D41–D46). Fraction D45 (667 mg) was separated by HPLC [ODS, MeOH–MeCN–H_2O (4:4:10)] to afford six additional fractions (D451–D456), and D452 gave **5** (164.5 mg, 0.00084 per cent). The fraction DD5-3 (86.5 mg) was further separated by HPLC [ODS, MeOH–MeCN–H_2O (1:1:3)] to give **6** [24.7 mg (0.00014 per cent)]. The *n*-BuOH extracts were dried and concentrated to give an oily residue (244 g). A part of the *n*-BuOH extract (6.02 g) was separated by column chromatography on silica gel (539 g) in 14 fractions, A–N, using a gradient of $CHCl_3$ and MeOH. Fraction I [$CHCl_3$–MeOH (7:3)] gave on drying a viscous oil (896 mg), which was further separated by HPLC [ODS, MeOH–MeCN–H_2O (1:4:11)] into seven fractions (I-1–I-7). Fraction I-6 gave **8** [20.3 mg (0.0042 per cent)].

Air-dried leaves (9.91 kg) were extracted two times with MeOH (66 and 39 l) for 3 and 4 days. The MeOH extract was concentrated to 10 l and extracted with hexane (5 × 5 l). Water (4 × 10 l) was added to the MeOH layer and extracted with EtOAc (5 × 5 l). Then saturated NaCl aqueous solution (10 l) was added to the MeOH layer and extracted with *n*-BuOH (4 × 10 l). The *n*-BuOH extracts were dried and concentrated to give an oily material (528 g). To a part of the *n*-BuOH extract (53.76 g), 150 ml of MeOH was added, stirred for 1 h, and filtered. The filtrate was concentrated to give on drying a viscous oil, which was dissolved in MeOH (150 ml). $CHCl_3$ (990 ml) was added into the MeOH solution,stirred for 1 h, and filtered. The filtrate was concentrated to give a viscous oil, NB1 (18.75 g), which was dissolved with 200 ml of water, and extracted with $CHCl_3$ (5 × 200 ml). The $CHCl_3$ extracts were concentrated to give a semisolid, BC (5.54 g), which was separated by column chromatography on silica gel (275 g) in 11 fractions, BC-1–BC-11, using a gradient of $CHCl_3$ and MeOH. Fraction BC-4 [$CHCl_3$–MeOH (9:1)] gave 183.1 mg of a semisolid, which was further separated by HPLC [ODS, MeOH–H_2O (8:2)] into three fractions (BC4-1–BC4-3). Fraction BC4-1 gave a viscous oil (142.7 mg), which was separated by HPLC [ODS, MeOH–H_2O (6:4)] into five fractions (BC41-1–BC41-5). Fraction BC41-2 (88.2 mg) was separated by HPLC [ODS, MeOH–MeCN–H_2O (1:2:7)] to give **7** [32.2 mg (0.0032 per cent)].

21-Hydroxypregna-4,6-diene-3,12,20-trione (1)

Colorless microcrystals; mp 161–163 °C; $[\alpha]^{24}_{D}$+90.6 (*c* 0.223, MeOH); UV ($CHCl_3$) λ_{max}(log ε) 265 (4.23) nm; IR ($CHCl_3$) ν_{max} 3500, 1709, 1663, 1630, 1618 cm^{-1}; ^{1}H ($CdCl_3$, 500 MHz) and ^{13}C NMR ($CdCl_3$, 125 MHz) data, see Tables 1.1 and 1.2; HREIMS *m/z* 342.1832 (calcd for $C_{21}H_{26}O_4$ 342.1831); HRFABMS *m/z* 343.1906 $[M+H]^+$ (calcd for $C_{21}H_{27}O_3$, 343.1909).

Table 1.1: ^{13}C NMR spectroscopic data of compounds. **1**–**3** (125 MHz, δ in ppm, $CDCl_3$)

Position	*1*	*2*	*3*
1	33.6 (CH_2)	33.5 (CH_2)	33.5 (CH_2)
2	33.6 (CH_2)	33.6 (CH_2)	33.9 (CH_2)
3	198.7 (qC)	198.8 (qC)	199.3 (qC)
4	124.8 (CH)	124.7 (CH)	124.3 (CH)
5	161.1 (qC)	161.4 (qC)	162.4 (qC)
6	129.2 (CH)	129.0 (CH)	129.1 (CH)
7	137.7 (CH)	138.1 (CH)	138.1 (CH)
8	36.6 (CH)	36.3 (CH)	34.9 (CH)
9	51.5 (CH)	51.0 (CH)	48.6 (CH)
10	36.2 (qC)	36.2 (qC)	36.0 (qC)
11	37.2 (CH_2)	37.4 (CH_2)	28.7 (CH_2)
12	211.6 (qC)	216.6 (qC)	72.2 (CH)
13	59.1 (qC)	57.7 (qC)	49.7 (qC)
14	54.2 (CH)	52.7 (CH)	58.2 (CH)
15	23.0 (CH_2)	22.9 (CH_2)	28.4 (CH_2)
16	23.5 (CH_2)	24.8 (CH_2)	67.1 (CH)
17	49.5 (CH)	50.7 (CH)	74.8 (qC)
18	13.5 (CH_3)	12.1 (CH_3)	10.1 (CH_3)
19	15.9 (CH_3)	15.9 (CH_3)	16.0 (CH_3)
20	210.8 (qC)	68.0 (CH)	208.2 (qC)
21	69.5 (CH_2)	23.1 (CH_3)	25.3 (CH_3)

@20R-Hydroxypregna-4,6-diene-3,12-dione (2)

Colorless microcrystals; mp 167–170 °C; $[\alpha]^{20}_{D}$ +85.3 (*c* 0.346, $CHCl_3$); UV ($CHCl_3$) λ_{max}(log ε) 278 (4.19) nm; IR ($CHCl_3$) ν_{max} 3416, 1694, 1663, 1653, 1618 cm^{-1}; ^{1}H ($CHCl_3$, 500 MHz) and ^{13}C NMR ($CHCl_3$, 125 MHz) data, see Tables 1.1 and 1.2; HRFABMS *m/z* 329.2133 $[M+H]^+$ (calcd for $C_{21}H_{29}O_3$, 329.2117).

16β,17β-Epoxy-12β-hydroxypregna-4,6-diene-3,20-dione (3)

Colorless microcrystals; mp 169–172 °C; $[\alpha]^{20}_{D}$ –2.4 (*c* 0.415, $CHCl_3$); UV ($CHCl_3$) λ_{max}(log ε) 276 (3.98) nm; IR (KBr) ν_{max} 3440, 1694, 1650, 1615 cm^{-1}; ^{1}H ($CHCl_3$, 500

MHz) and ^{13}C NMR ($CHCl_3$, 125 MHz) data, see Tables 1.1 and 1.2; HREIMS *m/z* 342.1831 (cal Cd for $C_{21}H_{26}O_4$ 342.1831).

Table 1.2: ^{1}H NMR spectroscopic data of compounds **1-3** (500 MHz, δ in ppm and *J* in Hz, $CDCl_3$)

Position	*1*	*2*	*3*
1	α) 1.76 (1H, m)	α) 1.74 (1H, ddd, 13.9, 13.5, 5.4)	α) 1.75 (1H, m)
	β) 1.89 (1H, ddd, 13.2, 5.4, 2.2)	β) 1.88 (1H, ddd, 13.5, 5.4, 2.2)	β) 2.00 (1H, ddd, 13.4, 5.4, 2.2)
2	α) 2.47 (1H, m)	α) 2.47 (1H, m)	α) 2.45 (1H, brdd, 18.1, 4.4)
	β) 2.60 (1H, ddd, 13.9, 13.9, 5.4)	β) 2.58 (1H, ddd, 13.9, 12.7, 5.4)	β) 2.56 (1H, ddd, 18.1, 14.4, 5.4)
4	5.75 (1H, s)	5.75 (1H, s)	5.68 (1H, s)
6	6.21 (1H, dd, 9.8, 2.7)	6.21 (1H, dd, 9.8, 2.7)	6.12 (1H, dd, 9.8, 2.7)
7	6.12 (1H, brd, 9.8)	6.14 (1H, dd, 9.8, 1.5)	5.93 (1H, dd, 9.8, 1.7)
8	2.65 (1H, brt, 10.0)	2.65 (1H, brt, 10.8)	2.19 (1H, m)
9	1.65 (1H, ddd, 13.6, 10.0, 4.4)	1.64 (1H, m)	1.32 (1H, ddd, 13.3, 9.6, 4.2)
11	α) 2.33 (1H, dd, 13.7, 4.4)	α) 2.37 (1H, dd, 14.2, 4.4)	α) 1.91 (1H, ddd, 13.2, 4.4, 4.2)
	β) 2.56 (1H, dd, 13.7, 13.6)	β) 2.56 (1H, dd, 14.2, 13.9)	β) 1.57 (1H, ddd, 13.2, 13.2, 11.0)
12	α) 4.29 (1H, br dd, 11.0, 4.4)		
14	1.68 (1H, m)	1.62 (1H, dd, 12.0, 6.1)	1.94 (1H, dd, 12.7, 5.6)
15	α) 2.07 (1H, m) β) 1.69 (1H, m)	α) 1.99 (1H, m) β) 1.58 (1H, m)	α) 2.15 (1H, m) β) 1.71 (1H, m)
16	α) 1.84 (1H, m) β) 2.31 (1H, m)	α) 1.84 (1H, m) β) 1.34 (1H, m)	3.91 (1H, s)
17	3.3 (1H, dd, 9.3, 9.5)	2.03 (1H, dd, 9.8, 9.8)	
18	1.07 (3H, s)	1.18 (3H, s)	0.99 (3H, s)
19	1.20 (3H, s)	1.21 (3H, s)	1.09 (3H, s)
20		3.55 (1H, m)	
21	4.27 (1H, d, 19.8) 4.58 (1H, d, 19.8)	1.17 (3H, d, 6.11)	2.04 (3H, s)

12β-Hydroxypregna-4,6,16-triene-3,20-dione (neridienone A, 4)

The structure of compound **4** was confirmed by analysis of its NMR spectra (^{1}H NMR, ^{13}C NMR, H-H COSY, DEPT, HMQC, HMBC, and NOESY), and the physical and spectroscopic data were in general agreement with those reported in the literature (Abe and Yamauchi, 1976): The ^{13}C NMR data of **4** have been reported (Huq *et al.*, 1999) but the assignment there is wrong. The ^{13}C NMR ($CdCl_3$, 125 MHz): d 199.4 (C-3), 198.9 (C-20), 162.7 (C-5), 155.2 (C-17), 149.0 (C-16), 138.6 (C-7), 129.1 (C-6), 124.3 (C-4), 73.2 (C-12), 52.8 (C-13), 51.6 (C-14), 49.0 (C-9), 36.1 (C-10), 34.8 (C-8), 33.9 (C-2), 33.6 (C-1), 31.7 (C-15), 28.6 (C-11), 26.8 (C-21), 16.2 (C-19), 11.5 (C-18).

Table 1.3: ^{13}C and ^{1}H NMR data of **6** (Pyridine-d_5, 125 MHz for ^{13}C NMR and 500 MHz for ^{1}H NMR, δ in ppm *J* in Hz)

Position	$^{13}C^a$	*Connected* $^{1}H^b$
1	35.5 (CH_2)	α: 1.42 (1H, ddd, 13.7, 13.7, 5.1)
		β: 1.63 (1H, m)
2	34.1 (CH_2)	α: 2.30 (1H, m)
		β: 2.36 (1H, m)
3	197.8 (qC)	
4	124.8 (CH)	5.83 (1H, s)
5	168.3 (qC)	
6	32.4 (CH_2)	α: 2.13 (1H, m)
		β: 2.28 (1H, m)
7	31.3 (GH_2)	α: 0.86 (1H, m)
		β: 1.68 (1H, ddd, m)
8	34.5 (CH)	1.78 (1H, m)
9	55.1 (CH)	1.21 (1H, ddd, 13.6, 11.2, 5.1)
10	38.9 (qC)	
11	37.8 (CH_2)	α: 2.24 (1H, dd, 14.0, 5.1)
		β: 2.51 (1H, dd, 14.0, 13.6)
12	217.5 (qC)	
13	57.0 (qC)	
14	54.9 (CH)	1.28 (1H, m)
15	23.8 (CH_2)	α: 1.59 (1H, m)
		β 1.29 (1H, m)
16	24.5 (CH_2)	α: 1.80 (1H, m)
		β: 1.30 (1H, m)
17	45.4 (CH)	2.58 (1H, dd, 9.6, 9.5)
18	12.3 (CH_3)	1.12 (3H, s)
19	16.5 (CH_3)	1.07 (3H, s)
20	73.8 (CH)	3.64 (1H, ddd, 9.6, 4.3, 2.9)
21	66.3 (CH_2)	a: 4.02 (1H, dd, 11.2, 2.9)
		b: 3.75 (1H, dd, 11.2, 4.3)

a) Multiplicity were determined by DEPT; *b*) Connection were determined by HMQC.

20S,21-Dihydroxypregna-4,6-diene-3,12-dione (neridienone B, 5)

The structure of compound **5** was confirmed by analysis of its NMR spectra (^1H NMR, ^{13}C NMR, H-H COSY, DEPT, HMQC, HMBC, and NOESY), and the physical and spectroscopic data of **5** were in good agreement with those reported in the literature (Abe and Yamauchi, 1976): The ^{13}C NMR data of **5** have not yet been reported: ^{13}C NMR ($CdCl_3$, 125 MHz) δ 216.8 (C-12), 198.7 (C-3), 161.2 (C-5), 137.9 (C-7), 129.1 (C-6), 124.7 (C-4), 72.1 (C-20), 65.9 (C-21), 57.6 (C-13), 52.5 (C-9), 51.0 (C-14), 44.9 (C-17), 37.3 (C-11), 36.3 (C-8), 36.2 (C-10), 33.6 (C-2), 33.5 (C-1), 23.8 (C-16), 22.9 (C-15), 15.9 (C-19), 12.2 (C-18).

20S,21-Dihydroxypregn-4-ene-3,12-dione (6)

Colorless microcrystals, mp 207–208 °C (acetone–hexane); $[\alpha]^{20}_D$ +185.3 (*c* 0.246, $CHCl_3$); IR (KBr) cm^{-1}:3424, 2920, 1689, 1670, 1620; UV (MeOH) nm (log ε): 234 (3.99); ^1H and ^{13}C NMR data are shown in Table 1.3; HR-FAB-MS *m/z* 347.2229 $[M + H]^+$ (Calcd for $C_{21}H_{31}O_4$, 347.2223).

Extraction, Isolation, and Identification of Less Polar Cardenolides and Cardenolide Monoglycosides 9–21

The air-dried stems and twigs (19.5 kg) were combined and extracted with MeOH (85 l) for 20 days. The MeOH extract was concentrated to 4 l and extracted with hexane (8 × 1.0 l). Water (1.3 l) was added to the MeOH layer, extracted with EtOAc (3 × 3.0 l), dried (Na_2SO_4), and concentrated to give an oily residue (96.5 g). This material was separated by column chromatography [silica gel (1.1 kg), gradient mixture of hexane, EtOAc, and MeOH] into five fractions, A–E. Fraction B [hexane–EtOAc (1:1), EtOAc] and fraction C (EtOAc) gave on drying viscous oils, 29.58 g and 23.33 g, respectively. Fraction B was dissolved in EtOAc (200 ml), stirred for 1 h, filtered, and concentrated to give 19.86 g of a viscous oil, which was further separated by column chromatography [silica gel (1 kg), gradient mixture of hexane, EtOAc, and MeOH] into nine fractions, B1–B9. Fractions B5 [hexane–EtOAc (40:60)], and B6 and B7 [hexane–EtOAc (0:100)] gave on drying viscous oils (B5 0.451g, B6; 9.00 g, B7; 1.76 g). B5 afforded compounds **13*** (12.6 mg, 0.00006 per cent), **9** (8.9 mg, 0.00005 per cent), and **10** (23.5 mg, 0.00012 per cent) by separation using silica gel HPLC [hexane–EtOAc (4:6)], followed by ODS HPLC [MeOH–MeCN– H_2O (1:9:10)]. B6 was subjected to silica gel column chromatography [silica gel (1 kg), a gradient of hexane, EtOAc, and MeOH] to give seven fractions, B61–B67. B64 (7.73 g) was further separated by HPLC [ODS, MeOH–MeCN–H_2O (1:6:9)] to give sub-fraction B643 (5.310 g), B644 **14****, 1.880 g (0.0096 per cent)], B645 [**17**, (392 mg, 0.0020 per cent)], and B646 (623 mg). B643 was further separated by HPLC [ODS, MeOH–MeCN–H_2O (1:9:10)] to give **13*** [31.1 mg (0.00016 per cent)], **14**** [231.2 mg (0.00119 per cent)], **19** [52.7 mg (0.00027 per cent)], and **20** [39.5 mg (0.00020 per cent). B646 was further separated by HPLC [ODS, MeOH–MeCN–H_2O (1:9:10)] to give compounds **11** [46.7 mg (0.00024 per cent)] and **16** [295.9 mg (0.00152 per cent)]. B7 was separated by column chromatography [silica gel (300 g), gradient mixture of hexane, EtOAc, and MeOH] into five fractions, B71–B75. B72 (157 mg) was further separated by HPLC [ODS, MeOH–MeCN–H_2O (1:6:9)] to give compound**14**** [21.0 mg (0.00011 per cent)]. B73 (1.31 g) was separated by HPLC [ODS, MeOH–MeCN–H_2O (1:6:9)] to give compounds

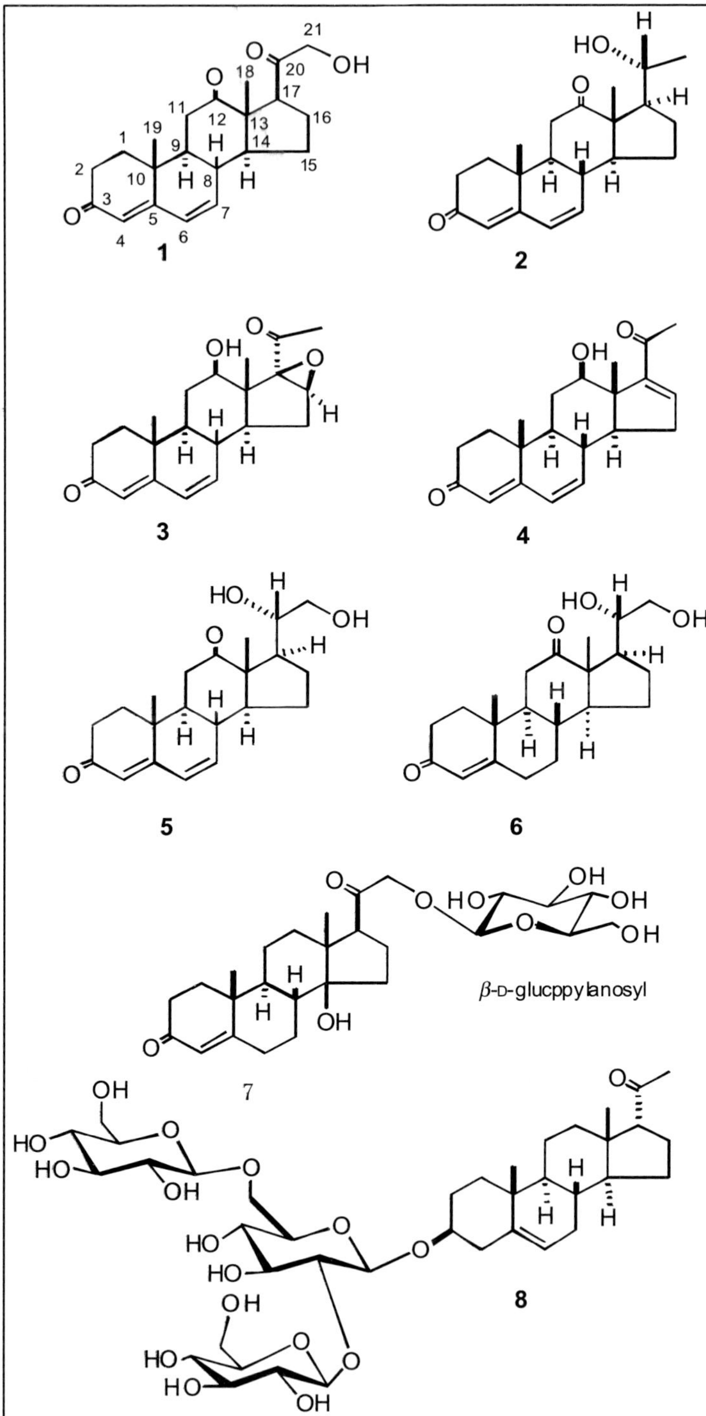

Figure 1.1: The structures of pregnanes **1-6** and pregnane glycosides **7** and **8**.

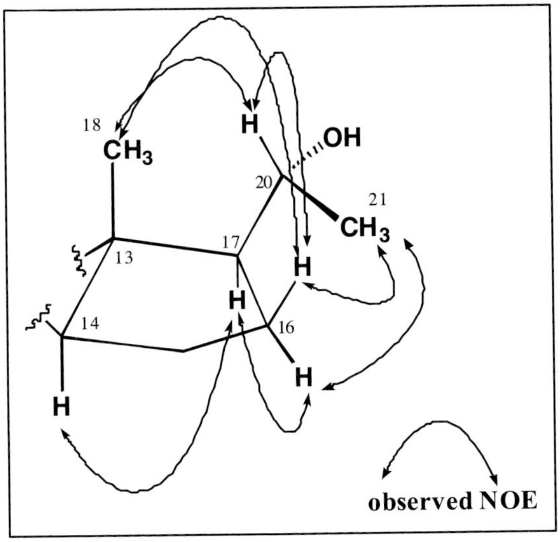

Figure 1.2: NOE correlations of the D ring and C-17 side chain of compound **2**.

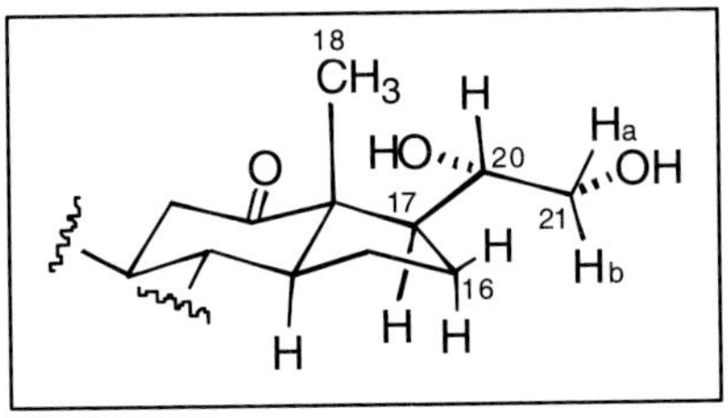

Figure 1.3: 20*S* Stereostructure of C-17 side chain of compound **6**.

15 [338.4 mg (0.00173 per cent)], **18** [27.8 mg (0.00014 per cent)], and **21** [308 mg (0.00158 per cent)]. B74 (127 mg) was separated by HPLC [ODS, MeOH–MeCN–H_2O (1:6:8)] to give three fractions (B741, B742, and B743). B742 (73.5 mg) was further purified by HPLC [ODS, MeOH–MeCN–H_2O (1:6:9)] to give compound **12** (18.7 mg, 0.00010 per cent)]. Fraction C was separated by flash column chromatography [silica gel, hexane–EtOAc (1:59)] into six fractions, C1–C6. Fraction C3 (9.32 g) was separated further by flash column chromatography [silica gel, hexane–EtOAc (3:7)] into four fractions, C31–C34. Fraction C31 (1.410 g, 0.00723 per cent) was identified as compound **14****.

*The combined yield of **13** is 43.7 mg (0.00022 per cent).

The combined yield of **14 is 3.542 g (0.01816 per cent).

3β-O-(D-Sarmentosyl)-14-hydroxy-5β,14β-card-20(22)-enolide (9)

Colorless microcrystals; mp 110 °C (acetone–hexane); $[\alpha]^{20}_D$ −1.3 (*c* 0.231, $CHCl_3$); IR ($CHCl_3$) ν_{max} 3613, 3591, 3009, 1784, 1745 cm^{-1}; ^1H and ^{13}C NMRdata, see Table 1.4; HRESI *m/z* 541.3156 (calcd for $C_{30}H_{46}O_7Na$ 541.3156). Since only D-sarmentose is known in *N. oleander*, the sugar moiety in **9** and **10** is regarded as D-sarmentose.

3β-O-(D-Sarmentosyl)-8,14-epoxy-5β,14β-card-16,20(22)-dienolide (10)

Colorless microcrystals; mp 114 °C (acetone–hexane); $[\alpha]^{20}_D$ +52.9 (*c* 0.662, $CHCl_3$); IR ($CHCl_3$) ν_{max} 3572, 3011, 1749, 1626 cm^{-1}; ^1H and ^{13}C NMR data, see Table 1.4; HRFABMS *m/z* 515.3005 (calcd for $C_{30}H_{43}O_7$ $[M+1]^+$, 515.3009).

3β-O-(D-Diginosyl)-8,14,16α,17-diepoxy-5β,14β-card-20(22)-enolide (11)

Colorless microcrystals; mp 123 °C (acetone–hexane); $[\alpha]^{20}_D$ +95.7 (*c* 0.277, $CHCl_3$); IR ($CHCl_3$) n_{max} 3555, 3030, 1788, 1755 cm^{-1}; ^1H and ^{13}C NMR data, see Table 1.4;

Table 1.4: ^{13}C and ^{1}H NMR data of **9**–**12** ($CdCl_3$, 125 MHz for ^{13}C NMR and 500 Hz for ^{1}H NMR, δ in ppm *J* in Hz)[a]

Compound →	**9**		**10**		**11**		**12**	
Position →	^{13}C	^{1}H	^{13}C	^{1}H	^{13}C	^{1}H	^{13}C	^{1}H
1	30.2 (t)	1.48 (1H, m)	30.2 (t)	1.46 (1H, m)	30.2 (t)	1.44 (1H, m)	37.1 (t)	β) 1.70 (1H, m)
		1.46 (1H, m)		1.43 (1H, m)		1.41 (1H, m)		α) 0.97 (1H, m)
2	26.7 (t)	α) 1.66 (1H, m)	26.9 (t)	α) 1.71 (1H, m)	26.8 (t)	α) 1.74 (1H, m)	29.1 (t)	α) 1.92 (1H, m)
		β) 1.46 (1H, m)		β) 1.46 (1H, m)		β) 1.44 (1H, m)		β) 1.48 (1H, m)
3	72.6 (d)	4.03 (1H, br s, $W_{h/2}$=7.5)	72.5 (d)	4.03 (1H, br s, $W_{h/2}$=7.5)	72.6 (d)	4.05 (1H, br s, $W_{h/2}$=7.5)	76.6 (d)	3.67 (1H, m)
4	29.9 (t)	α) 1.73 (1H, m)	29.9 (t)	α) 1.73 (1H, m)	29.9 (t)	α) 1.76 (1H, m)	34.1 (t)	α)1.63 (1H, m)
		β) 1.43 (1H, m)		β) 1.52 (1H, brd, 13.4)		β) 1.50 (1H, m)		β) 1.28 (1H, m)
5	36.3 (d)	1.65 (1H, m)	36.4 (d)	1.79 (1H, m)	36.3 (d)	1.77 (1H, m)	44.2 (d)	1.06 (1H, m)
6	26.6 (t)	β) 1.87 (1H, m)	24.7 (t)	β) 2.17 (1H, tt, 13.9, 4.6)	24.6 (t)	β) 2.11 (1H, tt, 14.0, 4.2)	28.4 (t)	β) 1.37 (1H, m)
		α) 1.26 (1H, m)		α) 1.30 (1H, m)		α) 1.26 (1H, m)		α) 1.24 (1H, m)
7	21.4 (t)	β) 1.73 (1H, m)	26.9 (t)	α) 1.83 (1H, m)	26.3 (t)	α) 1.82 (1H, td, 14.0, 5.1)	27.0 (t)	β) 1.97 (1H, m)
		α) 1.66 (1H, m)		β) 1.16 (1H, brd, 14.0)		β) 1.12 (1H, brd, 14.0)		α) 1.03 (1H, m)
8	41.9 (d)	1.56 (1H, m)	65.2 (s)		65.6 (s)		41.6 (d)	1.49 (1H, m)
9	35.8 (d)	1.60 (1H, m)	36.2 (d)	1.94 (1H, brdd, 10.5, 5.1)	36.3 (d)	1.90 (1H, dd, 11.7, 4.2)	49.7 (d)	0.87 (1H, m)
10	35.2 (s)		36.8 (s)		36.7 (s)		35.8 (s)	
11	21.2 (t)	α) 1.43 (1H, m)	15.7 (t)	1.30 (2H, m)	14.7 (t)	α) 1.30 (1H, m)	20.8 (t)	α) 1.55 (1H, m)
		β) 1.20 (1H, m)				β) 1.18 (1H, m)		β) 1.26 (1H, m)

Contd...

Table 1.4–*Contd...*

Compound →	**9**		**10**		**11**		**12**	
Position →	^{13}C	^{1}H	^{13}C	^{1}H	^{13}C	^{1}H	^{13}C	^{1}H
12	40.1 (t)	β) 1.52 (1H, m)	33.4 (t)	β) 1.84 (1H, m)	30.0 (t)	β) 1.51 (1H, m)	39.1 (t)	β) 1.52 (1H, m)
		α) 1.39 (1H, m)		α) 1.28 (1H, m)		α) 1.48 (1H, m)		α) 1.31 (1H, m)
13	49.6 (s)		44.8 (s)		41.9 (s)		49.9 (s)	
14	85.6 (s)		70.1 (s)		67.4 (s)		84.2 (s)	
15	33.2 (t)	α) 2.12 (1H, m)	33.1 (t)	α) 2.61 (1H, dd, 20.0, 2.8)	29.5 (t)	α) 2.23 (1H, brd, 15.1)	41.0 (t)	α) 2.67 (1H, dd, 15.6, 9.8)
		β) 1.68 (1H, m)		β) 2.57 (1H, dd, 20.0, 2.8)		β) 2.07 (1H, brd, 15.1)		β) 1.75 (1H, dd, 15.6, 2.5)
16	26.9 (t)	α) 2.15 (1H, m)	132.1 (d)	6.07 (1H, br t, 2.8)	63.2 (d)	3.69 (1H, brs)	73.9 (d)	5.45 (1H, ddd, 9.8, 8.5, 2.5)
		β) 1.87 (1H, m)						
17	50.9 (d)	2.77 (1H, brd, 8.3, 4.9)	143.1 (s)		66.7 (s)		56.0 (d)	3.17 (1H, d, 8.5)
18	15.8 (q)	0.87 (3H, s)	19.9 (q)	1.22 (3H, s)	18.0 (q)	1.21 (3H, s)	15.9 (q)	0.93 (3H, s)
19	23.6 (q)	0.93 (3H, s)	24.5 (q)	1.03 (3H, s)	24.6 (q)	0.98 (3H, s)	12.1 (q)	0.79 (3H, s)
20	174.4 (s)		157.6 (s)		162.6 (s)	167.5 (s)		
21	73.4 (t)	α) 4.97 (1H, brd, 18.1)	71.4 (t)	α) 4.97 (1H, dd, 16.2, 1.6)	71.7 (t)	α) 4.79 (1H, dd, 17.8, 1.7)	75.6 (t)	α) 4.95 (1H, dd, 18.1, 1.7)
		β) 4.81 (1H, brd, 18.1)		β) 4.91 (1H, dd, 16.2, 1.6)		β) 4.71 (1H, dd, 17.8, 1.7)		β) 4.84 (1H, dd, 18.1, 1.7)
22	117.7 (d)	5.87 (1H, brs)	112.9 (d)	5.95 (1H, br s)	119.5 (d)	6.23 (1H, t, 1.7)	121.4 (d)	5.97 (1H, t, 1.7)
23	174.4 (s)		174.2 (s)		172.8 (s)	174.0 (s)		

Contd...

Table 1.4–*Contd...*

Compound →	**9**		**10**		**11**		**12**	
Position →	^{13}C	^{1}H	^{13}C	^{1}H	^{13}C	^{1}H	^{13}C	^{1}H
16-OAc							21.0 (q)	1.96 (3H, s)
							170.4 (s)	
1'	96.5 (d)	4.71 (1H, dd, 9.5, 2.4)	96.9 (d)	4.72 (1H, dd, 9.5, 2.4)	98.0 (d)	4.46 (1H, dd, 9.8, 2.0)	97.5 (d)	4.53 (1H, dd, 9.8, 2.2)
2'	31.5 (t)	α) 1.84 (1H, m)	31.5 (t)	α) 1.86 (1H, m)	32.1 (t)	α) 1.95 (1H, br dd, 12.2, 4.9)	32.0 (t)	α) 1.94 (1H, m)
		β) 1.76 (1H, m)		β) 1.78 (1H, m)		β) 1.71 (1H, ddd, 12.2, 12.2, 9.8)		β) 1.68 (1H, ddd, 12.0, 12.0, 9.8)
3'	78.5 (d)	3.58 (1H, q, 2.9)	78.5 (d)	3.58 (1H, q, 3.2)	78.0 (d)	3.34 (1H, ddd, 12.2, 4.9, 3.2)	77.9 (d)	3.33 (1H, ddd, 12.0, 4.9, 3.2)
4'	67.9 (d)	3.39 (1H, m)	67.9 (d)	3.40 (1H, m)	67.2 (d)	3.68 (1H, m)	67.1 (d)	3.69 (1H, brs)
5'	69.0 (d)	3.91 (1H, q, 6.6)	69.1 (d)	3.91 (1H, br q, 6.6)	70.4 (d)	3.43 (1H, q, 6.3)	70.4 (d)	3.44 (1H, q, 6.6)
6'	16.6 (q)	1.23 (3H, d, 6.6)	16.6 (q)	1.23 (3H, d, 6.6)	16.8 (q)	1.34 (3H, d, 6.3)	16.8 (q)	1.35 (3H, d, 6.6)
3'-OMe	57.1 (q)	3.38 (3H, s)	57.1 (q)	3.38 (3H, s)	55.7 (q)	3.40 (3H, s)	55.7 (q)	3.39 (3H, s)

a: Assignments are based on DEPT, ^{1}H-^{1}H COSY, HMQC, and HMBC experiments.

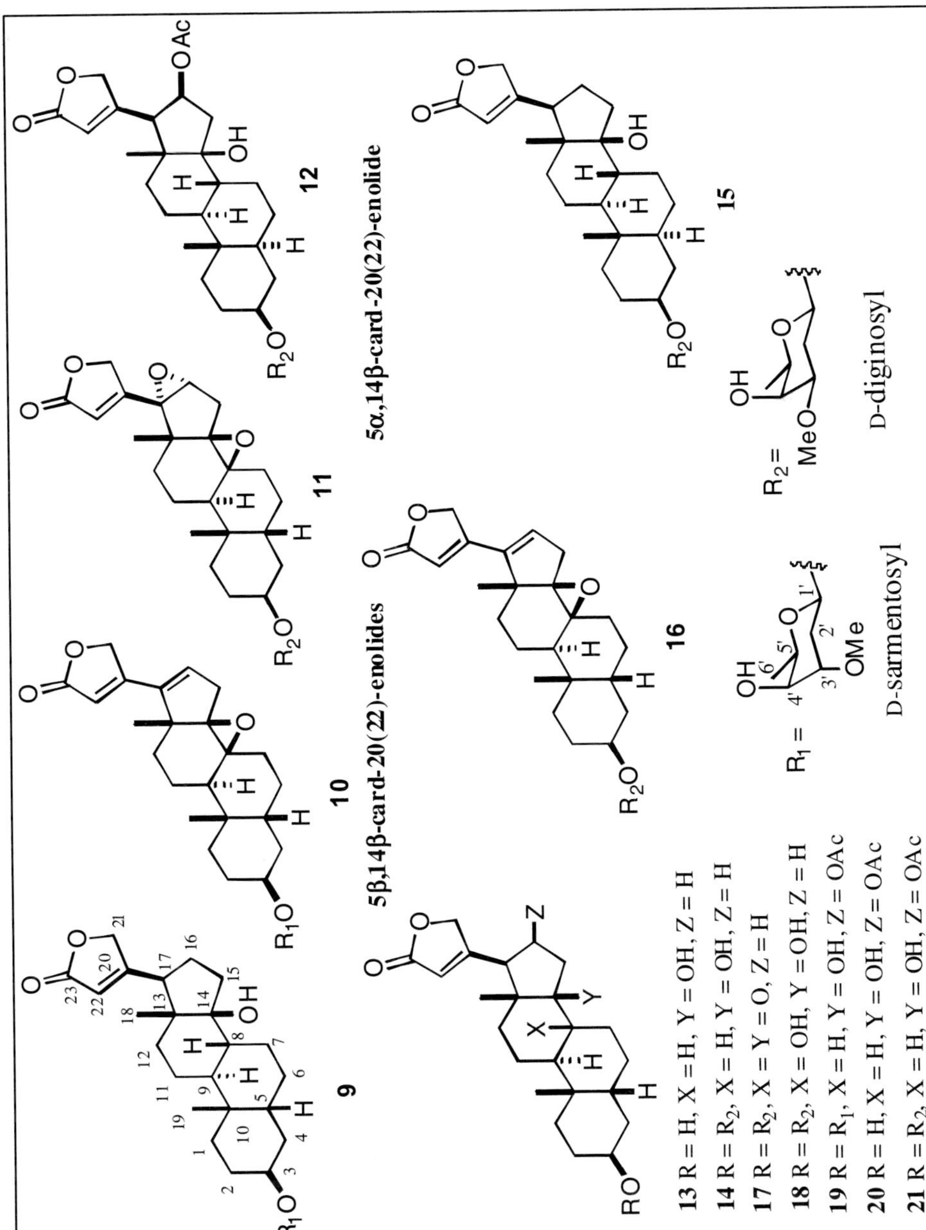

Figure 1.4: Less polar cardenolides and cardenolide monoglycosides isolated from *Nerium oleander*.

HRFABMS *m/z* 531.2968 [calcd for $C_{30}H_{43}O_8$ $[M+1]^+$, 531.2958]. Since only D-diginose is known in *N. oleander*, the sugar moiety in **11** and **12** is regarded as D-diginose.

3β-O-(D-Diginosyl)-16β-acetoxy-14-hydroxy-5α,14β-card-20(22)-enolide (12)

Colorless microcrystals; mp 201 °C (acetone–hexane); $[\alpha]^{20}_D$ −21.4 (*c* 0.42, $CHCl_3$); IR ($CHCl_3$) ν_{max} 3516, 3439, 1743 cm^{-1}; ^1H and ^{13}C NMR data, see Table 1.4; HRESI *m/z* 599.3197 (calcd for $C_{32}H_{48}O_9Na$ 599.3196).

Extraction, Isolation, and Identification of More Polar Cardenolide and Cardenolide Monoglycosides 22–34

The air-dried stems and twigs (19.5 kg) were combined and extracted with MeOH (85 l) for 20 days. The MeOH extract was concentrated to 4 l and extracted with hexane (8 × 1000 ml). Water (1.3 l) was added to the MeOH layer, extracted with EtOAc (3 × 3000 ml), dried (Na_2SO_4), and concentrated to give an oily material (96.5 g). The water layer was further extracted with *n*-BuOH (3 × 500 ml), dried (Na_2SO_4), and concentrated to give an oily residue (53.76 g).

The EtOAc extract (96.5 g) was separated by column chromatography [silica gel (1.1 kg), a gradient of hexane, EtOAc, and MeOH] into five fractions, A–E. Fraction B [hexane–EtOAc (1:1), EtOAc], fraction C (EtOAc), and fraction D [EtOAc–MeOH (1:1)] gave on drying viscous oils, weighing 29.58 g, 23.33g, and 32.15g, respectively. The fraction B was dissolved in EtOAc (200 ml), stirred for 1 h, filtered, and concentrated to give viscous oil (19.86 g), which was further separated by column chromatography [silica gel (1 kg), a gradient of hexane, EtOAc, and MeOH] into 9 fractions, B1–B9. Fractions B7 [EtOAc (100 per cent)], and B8 [EtOAc(100 per cent)] gave on drying viscous oils [B7 (1.76 g), B8 (0.84 g)]. Fraction B7 was subjected to column chromatography [silica gel (300 g), gradient of hexane, EtOAc, and MeOH] to give five fractions, B71–B75. B73 (1.31 g) afforded compound **27** [53.51 mg (0.00027 per cent)] by separation using HPLC [ODS, MeOH–MeCN–H_2O (1:1:2)]. B8 was subjected to column chromatography [silica gel (80 g), gradient of hexane, EtOAc, and MeOH] to give five fractions, B81–B85. B83 (296.0 mg) afforded compound **29** [9.7 mg (0.00005 per cent)] by separation using HPLC [ODS, MeOH–MeCN–H_2O (1:3:5)]. Fraction C was subjected to flash column chromatography [silica gel (1 kg), hexane–EtOAc (1:59)] to give six fractions, C1–C6. Fraction C3 (8.65 g) was further separated by flash column chromatography [silica gel (800 g), hexane–EtOAc (3:7)] into four fractions, C31–C34. Fraction C33 (3.8 g) afforded compounds **24** [10.2 mg (0.000052 per cent)] and **33** [132.3 mg (0.00068 per cent)] by successive separation using HPLC [ODS, MeOH–MeCN–H_2O (1:6:9)], [ODS, MeOH–MeCN–H_2O (4:4:9)], and [ODS, MeOH–MeCN–H_2O (3:4:10)]. Fraction C34 (1.134 g) was divided into $CHCl_3$-soluble (C341) and $CHCl_3$-insoluble (C342) fractions. C342 (0.80 g) afforded compound **23** [13.9 mg (0.000071 per cent)] by separation using HPLC [ODS, MeOH–MeCN–H_2O (4:4:10)]. Fraction C4 (0.96 g) was separated by flash column chromatography [silica gel (100 g), hexane–EtOAc (2:8)] into eight fractions, C41–C48. C47 was compound **25** [81.7 mg (0.00042 per cent)]. Compound **32** [93.7 mg (0.00048 per cent)] was obtained by crystallization of C43 from EtOAc. Fraction C5 (9.06 g) was separated by flash column chromatography [silica gel (900 g), hexane–EtOAc (1:10)] into three fractions, C51–

C53. C51 was compound **25** [575.1 mg (0.00295 per cent)]. Additional compound **25** [165.7 mg (0.00085 per cent)] was obtained from C52 by crystallization from MeOH. Fraction C53 (2.16 g) was separated by HPLC [ODS, MeOH–MeCN–H_2O (4:4:10)] to give compounds **25** [704.0 mg (0.00362 per cent)] and **26** [451.5 mg (0.00232 per cent)]. Fraction C6 (851 mg) was separated by flash column chromatography [silica gel (90 g), EtOAc] into four fractions, C61–C64. Fraction C62 was crystallized from EtOAc to give compound **30** [107.2 mg (0.00055 per cent)]. Fraction D was dissolved in EtOAc (200 mL), stirred for 1 h, filtered, and concentrated to give viscous oil (17.059 g), which was separated by column chromatography [silica gel (620 g), gradient of $CHCl_3$ and MeOH] into 12 fractions, D1–D12. Fraction D4 [$CHCl_3$–MeOH (98:2), 1.56 g] was further separated by flash column chromatography [silica gel (160 g), EtOAc] into six fractions, D41–D46. D42 (178 mg) was separated by silica gel HPLC [silica gel (20 g), EtOAc], followed by HPLC [ODS, MeOH–H_2O (55:45)] to give compound **34** [18.6mg (0.00095 per cent)]. The soluble portion of D43 (0.385 g) in EtOAc (D431, 0.314 g) was separated by HPLC [ODS, MeOH–H_2O (55:45)] to give compounds **25** [40.2 mg (0.00021 per cent)], **26** [56.2 mg (0.00029 per cent)], and **31** [46.7mg (0.00024 per cent)]. The insoluble portion of D43 in EtOAc (D432, 68 mg) was subjected to HPLC [ODS, MeOH–H_2O (55:45)] to give D4323 [**22**, 4.2mg (0.00002 per cent)], D4324, and D4325 [**31**, 9.6 mg (0.000049 per cent)]. Separation of D4324 by HPLC [ODS, MeOH–MeCN–H_2O (1:1:2.5)] gave compounds **22** [5.4 mg (0.000028 per cent)] and **31** [6.8 mg (0.000035 per cent)].

Compound **28** (17.4 mg, 0.000089 per cent) was obtained from the *n*-BuOH extract (53.76 g) by separation using column chromatography [silica gel, a gradient of $CHCl_3$ and MeOH], followed by HPLC [ODS, MeOH–MeCN–H_2O (1:2:7)].

Cardenolide monoglycosides named cardenolide B-1 (**22**), cardenolide B-2 (**23**) and oleagenin (**24**) were the first isolated compounds from natural sources by us. Their physical constants, nuclear magnetic resonance (NMR), infra red (IR), ultra violet (UV), and high resolution fast atom bombardment mass (HR FAB-MS) spectrometric data are given below.

3β-O-(β-D-Digitalosyl)-8,14-epoxy-5β,14β-card-20(22)-enolide (22)

Colorless microcrystals, mp 203–206 oC (acetone–hexane); $[\alpha]^{20}_D$ +28.57 (*c* 0.392, $CHCl_3$); IR ($CHCl_3$) cm^{-1}: 3539, 2936, 1786, 1751, 1631; UV (MeOH) nm (log *e*): 222 (4.05); ^1H and ^{13}C NMR data are shown in Table 1.5; HRFABMS *m/z* 533.3104 [M + H]$^+$ (Calcd for $C_{30}H_{45}O_8$, 533.3115).

3β-O-(β-D-Diginosyl)-7β,8-epoxy-14-hydroxy-5β,14β-card-20(22)-enolide (23)

Colorless microcrystals, mp 167–171°C (acetone–hexane); $[\alpha]^{20}_D$ –6.06 (*c* 0.330, $CHCl_3$); IR ($CHCl_3$) cm^{-1}: 3537, 3010, 2932, 1765, 1746; UV (MeOH) nm (log ε): 218 (4.20); ^1H and ^{13}C NMR data are shown in Table 1.5; HRFABMS *m/z* 533.3113 [M + H]$^+$, (Calcd for $C_{30}H_{45}O_8$, 533.3115).

(8R)-3β-Hydrxy-14-oxo-15(14→8)abeo-5β-card-20(22)-enolide (24)

Colorless prisms, mp 278–285°C (MeOH); $[\alpha]^{20}_D$ +49.60 (*c* 0.254, MeOH); IR (KBr) cm^{-1}: 3399, 2937, 1748, 1692; UV (MeOH) nm (log ε): 207 (4.32); ^1H and ^{13}C NMR data

Table 1.5: ^{13}C and ^{1}H NMR data of **22–24** (125 MHz for ^{13}C NMR and 500 MHz for ^{1}H NMR, δ in ppm *J* in Hz)[a].

Position	**22** *(in $CDCl_3$)*		**23** *(in $CDCl_3$)*		**24** *(in C_5D_5N)*	
	δ_C *mult.*	δ_H *(mult., J)*	δ_C *mult.*	δ_H *(mult., J)*	δ_C *mult.*	δ_H *(mult., J)*
1	30.4, CH_2	1.45 (1H, m) 1.49 (1H, m)	31.1, CH_2	1.43 (1H, m) 1.09 (1H, m)	31.6, CH_2	1.79 (1H, m) 1.58 (1H, m)
2	26.6, CH_2	α: 1.47 (1H, m) β: 1.82 (1H, m)	27.1, CH_2	α: 1.58 (1H, m) β: 1.80 (1H, m)	28.9, CH_2	α: 1.62 (1H, m) β: 1.70 (1H, m)
3	73.7, CH	4.07 (1H, br s, $W_{h/2}$ = 7.5)	71.9, CH	4.01 (1H, br s, $W_{h/2}$ = 7.5)	65.8, CH	4.32 (1H, br s, $W_{h/2}$ = 8.0)
4	30.0, CH_2	α: 1.80 (1H, m) β: 1.60 (1H, m)	32.7, CH_2	α: 1.35 (1H, m) β: 1.48 (1H, m)	34.5, CH_2	α: 1.85 (1H, m) β: 1.52 (1H, br dd 14.2, 3.2)
5	36.6, CH	1.79 (1H, m)	33.6, CH	1.62 (1H, m)	37.1, CH	2.08 (1H, br d, 13.2)
6	24.5, CH_2	α: 1.30 (1H, m) β: 2.15 (1H, m)	27.9, CH_2	α: 1.47 (1H, m) β: 2.30 (1H, m)	24.8, CH_2	α: 1.12 (1H, m) β: 2.35 (1H, m)
7	26.7, CH_2	α: 1.78 (1H, m) β: 1.14 (1H, m)	51.2, CH	3.21 (1H, d, 5.9)	29.5, CH_2	α: 1.06 (1H, ddd, 13.9, 13.9, 4.6) β: 1.98 (1H, m)
8	65.3, qC		63.9, qC		49.1, qC	
9	36.7, CH	1.90 (1H, dd, 11.0, 4.6)	31.6, CH	2.23 (1H, m)	46.0, CH	2.51 (1H, br d, 8.3)
10	36.7, qC		33.6, qC		37.9, qC	
11	16.1, CH_2	α: 1.15 (1H, m) β: 1.26 (1H, m)	20.3, CH_2	α: 1.41 (1H, m) β: 1.56 (1H, m)	21.4, CH_2	α: 2.32 (1H, m) β: 1.72 (1H, m)
12	37.0, CH_2	α: 1.16 (1H, m) β: 1.58 (1H, m)	41.0, CH_2	α: 1.54(1H, m) β: 1.75 (1H, m)	42.7, CH_2	1.96(2H, m)
13	41.8, qC		52.2, qC		47.5, qC	
14	70.5, qC	81.0, qC		2.37 (14-OH)		221.3, qC

Contd...

Table 1.5–*Contd...*

Position	**22** (*in* $CDCl_3$)		**23** (*in* $CDCl_3$)		**24** (*in* C_5D_5N)	
	δ_C *mult.*	δ_H (*mult., J*)	δ_C *mult.*	δ_H (*mult., J*)	δ_C *mult.*	δ_H (*mult., J*)
15	25.7, CH_2	α: 2.00 (1H, m) β: 1.74 (1H, m)	34.4, CH_2	α: 2.24 (1H, m) β: 1.77 (1H, m)	44.1, CH_2	α: 1.88 (1H, dd, 14.4, 6.1) β: 1.68 (1H, ddd, 14.4, 14.4, 6.8)
16	27.0, CH_2	α: 1.88 (1H, m) β: 1.98 (1H, m)	28.4, CH_2	α: 2.26 (1H, m) β: 1.96 (1H, m)	26.9, CH_2	α: 2.68 (1H, dddd, 15.1, 14.4, 7.1, 6.8) β: 1.38 (1H, br dd, 15.1, 6.8)
17	51.5, CH	2.57 (1H, dd, 11.2, 6.6)	50.6, CH	2.81 (1H, dd, 8.3, 5.7)	53.0, CH	2.97 (1H, br d, 7.1)
18	16.1, CH_3	0.85 (3H, s)	17.1, CH_3	0.90 (3H, s)	23.4, CH_3	0.91 (3H, s)
19	24.7, CH_3	1.01 (3H, s)	24.0, CH_3	0.95 (3H, s)	26.6, CH_3	0.81 (3H, s)
20	169.5, qC	173.6, qC	171.9, qC			
21	73.2, CH_2	α: 4.71 (1H, dd, 17.4, 1.0) β: 4.81 (1H, dd, 17.5, 1.7)	73.3, CH_2	α: 4.79 (1H, dd, 18.1, 1.2) β: 4.94 (1H, dd, 18.1, 1.2)	73.4, CH_2	α: 4.80 (1H, dd, 17.6, 1.7) β: 4.72 (1H, dd, 17.6, 1.7)
22	116.9, CH	5.88 (1H, br s)	117.8, CH	5.88 (1H, br s)	116.4 (d)	5.89 (1H, br s)
23	173.6, qC	174.2, qC	173.8, qC			
1'	101.3, CH	4.27 (1H, d, 7.8)	97.9, CH	4.43 (1H, dd, 9.8, 1.7)		
2'	70.8, CH	3.66 (1H, dd, 9.5, 7.8)	32.0, CH_2	α: 1.94 (1H, m) β: 1.69 (1H, m)		
3'	82.8, CH	3.22 (1H, dd, 9.5, 3.4)	78.0, CH	3.34 (1H, ddd, 12.1, 4.8, 3.2)		
4'	68.2, CH	3.85 (1H, br s)	67.2, CH	3.70 (1H, br s)		
5'	70.4, CH	3.57 (1H, br q, 6.3)	70.4, CH	3.42 (1H, q, 6.6)		
6'	16.2, CH_3	1.36 (3H, d, 6.3)	16.8, CH_3	1.32 (3H, d, 6.6)		
OMe	57.6, CH_3	3.53 (3H, s)	55.7, CH_3	3.40 (3H, s)		

a: Assighnment are based on DEPT, ^{1}H-^{1}H COSY, HMQC, and HMBC spectra.

are shown in Table 1.5; HRFABMS *m/z* 373.2376 [M + H] $^{+}$ (Calcd for $C_{23}H_{33}O_4$, 373.2378).

The structures of the known compounds **25-34** were confirmed by the analyses of their NMR, IR, UV, and HRFABMS spectrometric data and by comparison of their physical constants indicated here with those in literatures.

Odoroside H [3β-O-(D-Digitalosyl)-14-hydroxy-5β,14β-card-20(22)-enolide] (Cabrera et al., 1993)

25 was obtained as colorless microcrystals; mp 231–234°C (MeOH); $[\alpha]^{20}_D$ +5.57o (*c* 0.556, MeOH). ^{13}C NMR: see Table 1.9. IR ($CHCl_3$): ν_{max} cm^{-1} 3539, 3462, 2880, 1780, 1728, 1620. UV (MeOH): λ_{max} nm (log ε) 218 (4.08). HR FAB-MS *m/z*: 535.3271 [calcd for $C_{30}H_{47}O_8$ (M+H)$^+$, 535.3271].

Neritaloside [3β-O-(D-Digitalosyl)-16β-acetoxy-14-hydroxy-5β,14β-card-20(22)-enolide] (Cabrera et al., 1993; Yamauchi and Abe, 1990)

26 was obtained as colorless microcrystals; mp 143–146°C (acetone-hexane); $[\alpha]^{20}_D$ +6.78o (*c* 1.046, $CHCl_3$). ^{13}C NMR: see Table 1.9. IR ($CHCl_3$): ν_{max} cm^{-1} 3516, 3456, 3013, 2939, 1743. UV (MeOH): λ_{max} nm (log ε) 217 (4.04). HR FAB-MS *m/z*: 593.3326 [calcd for $C_{32}H_{49}O_{10}$ (M+H)$^+$, 593.3326].

Oleandrin [3β-O-(L-oleandrosyl)-16β-aceoxy-14-hydroxy-5β,14β-card-20(22)-enolide] (Abe et al., 1996; Yamauchi and Abe, 1978)

27 was obtained as colorless microcrystals; mp 243–249°C (MeOH); $[\alpha]^{20}_D$ −12.90° (*c* 0.062, MeOH). ^{13}C NMR: see Table 1.9. IR ($CHCl_3$): ν_{max} cm^{-1} 3539, 3462, 2944, 1746. HR FAB-MS *m/z*: 577.3377 [calcd for $C_{32}H_{49}O_9$ (M+H)$^+$, 577.3377].

3β-O-(D-Glucosyl)-16β-acetoxy-14-hydroxy-5β,14β-card-20(22)-enolide (Yamauchi et al., 1975; Paper and Franz, 1989)

28 was obtained as colorless microcrystals; mp 151–153°C (acetone-hexane); $[\alpha]^{20}_D$ −18.05° (*c* 0.670, MeOH). ^{13}C NMR: see Table 1.9. IR (KBr): ν_{max} cm^{-1} 3429, 2939, 1738.

3β-O-(D-Diginosyl)-14,16β-dihydroxy-5β,14β-card-20(22)-enolide] (Hanada et al., 1992; Jäger and Reichstein, 1959)

29 was obtained as an amorphous compound; $[\alpha]^{21}_D$ +5.55° (*c* 0.54, MeOH). ^{13}C NMR: see Table 1.9. IR ($CHCl_3$): ν_{max} cm^{-1} 3605, 3499, 3026, 2878, 1782, 1745. HR FAB-MS *m/z* 535.3281 [calcd for $C_{30}H_{47}O_8$ (M+H)$^+$, 535.3271].

3β-O-(D-Digitalosyl)-14-hydroxy-5α,14β-card-20(22)-enolide (Yamauci et al., 1976; Hanada et al., 1992)

30 was obtained as colorless microcrystals; mp 230–234°C (MeOH); $[\alpha]^{20}_D$ +0.86° (*c* 1.153, MeOH). ^{13}C NMR: see Table 1.9. IR ($CHCl_3$): ν_{max} cm^{-1} 3518, 3011, 2940, 1788, 1746. UV (MeOH): λ_{max} nm (log ε) 218 (3.96).

3β-O-(D-Digitalosyl)-8,14-epoxy-5β,14β-card-16,20(22)-dienolide (Hanada et al., 1992; Yamauchi et al., 1973)

31 was obtained as colorless microcrystals; mp 217–220oC (acetone–hexane);

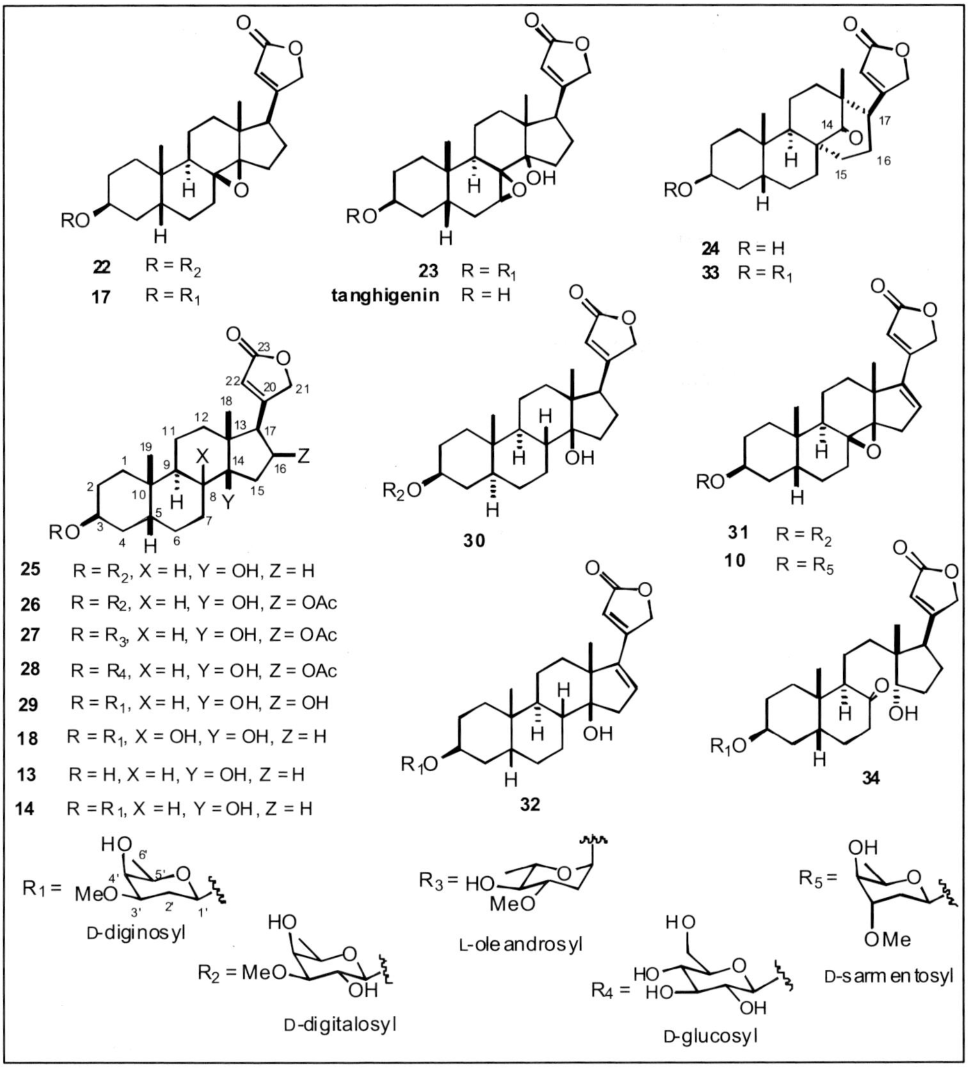

Figure 1.5: Structure of compounds **10**, **13**, **14**, tanghigenin, **17**, **18**, and **22–34**.

$[\alpha]^{20}_{D}$ +13.36° (*c* 0.546, $CHCl_3$). ^{13}C NMR: see Table 1.9. IR ($CHCl_3$): ν_{max} cm^{-1} 3480, 2944, 1782, 1743, 1631. UV (MeOH): λ_{max} nm (log ε) 219 (3.19).

3β-O-(D-Diginosyl)-14-hydroxy-5β,14β-card-16,20(22)-dienolide (Jäger and Reichstein, 1959)

32 was obtained as colorless microcrystals; mp 187–190°C (acetone–hexane); $[\alpha]^{20}_{D}$ +26.87° (*c* 1.256, $CHCl_3$). ^{13}C NMR: see Table 1.9. IR ($CHCl_3$): n_{max} cm^{-1} 3507, 3362, 2943, 1782, 1730, 1697, 1622; UV (MeOH): λ_{max} nm (log ε) 217 (4.12).

Oleaside A [(8R)-3β-O-(D-Diginosyl)-14-oxo-15(14→8)abeo-5β-card-20(22)-enolide] (Abe and Yamauchi, 1979)

33 was obtained colorless prisms; mp 242–245°C (MeOH); $[\alpha]^{20}_{D}$+27.60 (*c* 0.920, $CHCl_3$). ^{13}C NMR: see Table 1.9. IR (KBr) ν_{max} cm^{-1} 3420, 2961, 1788, 1745; UV (MeOH): λ_{max} nm (log ε) 213 (4.10); HR FAB-MS *m/z*: 517.3165 [calcd for $C_{30}H_{45}O_7$ $(M+H)^+$, 517.3166].

Neriaside [3β-O-(D-Diginosyl)-8,14-seco-14α-hydroxy-8-oxo-5β-card-20(22)-enolide] (Abe et al., 1996; Yamauchi and Abe, 1978)

34 was obtained colorless prisms; mp 159–163°C (MeOH); $[\alpha]^{20}_{D}$+21.42° (*c* 0.462, $CHCl_3$). ^{13}C NMR: see Table 1.9. IR (KBr) ν_{max} cm^{-1} 3483, 3478, 2959, 1782, 1751, 1693, 1626. HR FAB-MS *m/z*: 535.3274 [calcd for $C_{30}H_{47}O_8$ $(M+H)^+$, 535.3271].

Extraction, Isolation, and Identification of Cardenolide Diglycosides 35–45

Air-dried leaves (9.91 kg) were extracted twice with MeOH (66 and 39 l) for 3 and 4 days. The MeOH extract was concentrated to 10 l and extracted with hexane (5 × 5 l). Water (4 × 10 l) was added to the MeOH layer, extracted with EtOAc (5 × 5 l). Then saturated NaCl aqueous solution (10 l) was added to the MeOH layer and extracted with *n*-BuOH (4 × 10 l). The *n*-BuOH extracts were dried and concentrated to give an oily material (528 g). To a part of the *n*-BuOH extract (53.76 g), 150 ml of MeOH was added, stirred for 1 h, and filtered. The filtrate was concentrated to give on drying a viscous oil, which was dissolved with 110 ml of MeOH, and added 990 ml of $CHCl_3$, stirred for 1 h, and filtered. The filtrate was concentrated to give a viscous oil, NB1 (18.75 g), which was dissolved with 200 ml of water, and extracted with $CHCl_3$ (5 × 200 ml). The $CHCl_3$ extracts were concentrated to give a semisolid, BC (5538.7 mg), which was separated by column chromatography on silica gel (275 g) in 11 fractions, BC-1–BC-11, using a gradient of $CHCl_3$ and MeOH. Fraction BC-3 [$CHCl_3$–MeOH (9:1)] gave 606.7 mg of a semisolid, which was further separated by HPLC [ODS, MeOH–H_2O (9:1)] into three fractions (BC3-1–BC3-3). Fraction BC3-1 gave a powder (542.8 mg), which was separated by HPLC [ODS, MeOH–H_2O (65:35)] into five fractions (BC31-1–BC31-5). Fraction BC31-2 (143.3 mg) was separated by HPLC [ODS, MeOH–H_2O (5:5)] to give **35** [23.9 mg (0.0024 per cent)], **36** [67.5 mg (0.0067 per cent)] and **44** [16.5 mg (0.0016 per cent)]. Fraction BC31-3 (71.7 mg) was separated by HPLC [ODS, MeOH–MeCN–H_2O (1:6:12)] to give **39** [41.2 mg (0.0041 per cent)] and **37** [16.8 mg (0.0017 per cent)]. Fraction BC-5 [$CHCl_3$–MeOH (9:1 and 8:2)] gave 288.8 mg of a semisolid, which was further separated by HPLC [ODS, MeOH–H_2O (8:2)] into three fractions (BC5-1–BC5-3). Fraction BC5-1 gave a powder (228.0 mg), which was separated by HPLC [ODS, MeOH–H_2O (6:4)] into five fractions (BC51-1–BC51-5). Fraction BC51-3 (29.2 mg) was separated by HPLC [ODS, MeOH–MeCN–H_2O (1:2:7)] to give **38** [14.9 mg (0.0015 per cent)] and **45** [3.2 mg (0.0003 per cent)]. Fraction BC51-4 (36.1 mg) was separated by HPLC [ODS, MeCN–H_2O (28:72)] to give **41** [9.0 mg (0.0009 per cent)] and **42** [10.6 mg (0.0010 per cent)]. The yield of each compound in parentheses is based on the weight of air-dried leaves.

Air-dried stems and twigs (19.46 kg) were combined and extracted with MeOH (85 l) for 20 days. The MeOH extract was concentrated to 4 l and extracted with hexane (8 × 1 l). Water (1 l) was added to the MeOH layer, and extracted with EtOAc (3 × 3 l) and *n*-BuOH (4 × 2 l), successively. The *n*-BuOH extracts were dried and concentrated to give an oily residue (244 g). A part of the *n*-BuOH extract (6.02) was separated by column chromatography on silica gel (539 g) in 14 fractions, A–N, using a gradient of $CHCl_3$ and MeOH. Fraction D [$CHCl_3$–MeOH (8:2)] gave on drying a viscous oil (374.6 mg), which was further separated by HPLC [ODS, MeOH–MeCN–H_2O (1:2:5)] into five fractions (D-1–D-5). Fraction D-2 gave 42.4 mg of a semisolid, which was separated by HPLC [ODS, MeOH–MeCN–H_2O (1:2:7)] to give **38** [14.7 mg (0.0030 per cent)] and **45** [(4.5 mg (0.0009 per cent)). Fraction D-5 (30.3 mg) was separated by HPLC [ODS, MeOH–MeCN–H_2O (1:2:6)] to give **43** [14.5 mg (0.0030 per cent)]. Fraction E gave on drying a viscous oil (91.8 mg), which was separated by HPLC [ODS, MeOH–MeCN–H_2O (1:3:9)] to give **38** [2.5 mg (0.0005 per cent)], **43** [4.4 mg (0.0009 per cent)], and **40** [3.8 mg (0.0008 per cent)]. The yield of each compound in parentheses is based on the weight of air-dried stems and twigs.

3β-O-[β-D-glucopyranosyl-(1→4)-β-D-diginopyranosyl]-14α-hydroxy-8-oxo-8,14-seco-5β-card-20(22)-enolide (35)

Colorless microcrystals, mp 138–143 °C (acetone–hexane); $[\alpha]^{20}_{D}$ –28.56° (*c* 1.362, MeOH); IR (KBr) cm^{-1}: 3467, 2938, 1736, 1698, 1626, 1453, 1192; UV (MeOH) nm (log ε): 215 (4.05); ^{1}H and ^{13}C NMR data are shown in Table 1.6; HRFABMS *m/z* 719.3615 $[M + Na]^+$ (Calcd for $C_{36}H_{56}O_{13}Na$, 719.3619).

Extraction, Isolation, and Identification of Cardenolide Triiglycosides 46–61

Isolation from Stems and Twigs

The *n*-butanol extract (244 g) was obtained from air-dried stems and twigs (19.46 kg) of *N. oleander* by the extraction procedures in Scheme 1.1. This material was separated by the combination of column chromatography [silica gel, gradient ($CHCl_3$–MeOH)] and reversed phase HPLC [ODS, gradient (MeOH–CH_3CN–H_2O)] by the separation procedures in Scheme 1.2. The isolated compounds and their yields are shown as following: **46** [7.280g (0.0374 per cent)], **47** [12.630 g (0.0649 per cent)], **48** [1.627 g (0.0084 per cent)], **49** [2.307 g (0.0119 per cent)], **50** [0.717 g (0.0037 per cent)], **51** [1.036 g (0.0053 per cent)], **52** [0.454 g (0.0023 per cent)], **53** [2.860 g (0.0147 per cent)], **54** (0.450 g (0.0023 per cent)), **55** [0.482 g (0.0025 per cent)], **56** [0.510 g (0.0026 per cent)], **59** [0.741 g, (0.0038 per cent)], **60** [1.977 g, (0.0102 per cent)], **61** [0.162 g (0.0008 per cent)].

Isolation from Leaves

The *n*-butanol extract (244 g) was obtained from air-dried leaves (9.91 kg) of *N. oleander* by extraction procedures in Scheme 1.3. This material was separated by the combination of column chromatography [silica gel, gradient ($CHCl_3$–MeOH–H_2O)] and reversed phase HPLC [ODS, gradient (MeOH-CH_3CN-H_2O)] by the separation procedures in Scheme 1.4. The isolated compounds and their yields are shown as following: **46** [280 mg (0.0028 per cent)], **47** [142 mg (0.0014 per cent)], **48** [277 mg

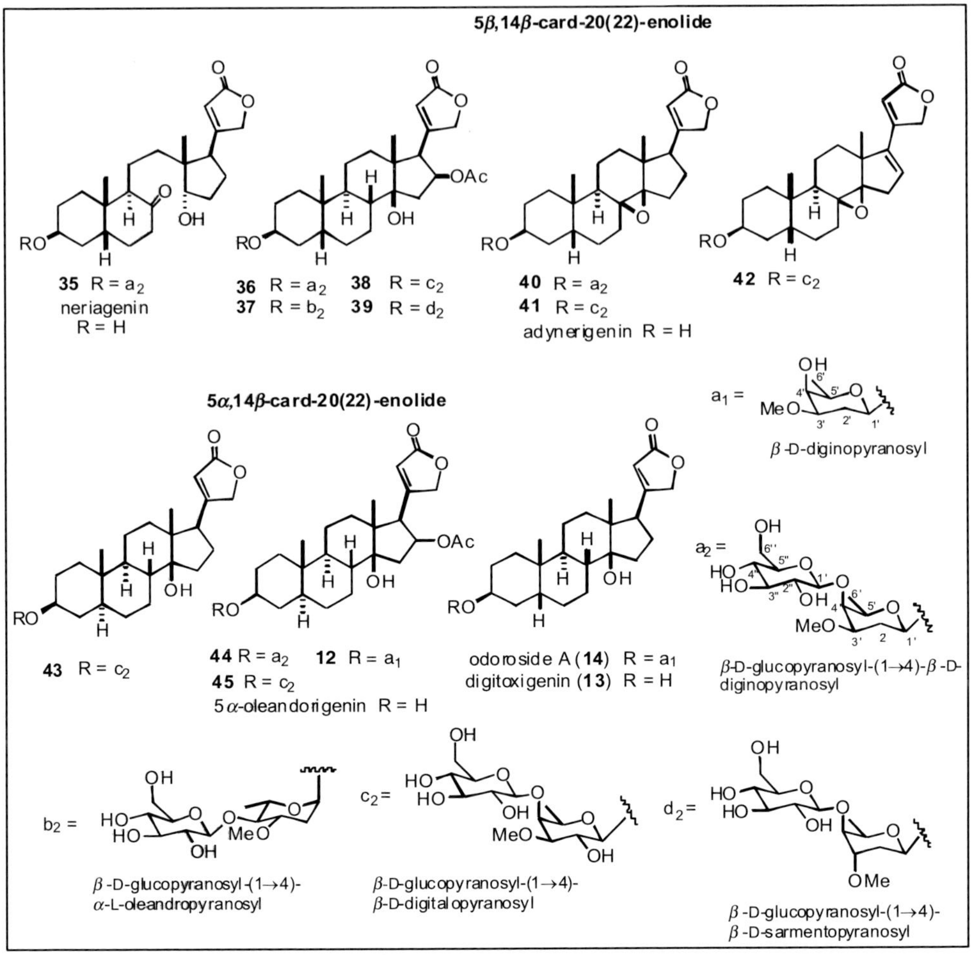

Figure 1.6: Structure of compounds **12** and **35–45,** neriagenin, adynerigenin, 5α-oleandorigenin, odoroside A (**14**), and digitoxigenin (**13**).

(0.0028 per cent)], **50** [1408 mg (0.0142 per cent)], **53** [1166.2 mg (0.0118 per cent)], **56** [60 mg (0.0006 per cent)], **57** [115 mg (0.0012 per cent)], **58** [147 mg (0.0015 per cent)], **59** [237 mg, (0.0024 per cent)], **60** [786 mg, (0.0079 per cent)].

Identification of Isolated Compounds 46–61

Cardenolide B-3 (**61**) was the first isolated compounds from natural sources by us and its physical constant, NMR, IR, UV, CD, and HRFABMS spectroscopic data are given below. Although structures of **53** and **55** have already been reported by Yamauchi et al., their structure elucidation were based the products by acid and enzymatic hydrolyses of a mixture of **53** and **55**. Since we isolated **53** and **55** in pure form in this work, their structures were confirmed by the analyses of ^{1}H- and ^{13}C-

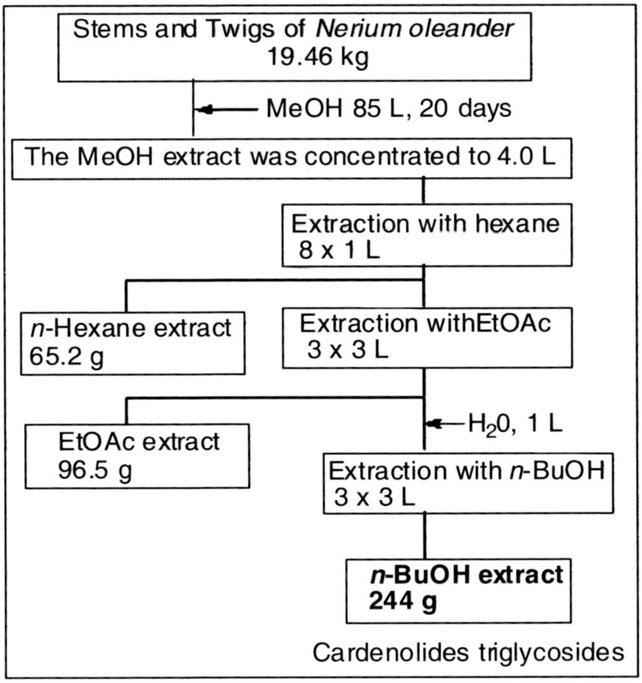

Scheme 1.1: Extraction procedures of the stem and twings of *Nerium oleander.*

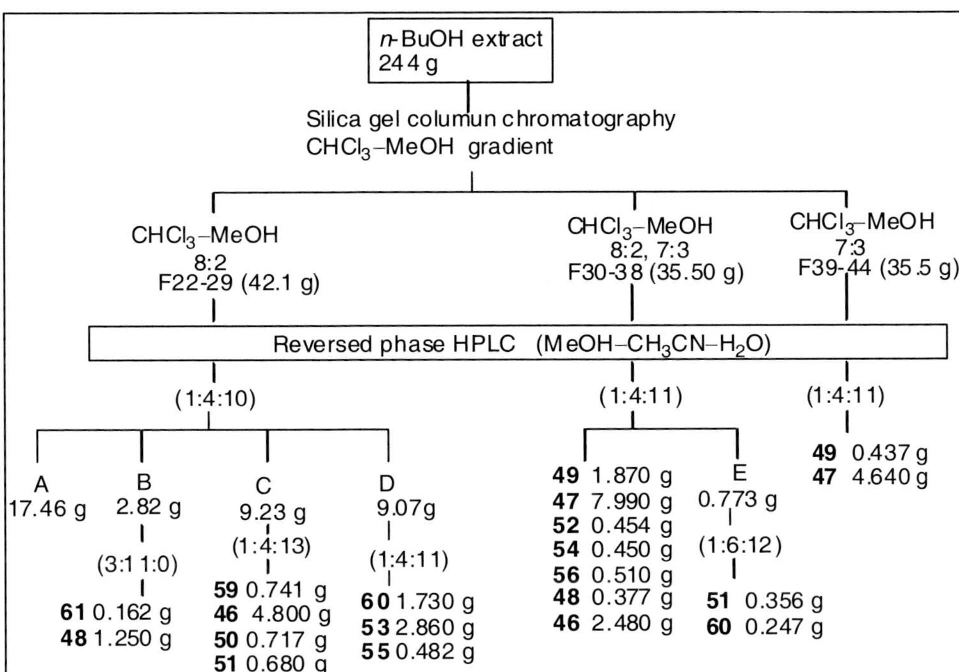

Scheme 1.2: Separation procedures of *n*-butanol extract of the stem and twings of *Nerium oleander.*

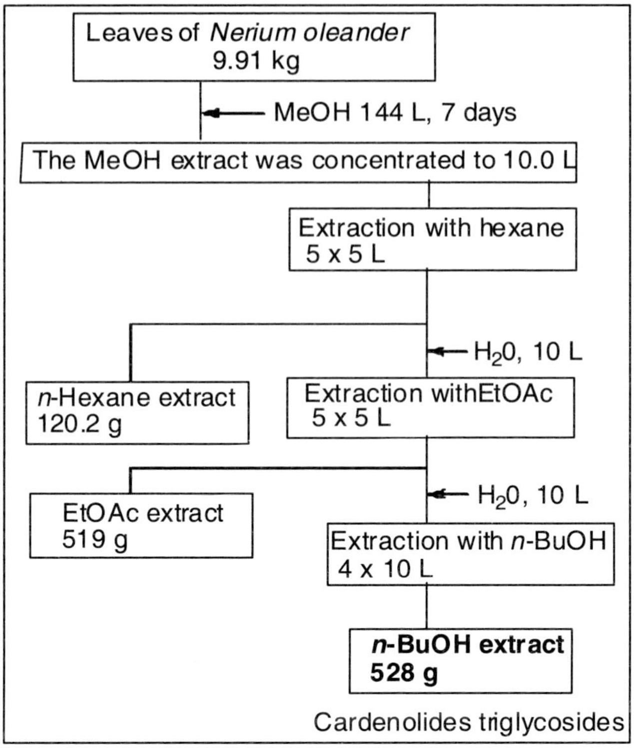

Scheme 1.3: Extraction procedures of the leaves of *Nerium oleander.*

Table 1.6: ^{13}C and ^{1}H NMR data of **35** (pyridine-d_5, 125 MHz for ^{13}C NMR and 500 MHz for ^{1}H NMR, δ in ppm J in Hz)

Position	$^{13}C^a$	*Connected* $^1H^b$
1	31.0 (CH_2)	β 1.56 (1H, m)
		α 1.70 (1H, m)
2	27.7 (CH_2)	β 1.93 (1H, m)
		α 1.68 (1H, m)
3	72.8 (CH)	4.28 (1H, br s, $W_{h/2}$ = 8.0)
4	30.1 (CH_2)	α 2.08 (1H, m)
		β 1.73 (1H, m)
5	36.8 (CH)	1.90 (1H, m)
6	28.7 (CH_2)	β 2.05 (1H, m)
		α 1.50 (1H, m)
7	38.2 (CH_2)	α 2.50 (1H, td, 13.4, 6.8)
		β 2.28 (1H, ddd, 13.4, 4.9, 2.7)
8	216.2 (qC)	

Contd...

Table 1.6–*Contd...*

Position	$^{13}C^{a}$	*Connected* $^{1}H^{b}$
9	52.0 (CH)	2.79 (1H, d, 10.0)
10	42.7 (qC)	
11	18.4 (CH_2)	a 1.76 (1H, m)
		b 1.45 (1H, m)
12	35.3 (CH_2)	a 1.65 (1H, m)
		b 1.29 (1H, ddd, 12.5, 12.5, 6.1)
13	51.3 (qC)	
14	79.5 (CH)	4.15 (1H, m)
15	27.3 (CH_2)	β 2.03 (1H, m)
		α 1.70 (1H, m)
16	30.8 (CH_2)	α 2.03 (1H, m)
		β 1.84 (1H, m)
17	46.3 (CH)	3.00 (1H, t, 9.3)
18	17.7 (CH_3)	0.68 (3H, s)
19	23.9 (CH_3)	0.74 (3H, s)
20	172.4 (qC)	
21	74.0 (CH_2)	a 4.89 (1H, dd, 17.6, 2.0)
		b 4.71 (1H, dd, 17.6, 1.5)
22	116.8 (CH)	6.01 (1H, br d, 1.0)
23	174.1 (qC)	
1'	99.1 (CH)	4.71 (1H, dd, 9.8, 2.2)
2'	33.2 (CH_2)	β 2.34 (1H, td, 12.2, 9.8)
		α 2.13 (1H, d, 12.2, 4.4)
3'	80.1 (CH)	3.45 (1H, ddd, 12.2, 4.4, 2.7)
4'	74.1 (CH)	4.14 (1H, m)
5'	70.9 (CH)	3.52 (1H, br q, 6.4)
6'	17.9 (CH_3)	1.51 (3H, d, 6.4)
3'-OMe	56.2 (CH_3)	3.36 (3H, s)
1"	105.0 (CH)	5.11 (1H, d, 7.8)
2"	76.0 (CH)	3.91 (1H, dd, 8.8, 7.8)
3"	78.4 (CH)	4.17 (1H, t, 8.8)
4"	72.0 (CH)	4.11 (1H, t, 8.8)
5"	78.5 (CH)	3.90 (1H, m)
6"	63.2 (CH_2)	b 4.51 (1H, dd, 11.7, 2.4)
		a 4.30 (1H, dd, 11.7, 5.6)

a) Multiplicity were determined by DEPT.

b) Connection were determined by HMQC.

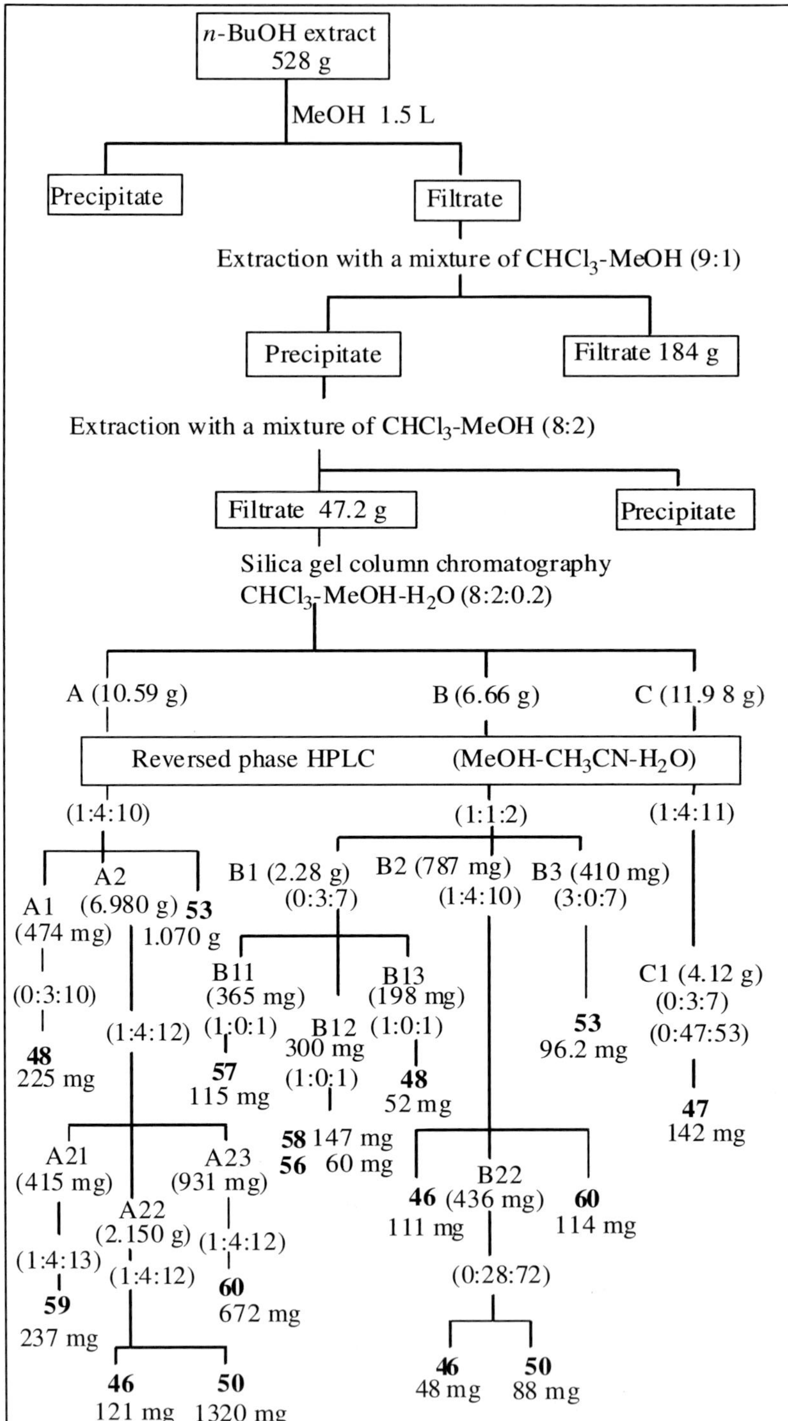

Scheme 1.4: Separation procedures of *n*-butanol extract of the leaves of *Nerium oleander*.

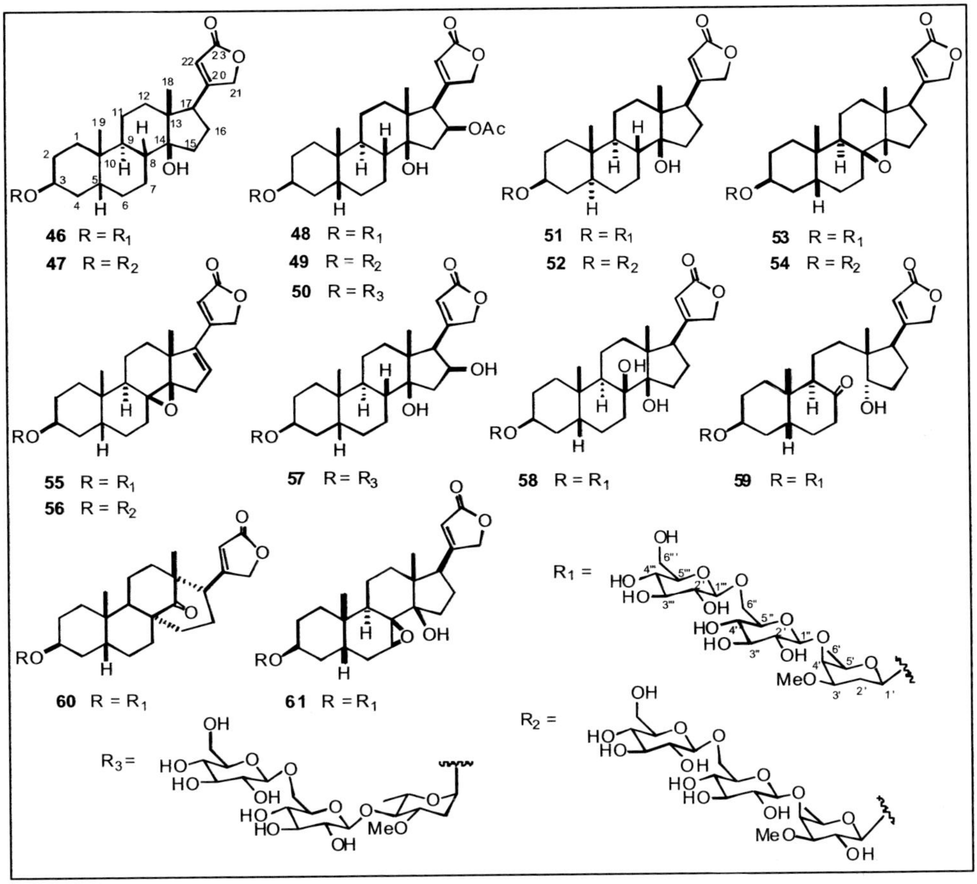

Figure 1.7: Cardenolide triglycoside from *Nerium oleander.*

NMR spectra including H-H COSY, DEPT, HMQC, HMBC, and NOESY experiments. The physical constants, NMR and IR spectroscopic data of **53** and **55** are given below.

Cardenolide B-3

61 was obtained as colorless microcrystals; mp 169–171 °C (acetone-hexane); $[\alpha]^{20}_D$ -1.62° (*c* 0.308, MeOH). ^{1}H NMR (C_5D_5N) δ6.11 (1H, br s, H-22), 5.17 (1H, br dd, *J* = 17.8, 1.7 Hz, 21b-H), 5.15 (1H, d, *J* = 7.6 Hz, 1'''-H), 5.09 (1H, d, *J* = 7.8 Hz, 1''-H), 4.97 (1H, dd, *J* = 17.8, 1.2 Hz, 21a-H), 4.80 (1H, br dd, *J* = 11.7, 2.5 Hz, 6''b-H), 4.64 (1H, br dd, *J* = 8.3 Hz, 1'-H), 4.50 (1H, *J* = 11.8, 5.4 Hz, 6'''b-H), 4.35 (1H, *J* = 11.8, 2.4 Hz, 6'''a-H), 4.31 (1H, m, 4'-H), 4.27 (1H, dd, *J* = 11.7, 6.8 Hz, 6''a-H), 4.21 (1H, m, 4'''-H), 4.20 (1H, br s $W_{h/2}$ = 7.5 Hz, 3-H), 4.19 (1H, m, 3'''-H), 4.12 (1H, dd, *J* = 9.0, 9.0 Hz, 3''-H), 4.06 (1H, m, 5''-H), 4.02 (1H, m, 2'''-H), 3.97 (1H, m, 4''-H), 3.92 (1H, m, 5'''-H), 3.88 (1H, m, 2''-H), 3.52 (1H, q, *J* = 6.4 Hz, 5'-H), 3.42 (1H, d, *J* = 5.9 Hz, 7-H), 3.39 (1H, m, 3'-H), 3.35 (3H, s), 2.80 (1H, dd, *J* = 5.6, 4.6 Hz, 17-H), 2.40 (1H, m, 15a-H), 2.37 (14-OH), 2.36 (1H, m, 9-H), 2.32 (1H, m, 2'b-H), 2.29 (1H, m, 16b-H), 2.19 (1H, m, 16a-H), 2.09 (1H, m,

2′a-H), 2.04 (1H, m, 16b-H), 1.90 (1H, m, 2b-H), 1.86 (1H, m, 15b-H), 1.74 (1H, m, 5b-H), 1.69 (1H, m, 2a-H), 1.66 (1H, d, *J* = 6.4 Hz, 6'-H), 1.63 (1H, m, 12b-H), 1.60 (1H, m, 4b-H), 1.56 (1H, m, 12a-H), 1.53 (1H, m, 1a-H), 1.50 (1H, m, 4a-H), 1.48 (1H, m, 6a-H), 1.45 (1H, m, 1b-H), 1.06 (3H, s, 18-CH_3), 1.05 (3H, s, 19-CH_3). ^{13}C NMR (C_5D_5N): see Table 1.10. IR (KBr) ν_{max} 3389, 2973, 1745, 1642, 1100, 1028 cm^{-1}. UV (MeOH) λ_{max}(log ε): 216 (4.05) nm. CD (MeOH) $[\theta]_{289}$ -900, $[\theta]_{238}$ +9170. HRFABMS *m/z* 855.4024 (calcd for $C_{42}H_{63}O_{18}$ [M–H]$^-$, 855.4015).

3β-O-(4-O-Gentiobiosyl-D-dignosyl)-8,14-epoxy-5β,14β-card-20(22)-enolide (Yamauchi et al., 1975)

53 was obtained as colorless microcrystals; mp 201–203 °C (acetone-hexane); $[\alpha]^{20}_D$ +14.6° (*c* 0.125, MeOH). ^{1}H NMR (C_5D_5N) δ 6.04 (1H, br s, 22-H), 5.14 (1H, d, *J* = 7.8 Hz, 1'''-H), 5.05 (1H, d, *J* = 7.8 Hz, 1''-H), 4.91 (1H, dd, *J* = 17.5, 1.7 Hz, 21b-H), 4.81 (1H, dd, *J* = 17.5, 2.0 Hz, 21a-H), 4.77 (1H, m, 6''b-H), 4.64 (1H, dd, *J* = 9.6, 1.7 Hz, 1'-H), 4.48 (1H, m, 6'''b-H), 4.34 (1H, m, 6'''a-H), 4.31 (1H, m, 3-H), 4.28 (1H, m, 4'-H), 4.26 (1H, m, 6''a-H), 4.19 (1H, m, 4'''-H), 4.18 (1H, m, 3'''-H), 4.11 (1H, m, 3''-H), 4.04 (1H, m, 5''-H), 4.00 (1H, m, 2'''-H), 3.98 (1H, m, 4''-H), 3.91 (1H, m, 5'''-H), 3.87 (1H, m, 2''-H), 3.53 (1H, q, *J* = 6.3 Hz, 5'-H), 3.42 (1H, m, 3'-H), 3.35 (3H, s, OMe), 2.46 (1H, m, 17-H), 2.35 (1H, m, 2′b-H), 2.12 (1H, m, 2′a-H), 1.95 (1H, m, 5-H), 1.64 (1H, d, *J* = 6.3 Hz, 6'-H), 1.07 (3H, s, 19-H), 0.80 (3H, s, 18-H). ^{13}C NMR (C_5D_5N): see Table 1.10. IR (KBr): ν_{max} cm^{-1} 3404, 1747.

3β-O-(4-O-gentiobiosyl-D-dignosyl)-8,14-epoxy-5β,14β-card-16,20(22)-enolide (Yamauchi et al., 1975)

55 was obtained as colorless microcrystals; mp 160-163 °C (acetone-hexane); $[\alpha]^{20}_D$ 22.8° (*c* 0.785, MeOH). ^{1}H NMR(C_5D_5N) δ 6.28 (1H, m, 22-H), 6.08 (1H, br t, *J* = 2.8 Hz, 16-H), 5.15 (1H, d, *J* = 7.6 Hz, 1'''-H), 5.09 (1H, d, *J* = 7.8 Hz, 1''-H), 5.09 (1H, br dd, *J* = 16.2, 1.7 Hz, 21b-H), 5.05 (1H, br dd, *J* = 16.2, 1.7 Hz, 21a-H), 4.79 (1H, dd, *J* = 11.8, 1.7 Hz, 6''b-H), 4.68 (1H, br dd, *J* = 9.5, 2.0, 1'-H), 4.50 (1H, dd, *J* = 11.6, 2.4 Hz, 6'''b-H), 4.34 (1H, dd, *J* = 11.7, 5.4 Hz, 6'''a-H), 4.31 (1H, m, 4'-H), 4.29 (1H, m, 3-H), 4.27 (1H, m, 6''a-H), 4.21 (1H, m, 4'''-H), 4.18 (1H, m, 3'''-H), 4.12 (1H, m, 3''-H), 4.07 (1H, m, 5''-H), 4.02 (1H, m, 2'''-H), 3.98 (1H, m, 4''-H), 3.92 (1H, m, 5'''-H), 3.88 (1H, m, 2''-H), 3.52 (1H, q, *J* = 6.4 Hz, 5'-H), 3.42 (1H, m, 3'-H), 3.36 (3H, s, 3'-OMe), 2.36 (1H, m, 2′b-H), 2.12 (1H, m, 2′a-H), 1.95 (1H, m, 9-H), 1.92 (1H, m, 5-H), 1.65 (3H, d, *J* = 6.4 Hz, 6'-H), 1.24 (3H, s, 18-H), 1.10 (3H, s, 19-H). ^{13}C NMR (C_5D_5N): see Table 1.10. IR (KBr): ν_{max} cm^{-1} 3452, 1746.

Identification of Known Compounds

Compounds **46–52**, **54**, **56–60** were confirmed by the analyses of ^{1}H- and ^{13}C-NMR spectra including H-H COSY, DEPT, HMQC, HMBC, and NOESY experiments as well as by comparison of their spectral data and physical data with those reported previously. Their physical constants, IR spectroscopic data and references are given below. For the convenience for the identification of the compounds, ^{13}C NMR spectroscopic data of compounds **46–61** were summarized in Table 1.10.

Table 1.7: NMR data of the sugar moiety and C-1–C-5 of **35**, **36**, and **40** in C_5D_5N.

Position	**35**		**36**		**40**
	^{13}C	^{1}H	^{13}C	^{1}H	^{13}C
1	31.0 (CH_2)	β 1.56 (1H, m)	30.7 (CH_2)	β 1.62 (1H, m)	31.0 (CH_2)
		α 1.70 (1H, m)		α 1.48 (1H, m)	
2	27.7 (CH_2)	β 1.93 (1H, m)	27.7 (CH_2)	β 1.86 (1H, m)	27.4 (CH_2)
		α 1.68 (1H, m)		α 1.62 (1H, m)	
3	72.8 (CH)	4.28 (1H, br s, $W_{h/2}$ = 8.0)	73.1 (CH)	4.26 (1H, br s)	72.7 (CH)
4	30.1 (CH_2)	α 2.08 (1H, m)	30.5 (CH_2)	α 1.82 (1H, m)	30.2 (CH_2)
		β 1.73 (1H, m)		β 1.58 (1H, m)	
5	36.8 (CH)	1.90 (1H, m)	37.0 (CH)	1.82 (1H, m)	37.1 (CH)
1'	99.1 (CH)	4.71 (1H, dd, 9.8, 2.2)	98.9 (CH)	4.69 (1H, dd, 9.8, 9.7)	98.8 (CH)
2'	33.2 (CH_2)	β 2.34 (1H, td, 12.2, 9.8)	33.2 (CH_2)	2.33 (1H, ddd, 12.2, 12.0, 9.8)	33.3 (CH_3)
		α 2.13 (1H, d, 12.2, 4.4)		2.11 (1H, m)	
3'	80.1 (CH)	3.45 (1H, ddd, 12.2, 4.4, 2.7)	80.1 (CH)	3.42 (1H, ddd, 12.2, 4.4, 2.7)	80.2 (CH)
4'	74.1 (CH)	4.14 (1H, m)	74.2 (CH)	4.13 (1H, m)	73.3 (CH)
5'	70.9 (CH)	3.52 (1H, br q, 6.4)	70.8 (CH)	3.50 (1H, br q, 6.3)	70.9 (CH)
6'	17.9 (CH_3)	1.51 (3H, d, 6.4)	17.9 (CH_3)	1.51 (3H, d, 6.3)	18.2 (CH_3)
3'-OMe	56.2 (CH_3)	3.36 (3H, s)	56.1 (CH_3)	3.35 (3H, s)	56.2 (CH_3)
1"	105.0 (CH)	5.11 (1H, d, 7.8)	105.0 (CH)	5.09 (1H, d, 7.8)	104.6 (CH)
2"	76.0 (CH)	3.91 (1H, dd, 8.8, 7.8)	76.0 (CH)	3.91 (1H, m)	75.7 (CH)
3"	78.4 (CH)	4.17 (1H, t, 8.8)	78.4 (CH)	4.17 (1H, t, 8.8)	78.6 (CH)
4"	72.0 (CH)	4.11 (1H, t, 8.8)	72.0 (CH)	4.12 (1H, m)	71.9 (CH)
5"	78.5 (CH)	3.90 (1H, m)	78.5 (CH)	3.89 (1H, m)	78.4 (CH)
6"	63.2 (CH_3)	β 4.51 (1H, dd, 11.7, 2.4)	63.2 (CH_3)	4.51 (1H, dd, 11.5, 2.4)	62.8 (CH_3)
		α 4.30 (1H, dd, 11.7, 5.6)		4.30 (1H, dd, 11.5, 5.6)	

Table 1.8: ^{13}C NMR spectroscopic data (125 MHz, C_5H_5N) of **61**, **46**, **48**, and **53**[a]

Position	***61***	***46***	***48***	***53***
	δ_C, mult.	δ_C, mult.	δ_C, mult.	δ_C, mult.
1	31.9 (t)	30.7 (t)	30.7 (t)	31.0 (t)
2	27.6 (t)	27.0 (t)	27.1 (t)	27.4 (t)
3	72.4 (d)	73.0 (d)	73.6 (d)	73.6 (d)
4	33.1 (t)	30.3 (t)	30.5 (t)	30.3 (t)
5	32.0 (d)	35.8 (d)	37.0 (d)	36.7 (d)
6	28.4 (t)	27.3 (t)	27.0 (t)	27.3 (t)
7	51.1 (d)	22.0 (t)	21.7 (t)	25.2 (t)
8	64.5 (s)	41.8 (d)	42.0 (d)	65.2 (s)
9	34.4 (d)	37.0 (d)	35.9 (d)	37.1 (d)
10	34.0 (s)	35.5 (s)	35.5 (s)	37.1 (s)
11	21.0 (t)	21.5 (t)	21.2 (t)	16.5 (t)
12	40.9 (t)	39.8 (t)	39.0 (t)	36.7 (t)
13	52.7 (s)	50.1 (s)	50.5 (s)	41.8 (s)
14	81.8 (s)	84.6 (s)	83.5 (s)	70.8 (s)
15	35.4 (t)	33.1 (t)	41.3 (t)	26.9 (t)
16	28.8 (t)	27.2 (t)	75.0 (d)	25.9 (t)
17	51.0 (d)	51.4 (d)	56.8 (d)	51.4 (d)
18	17.4 (q)	16.2 (q)	16.3 (q)	16.3 (q)
19	24.5 (q)	23.9 (q)	23.9 (q)	25.0 (q)
20	175.1 (s)	176.0 (s)	170.2 (s)	170.6 (s)
21	73.7 (t)	73.7 (t)	76.2 (t)	73.6 (t)
22	117.8 (d)	117.6 (d)	121.6 (d)	116.9 (t)
23	174.4 (s)	174.5 (s)	174.1 (s)	173.8 (s)
OAc			170.0 (s)	
			20.7 (q)	
1'	98.9 (d)	98.7 (d)	98.9 (d)	98.8 (d)
2'	33.3 (t)	33.2 (t)	33.3 (t)	33.3 (t)
3'	80.2 (d)	80.1 (d)	80.2(d)	80.2 (d)
4'	73.6 (d)	73.2 (d)	73.1(d)	73.6 (d)
5'	71.0 (d)	70.8 (d)	70.9 (d)	70.9 (d)
6'	18.2 (q)	18.1 (q)	18.1 (q)	18.1 (q)
OMe	56.2 (q)	56.1(q)	56.2 (q)	56.2 (q)
1"	104.7 (d)	104.5 (d)	104.6 (d)	104.7 (d)
2"	75.8 (d)	75.6 (d)	75.7 (d)	75.7 (d)
3"	78.4 (d)	78.2 (d)	78.5 (d)	78.3 (d)

Contd...

Table 1.8–*Contd...*

Position	*61*	*46*	*48*	*53*
	δ_C, *mult.*	δ_C, *mult.*	δ_C, *mult.*	δ_C, *mult.*
4''	72.0 (d)	71.8 (d)	71.8 (d)	71.9 (d)
5''	77.7 (d)	77.6 (d)	77.6 (d)	77.6 (d)
6''	70.5 (t)	70.3 (t)	70.5 (t)	70.5 (t)
1'''	105.6 (d)	105.5 (d)	105.6 (d)	105.6 (d)
2'''	75.3 (d)	75.1 (d)	75.2 (d)	75.2 (d)
3'''	78.6 (d)	78.4 (d)	78.4 (d)	78.5 (d)
4'''	71.9 (d)	71.6 (d)	71.9 (d)	71.8 (d)
5'''	78.5 (d)	78.4 (d)	78.3 (d)	78.4 (d)
6'''	62.9 (t)	62.7 (t)	62.8 (t)	62.8 (t)

a: Signals were assigned from ^{1}H-^{1}H COSY, HMQC, and HMBC spectra.

3β-O-(4-O-Gentiobiosyl-D-diginosyl)-14-hydroxy-5β,14β-card-20(22)-enolide (Yamauchi et al., 1975; Hill et al., 1991)

46 was obtained as colorless powder; mp 175–179 °C (acetone–hexane); $[\alpha]^{20}_D$ -23.5° (*c* 0.625, MeOH). IR (KBr): ν_{max} cm^{-1} 3508, 1742.

3β-O-(4-O-Gentiobiosyl-D-digitalosyl)-14-hydroxy-5β,14β-card-20(22)-enolide (Yamauchi et al., 1975; Hanada et al., 1992; Rangaswami and Reichstein, 1949)

47 was obtained as colorless powder; mp 172–175 °C (acetone–hexane); $[\alpha]^{20}_D$ -18.9° (*c* 0.730, MeOH). IR (KBr): ν_{max} cm^{-1} 3408, 1745.

3β-O-(4-O-Gentiobiosyl-D-diginosyl)-16-β-acetoxy-14-hydroxy-5β,14β-card-20(22)-enolide (Abe and Yamauchi, 1992)

48 was obtained as colorles powder; mp 180–183 °C (acetone–hexane); $[\alpha]^{20}_D$ -28.0° (*c* 0.596, MeOH). IR (KBr): ν_{max} cm^{-1} 3408, 1745.

3β-O-(4-O-Gentiobiosyl-D-digitalosyl)-16-β-acetoxy-14-hydroxy-5β,14β-card-20(22)-enolide (Yamauchi et al.,1976)

49 was obtained as colorless powder; mp 185–190 °C (acetone–hexane); $[\alpha]^{20}_D$ -18.3° (*c* 0.769, MeOH). IR (KBr): ν_{max} cm^{-1} 3418, 1738.

3β-O-(4-O-Gentiobiosyl-L-oleandrosyl)-16-β-acetoxy-14-hydroxy-5β,14β-card-20(22)-enolide (Yamauchi et al., 1975)

50 was obtained as colorless powder; mp 169–173 °C (acetone–hexane); $[\alpha]^{20}_D$ -60.9° (*c* 0.465, MeOH). IR (KBr): ν_{max} cm^{-1} 3354, 1738.

3β-O-(4-O-Gentiobiosyl-D-diginosyl)-14-hydroxy-5α,14β-card-20(22)-enolide (odoroside K) (Hill et al., 1991; Rittel and Reichstein, 19954)

51 was obtained as colorless powder; mp 166–168 °C (acetone–hexane); $[\alpha]^{20}_D$ -22.8° (*c* 0.654, MeOH); IR (KBr): ν_{max} cm^{-1} 3250, 1740.

Table 1.9: ^{13}C NMR data of **22–34** (125 MHz, d in ppm *J* in Hz)

Position	**22**	**23**	**24**		**25**	**26**	**27**	**28**	**29**	**30**	**31**	**32**	**33**	**34**
	$CDCl_3$	$CDCl_3$	$CDCl_3$	C_5D_5N	$CDCl_3$	$CDCl_3$	$CDCl_3$	C_5D_5N	$CDCl_3$	$CDCl_3$	$CDCl_3$	$CDCl_3$	$CDCl_3$	$CDCl_3$
1	30.4, CH_2	31.1, CH_2	30.9, CH_2	31.6, CH_2	30.2, CH_2	30.0, CH_2	26.6, CH_2	30.8, CH_2	26.6, CH_2	37.1, CH_2	30.1, CH_2	30.2, CH_2	31.5, CH_2	30.3, CH_2
2	26.6, CH_2	27.1, CH_2	28.1, CH_2	28.9, CH_2	26.5, CH_2	26.4, CH_2	26.5, CH_2	27.1, CH_2	29.9, CH_2	29.2, CH_2	26.6, CH_2	26.5, CH_2	27.0, CH_2	28.3, CH_2
3	73.7, CH	71.9, CH	66.6, CH	65.8, CH	73.9, CH	73.9, CH	71.3, CH	74.2, CH	72.5, CH	77.7, CH	73.8, CH	72.6, CH	72.2, CH	72.6, CH
4	30.0, CH_2	32.7, CH_2	33.5, CH_2	34.5, CH_2	30.0, CH_2	30.0, CH_2	34.5, CH_2	30.4, CH_2	30.1, CH_2	34.2, CH_2	30.0, CH_2	29.9, CH_2	29.9, CH_2	30.8, CH_2
5	36.6, CH	33.6, CH	36.4, CH	37.1, CH	36.5, CH	36.4, CH	36.4, CH	36.7, CH	36.2, CH	44.2, CH	36.5, CH	36.5, CH	36.8, CH	36.1, CH
6	24.5, CH_2	27.9, CH_2	23.9, CH_2	24.8, CH_2	26.6, CH_2	26.4, CH_2	30.4, CH_2	27.1, CH_2	26.6, CH_2	28.5, CH_2	24.6, CH_2	26.6, CH_2	24.2, CH_2	30.9, CH_2
7	26.7, CH_2	51.2, CH	29.0, CH_2	29.5, CH_2	21.2, CH_2	20.7, CH_2	21.0, CH_2	21.7, CH_2	21.8, CH_2	27.4, CH_2	27.0, CH_2	21.2, CH_2	29.1, CH_2	37.8, CH_2
8	65.3, qC	63.9, qC	48.8, qC	49.1, qC	41.9, CH	41.7, CH	41.8, CH	42.0, CH	42.1, CH	41.6, CH	65.1, qC	41.0, CH	48.8, qC	216.7, qC
9	36.7, CH	31.6, CH	45.7, CH	46.0, CH	35.8, CH	35.6, CH	35.6, CH	35.9, CH	35.7, CH	49.8, CH	36.2, CH	36.3, CH	46.0, CH	50.9, CH
10	36.7, qC	33.6, qC	37.5, qC	37.9, qC	35.2, qC	35.0, qC	35.1, qC	35.4, qC	35.2, qC	35.9, qC	36.7, qC	35.1, qC	37.3, qC	42.5, qC
11	16.1, CH_2	20.3, CH_2	21.3, CH_2	21.4, CH_2	21.4, CH_2	21.0, CH_2	20.8, CH_2	21.2, CH_2	21.0, CH_2	21.1, CH_2	15.6, CH_2	19.8, CH_2	21.4, CH_2	27.2, CH_2
12	37.0, CH_2	41.0, CH_2	42.6, CH_2	42.7, CH_2	40.1, CH_2	39.2 CH_2	39.3 CH_2	39.0, CH_2	41.7 CH_2	39.8, CH_2	33.3, CH_2	38.4, CH_2	42.6, CH_2	34.7, CH_2
13	41.8, qC	52.2, qC	47.3, qC	47.5, qC	49.6, qC	49.9, qC	50.0, qC	50.5, qC	49.6, qC	49.5, qC	44.7, qC	52.2, qC	47.4, qC	51.4, qC
14	70.5, qC	81.0, qC	220.8, qC	221.3, qC	85.5, qC	84.2, qC	84.3, qC	83.5, qC	86.3, qC	85.4, qC	70.1, qC	85.6, qC	220.7, qC	78.9, qC
15	25.7, CH_2	34.4, CH_2	44.1, CH_2	44.1, CH_2	33.2, CH_2	41.2, CH_2	41.3, CH_2	41.3, CH_2	41.9, CH_2	33.0, CH_2	33.0, CH_2	40.4, CH_2	44.1, CH_2	26.8, CH_2
16	27.0, CH_2	28.4, CH_2	26.9, CH_2	26.9, CH_2	27.0, CH_2	74.0, CH	73.9, CH	75.0, CH	73.3, CH	26.8, CH_2	132.2, CH	132.1, CH	26.9, CH_2	17.5, CH_2
17	51.5, CH	50.6, CH	53.3, CH	53.0, CH	50.9, CH	56.1, CH	56.1, CH	56.9, CH	58.1, CH	50.8, CH	143.0, qC	144.0, qC	53.1, CH	45.8, CH
18	16.2, CH_3	17.1, CH_3	23.3, CH_3	23.4, CH_3	15.8, CH_3	15.9, CH_3	15.9, CH_3	16.3, CH_3	16.7, CH_3	15.7, CH_3	19.9, CH_3	16.8, CH_3	23.4, CH_3	17.3, CH_3
19	24.7, CH_3	24.0, CH_3	26.4, CH_3	26.6, CH_3	23.7, CH_3	23.6, CH_3	23.8, CH_3	23.7, CH_3	23.6, CH_3	12.1, CH_3	24.5, CH_3	23.8, CH_3	26.3, CH_3	23.9, CH_3
20	169.5, qC	173.6, qC	170.5, qC	171.9, qC	174.4, qC	170.4, qC	167.6, qC	169.7, qC	168.5, qC	174.5, qC	157.6, qC	158.3, qC	170.4, qC	171.4, qC
21	73.2, CH_2	73.3, CH_2	72.8, CH_2	73.4, CH_2	73.4, CH_2	75.6, CH_2	75.6, CH_2	76.2, CH_2	75.4, CH_2	73.4, CH_2	71.4, CH_2	71.7, CH_2	72.8, CH_2	73.8, CH_2
22	116.9, CH	117.8, CH	116.7, CH	116.4 (d)	117.1, CH	121.3, CH	121.4, CH	121.6, CH	119.8, CH	117.6, CH	112.8, CH	112.4, CH	116.4 (d)	116.7, CH
23	173.6, qC	174.2, qC	173.5, qC	173.8, qC	174.4, qC	174.1, qC	174.0, qC	174.1, qC	174.2, qC	174.5, qC	174.2, qC	174.4, qC	173.5, qC	174.0, qC

Contd...

Table 1.9–*Contd...*

Position	**22**	**23**	**24**		**25**	**26**	**27**	**28**	**29**	**30**	**31**	**32**	**33**	**34**
	$CDCl_3$	$CDCl_3$	$CDCl_3$	C_5D_5N	$CDCl_3$	$CDCl_3$	$CDCl_3$	C_5D_5N	$CDCl_3$	$CDCl_3$	$CDCl_3$	$CDCl_3$	$CDCl_3$	$CDCl_3$
16-OAc						21.0, CH_3	21.04, CH_3	20.7, CH_3						
						167.8, qC	170.4, qC	170.2, qC						
1'	101.3, CH	97.9, CH			101.1, CH	101.3, CH	95.5, CH	103.1, CH	97.8, CH	100.8, CH	100.3, CH	97.8, CH	97.5, CH	98.4, CH
2'	70.8, CH	32.0, CH_2			70.8, CH	70.7, CH	29.8, CH	75.4, CH	32.1, CH_2	70.5, CH	70.7, CH	32.1, CH_2	32.1, CH_2	32.1, CH_2
3'	82.8, CH	78.0, CH			82.8, CH	82.8, CH	78.4, CH	78.8, CH	78.0, CH	82.9, CH	82.8, CH	78.0, CH	77.9, CH	77.9, CH
4'	68.2, CH	67.2, CH			68.2, CH	68.1, CH	67.6, CH	72.0, CH	67.2, CH	67.9, CH	68.1, CH	67.2, CH	67.2, CH	66.9, CH
5'	70.4, CH	70.4, CH			70.3, CH	70.4, CH	76.3, CH	78.4, CH	70.4, CH	70.3, CH	70.3, CH	70.4, CH	70.3, CH	70.4, CH
6'	16.2, CH_3	16.8, CH_3			16.4, CH_3	16.4, CH_3	17.8, CH_3	63.0, CH_3	16.8, CH_3	16.5, CH_3	16.4, CH_3	16.6, CH_3	16.9, CH_3	16.8, CH_3
3'-OMe	57.6, CH_3	55.7, CH_3			57.5, CH_3	57.6, CH_3	56.4, CH_3		55.7, CH_3	57.4, CH_3	57.5, CH_3	55.7, CH_3	55.8, CH_3	55.7, CH_3

Table 1.10: ^{13}C NMR data of **46–61** (C_6D_5N, 125 MHz, δ in ppm, J in Hz)[a,b].

Position	***46***	***47***	***48***	***49***	***50***	***51***	***52***	***53***	***54***	***55***	***56***	***57***	***58***	***59***	***60***	***61***
1	30.7 (t)	30.5 (t)	30.7 (t)	30.6 (t)	31.1 (t)	37.4 (t)	37.4 (t)	31.0 (t)	30.9 (t)	30.8 (t)	30.7 (t)	31.1 (t)	32.4 (t)	30.8 (t)	31.9 (t)	31.9 (t)
2	27.0 (t)	27.1 (t)	27.1 (t)	27.0 (t)	26.8 (t)	30.1 (t)	30.0 (t)	27.4 (t)	27.4 (t)	27.3 (t)	27.3 (t)	26.9 (t)	27.5 (t)	27.2 (t)	27.2 (t)	27.6 (t)
3	73.0 (d)	74.4 (d)	73.6 (d)	74.4 (d)	72.0 (d)	78.5 (d)	77.3 (d)	73.6 (d)	74.2 (d)	72.9 (d)	74.2 (d)	72.0 (d)	72.8 (d)	74.5 (d)	72.8 (d)	72.4 (d)
4	30.3 (t)	30.7 (t)	30.5 (t)	30.5 (t)	30.5 (t)	34.9 (t)	34.7 (t)	30.3 (t)	30.4 (t)	30.4 (t)	30.4 (t)	30.1 (t)	30.5 (t)	30.6 (t)	30.5 (t)	33.1 (t)
5	35.8 (d)	36.7 (d)	37.0 (d)	36.6 (d)	35.8 (d)	44.5 (d)	44.5 (d)	36.7 (d)	36.7 (d)	37.2 (d)	36.7 (d)	37.1 (d)	37.4 (d)	36.7 (d)	37.4 (d)	32.0 (d)
6	27.3 (t)	27.2 (t)	27.0 (t)	27.0 (t)	27.1 (t)	30.0 (t)	29.2 (t)	27.3 (t)	27.4 (t)	25.3 (d)	27.1 (t)	27.2 (t)	28.6 (t)	27.2 (t)	24.6 (t)	28.4 (t)
7	22.0 (t)	21.6 (t)	21.7 (t)	21.6 (t)	21.2 (t)	28.1 (t)	28.0 (t)	25.2 (t)	25.1 (t)	27.2 (t)	25.1 (t)	22.0 (t)	23.4 (t)	38.2 (t)	29.3 (t)	51.1 (d)
8	41.8 (d)	42.0 (d)	42.0 (d)	42.0 (d)	41.8 (d)	41.8 (d)	41.7 (d)	65.2 (s)	65.2 (s)	65.1 (s)	65.1 (s)	42.2 (d)	76.8 (s)	216.4 (s)	48.9 (s)	64.5 (s)
9	37.0 (d)	36.0 (d)	35.9 (d)	35.9 (d)	37.1 (d)	50.0 (d)	50.0 (d)	37.1 (d)	37.0 (d)	36.3 (d)	36.3 (d)	35.8 (d)	36.8 (d)	51.3 (d)	46.0 (d)	34.4 (d)
10	35.5 (s)	35.5 (s)	35.5 (s)	35.4 (s)	35.5 (s)	36.1 (s)	36.1 (s)	37.1 (s)	37.0 (s)	31.7 (s)	37.0 (s)	35.5 (s)	35.8 (s)	42.7 (s)	37.6 (s)	34.0 (s)
11	21.5 (t)	22.0 (t)	21.2 (t)	21.4 (t)	21.7 (t)	21.6 (t)	21.5 (t)	16.5 (t)	16.5 (t)	16.1 (t)	16.0 (t)	21.4 (t)	18.3 (t)	27.7 (t)	21.3 (t)	21.0 (t)
12	39.8 (t)	40.0 (t)	39.0 (t)	39.0 (t)	39.0 (t)	39.7 (t)	39.7 (t)	36.7 (t)	36.8 (t)	33.4 (t)	33.4 (t)	40.2 (t)	40.7 (t)	35.2 (t)	42.6 (t)	40.9 (t)
13	50.1 (s)	50.2 (s)	50.5 (s)	50.5 (s)	50.5 (s)	50.1 (s)	50.0 (s)	41.8 (s)	41.5 (s)	45.0 (s)	45.0 (s)	50.6 (s)	50.9 (s)	51.3 (s)	47.5 (s)	52.7 (s)
14	84.6 (s)	84.7 (s)	83.5 (s)	83.4 (s)	83.5 (s)	84.6 (s)	84.6 (s)	70.8 (s)	70.7 (s)	70.3 (s)	70.3 (s)	84.2 (s)	85.9 (s)	79.4 (d)	221.3 (s)	81.8 (s)
15	33.1 (t)	33.2 (t)	41.3 (t)	41.3 (t)	41.3 (t)	33.2 (t)	33.2 (t)	26.9 (t)	26.8 (t)	33.4 (t)	33.3 (t)	44.0 (t)	35.3 (t)	27.2 (t)	44.0 (t)	35.4 (t)
16	27.2 (t)	27.4 (t)	75.0 (d)	74.9 (d)	75.0 (d)	27.3 (t)	27.3 (t)	25.9 (t)	25.9 (t)	132.9 (d)	132.9 (d)	72.4 (d)	27.5 (t)	18.3 (t)	26.9 (t)	28.8 (t)
17	51.4 (d)	51.5 (d)	56.8 (d)	56.8 (d)	56.8 (d)	51.5 (d)	51.5 (d)	51.4 (d)	51.4 (d)	143.3 (s)	143.3 (s)	59.4 (t)	52.3 (d)	46.3 (d)	52.9 (d)	51.0 (d)
18	16.2 (q)	16.2 (q)	16.3 (q)	16.3 (q)	16.3 (q)	16.2 (q)	16.2 (q)	16.3 (q)	16.3 (q)	20.1 (q)	20.1 (q)	17.0 (q)	18.6 (q)	17.6 (q)	23.3 (q)	17.4 (q)
19	23.9 (q)	23.7 (q)	23.9 (q)	23.7 (q)	24.0 (q)	12.2 (q)	12.2 (q)	25.0 (q)	24.8 (q)	24.9 (q)	24.7 (q)	24.1 (q)	26.2 (q)	23.8 (q)	26.4 (q)	24.5 (q)
20	176.0 (s)	175.9 (s)	170.2 (s)	169.7 (s)	169.7 (s)	175.9 (s)	174.5 (s)	170.6 (s)	170.6 (s)	158.5 (s)	158.5 (s)	172.4 (s)	175.7 (s)	172.5 (s)	171.8 (s)	175.1 (s)
21	73.7 (t)	73.7 (t)	76.2 (t)	76.2 (t)	76.2 (t)	73.7 (t)	73.7 (t)	73.6 (t)	73.6 (t)	71.8 (t)	74.2 (t)	76.7 (t)	73.7 (t)	76.4 (t)	73.4 (t)	73.7 (t)
22	117.6 (d)	117.7 (d)	121.6 (d)	121.6 (d)	121.7 (d)	117.7 (d)	117.7 (d)	116.9 (d)	116.9 (d)	113.2 (d)	113.1 (d)	120.2 (d)	117.7 (d)	116.8 (d)	116.3 (d)	117.8 (d)
23	174.5 (s)	174.5 (s)	174.1 (s)	174.1 (s)	174.1 (s)	174.5 (s)	175.9 (s)	173.8 (s)	173.9 (s)	174.5 (s)	174.5 (s)	174.6 (s)	174.4 (s)	174.1 (s)	173.8 (s)	174.4 (s)

Contd...

Table 1.10–*Contd...*

Position	***46***	***47***	***48***	***49***	***50***	***51***	***52***	***53***	***54***	***55***	***56***	***57***	***58***	***59***	***60***	***61***
16-OAc			170.0 (s)	170.2 (s)	170.2 (s)											
			20.7 (q)	20.7 (q)	20.7 (q)											
1'	98.7 (d)	103.4 (d)	98.9 (d)	103.4 (d)	96.0 (d)	98.3 (d)	102.4 (d)	98.8 (d)	103.5 (d)	98.9 (d)	103.5 (d)	95.7 (d)	98.7 (d)	99.0 (d)	98.8 (d)	98.9 (d)
2'	33.2 (t)	70.6 (d)	33.3 (t)	70.6 (d)	35.8 (t)	33.3 (t)	70.6 (d)	33.3 (t)	71.4 (d)	33.3 (t)	71.3 (d)	35.8 (t)	33.3 (t)	33.2 (t)	33.3 (t)	33.3 (t)
3'	80.1 (d)	85.7 (d)	80.2 (d)	85.6 (d)	79.4 (d)	80.2 (d)	85.6 (d)	80.2 (d)	85.7 (d)	80.2 (d)	85.7 (d)	79.4 (d)	80.2 (d)	80.2 (d)	80.1 (d)	80.2 (d)
4'	73.2 (d)	76.0 (d)	73.1 (d)	75.9 (d)	82.2 (d)	73.4 (d)	75.8 (d)	73.6 (d)	75.8 (d)	73.6 (d)	75.8 (d)	82.2 (d)	73.5 (d)	73.1 (d)	73.6 (d)	73.6 (d)
5'	70.8 (d)	71.4 (d)	70.9 (d)	71.3 (d)	67.8 (d)	70.9 (d)	71.4 (d)	70.9 (d)	70.6 (d)	71.0 (d)	70.6 (d)	67.8 (d)	70.9 (d)	70.9 (d)	70.9 (d)	71.0 (d)
6'	18.1 (q)	18.0 (q)	18.1 (q)	18.0 (q)	18.9 (q)	18.2 (q)	18.0 (q)	18.1 (q)	18.0 (q)	18.2 (q)	18.0 (q)	18.8 (q)	18.1 (q)	18.1 (q)	18.1 (q)	18.2 (q)
OMe	56.1 (q)	58.9 (q)	56.2 (q)	58.9 (q)	56.9 (q)	56.3 (q)	58.9 (q)	56.2 (q)	58.9 (q)	56.2 (q)	58.9 (q)	56.7 (q)	56.2 (q)	56.2 (q)	56.2 (q)	56.2 (q)
1''	104.5 (d)	105.2 (d)	104.6 (d)	105.1 (d)	105.0 (d)	104.6 (d)	105.1 (d)	104.7 (d)	105.1 (d)	104.7 (d)	105.1 (d)	105.0 (d)	104.6 (d)	104.5 (d)	104.7 (d)	104.7 (d)
2''	75.6 (d)	75.8 (d)	75.7 (d)	75.7 (d)	75.8 (d)	75.8 (d)	75.8 (d)	75.7 (d)	75.2 (d)	75.7 (d)	75.2 (d)	75.8 (d)	75.7 (d)	75.7 (d)	75.7 (d)	75.8 (d)
3''	78.2 (d)	78.4 (d)	78.5 (d)	78.3 (d)	78.4 (d)	78.4 (d)	78.6 (d)	78.3 (d)	78.4 (d)	78.4 (d)	78.5 (d)	78.3 (d)	78.3 (d)	78.3 (d)	78.4 (d)	78.4 (d)
4''	71.8 (d)	71.9 (d)	71.8 (d)	71.8 (d)	72.1 (d)	72.0 (d)	71.9 (d)	71.9 (d)	71.9 (d)	71.8 (d)	71.8 (d)	72.1 (d)	71.9 (d)	71.9 (d)	71.8 (d)	72.0 (d)
5''	77.6 (d)	77.7 (d)	77.6 (d)	77.7 (d)	77.3 (d)	77.7 (d)	77.7 (d)	77.6 (d)	77.7 (d)	77.7 (d)	77.7 (d)	77.3 (d)	77.6 (d)	77.7 (d)	77.6 (d)	77.7 (d)
6''	70.3 (t)	70.5 (t)	70.5 (t)	70.4 (t)	70.7 (t)	70.5 (t)	70.5 (t)	70.5 (t)	70.5 (t)	70.5 (t)	70.5 (t)	70.7 (t)	70.4 (t)	70.4 (t)	70.5 (t)	70.5 (t)
1'''	105.5 (d)	105.6 (d)	105,6 (d)	105.6 (d)	105.6 (d)	105.6 (d)	105.6 (d)	105.6 (d)	105.6 (d)	105.6 (d)	105.6 (d)	105.6 (d)	105.6 (d)	105.6 (d)	105.6 (d)	105.6 (d)
2'''	75.1 (d)	75.2 (d)	75.2 (d)	75.2 (d)	75.3 (d)	75.3 (d)	75.2 (d)	75.2 (d)	75.2 (d)	75.3 (d)	75.2 (d)	75.3 (d)	75.2 (d)	75.2 (d)	75.2 (d)	75,3 (d)
3'''	78.4 (d)	78.5 (d)	78.4 (d)	78.5 (d)	78.5 (d)	78.6 (d)	78.5 (d)	78.5 (d)	78.5 (d)	78.6 (d)	78.4 (d)	78.5 (d)	78.5 (d)	78.5 (d)	78.5 (d)	78.6 (d)
4'''	71.6 (d)	71.8 (d)	71.9 (d)	71.8 (d)	71.8 (d)	71.8 (d)	71.8 (d)	71.8 (d)	71.8 (d)	72.0 (d)	71.9 (d)	71.8 (d)	71.8 (d)	71.7 (d)	71.8 (d)	71.9 (d)
5'''	78.4 (d)	78.5 (d)	78.3 (d)	78.4 (d)	78.5 (d)	76.6 (d)	78.4 (d)	78.4 (d)	78.6 (d)	78.5 (d)	78.6 (d)	78.4 (d)	78.5 (d)	78.3 (d)	78.5 (d)	78.5 (d)
6'''	62.7 (t)	62.9 (t)	62.8 (t)	62.8 (t)	62.9 (t)	62.9 (t)	62.9 (t)	62.8 (t)	62.9 (t)	62.9 (t)	62.9 (t)	62.9 (t)	62.8 (t)	62.8 (t)	62.9 (t)	62.9 (t)

a: Multiplicities were determined by the Dept.

b: Signals were assigned from the HMQC and HMBC spectra.

3β-O-(4-O-Gentiobiosyl-D-digitalosyl)-14-hydroxy-5α,14β-card-20(22)-enolide (Hanada et al., 1992)

52 was obtained as colorless powder; mp 170–173 °C (acetone–hexane); $[\alpha]^{29}{}_{D}$ -23.6° (*c* 0.585, MeOH). IR (KBr): ν_{max} cm^{-1} 3474, 1726.

3β-O-(4-O-gentiobiosyl-D-digitalosyl)-8,14-epoxy-5β,14β-card-20(22)-enolide (Abe and Yamauchi, 1992)

54 was obtained as colorless powder; mp 170–172 °C (acetone–hexane); $[\alpha]^{28}{}_{D}$ -20.6° (*c* 0.631, MeOH). IR (KBr): ν_{max} cm^{-1} 3303, 1746.

3β-O-(4-O-Gentiobiosyl-D-digitalosyl)-8,14-epoxy-5β,14β-card-16,20(22)-enolide (Abe and Yamauchi, 1992)

56 was obtained as colorless powder; mp 181–184 °C (acetone–hexane); $[\alpha]^{20}{}_{D}$ +28.5° (*c* 0.260, MeOH). IR (KBr): ν_{max} cm^{-1} 3344, 1746.

3β-O-(4-O-Gentiobiosyl-L-oleandrosyl)-14,16β-dihydroxy-5β,14β-card-20(22)-enolide (Abe and Yamauchi, 1992)

57 was obtained as colorless powder (acetone–hexane); mp 208–211 °C; $[\alpha]^{20}{}_{D}$ -41.0° (*c* 0.315, MeOH). IR (KBr): ν_{max} cm^{-1} 3431, 1728.

3β-O-(4-O-Gentiobiosyl-D-deginosyl)-8β,14-dihydroxy-5β,14β-card-20(22)-enolide (Abe and Yamauchi, 1992)

58 was obtained as colorless powder (acetone–hexane); mp 181–184 °C; $[\alpha]^{20}{}_{D}$ -21.5° (*c* 0.455, MeOH). IR (KBr): ν_{max} cm^{-1} 3430, 1738.

3β-O-(4-O-Gentiobiosyl-D-deginosyl)-14α-hydroxy-8-oxo-8,14-seco-5β-card-20(22)-enolide (Yamauchi and Abe, 1978)

59 was obtained as colorless powder; mp 185–189 °C (acetone–hexane); $[\alpha]^{20}{}_{D}$ -11.3° (*c* 0.515, MeOH). IR (KBr): ν_{max} cm^{-1} 3514, 1745.

3β-O-(4-O-gentiobiosyl-D-deginosyl)-14-oxo-15(15Õ8)abeo-card-20(22)-enolide (Abe and Yamauchi, 1979):

60 was obtained as colorless powder; mp 184–186 °C (acetone–hexane); $[\alpha]^{20}{}_{D}$ +14.6° (*c* 0.125, MeOH); IR (KBr): ν_{max} cm^{-1} 3403, 1747.

Inhibitory Activity on Induction of Intercellular Adhesion Molecule-1 (ICAM-1)

Cells

Human lung carcinoma A 549 cells were provided by the Heath Science research resources Bank (Tokyo, Japan). A549 cells were maintained in RPMI 1640 medium (Invitrogen, Carlsbad, CA) supplemented with 10 per cent (v/v) fetal calf serum (JRH Bioscience Lenexa, KS) and a penicillin–streptomycin–neomycin antibiotic mixture (Invitrogen).

Reagent

Mouse anti-human ICAM-1 antibody (clone 15.2) was purchased from Leinco Technologies, Inc. (St. Louis, MO), and horseradish peroxidase-conjugated goat anti-mouse IgG antibody was obtained from Jackson Immuno Research Laboratories, Inc. (West-Grove, PA). Recombinant human IL-1α and TNF-α were kindly provided by Dainippon Pharmaceutical Co Ltd. (Osaka Japan).

Procedures

A 549 cells, were seeded in a microtiter plate at 2 × 10^4 cell/well the day before the assay. After A549 cells were pretreated with or without test compounds in 75 *m*l for 1 h, 25*m*l of IL-1α (1 ng/ml) or TNF-α (10 ng/ml) were added to the culture, and the cells were further incubated for 6 h. The cells were washed once with phosphate-buffered saline (PBS) and fixed by incubation with 1 per cent paraformaldehyde–PBS for 15 min and then washed once with PBS. After blocking with 1 per cent bovine serum albumin–PBS overnight, the fixed cells were treated with mouse anti-human ICAM-1 antibody for 60 min. After being washed three times with 0.02 per cent Tween 20-PBS, the cells were treated with horseradish peroxidase-linked anti-mouse IgG antibody for 60 min. The cells were washed three times with 0.02 per cent Tween 20–PBS. The cells were incubated with the substrate (0.1 per cent *o*-phenylenediamine dihydrochloride and 0.02 per cent H_2O_2 in 0.2 M sodium citrate buffer, pH 5.3) for 20 min at 37°C in the dark and assayed for the absorbance at 415 nm by using a microplate reader. Expression of ICAM-1 was calculated as follows:

Expression of ICAM-1 (per cent of control) = [(absorbance with sample and cytokine treatment – absorbance without cytokine treatment)/(absorbance with IL-1α treatment – absorbance without cytokine treatment)] × 100

Cell Viability

A549 cells (2 × 10^4 cell/well) were seeded in a microtiter plate the day before the assay and incubated in the presence or absence of test compounds for 24 h. At the last 4 h of induction, the cell were pulsed with 500 *m*g/ml of 3-(4,5-dimethylthiazo-2-yl)-2,5-diphenyl tetrazolium bromide (MTT) for 4 h. MTT formazan was solubilized with 5 per cent sodium dodecyl sulfate (SDS) overnight. Absorbance at 595 nm was measured. Cell viability (per cent) was calculated as follows:

Cell viability (per cent) = [(experimental absorbance – background absorbance)/(control absorbance – background absorbance)] × 100

Cell Growth Inhibitory Activity of Compounds to WI-38 Fibroblast Cell, VA-13 Malignant Tumor Cell, and HepG2 Human Liver Tumor Cell in vitro

Cells

WI-38 is the normal human fibroblast derived from female human lung. VA-13 is malignant tumor cells induced from WI-38 by infection of SV-40 virus. HepG2 is Human liver tumor cells. These cell lines are available from the Institute of Physical and Chemical Research (RIKEN), Tukuba, Ibaraki, Japan. WI-38 and VA-13 cells were maintained in Eagle's MEM medium (Nissui Pharmaceutical Co., Tokyo, Japan) and RITC 80-7 medium (Asahi Technoglass Co., Chiba, Japan), respectively, both supplemented with 10 per cent (v/v) fetal bovine serum (FBS) (Filtron PTY LTD.,

Australia) with 80 μg/ml of kanamycin. HepG2 cells were maintained in D-MEM medium (Invitrogen) supplemented with 10 per cent (v/v) FBS (Filtron PTY LTD., Australia) with 80 μg/ml of kanamycin.

Procedures

Medium (100 μl) containing ca. 5, 000 cells (WI-38, VA-13, HepG2) were incubated at 37 °C in humidified atmosphere of 5 per cent CO_2 for 24 h in microtiter plate. Then test samples dissolved in dimethyl sulfoxide (DMSO) were added to the medium and incubation was continued further for 48 h in the same conditions. Coloration substrate, WST-8 [2-(2-methyl-4-nitrophenyl)-3-(4-nitrophenyl)-5-(2,4-disulfophenyl)-2H-tetrazolium, monosodium salt] was added to the medium. The resulting formazan concentration was determined by the absorption at 450 nm. Cell viability (per cent) was calculated as [(experimental absorbance – background absorbance)/(control absorbance – background absorbance)]×100. Cell viability at different concentration of compounds was plotted and 50 per cent inhibition of growth was calculated as IC_{50}.

Cellar Accumulation of Calcein

Cells

Adriamycin-resistant human ovarian cancer A2780 cells (AD10) were maintained in RPMI-1640 medium (Invitrogen) supplemented with 10 per cent (v/v) FBS (Fitron PTY Ltd., Australia) with 80 μg/ml kanamycin.

Procedures

Medium (100 μl) containing ca. 1×10^6 cells was incubated at 37°C in a humidified atmosphere containing 5 per cent CO_2 for 24 h. Test compounds were dissolved in DMSO and diluted with PBS (–). Test sample (50 μl) were added to the medium and incubated for 15 min. Then, 50 μl of the fluorogenic dye calcein AM [1 μl in PBS (–)] was added to the medium, and incubation was continued for a further 60 min. After removing the supernatant, each microplate was washed with 200 μl of cold PBS (–). The washing step was repeated twice and 200 ml of cold PBS (–) was added. Retention of the resulting calcein was measured as calcein-specific fluorescence. The absorption maximum for calcein is 494 nm, and emission maximum is 517 nm.

Results and Discussion

Structure Determination of New Pregnanes 1–3 and 6.

A methanol extract of air-dried stems and twigs of *N. oleander* was partitioned successively with hexane, ethyl acetate, and butanol. The ethyl acetate-soluble portion was separated by silica gel column chromatography and normal- and reverse-phase HPLC. Three new pregnanes, 21-hydroxypregna-4,6-diene-3,12,20-trione (**1**), 20*R*-hydroxypregna-4,6-diene-3,12-dione (**2**), 16β,17β-epoxy-12β-hydroxypregna-4,6-diene-3,20-dione (**3**), and 20*S*,21-dihydroxypregn-4-ene-3,12-dione (**6**) were isolated together with two known derivatives, 12β-hydroxypregna-4,6,16-triene-3,20-dione (neridienone A, **4**) (Abe and Yamauchi, 1976; Huq *et al.*, 1999) and 20*S*,21-dihydroxypregna-4,6-diene-3,12-dione (neridienone B, **5**)(Abe and Yamauchi, 1976).

21-*O*-(β-D-gulucopyranosyl)-14β-hydroxypregn-4-ene-3,20-dione (**7**) (Abe and Yamauchi, 1992) was isolated from *n*-BuOH extract of leaves and 3β-*O*-{β-D-gulucopyranosyl-(1→2)-[β-D-gulcopyranosyl-(1→6)]-β-D-glucopyranosy}-17α-pregn-5-ene-20-one (**8**)(Yamauchi *et al.*, 1972) was isolated from *n*-BuOH extract of a mixture of stems and twigs. Compound **1** gave the elemental composition, $C_{21}H_{26}O_4$, which was determined by a combination of an analysis of the HREIMS and ^{1}H and ^{13}C NMR data. The IR spectrum of **1** indicated the presence of hydroxyl (3500 cm^{-1}), carbonyl (1709 cm^{-1}), and conjugated carbonyl (1663, 1630, and 1618 cm^{-1}) groups. The UV spectrum of **1** was consistent with the presence of a conjugated dienone chromophore [265 nm (log *e* 4.23)]. The ^{13}C NMR spectrum displayed 21 carbon signals (Table 1.1). Three carbonyl carbon signals appeared at δ 198.7, 210.8, and 211.6 and four olefin carbon resonances were located at δ 124.8 (CH), 129.2 (CH), 137.7 (CH), and 161.1 (qC). A signal for one carbon-bearing oxygen was observed at δ 69.5 (CH_2). Judging from the DEPT and HMQC spectra, the remaining carbon resonances were two methyl carbons, five methylene carbons, four methine carbons, and two quaternary carbons. The ^{1}H NMR spectra showed two singlet methyls (δ 1.07 and 1.20) (Table 1.2). The connectivity of the protonated carbons (C-1 to C-2; C-6 to C-7, C-7 to C-8, C-8 to C-9, C-9 to C-11; C-8 to C-14, C-14 to C-15, C-15 to C-16) was determined from the ^{1}H-^{1}H COSY spectrum. A HMBC experiment was used to determine the carbon-carbon connections through the non-protonated carbon atoms [HMBC correlations: C-10 (δ 36.2) with H_2-1, H_2-2, H-4, H-9, H_2-11, Me-19; C-13 (d 59.1) with H-11α, H-14, H_2-15, H_2-16, H-17, Me-18]. Interpretation of these results suggested that compound **1** has steroid A, B, C, and D rings (Ahmed *et al.*, 2006; Wang *et al.* 2006). HMBC correlations [the carbonyl carbon at δ 198.7 with H-1β and H_2-2; the disubstituted olefin carbon at δ 161.1 with H-1β, Me-19, and the olefin protons H-4, H-6, and H-7] were used to place the carbonyl group at C-3 and a conjugated double bond at the C-4 and C-6 positions. The HMBC correlations [the carbonyl carbon at δ 211.6 with H-11α and Me-18; the carbonyl carbon at d 210.8 with the oxygenated methylene protons at C-21 (δ 4.27 and 4.58) and the methine proton at C-17 (δ 3.30)] showed that two carbonyl carbons and one oxygenated primary carbon are located at C-12, C-20, and C-21, respectively, and the hydroxy acetyl side chain is connected at C-17. Thus, the planar structure of **1** was established as 21-hydroxypregna-4,6-diene-3,12,20-trione (**1**). NOESY NMR experiments were used for assignment of the relative configuration of **1**. The NOESY correlations [H-2β with Me-19; Me-19 with H-8 and H-11β; H-8 and H-11β with Me-18; Me-18 with H-15β and H-16β; H-14 with H-17 and H-15α; H-15α with H-16α; H-21a with H-17; H-21b with Me-18 and H-17; H-9 with H-11α] indicated the full stereostructure of the molecule **1**. Thus, 10β-Me, 8β-H, 9α-H, 13β-Me, 14α-H, and 17β-hydroxyacetyl substituents were confirmed for **1**. Compound **2** was assigned the elemental composition, $C_{21}H_{28}O_3$, which was determined from the HRFABMS and ^{1}H and ^{13}C NMR spectroscopic data. Similar IR and UV data were obtained for compound **2** as compared to compound **1**. The ^{13}C NMR spectrum displayed 21 carbon signals with two carbonyl carbons located at δ 198.8 and 216.6, one hydroxylated methine carbon at δ 68.0, and four olefin carbons at δ 124.7 (δ), 129.0 (δ), 138.1 (d), and 161.4 (s). As judged from the DEPT and HMQC spectra, the remaining carbon resonances were three methyl carbons, five methylene carbons, four methine carbons, and two quaternary carbons. The ^{1}H NMR spectrum showed two singlet methyls (δ1.18 and 1.21) and one doublet methyl (δ1.17). Compound **2** showed very similar ^{13}C and ^{1}H NMR spectra to those of **1** except in the vicinity of the side chain at C-17 (Tables 1.1 and 1.2). The connectivity of the protonated carbons determined by analysis of the ^{1}H-^{1}H COSY spectrum and the carbon-carbon connections through the non-protonated carbon atoms determined by the HMBC experiment indicated that compound **2** has a pregna-4,6-diene-3,12-dione structure like **1**. The chemical shifts of C-1 through C-11, C-15, and C-19 in the ^{13}C NMR spectrum of **2** were superimposable on those of **1**, with differences observed in the values of C-20 and C-21. HMBC correlations [the carbonyl carbon at δ216.6 with H-9, H_2-11, H-17, and Me-18; the quaternary carbon at *d* 57.7 with H-11α, H-15α, H-16α, H-17, and Me-18; and the hydroxylated methine carbon at d 68.0 with the protons of Me-21 (δ 1.17) and methine proton at C-17 (δ 2.03)] showed that one carbonyl carbon and one hydroxylated methine carbon are located at C-12 and C-20, respectively, and that an acetyl side chain is connected at C-17. Thus, the planar structure of **2** was established as 20-hydroxypregna-4,6-diene-3,12-dione (**2**). Compound **2** showed similar NOESY correlations to those of **1** except for H-20 and Me-21 of the side chain at C-17. Thus, the 10β-Me, 8β-H, 9α-H, 13β-Me, 14α-H, and 17β-hydroxyethyl configurations in **2** could be confirmed. Additional NOESY correlations in the vicinity of H-20 [H-20 with Me-18 and H-16β; Me-21 with H-16α,β] indicated that the configuration of C-20 is *R* (Figure 1.2). Thus, the structure of compound **2** was determined as 20*R*-hydroxypregna-4,6-diene-3,12-dione. Compound **3** was assigned the molecular composition, $C_{21}H_{26}O_4$, determined by HREIMS and from the ^{1}H and ^{13}C NMR spectroscopic data. Similar IR and UV data were obtained for compound **3** as compared to compounds **1** and **2**. The ^{1}H and ^{13}C NMR spectra of **3** were also similar to those of **1**, with differences observed in the values for H- and C-12, 16, 17, and 21. HMBC correlations [the hydroxylated methine carbon at C-12 (δ72.2) with H_2-11, H-14, and Me-18; the quaternary carbon at C-13 (δ49.7) with H-8, H-11α, H-14, H_2-15, and Me-18; the oxygenated tertiary carbon at C-17 (δ74.8) with H-15β, Me-18, and Me-21; the oxygenated methine carbon at C-16 (δ 67.1) with H-14 and H-15*b*; the carbonyl carbon at d 208.2 with Me-21 (acetyl methyl)] were used to place one hydroxyl group at C-12, one carbonyl group at C-20, and an epoxy group between the C-16 and C-17 positions. Thus, the planar structure of **3** was assighed as 16,17-epoxy-12-hydroxypregna-4,6-diene-3,20-dione (**3**). Compound **3** showed very similar NOESY correlations to those of **1** except for H-12, H-16, and Me-21 of the side chain at C-17. NOESY correlations [H-11α for H-12;H-14 with H-12 and H-15α; H-15α ?with H-16; H-16 with Me-21] indicated the full stereostructure of **3**. Thus, the structure of compound **3** was determined as 16β,17β-epoxy-12β-hydroxypregna-4,6-diene-3,20-dione.

Compound **6** has the composition $C_{21}H_{30}O_4$, which was determined by HR-FAB-MS analysis. The IR spectrum of compound **6** indicated the existence of hydroxyl (3424 cm^{-1}), carbonyl (1689 cm^{-1}), and α,β-unsaturated-carbonyl (1670, 1620 cm^{-1}) groups. The UV spectrum indicated the existence of α,β-unsaturated ketone [234 nm (log ε 3.99)]. The ^{13}C NMR displayed 21 carbon signals (Table 1.3). Two carbonyl carbons resonated at δ217.5 and 197.8, and two olefin carbons were located at δ168.3 (qC) and 124.8 (CH). Two signals for carbons bearing oxygen were observed at α 73.8

(CH) and 66.3 (CH_2). From the DEPT and HMQC spectra, the remaining carbon resonances were two methyl, seven methylene, four methine, and two quaternary carbons. The ^{1}H NMR spectra showed two methyl singlets (δ 1.12 and 1.07). The connectivity of the protonated carbons (C-1 to C-2, C-6 through C-9, C-9 to C-11, C-8 to C-14, C-14 through C-17, C-17 to C-20, and C-20 to C-21) was determined by the ^{1}H-^{1}H COSY spectrum. HMBC experiment was used to determine the carbon-carbon connection through the nonprotonated carbon atoms [HMBC correlations: H-17 (δ 2.58) to C-13 (δ 57.0, qC), C-15, C-18, C-20 (δ 73.8, CH), and C-21 (δ 66.3, CH_2); CH_3-18 (δ 1.12) to C-12 (δ 217.5, qC), C-13 (δ 57.0, qC), C-14, and C-17; CH_3-19 (δ 1.07) to C-1, C-5 (δ 168.3, qC), C-9, and C-10 (δ 38.9, qC); H-1 (δ 1.42 and 1.63) to C-2, C-3 (δ 197.8, qC), C-9, C-10 (δ, 38.9, qC), C-19; H-4 (δ 5.83) to C-2, C-6, and C-10 (δ 38.9, qC); H-6 (δ 2.13 and 2.28) to C-4 (δ 124.8, CH), C-5 (δ 168.3, qC), C-7, C-8, and C-10 (δ 38.9, qC); H-9 (δ 1.21) to C-7, C-8, C-10 (δ 38.9, qC), C-11, and C-19; H-11 (δ 2.24 and 2.51) to C-8, C-9, and C-12 (δ 217.5, qC); H-14(δ 1.28) to C-7, C-9, C-12 (δ 217.5, qC), C-15, C-16, and C-18]. Interpretation of these results suggests that compound **6** has the pregnane skeleton bearing two carbonyl groups at C-3 and C-12, two hydroxyl groups at C-20 and C-21, and two olefin carbons of α,β-unsaturated ketone moiety at C-4 and C-5.

NOESY NMR experiments were used for assignment of the relative configuration of **6**. The NOESY correlations [CH_3-19 with H-1β, H-2β, H-6β, H-8 and H-11β; CH_3-18 with H-8, H-11β, H-15β, H-16β, and H-20; H-9 with H-1α, H-7α, H-11α, H-14; H-14 with H-9, H-7α, H-15α, H-17; H-17 with H-14, and H-16α] indicated the stereochemistry of the molecule **6**. Thus, 10β-Me, 8β-H, 9α-H, 13β-Me, 14α-H, and 17β-1,2-dihydroxyethyl substituents were confirmed for **1**. Additional NOESY correlations in the vicinity of H-20 [H-20 with H-16β, Me-18 and H-21a,b; H-21a with H-16α,β and H-20; H-21b with H-16α,β, H-17, and H-20] indicated that the configuration of C-20 is *S* (Figure 1.3). Thus, the structure of compound **1** was determined as 20*S*,21-dihydroxypregn-4-ene-3,12-dione.

Structure Determination of New Cardenolides Monoglycosides, Cardenolides N-1 (9), N-2 (10), N-3 (11), and N-4 (12)

A methanol extract of air-dried stems and twigs of *N. oleander* was partitioned successively with hexane, EtOAc, and *n*-BuOH. From the EtOAc soluble-portion, four new cardenolide monoglycosides, cardenolides N-1 (**9**), N-2 (**10**), N-3 (**11**), and N-4 (**12**) were isolated together with nine known cardenolides and cardenolide monoglycosides (**13–21**) using silica gel column chromatography and reverse-phase HPLC.

Cardenolide N-1 (**9**) gave the elemental composition, $C_{30}H_{46}O_7$, which was determined by HRESIMS analysis. The IR spectrum indicated the presence of hydroxy (3613 and 3591 cm^{-1}) and α,β-unsaturated-γ-lactone (1784 and 1745 cm^{-1}) groups. The ^{13}C NMR spectrum displayed 30 carbon resonances (Table 1.4). A carbonyl carbon resonated at δ 174.4 and two olefin carbon resonances were located at δ 174.4 (s) and 117.7 (d). Three resonances for carbons bearing oxygen were observed at δ 73.4 (t), 72.6 (d), and 85.6 (s) in addition to one methoxy methyl and four oxygenated carbon resonances of a 2,6-dideoxyhexose sugar. From the DEPT and HMQC spectra, the remaining carbon resonances were three methyl, 11 methylene, four methine, and two quaternary carbons. The ^{1}H NMR spectra showed two methyl singlets (δ 0.93 and 0.87) and one additional methyl doublet from the sugar portion at d 1.23 (δ, *J* = 6.6 Hz). The connectivity of the protonated carbons (C-1 through C-9; C-9, C-11, and C-12; C-15 through C-17) was determined from the ^{1}H-^{1}H COSY spectrum. An HMBC experiment was used to determine the carbon-carbon connection through the nonprotonated carbon atoms [HMBC correlations: C-10 (δ35.2) with H-6α and CH_3-19; C-13 (δ49.6) with H-11α, H-15α, H-17, and CH_3-18; C-14 (δ85.6) with H-12β, H-15α, H-17, and CH_3-18]. Interpretation of these results suggest that compound **9** has steroidal A, B, C, and D rings (Ahmed *et al.*, 2006; Wang *et al.*, 2006) bearing a hydroxy group at C-14 (Hanada, 1992). The HMBC correlation of the methine carbon bearing a glycosyl oxygen at δ72.6 with H-1' and H-2β, and COSY correlation of H-3 with H_2-2 and H_2-4 were used to place a *O*-glycosyl bond at C-3. The HMBC correlations [carbonyl carbon at δ174.4 with olefinic H-22 (δ5.87); olefinic methine carbon C-22 (δ 117.7) with H-17 and H_2-21; quaternary olefinic C-20 (δ174.4) with H-17 and H_2-21] showed the structure of the γ-lactone moiety and the connection of its C-20 position at C-17 of the steroid D-ring.

The sugar portion of **9** was assigned as sarmentose on the basis of comparisons of the ^{13}C and ^{1}H NMR data with those of analogous compounds (Abe and Yamauchi, 1978; Abe and Yamauchi, 1996; Hanada, 1992). This is supported by the NOESY correlations (H-1' with H-5' and H-2'α; H-3' with H-4'; H-4' with H-3', H-5', and CH_3-6') as well as a small coupling constant of H-3' (q, *J* = 2.9 Hz). Since only D-sarmentose is known in *N. oleander*, the sugar in **9** is regarded as D-sarmentose.

NOESY correlations [CH_3-19 with H-5 and H-12α with H-15α] suggested AB-*cis* and CD-*cis* ring junctions of **9**. In the ^{1}H-NMR-spectra, the small coupling constant of H-3 ($W_{h/2}$ = 7.5 Hz) was in good agreement with that of α(*eq*)-H at C-3 of 5β-steroids. The spectroscopic analyses and NOESY correlations [CH_3-19 with H-6β, H-8, and H-11β; H-12β with CH_3-18; CH_3-18 with H-22; H-12α with H-17; H-17 with H-16α; H-16β with H-22] indicated the structure and relative configuration of **9** as 3β-*O*-(D-sarmentosyl)-14-hydroxy-5β,14β-card-20(22)-enolide.

Cardenolide N-2 (**10**) had the composition, $C_{30}H_{42}O_7$, which was determined by HRFABMS analysis. The IR spectrum indicated the presence of hydroxy (3572 cm^{-1}) and α,β-unsaturated-γ-lactone (1749 cm^{-1}) groups. The ^{13}C NMR spectrum displayed 30 carbon resonances. ^{1}H and ^{13}C NMR data of the sugar part and A-ring are in good accordance with those of **9**. Thus, the partial structures of the sugar moiety and the A-ring of **9** and **10** are the same. The 3β-*O*-(D-sarmentosyl)-5β, 14β-card-20(22)-enolide structure of **10** was confirmed by analogous NMR analysis of **10** with that of **9**. Since only D-sarmentose is known in *N. oleander* as mentioned above, the sugar moiety in **10** is also regarded as D-sarmentose. The unsaturated γ-lactone structure, its position at C-17, and the existence of an additional double bond between C-16 and C-17 were confirmed by HMBC correlations [C-23 (δ174.2) with H_2-21 and H-22; C-20 (δ157.6) with H_2-15, H-16 (d 6.07), H_2-21, and H-22]. HMBC correlations of two oxymethine carbons [C-8 (δ65.2) with H-7β, H-9, and H_2-15; C-14 (δ70.1) with H-7α, H_2-15, H-16, and CH_3-18] indicated the existence of an 8,14-epoxide ring. Analysis of NOESY correlations [H-3 with H-1'; H-4α with H-7α and H-9; H-9 with H-12α; CH_3-19 with H-5 and H-6β; H-12β with H-22; H-15α with H-7β and H-16; CH_3-18 with H-22] indicated the structure and relative configuration of **10** to be 3β-*O*-(D-sarmentosyl)-8,14-epoxy-5β,14β-card-16,20(22)-dienolide. The β-orientation of the 8,14-epoxide ring was supported by NOE correlation of H-15α with H-7β (*Note 1*) and the observed 0.35 ppm downfield shift of CH_3-18 of **10** (*Note 2*; Paquette, 1979; Ando, 1982; Ando, 1993) compared with that of **9**.

Cardenolide N-3 (**11**) had the composition, $C_{30}H_{42}O_8$, as determined by HRFABMS. Similar IR data were obtained for compound **11** as compared to compounds **9** and **10**. The ^{13}C NMR spectrum displayed 30 carbon resonances. ^{1}H- and ^{13}C NMR spectra of the sugar part of **11** are different from those of **9** and **10**. Chemical shifts in the ^{13}C NMR spectrum of the sugar portion, C-1'–C-6' and OCH_3 of **11** in $CDCl_3$ are in good accordance with those of neridiginoside[8], oleandrigenin 3-O-β-D-diginoside (Cabrera, 1993), and digitoxigenin 3-O-β-D-diginoside (Cabrera, 1993). The coupling constants ($J_{3',2'\beta}$ = 12.2 Hz, $J_{3',2'\alpha}$ = 4.9 Hz, and $J_{3',4'}$ = 3.2 Hz) of H-3' and NOESY correlations (H-3 with H-1'; H-1' with H-3' and 5') of the sugar part of **11** indicated it to be diginose. Since only D-diginose is known in *N. oleander*, the sugar moiety in **11** is regarded as D-diginose.

Chemical shifts in the ^{1}H and ^{13}C NMR spectra of the A- and B-rings of **11** are in good accordance with those of **10**. Thus, **11** is suggested to possess a 3β-*O*-(D-diginosyl)-8,14-epoxy-5β,14β-card-20(22)-enolide structure, which was confirmed by analysis of ^{1}H and ^{13}C NMR spectra a method analogous with that of **10**. The unsaturated γ-lactone structural moiety, its position at C-17, and existence of an additional epoxide ring between C-16 and C-17 were confirmed by HMBC correlations [C-23 (δ 172.8) with H-22; C-20 (δ 162.6) with H_2-21 and H-22; C-17 (δ 66.7) with H_2-15, CH_3-18, and H-22; C-16 (δ 63.2) with H_2-15]. NOESY correlations (H-12β with CH_3-18 and H-22; CH_3-18 with H-22 and H-15β) indicated the existence of a 17β-unsaturated γ-lactone and 16α,17α-epoxide ring. Thus, the full structure and relative configuration of **11** is 3β-*O*-(D-diginosyl)-8, 14;16α,17-diepoxy-5β, 14β-card-20(22)-enolide.

Cardenolide N-4 (**12**) had the composition $C_{32}H_{48}O_9$, as determined by HRESIMS. Similar IR data were obtained for compound **12** when compared to compounds **9**, **10** and **11**. The ^{13}C NMR displayed 32 carbon resonances. Chemical shifts in the ^{1}H and ^{13}C NMR spectra of the sugar part of **12** are in good accordance with those of **11** but different from those of **9** and **10**. Thus, the sugar part of **12** is diginose. Chemical shifts in ^{1}H- and ^{13}C NMR spectrum of the A-ring of **12** are different from those of **9–11**. NOESY correlations (H-1' with H-3', H-5', and H-3; H-5 with H-3 and H-9; CH_3-19 with H-8) indicated 5α-H orientation, A,B-trans ring fusion, and a 3β(*eq*)-*O*-glycosyl bond in **12**. Thus, **12** possesses a 3β-*O*-(diginosyl)-5α-card-20(22)-enolide structure. The A,B-*trans* and A,B-*cis* ring junctions in **12**, and in **9–11**, respectively are also indicated by the chemical shifts of C-19 (d 12.1 for *trans*-derivative **12** and d 23.6, 24.5,

---

Note 1: The investigation of a molecular model indicated that NOE correlation of **10** with the 8β,14β-epoxide ring should exist between H-7β and H-15α, on the contrary that of the corresponding compound with the 8α,14α-epoxide ring should exist between H-7α and H-15α.

Note 2: The epoxide function deshields protons that are situated on the same side of oxygen.

24.6 for *cis*-derivatives **9–11**, respectively) (Ando *et al.*, 1994; Kesselmans *et al.*, 1991). The structure of the unsaturated γ-lactone moiety and its attachment position at C-17 were confirmed by similar HMBC correlation for **12** similar those for **9–11**. Existence of an acetoxy group at C-16 was confirmed by HMBC correlation [C-16 (δ 73.9) with H-15β and H-17] as well as the chemical shift and coupling constants of H-16 [d 5.45 ($J_{16, 15\alpha}$ = 9.8 Hz, $J_{16,15\beta}$ = 2.5 Hz, and $J_{16,17}$ = 8.5 Hz)]. HMBC correlation of tertiary carbons bearing a hydroxy group [C-14 (d 84.2) with H-15α, H-16, CH_3-18] indicated the existence of a C-14 hydroxy group. *Cis*-fusion in the C- and D-rings, β-orientations of 14-hydroxy and 16-acetoxy groups, and the β-orientatin of the unsaturated γ-lactone moiety at C-17 in **12** were confirmed by NOESY correlations (H-9 with H-15α; H-12α with H-16; CH_3-18 with H-12β and H- 22). Since only D-diginose is known in *N. oleander*, the sugar in **12** is also regarded as D-digiose. Thus, the full structure of **12** is 3β-*O*-(D-diginosyl)-16β-acetoxy-14-hydroxy-5α, 14β-card-20(22)-enolide.

We isolated a further nine related cardenolides (*Note 3*): 3β,14-dihydroxy-5β,14β-card-20(22)-enolide (**13**) (Jäger, 1959; Jolad, 1981), 3β-*O*-(D-diginosyl)-14-hydroxy-5β,14β-card-20(22)-enolide (**14**) (Cabrera, 1993), 3β-*O*-(D-diginosyl)-14-hydroxy-5α,14β-card-20(22)-enolide (**15**) (Abe, 1978; Rangaswami, 1949), 3β-*O*-(D-diginosyl)-8,14-epoxy-5β,14β-card-16,20(22)-dienolide (**16**) (Yamauchi, 1973), 3β-*O*-(D-diginosyl)-8,14-epoxy-5β,14β-card-20(22)-enolide (**17**) (Abe, 1996; Janiak, 1963), 3β-*O*-(D-diginosyl)-8,14-dihydroxy-5β,14β-card-20(22)-dienolide (**18**) (Abe, 1996), 3β-*O*-(D-sarmentosyl)-16β-acetoxy-14-hydroxy-5β,14β-card-20(22)-enolide (**19**) (Aebi, 1950), 16β-acetoxy-3β,14-dihydroxy-5β,14β-card-20(22)-enolide (**20**) (Tori, 1973), and 3β-*O*-(D-diginosyl)-16β-acetoxy-14-hydroxy-5β,14β-card-20(22)-enolide (**21**) (Cabrera, 1993).

Structure Determination of New Cardenolides Monoglycosides, Cardenolides B-1 (22), and B-2 (23), and Identification of Oleagenin (24)

A methanol extract of air-dried stems and twigs of *N. oleander* was partitioned successively with hexane, EtOAc, and *n*-BuOH. As mentioned in the previous section, we isolated three cardenolide sarmentosides and eight cardenolid diginosides including four new compounds, the major component of which was odoroside A (**14**) (0.018 per cent) (Zhao *et al.*, 2007). In this section, we describe the structure determination of two new cardenolide monoglycosides, cardenolides B-1 (**22**) and B-2 (**23**), and oleagenin (**24**), which were isolated from more polar fraction of the extract with EtOAc using silica gel column chromatography and reversed-phase HPLC.

Cardenolide B-1 (**22**) gave the elemental composition, $C_{30}H_{44}O_8$, which was determined by HRFABMS analysis. The IR spectrum of **22** indicated the presence of

---

Note 3: The structures, including configuration of the following 13 compounds, were confirmed by full analysis of their NMR spectra at 500 MHz (^{1}H-NMR, ^{1}H-^{1}H COSY, NOESY, HMQC, HMBC) and at 125 MHz (^{13}C-NMR, DEPT) as well as HREIMS or HRFABMS. The yield of each compound in parenthesis is based on the•@weight of air-dried stems and twigs of *N. oleander*.

hydroxyl (3539 cm^{-1}) and α,β-unsaturate-γ-lactone (1786, 1751 and 1631 cm^{-1}) groups. The ^{13}C NMR spectrum displayed 30 carbon signals (Table 1.5). A carbonyl carbon resonated at d 173.6 and two olefin carbon resonances were located at d 169.5 (qC) and 116.9 (CH). Four resonances for carbons bearing oxygen were observed at δ73.2 (CH_2), 73.7 (CH), 70.5 (qC), and 65.3 (qC) in addition to one methoxy methyl and five oxygenated carbon signals of a 6-deoxyhexose sugar. From the DEPT and HMQC spectra, the remaining carbon resonances were three methyl, nine methylene, three methine, and two quaternary carbons. The ^{1}H NMR spectra showed two methyl singlets (δ0.85 and 1.01) and one additional methyl doublet from the sugar portion at 1.36 (δ, *J* = 6.3 Hz). The connectivity of the protonated carbons (C-1 through C-7; C-9, C-11, and C-12; C-15 through C-17) was determined from the ^{1}H-^{1}H COSY spectrum. An HMBC experiment was used to determine the carbon-carbon connection through the nonprotonated carbon atoms [HMBC correlations: H-17 (δ 2.57) to C-12, C-13 (δ 41.8, qC), C-15, C-18, C-20 (δ 169.5, qC), C-21 (δ 73.2, CH_2), and C-22 (δ 116.9, CH); CH_3-18 (δ0.85) to C-12, C-13 (δ41.8, qC), C-14 (δ70.5, qC), and C-17; CH_3-19 (δ1.01) to C-1, C-5, C-9, and C-10 (δ36.7, qC); H-11α and β (δ1.15 and 1.26) to C-8 (δ65.3, qC), C-9, and C-12]. Interpretation of these results suggests that compound **22** has steroid A, B, C, and D rings (Wang *et al.*, 2006; Ahmed *et al.*, 2006) bearing an 8,14-epoxide ring, and an α,β-unsaturated γ-lactone moiety at C-17. The HMBC correlations [H-3 to C-2, C-5, and C-1'; H-1' to C-3] were used to place an *O*-glycosyl bond at C-3. The chemical shift values of C-8 (δ 65.3) and C-14 (δ 70.5) of **22** are in good accordance with those of analogous epoxides **10** (Zhao *et al.*, 2007) [C-8 (δ65.2) and C-14 (δ70.1)] and **17** (Abe *et al.*, 1996; Zhao *et al.*, 2007; Janika *et al.*, 1963) [C-8 (δ 65.3) and C-14 (δ 70.5)] but different from those of diol **18** (Abe *et al.*, 1996; Zhao *et al.*, 2007) [C-8 (δ77.2) and C-14 (δ 85.9)]. The sugar portion of **22** was assigned to digitalose on the basis of comparisons of the ^{13}C and ^{1}H NMR data of **22** (Table 1.5) with those of an analogous compound such as **25** (Cabrera,1993) [^{13}C NMR: *d* 73.9 (C-3), 101.1 (C-1'), 70.8 (C-2'), 82.8 (C-3'), 68.2 (C-4'), 70.3 (C-5'), 16.4 (C-6'), 57.5 (OMe); ^{1}H NMR: δ4.04 (H-3, br s, $W_{h/2}$ = 7.5 Hz), 4.24 (H-1', d, *J* = 7.6 Hz), 3.65 (H-2', dd, *J* = 10.3, 7.6 Hz), 3.21 (H-3', dd, *J* = 7.6, 3.3 Hz), 3.84 (H-4', br d, *J* = 3.3 Hz), 3.56 (H-5', br q, *J* = 6.6 Hz), 1.34 (H-6', d, *J* = 6.6 Hz), 3.52 (OCH_3, s)). Since only D-digitalose is known in *N. oleander*, the sugar in **22** is regarded as D-digitalose. The conclusion is supported by the coupling constants of ^{1}H NMR spectrum (Table 1.5) and the NOESY correlations (H-1' to H-3' and H-5'; H-3' to H-1', H-4', and H-5'; H-4' to H-3' and H-5'; H-5' to H-1', H-3', and H-4'; H-6' to H-4' and H-5') of sugar moiety of **22**. NOESY correlations [CH_3-19 with H-5; H-4α with H-7α and H-9] suggested AB-cis ring junction in **22**. The β-configuration of the 8,14-epoxide ring of **22** was strongly suggested by the fact that the chemical shits of C-8 and C-14 are in good accordance with those of known cardenolides with 8β,14β-epoxide ring as mentioned above. This was also supported by NOE correlation of H-15α with H-7α and H-7β. In ^{1}H-NMR-spectra, the small coupling constant of H-3 ($W_{h/2}$ = 7.5 Hz) was in good agreement with that of α(*eq*)-H at C-3 of 5β steroids. The above-mentioned spectroscopic analyses and NOESY correlations [CH_3-19 with H-6β, and 11β; H-11β with H-12β and CH_3-18; CH_3-18 with H-21a and H-22; H-12α with H-9 and H-17; H-17 with H-15α and H-16α; H-16β with H-22 and CH_3-18] indicated the relative stereochemistry of **22** to be 3β-*O*-(β-D-digitalosyl)-8, 14-epoxy-

5β, 14β-card-20(22)-enolide. Since all known cardenolides isolated from *N. oleander* possess the same absolute configuration in genin moiety as shown in structures **25**, **18**, **10** and **17**, the absolute configuration of **22** is regarded as (3S, 5R, 8S, 9R, 10S, 13R, 14R, 17R). This conclusion was also supported by the fact that $[\alpha]_D$ sign of **22**{$[\alpha]^{20}_D$ +28.57 (*c* 0.392, $CHCl_3$)} is the same as those of 3β-*O*-(β-D-digitalosyl)- and 3β-*O*-(β-D-diginosyl)-cardenolides with analogous structures such as **25** {$[\alpha]^{20}_D$ +5.57 (*c* 0.56, MeOH)} and **17** {$[\alpha]^{20}_D$ +13.4 (*c* 0.55, $CHCl_3$)}.

Cardenolide B-2 (**23**) had the composition, $C_{30}H_{44}O_8$, which was determined by HRFABMS analysis. Similar IR data were obtained for compound **23** as compared to compound **22**. The ^{13}C NMR spectrum displayed 30 carbon signals (Table 1.5). The 3β-*O*-(glycosyl)-5β,14β-card-20(22)-enolide structure of **23** was confirmed by analogous NMR analysis of **23** with that of **22**. ^{1}H and ^{13}C NMR spectra of the sugar portion of **23** are different from those of **22**. The coupling constants [H-1' ($J_{1',2'\beta}$ = 9.8 Hz and $J_{1',2'\alpha}$ = 1.7 Hz), H-3' ($J_{3',2'\beta}$ = 12.1 Hz, $J_{3',2'\alpha}$ = 4.8 Hz, and $J_{3',4'}$ = 3.2 Hz), and CH_3-6' (δ*J* = 6.6 Hz)] and NOESY correlations (H-1' with H-2'α, H-3' and H-5'; H-4' with H-3', H-5', 6' and 3'-OMe) of a 2,6-dideoxyhexose sugar of **23** suggested it to be diginose. The ^{13}C and ^{1}H NMR data of the sugar moiety of **23** were actually superimposable with 3β-*O*-(β-diginosyl)-moiety of **18** (Abe *et al*, 1996; Zhao *et al.*, 2007) [^{13}C NMR: δ 97.7 (C-1'), 32.0 (C-2'), 78.0 (C-3'), 67.2 (C-4'), 70.4 (C-5'), 16.8 (C-6'), 55.7 (OMe); ^{1}H NMR: *d* 4.45 (H-1', dd, *J* = 9.8, 1.7 Hz), 1.93 (H-2'α, m), 1.71 (H-2'β, m), 3.34 (H-3', ddd, *J* = 12.0, 4.9, 3.2 Hz), 3.69 (H-4', br s), 3.43 (H-5', q, *J* = 6.6 Hz), 1.32 (H-6', d, *J* = 6.6 Hz), 3.40 (OMe, s)] and **17** (Abe *et al.*, 1996; Zhao *et al.*, 2007; Janika *et al.*, 1963) [^{13}C NMR: *d* 97.7 (C-1'), 32.1 (C-2'), 78.0 (C-3'), 67. 1 (C-4'), 70. 3 (C-5'), 16. 9 (C-6'), 55.7 (OMe); ^{1}H NMR: *d* 4.47 (H-1', dd, *J* = 9.8, 2.0 Hz), 1.93 (H-2'α, m), 1.70 (H-2'β, m), 3.34 (H-3', ddd, *J* = 12.0, 4.9, 3.2 Hz), 3.69 (H-4', br s), 3.43 (H-5', q, *J* = 6.6 Hz), 1.34 (H-6', d, *J* = 6.6 Hz), 3.40 (OMe, s)]. Since only D-diginose is known in *N. oleander*, the sugar in **23** is regarded as D-diginose. The A-B cis ring junction of **23** was confirmed by NOE correlations [CH_3-19 with H-1β, H-5, H-6β, and 11β; H-2α with H-9]. Existence of an epoxide ring between C-7 and C-8, and a hydroxyl group at C-14 were suggested by their chemical shift values and HMBC correlation [H-7 (δ3.21) with C-6, C-8 (63.9, qC), C-14 (81.0, qC); H-6β (δ2.30) with C-4, C-5, C-7 (δ51.2, CH) and C8 (63.9, qC)]. The observed coupling constants of H-7 [H-7 with H-6α (*J* = 5.9 Hz) and H-7 with H-6β (*J* = 0 Hz)] are in good accordance with those deduced from the dihedral angles of H-7 with H-6α and H-6β. The β-olientation of the 7, 8-epoxide ring was also supported by NOE correlation (H-7 with H-15β, H-6α, and the proton of 14-OH). The observed NOE correlation of the proton of 14-OH [δ 2.37 (1H, s, $W_{h/2}$ = 5.0 Hz)] with CH_3-18 and H-7 indicated that the hydroxyl group at C-14 is fixed by intramolecular hydrogen bond with the oxygen of eopxide ring between C-7 and C-8. Thus, 7,8-epoxide ring, 14-hydroxyl group, and CH_3-18 are located in cis-β-olientation. The analysis of NOESY correlations [H-3 with H-1'; H-9 with H-2α, H-4α, H-11α, and H-12α; H-12α with H-17; 14-OH with CH_3-18 and H-7; CH_3-18 with 12β, H-21, and H_2-22] indicated the full stereochemistry of **23** to be the 3β-*O*-(β-D-diginosyl)-7β,8-epoxy-14-hydroxy-5β,14β -card-20(22)-enolide. The absolute configuration of **23** is regarded (3S, 5S, 7S, 8R, 9R,10S, 13R, 14R, 17R) by the same reason mentioned in the structure of **22.** This conclusion was also supported by the fact that observed and calculated $[\alpha]_D$ values of **23** showed same negative sign (*Note 4*).

Compound **24** gave the elemental composition, $C_{23}H_{32}O_4$, which was determined by HRFABMS analysis. The IR spectrum of **24** indicated the presence of hydroxyl (3399 cm^{-1}), α,β-unsaturate-γ-lactone (1748 cm^{-1}), and ketone (1692 cm^{-1}) groups. The ^{13}C NMR spectrum displayed 23 carbon signals (Table 1.15).

A carbonyl carbon resonated at δ221.3 and 173.8. Two olefin carbon resonances were located at δ 171.9 (qC) and 116.4 (CH). Two resonances for carbons bearing oxygen were observed at d 73.4 (CH_2) and 65.8 (CH). From the DEPT and HMQC spectra, the remaining carbon resonances were two methyl, nine methylene, three methine, and three quaternary carbons. The ^1H NMR spectra showed two methyl singlets (δ0.91 and 0.81). The connectivity of the protonated carbons (C-1 through C-7; C-9, C-11, and C-12; C-15 through C-17) was determined from the ^1H-^1H COSY spectrum. An HMBC experiment was used to determine the carbon-carbon connection through the nonprotonated carbon atoms [HMBC correlations: H-17 (δ2.97) to C-12, C-13 (δ47.5, qC), C-14 (δ221.3, qC), C-16, C-18, C-20 (δ171.9, qC), C-21 (δ73.4, CH_2), and C-22 (δ116.4, CH); CH_3-18 (δ0.91) to C-12, C-13 (δ47.5, qC), and C-14 (δ221.3, qC); CH_3-19 (δ0.81) to C-1, C-5, C-9, and C-10 (δ37.9, qC); H-11α and β (δ2.32 and 1.72) to C-9, and C-12; H-15α and β (δ1.88 and 1.68) to C-7 and C-9]. Interpretation of these results suggested that compound **24** was a rearranged cardenolide with a 14-oxo-15(14→8)*abeo*-card-20(22)-enolide skeleton. NOESY correlations [CH_3-19 with H-5, H-6, and H-12β; H-2α with H-9α; H-4α with H-7α; H-9 with H-15α; H-11α with H-16α; CH_3-18 with H12β and H-22; H-22 with H-15β] indicated full stereochemistry of **24** as (8*R*)-3β -hydroxy-14-oxo-15(14→8) *abeo*-5β-card-20(22)-enolide. Although the structure **24** is identical with that of aglycone of oleaside A that was obtained by acid hydrolysis (Abe and Yamauchi, 1979), this is the first isolation of **24** from natural sources.

We isolated a further related ten cardenolides monoglycosides: odoroside H [3β-*O*-(β-D-digitalosyl)-14-hydroxy-5β,14β-card-20(22)-enolide] (**25**) (Cabrer *et al.*, 1993), neritaloside [3β-*O*-(β-D-digitalosyl)-16β-acetoxy-14-hydroxy-5β, 14β-card-20(22)-enolide] (**26**) (Cabrer *et al.*, 1993; Yamauchi and Abe, 1990), oleandrin [3β-*O*-(α-L-oleandrosyl)-16β-aceoxy-14-hydroxy-5β,14β-card-20(22)-enolide] (**27**) (Abe *et al.*, 1996; Yamauchi and Abe, 1978), 3β-*O*-(β-D-glucosyl)-16β-acetoxy-14-hydroxy-5β, 14β-card-20(22)-enolide (**28**) (Yamauchi *et al.*, 1975; Paper and Franz, 1989), 3β-*O*-(β-D-diginosyl)-14,16β-dihydroxy-5β, 14β-card-20(22)- enolide] (**29**) (Hanada *et al.*, 1992; Jäger *et al.*, 1959), 3β-*O*-(β-D-digitalosyl)- 14-hydroxy-5α,14β-card-20(22)-enolide (**30**) (Yamauchi *et al.*, 1976; Hanada *et al.*, 1992), 3β-*O*-(β-D-digitalosyl)-8,14-epoxy-5β,14β-card-16,20(22)-enolide (**31**) (Hanada *et al.*, 1992; Yamauchi *et al.*, 1973), 3β-*O*-(β-D-

---

Note 4: The $[\alpha]_D$ value of cardenolide B-2 (**23**) was evaluated as following. The observed $[\alpha]_D$ values of digitoxigenin (**13**) (Zhao *et al.*, 2007) and odoroside A (**14**) (Zhao *et al.*, 2007) are +40.3 and +1.5, respectively. From these values, the contribution of diginosyl moity to $[\alpha]_D$ values of **14** is estimated to be –38.8. The $[\alpha]_D$ value of **23** was calculated to be –24.7 based on the observed and calculated $[\alpha]_D$ values of tannigenin and diginosyl moity, +14.1 and –38.8, respectively.

diginosyl)-14-hydroxy-5β, 14β-card-16,20(22)-enolide (**32**) (Jäger *et al.*, 1959), oleaside A [(8R)-3β-*O*-(β-D-diginosyl)- 14-oxo-15(14→8)*abeo*-5β-card-20(22)-enolide] (**33**) (Abe and Yamauchi, 1979), neriaside [3β-*O*-(β-D-diginosyl)-8, 14-seco-14α-hydroxy-8-oxo-5β-card-20(22)-enolide](**34**) (Abe *et al.*, 1996; Yamauchi and Abe, 1978). The most abundant component of this fraction is odoroside H (**25**) (0.008 per cent).

Structure Determination of A New Cardenolide Diglycoside (35) and Identification of Known Cardenolide Diglycosides 36–45

A methanol extract of air-dried leaves of the plant was partitioned with hexane, ethyl acetate, and butanol. Methanol-soluble portion of butanol extract was separated by silica gel column chromatography and reversed-phase HPLC. A new compound, 3β-*O*-[β-D-glucopyranosyl-(1→4)-β-D-diginopyranosyl]- 14α-hydroxy-8-oxo-8,14-seco-5β-card-20(22)-enolide (**35**) was isolated together with ten known cardenolide diglycosides: 3β-*O*-[β-D-glucopyranosyl-(1→4)- β-D-diginopyranosyl]-16β-acetoxy-14-hydroxy-5β,14β-card-20(22)-enolide (**36**) (Yamauchi *et al.*, 1975), 3β-*O*-(β-D-glucopyranosyl-(1→4)-α-L-oleandropyranosyl)- 16β-acetoxy-14-hydroxy-5β,14β-card-20(22)-enolide (**37**) (Yamauchi *et al.*, 1975), 3β-*O*-(β-D-glucopyranosyl-(1→4)-β-D-digitalopyranosyl)-16β-acetoxy-14-hydroxy-5β,14β-card-20(22)-enolide (**38**) (Miyatake *et al.*, 1959), 3β-*O*-(β-D-glucopyranosyl-(1→4)-β-D-sarmentopyranosyl)-16β-acetoxy-14-hydroxy-5β,14β-card-20(22)-enolide (**39**) (Abe and Yamauchi, 1992), 3β-*O*-(β-D-glucopyranosyl-(1→4)-β-D-diginopyranosyl)-8,14-epoxy-5β,14β-card-20(22)-enolide (**40**) (Bauer and Franz, 1985), 3β-*O*-(β-D-glucopyranosyl-(1→4)-β-D-digitalopyranosyl)-8,14-epoxy-5β,14β-card-20(22)-enolide (**41**) (Hanada *et al.*, 1992), 3β-*O*-(β-D-glucopyranosyl-(1→4)-β-D-digitalopyranosyl)-8,14-epoxy-5β,14β-card-16,20(22)-dienolide (**42**) (Yamauchi *et al.*, 1975), 3β-*O*-(β-D-glucopyranosyl-(1→4)-β-D-digitalopylanosyl)-14-hydroxy-5α,14β-card-20(22)-enolide (**43**) (Yamauchi *et al.*, 1976), 3β-*O*-(β-D-glucopyranosyl-(1→4)-β-D-diginopyranosyl)-16β-acetoxy-14-hydroxy-5α,14β-card-20(22)-enolide (**44**) (Hanada *et al.*, 1992), 3β-*O*-(β-D-glucopyranosyl-(1→4)-β-D-digitalopyranosyl)-16β-acetoxy-14-hydroxy-5α,14β-card-20(22)-enolide (**45**) (Hanada *et al.*, 1992).

Compound **35** has the composition $C_{36}H_{56}O_{13}$, which was determined by HR-FAB-MS analysis. The IR spectrum of compound **35** indicated the existence of hydroxyl (3467 cm^{-1}), α,β-unsaturated-γ-lactone (1736 cm^{-1}), and carbonyl (1698 cm^{-1}) groups. The ^{13}C NMR displayed 36 carbon signals (Table 1.6). Two carbonyl carbons resonated at d 216.2 and 174.1, and two olefin carbons were located at d 172.4 (qC) and 116.8 (CH_2). Three signals for carbons bearing oxygen were observed at d 74.0 (CH_2), 72.8 (CH), and 79.5 (CH) in addition to one methoxy methyl and ten oxygenated carbon signals of one 2,6-dideoxyhexose sugar and one hexose sugar moiety. From the DEPT and HMQC spectra, the remaining carbon resonances were three methyl, ten methylene, three methine, and two quaternary carbons. The ^{1}H NMR spectra showed two methyl singlets (d 0.68 and 0.74) and one additional methyl doublet from sugar portion at d 1.51 (δ, J = 6.4 Hz). The connectivity of the protonated carbons (C-1 through C-7, C-9 to C-11, C-11 to C-12, and C-14 through C-17) was determined by the ^{1}H-^{1}H COSY spectrum. HMBC experiment was used to determine the carbon-carbon connection through the nonprotonated carbon atoms [HMBC correlations: H-17 (δ 3.00) to C-12, C-13 (δ51.3, qC), C-15, C-18, C-20 (δ172.4, qC), C-21 (δ74.0, CH_2), and C-

22 (δ116.8, CH); CH_3-18 (δ0.68) to C-12, C-13 (δ51.3, qC), C-14 (δ79.5, qC), and C-17; CH_3-19 (δ0.74) to C-1, C-5, C-9, and C-10 (δ42.7, qC); H-11a and H-11b (δ1.76 and 1.45) to C-8 (δ216.2, qC), C-9, and C-12; H-14 (δ4.15) to C-13, C-15, C-17, and C-18]. Interpretation of these results suggests that compound **35** has the 8,14-secocardenolide skeleton bearing a carbonyl group at C-8, a hydroxyl group at C-14, and an α,β-unsaturated γ-lactone moiety at C-17. The HMBC correlations [H-3 with C-1'; H-1' with C-3] and the NOESY correlation [H-1' with H-3] were used to place an*O*-glycosyl bond at C-3. The HMBC correlation [H-1″ to C-4'] indicated that the second glycosyl bond exist at C-4'. The sugar portion of **35** was assigned to β-glucopyranosyl-(1→4)-β-diginopyranose on the basis of comparison of the ^{1}H and ^{13}C NMR data of **1** with those of known analogous compound such as**36** (Yamauchi *et al.*, 1975). The ^{13}C and ^{1}H NMR data of the sugar moiety of**35** were actually superimposable with 3 β-*O*-(β-D-glucopyranosyl-(1→4)-β-diginopyranosyl)-moiety of **36** (Table 1.7). This is supported by the NOESY correlation (H-1' with H-3, H-5' and H-2'α; H-3' with H-4' and H-5'; H-1" with H-4' and H-5"; H-2" with H-4"; H-3" with H-5") and the coupling constants of diginosyl moiety ($J_{1',2'\beta}$ = 9.8 Hz, $J_{2'\beta,3'}$ = 12.2 Hz, $J_{2'\alpha,3'}$ = 4.4 Hz, $J_{3',4'}$ = 2.7 Hz) and gulcosyl moiety ($J_{1'',2''}$ = 7.8 Hz, $J_{2'',3''}$ = 8.8 Hz, $J_{3'',4''}$ = 8.8 Hz). The small coupling constant of H-3 ($W_{1/2h}$ = 8.0 Hz) was in good agreement with that of α(*eq*)-H at C-3 of 5β-steriods. NOESY correlations [CH_3-19 with H-5; H-4α with H-9; CH_3-18 with H-14 and H-22] confirmed AB-cis ring fusion, α-configurations of 14-hydroxyl group, and β-configurations of unsaturated γ-lactone moiety at C_{17}. Although the relative stereochemistry between CH_3-19 and CH_3-18 was not determined by the NOESY experiment, the chemical correlation of the genin of **40**, adynerigenine with the genin of **35**, neriagenin was reported (Yamauchi and Abe, 1978) Thus, the relative stereochemistry of **35** is 3β-*O*-(β-*O*-glucopyranosyl-(1→4)-β-diginopyranosyl)-14α-hydroxy-8-oxo-8,14-seco-5β-card-20(22)-enolide.

Since only D-glucose and D-diginose are known in *N. oleander*, the sugar in **35** is regarded as β-D-glucopyranosyl-(1→4)-β-D-diginopyranose. Since all known cardenolides isolated from *N. oleander* possess the same absolute configuration in genin moiety as shown in structures **36–45**, the absolute configuration of 8,14-seco-cardenolide (**35**) is regarded as the same absolute configuration as those of **36–45** and (3S, 5R, 9R, 10S, 13R, 14S, 17R). Actually, the ^{13}C- and ^{1}H-NMR data of C-3 position of **35** [72.8 (CH), 4.28 (1H, br s)] are good accordance with those of **36** [73.1(CH), 4.26 (1H, br s)] and **40** [72.7 (CH), 4.33 (1H, br s)], which posses 3*S* configuration and the cis junction in A,B-ring (Note 5). In addition, δ values of ^{13}C NMR data of ring A (C-1 through C-5) and sugar moiety (C-1' through C-6' and C-1" through C-6") of **35** are superimpassable with those of **36** and **40**, which possess 3β-*O*-(β-D-glucopyranosyl-(1→4)-β-D-diginopyranosyl) and (3S, 5R, and 10S) configurations in A ring of genin moiety (Table 1.7) (*Note 5*). Thus, the structure of**35** regarded as 3β-*O*-[β-D-glucopyranosyl-(1→4)-β-D-diginopyranosyl]- 14α-hydroxy-8-

---

Note 5: C-1", C-4', C-1', and C-3 are enantiomeric centers and the change of a part of configurations on these carbons means that the compound was changed to diastereomer and different compound, whose NMR data are different. Since compound **35** showed the same ^{13}C NMR data with those of **36** and **40**, the configurations at C-1", C-4', C-1' of diglycosyl moiety and at C-3 of genin moiety are the same configuration or its enantiomer but not diastereomer.

oxo-8,14-seco-5β-card-20(22)-enolide (**35**) with (3S, 5R, 9R, 10S, 13R, 14S, 17R) configuration. This conclusion was also supported by the fact that observed and calculated $[\alpha]_D$ values of **35** showed same negative sign (*Note 6*).

Structure Determination of Cardenolide B-3 (61)

A methanol extract of air-dried stems and twigs of *N. oleander* was partitioned successively with hexane, EtOAc, and *n*-BuOH. The *n*-BuOH extract gave a new cardenolide triglycoside, cardenolide B-3 (**61**). Cardenolide B-3 (**61**) gave the elemental composition, $C_{42}H_{64}O_{18}$, which was determined by HRFABMS analysis. The IR spectrum of **61** indicated the presence of hydroxyl (3389 cm^{-1}) and α,β-unsaturated-γ-lactone (1745 and 1642 cm^{-1}) groups. The ^{13}C NMR spectrum displayed 42 carbon signals. A carbonyl carbon resonated at d 174.4 and two olefin carbon resonances were located at δ175.1 (s) and 117.8 (d). Five resonances for carbons bearing oxygen were observed at δ81.8 (s), 73.7 (t), 72.4 (d), 64.5 (s), and 51.1 (d) in addition to one methoxy methyl and sixteen oxygenated carbon signals of one 2,6-dideoxyhexose sugar and two hexose sugar moieties. From the DEPT and HMQC spectra, the remaining carbon resonances were three methyl, nine methylene, three methine, and two quaternary carbons. The ^1H NMR spectrum showed two methyl singlets (δ1.05 and 1.06) and one additional methyl doublet of 2,6-dideoxyhexose sugar at d 1.66 (δ, *J* = 6.4 Hz). The connectivity of the protonated carbons (C-1 through C-7; C-9, C-11, and C-12; C-15 through C-17) was determined from the ^1H-^1H COSY spectrum. An HMBC experiment was used to determine the carbon-carbon connection through the nonprotonated carbon atoms [HMBC correlations: H-17 (δ2.80) to C-12, C-13 (δ52.7, s), C-14 (δ81.8, s), C-15, C-16, C-18, C-20 (δ175.1, s), C-21 (δ73.7, t), and C-22 (δ117.8, d); H-18 (δ1.05) to C-12, C-13, C-14 (δ81.8, s), and C-17; H-19 (δ1.06) to C-1, C-5, C-9, and C-10 (δ34.0, s)]. Interpretation of these results suggests that compound **61** has steroid A, B, C, and D rings (Wang *et al.*, 2006; Ahmed *et al.* 2006), bearing an α,β-unsaturated γ-lactone moiety at C-17. The HMBC correlations [H-3 to C-2, C-5, and C-1'; H-1' to C-3] were used to place an *O*-glycosyl bond at C-3. The sugar portion of **61** were assigned as 3-*O*-β-glucopyranosyl-(1→6)-β-glucopyranosyl-(1→4)-β-diginopyranoside on the basis of comparisons of the ^{13}C NMR data (Table 1.8) with those of known analogous compounds**46** (Abe and Yamauchi, 1992; Yamauchi*etal.*, 1975), **48** (Abe and Yamauchi, 1992; Cabrela*et al.*, 1993), and **53** (Abe and Yamauchi, 1992; Yamauchi *et al.*, 1975) (Figure 1.8).

These assignments were supported by NOESY correlations [(H-1''' with H-6", H-3''', and H-5'''; H-2''' with H-4'''; H-3''' with H-1''' and H-5'''; H-4''' with H-2'''; H-5''' with H-1''' and H-3''');(H-1" with H-3" and H-5"; H-2" with H-4"; H-3" with H-1" and

Note 6: The $[\alpha]_D$ value of **35** was evaluated as following. The observed $[\alpha]_D$ values of digitoxigenin (Zhao *et al.*, 2007) and odoroside A (Zhao *et al.*, 2007) are +40.3 and +1.5, respectively. From these values, the contribution of diginosyl moity to $[\alpha]_D$ value of odoroside A is estimated to be –38.8. The observed $[\alpha]_D$ values of **12** (Zhao *et al.*, 2007) and the estimated $[\alpha]_D$ values of diginosyl moity are –21.4 and –38.8, respectively. From these values, the $[\alpha]_D$ values of 135α-oleandorigenin is estimated to be +17.4. Since the reported $[\alpha]_D$ value of **44** (Hanada *et al.*, 1992) is –27.4, the contribution of the (β-D-glucopyranosyl-(1→4)-β-D-diginopyranosyl)-moiety to $[\alpha]_D$ is estimated to be –44.8. Based on this value and the reported $[\alpha]_D$ value of neriagenin (-1.6), the $[\alpha]_D$ valu of **35** was estimated to be –46.4.

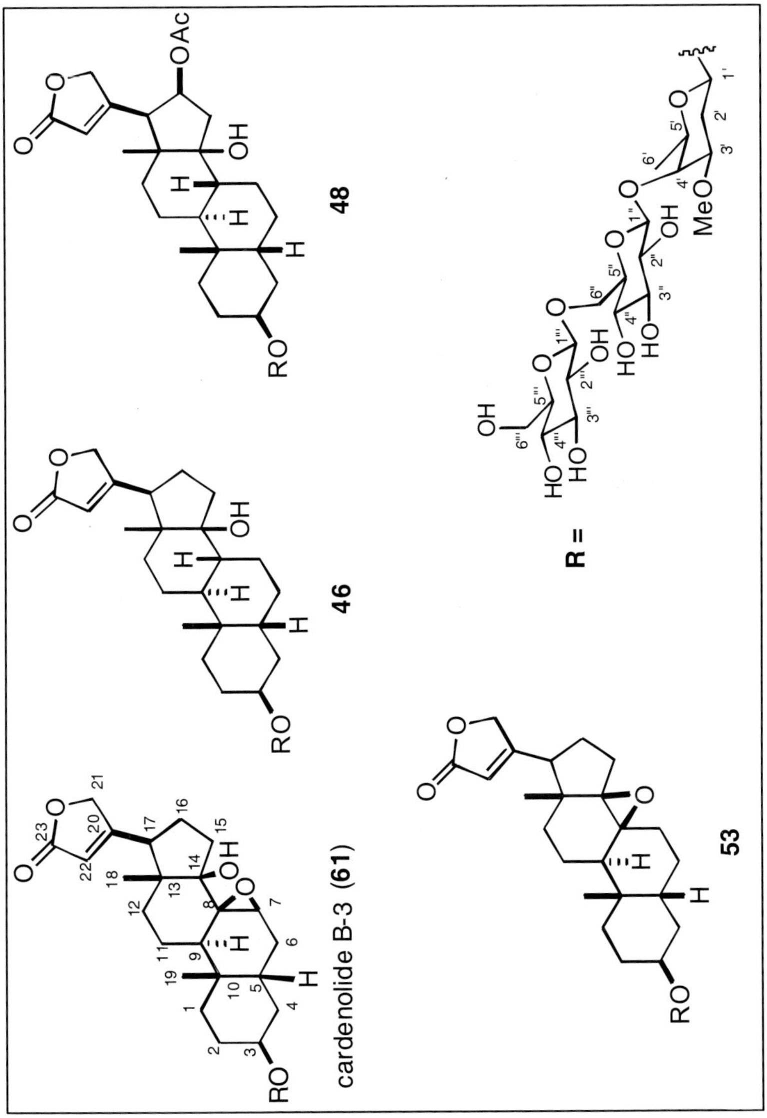

Figure 1.8

H-5"; H-4" with H-2"; H-5" with H-1" and H-3"); (H-1' with H-3', H-5', and H-3; H-3' with H-1' and H-5'; H-4' with H-3', H-5', and OMe; H-5' with H-1', H-3', and CH_3-6') as well as coupling constants observed [H-1''' (δ, *J* = 7.6 Hz); H-1" (δ, *J* = 7.8 Hz), H-1' (δ, *J* = 8.3 Hz)]. The C-1'''– C-6" linkage of glucose-glucose and the C-1"-C-4' linkage of glucose-diginose were determined by the analysis of HMBC correlations [(H-1''' to C-6" and H-6" to C-1''') and (H-1" to C-4' and H-4' and C-1"). Since only D-glucose and D-diginose are known in *N. oleander*, the sugar portion in **61** was assigned as 3-*O*-β-D-glucopyranosyl-(1→6)-β-D-glucopyranosyl-(1→4)-β-D-diginopyranoside. Existence of an epoxide ring between C-7 and C-8, and a hydroxyl group at C-14 were suggested by their chemical shift values and HMBC correlation [H-7(δ3.42) with C-6, C-8 (64.5, s), C-14 (81.8, s); H-6b (δ 2.29) with C-4, C-5, C-7 (δ 51.1, d) and C-8]. The observed coupling constants of H-7 [H-7 with H-6α (*J* = 5.9 Hz) and H-7 with H-6β (*J* = 0 Hz)] are in good accordance with those deduced from the dihedral angles of H-7 with H-6α and H-6β. The β-orientation of the 7,8-epoxide ring was also supported by NOE correlation [H-7 with H-15β, H-6α, and the proton of 14-OH (*δ*2.37)]. The observed NOE correlation of the proton of 14-OH with CH_3-18 and H-7 indicated that the hydroxyl group at C-14 is fixed by intramolecular hydrogen bond with the oxygen of 7,8-eopxide ring. The β-orientation of 14-OH was also supported by NOE correlation [H-12*a*?with H-9 and H-15α] that indicated *cis*-ring junction of C and D ring. Thus, 7,8-epoxide ring, 14-hydroxyl group, and CH_3-18 are located in*cis*-β-orientation. The analysis of NOESY correlations [CH_3-19 with H-1β, H-5, H-6β, and 11β; H-9 with H-2α, H-4α, H-11α, and H-12α; H-12α with H-17; CH_3-18 with 12β, H-21, and H-22] indicated the relative stereochemistry of **61** to be 3β-*O*-β-D-glucopyranosyl-(1→6)-β-D-glucopyranosyl-(1→4)-β-D-diginopyranosyl]-7β,8- epoxy-14-hydroxy-5β,14β -card-20(22)-enolide. Since all known cardenolides isolated from *N. oleander* possess same absolute configuration in genin moiety, the absolute configuration of **61** is regarded as 3*S*, 5*S*, 7*S*, 8*R*, 9*R*, 10*S*, 13*R*, 14*R*, and 17*R*.

Inhibitory Activity on Expression of Intercellular Adhesion Molecule-1 (ICAM-1) Induced by Interleukin-1 and Tumor Necrosis Factor-α (TNF)-α

Inflammatory cytokine, such as interleukin-1 (IL-1) and tumor necrosis factor-α (TNF)-α, play an essential role in inflammation and induce a variety of genes responsible for inflammatory responses, such as intercellular adhesion molecule-1 (ICAM-1). Expression of intercellular adhesion molecule-1 (ICAM-1) is induced by IL-1 and TNF-α on the surface of endothelial cells of blood vessels. ICAM-1 on the activated endothelial cells interacts with lymphocyte function-associated antigen-1 (LFA-1) on leucocytes in the blood stream, and the leucocytes begin rolling, adhere to the surface of endothelium, and finally migrate from the inside of the blood vessel to the inflammatory portion by chemo-taxis. The attack of leucocytes causes serious damage to the inflammatory tissue. Expression of excess amount of ICAM-1 on the surface of endothelial cells of a blood vessel plays an important role in the progress of inflammatory reaction. These facts suggest that the inhibitors of induction of ICAM-1 may turn out to yield a new type of antiinflammatory agent. With this in mind, we began to examine the compounds that were isolated from*N. oleander* for determining their inhibitory activity on the induction of ICAM-1 through bioassay.

Inhibitory Activity of Pregnanes on the Expression of ICAM-1 Induced by IL-1α

The *in vitro* anti-inflammatory activity of the isolated **2–4** was estimated by inhibition of the induction of ICAM-1 (Kawai *et al.*, 2000; Sugimoto *et al.*, 2000; Yuuya *et al.*, 1999; Higuchi *et al.*, 2003) using human cultured cell line A549 cells and the results are expressed as IC_{50} values. Cell viability was measured by an MTT assay (Table 1.11). Compound **4** showed potent inhibitory activity against the induction of ICAM-1 with weak inhibitory activity against cell growth of A549 cells (Figure 1.9).

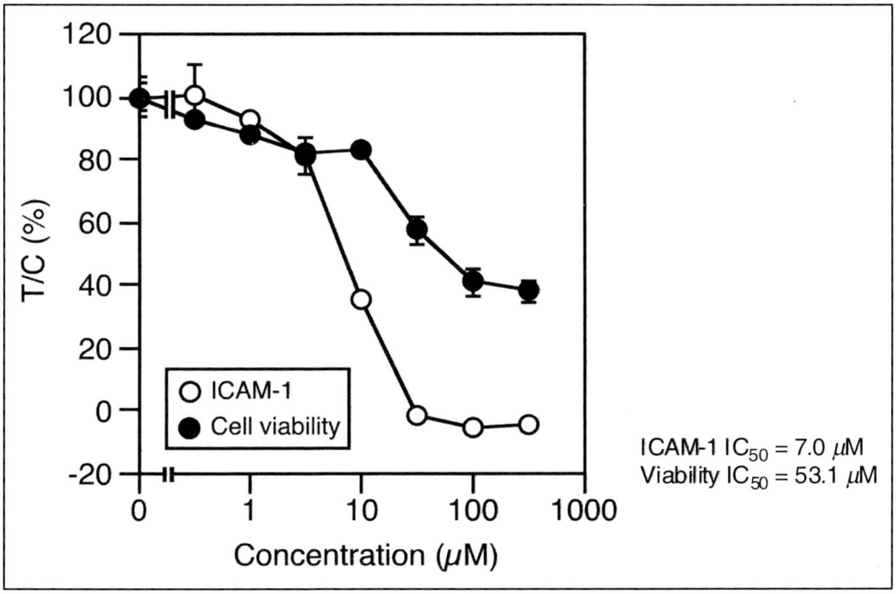

Figure 1.9: Effect of compound **4** on the induction of ICAM-1 in response to IL-1α open circles represent the ICAM-1 expression (mean±SD) of triplicate cultures). Cell viability was measured by a MTT assay (filled circles). Data points represents mean±SD of triplicate cultures.

Table 1.11: Effect of pregnanes **2–4** on induction of ICAM-1 and on ceil viability.

Compound	**2**	**3**	**4**
ICAM-1 IC_{50} (μM)[a]	>300	>100	7.0
MTT IC_{50} (μM)[b]	>300	>100	53.1

a: A549 cells were pretreated with various concentrations of test compound for 1 h and then incubated in the presence of IL-1α for 6 h. Absorbence at 415 nm was measured after treatment of the cells with primary and secondary antibodies and addition of the enzyme substrate. The experiments were carried out in triplicate cultures. b: A549 cells were incubated with serial dilutions of the compounds for 24 h. Cell viability (per cent) was measured by the MTT assay and used for determination of IC_{50} values. Experiments were carried out in triplicate cultures.

Inhibitory Activity of Less Polar Cardenolides and Cardenolide Monoglycosides 9–21 on the Expression of ICAM-1 Induced by IL-1α and TNF-α

The *in vitro* anti-inflammatory activity of the isolated compounds **9–21** was estimated by inhibition of the induction of ICAM-1 in the presence of IL-1α and TNF-α (Kawai *et al.*, 2000; Sugimoto *et al.*, 2000; Yuuya *et al.*, 1999; Higuchi *et al.*, 2003) using human cultured cell line A549 cells. Cell viability was measured by an MTT assay (Table 1.12). The assay results of **9–21** are summarized as follows: (1) The 5β,14β-card-20(22)-enolide structure is important for the inhibitory activity on the induction of ICAM-1. (2) Cardenolide N-1 (**9**) is the most effective compound. Since **9** showed very weak cytotoxic activity (IC_{50} > 100 μM), it is a desirable compound as an anti-inflammatory agent. (3) The structural change at C-3 of **9** from the 3β-*O*-(ᴅ-sarmentosyl)-group to the 3β-*O*-(ᴅ-diginosyl)- or 3β-hydroxyl groups did not show as great a change in the activities as that shown for **13** and **14**. (4) Introduction of an acetoxy group at C-16 in **9**, **13**, and **14** did not induce as great a change in the activities as shown in the corresponding compounds **19–21**. (5) Introduction of an additional hydroxy group at C-8 in **14** to **18** or a change of the 14-hydroxy group of **14** to the 8,14-epoxide ring of **17** decreased the activity. (6) Introduction of a double bond or an epoxide ring between C-16 and C-17 in **17** induced a further decrease of activity as shown in **16** and **11**. (7) The change of the 5β,14β-card-20(22)-enolide structure of **14** and **21** to the corresponding 5α,14β-card-20(22)-enolide structure of **15** and **12** led to a large decrease in activity. (8) Compounds **9–12**, **14**, **15**, **18**, **20**, and **21** showed inhibitory activities on the induction of ICAM-1 induced by IL-1α and TNF-α at the same level.

Inhibitory Activity of More Polar Cardenolides and Cardenolide Monoglycosides 22–34 on the Expression of ICAM-1 Induced by IL-1α and TNF-α

The *in vitro* anti-inflammatory activity of the isolated compounds **22–34** was estimated on the basis of inhibitory activity against the induction of the intercellular adhesion molecule-1 (ICAM-1) in the presence of IL-1α and TNF-α (Yuuya *et al.*, 1999; Kawai *et al.*, 2000; Sugimoto *et al.*, 2000; Higuchi *et al.*, 2003) using human cultured cell line A549 cells. Cell viability was measured by an MTT assay (Table 1.13). The assay results of **22–34** are summarized as follows: (1) The compounds **25–28** with 14-hydroxy-5β,14β-card-20(22)-enolide structure showed very strong inhibitory activity toward the induction of ICAM-1 at the IC_{50} values of less than 0.4 μM. Although the presence or absence of 16β-OAc at C-16 has no influence toward the activity, the presence of more polar hydroxyl group at C-16 reduced the activity as shown in that of **29**. (2) In them, cardenolide **28** is the most effective compound and the IC_{50} values are less than 0.2 μM. Since compound **28** showed very weak cytotoxic activity (IC_{50}>320 μM), it is a desirable compound as anti-inflammatory agents. (3) The structural changes of sugar moiety from the 3β-*O*-(ᴅ-digitalosyl) group in compound **26** to the 3β-*O*-(ʟ-oleandrosyl) group in compound **27** or 3β-*O*-(ᴅ-glucosyl) group in compound **28** gave a little influence toward the activities as shown in those of **26**, **27**, and **28**, respectively. (4) Change of 14-hydroxyl group of **25** to 8β,14β-epoxide ring induced

Table 1.12: Effect of cardenolides **9-21** on induction of ICAM-1 and on cell viability.

Compound	***9***	***10***	***11***	***12***	***13***	***14***	***15***	***16***	***17***	***18***	***19***	***20***	***21***
Assay							IC_{50} (μM)[a]						
ICAM-1[b]													
IL-1α	0.20	69.3	62.1	21.5	0.62	0.20	2.1	133	13.9	6.0	0.57	0.52	0.5
TNF-α	0.16	55.4	45.6	16.9	NT	0.48	1.8	NT	NT	5.9	NT	0.36	0.3
							IC_{50}(μM)[c]						
Cell viability by MTT assay[d]	>100	>100	>100	>100	>316	>316	>316	>316	>316	>100	>1000	>100	>316

a: IC_{50} values were calculated by using the following equation. Expression of ICAM-1 (per cent of control) = [(absorbance with sample and IL-1α/TNF-α treatment – absorbance without IL-1α/TNF-α treatment)/(absorbance with IL-1α/TNF-α treatment-absorbance without IL-1α/TNF-α treatment)] × 100. b: A549 cells (2 × 10^4 cells/well) were pretreated with various concentrations of the compounds for 1 h and then incubated in the presence of IL-1α or TNF-α for 6 h. Absorbance of 415 nm was measured after treatment of the cells with primary and secondary antibodies and addition of the enzyme substrate as described in Experimental section. The experiments were carried out in triplicate cultures. c: IC_{50} values were determined by using the following equation. Cell viability (%) = [(experimental absorbance – background absorbance)/(control absorbance – background absorbance)] × 100. d: A549 cells were incubated with serial dilutions of the compounds for 24 h. Cell viability (per cent) was measured by the MTT assay. The experiments were carried out in triplicate cultures.

the remarkable decrease of the activity as shown in that of cardenolide B-1 (**22**). (5) Introduction of a double bond at C-16 of 14-hydroxy-5β,14β-card-20(22)-enolide structure induced significant decrease of activity as shown in that of **32**. (6) The change of the 5β,14β-card-20(22)-enolide structure of **25** to the corresponding 5α,14β-card-20(22)-enolide structure of **30** induced large decrease of activity. (7) The skeletal rearrangement of the 5β,14β-cardenolide structure of **25** to 15(14→8)*abeo*-cardenolide derivatives **24** and **33**, and 8,14-seco-cardenolide derivative **34** induced large decrease of activity. (8) Compounds **22-24**, **26**, **28** and **30–33** showed inhibitory activity on the induction of ICAM-1 induced by IL-1α and TNF-α at nearly the same level.

Table 1.13: Effect of more polar cardenolide monoglycosides **22-34** on induction of ICAM-1 and on cell viability.

Compound	*ICAM-1[a] [IC_{50} (μM)][b]*		*Cell Viability by MTT Assay[c]*
	IL-1[d]	*TNF-α[d]*	*[IC_{50} (μM)]*
22	220	140	>320
23	6.6	5.7	>330
24	90	54	>320
25	0.20	NT	>1000
26	0.28	0.27	>320
27	0.39	NT	570
28	0.16	0.12	>320
29	5.2	NT	>1000
30	7.5	6.2	>320
31	31	20	>320
32	63	39	>320
33	81	57	>320
34	56	NT	>1000

a: A549 cells were pretreated with various concentrations of the compound for 1 h and then incubated in the presence of IL-1α or TNF-α for 6 h. Absorbancy of 415 nm was assayed after treatment of the cells with primary and secondary antibodies and addition of the enzyme substrate. b: The experiment were carried out in triplicate cultures. c: A549 cells were incubated with serial dilutions of the compounds for 24 h. Cell viability (per cent) was measured by MTT assay and used for determination of IC_{50}. The experiments were carried out in triplicate cultures. d: IC_{50} represent the means of two independent experiment except for **25**, **26**, **27**, and **28**.

Inhibitory Activity of Cardenolides and Cardenolide Diglycosides 35–45 on the Expression of ICAM-1 Induced by IL-1α and TNF-α

The *in vitro* anti-inflammatory activity of the isolated compounds **35–45** was estimated by inhibition of the induction of ICAM-1 in the presence of IL-1α and TNF-α using human cultured cell line A549 cells. Cell viability was measured by an MTT assay (Table 1.14). The assay results of **35–45** are summarized as follows: (1) 3β-*O*-(diglycosyl)-16β-acetoxy-14-hydroxy-5β,14β-card-20(22)-enolide structure is important for the inhibitory activity on the induction of ICAM-1 as shown in those of **36–39**. (2) 3β-*O*-(β-D-glucopyranosyl-(1→4)-α-L-oleandropyranosyl)- 16β-acetoxy-14-hydroxy-5β,14β-card-20(22)-enolide (**37**) is the most effective compound. Since **37** showed very weak cytotoxic activity (IC_{50} > 320 ¦ M), it is a desirable compound as an anti-inflammatory agents. (**37**) The structural change at C-3 of **37** from the 3 β-*O*-(β -D-glucopyranosyl-(1→4)-α-L-oleandropyranosyl)-group to the 3β-*O*-[β-D-glucopyranosyl-(1→4)-β-D-diginopyranosyl]-, 3 β-*O*-(β-D-glucopyranosyl- (1→4)-β-D-digitalopyranosyl), or 3β-*O*-(β -D-glucopyranosyl-(1→4)-β-D- sarmentopyranosyl) groups showed a decrease in the activities as that shown for **36**, **38**, and **39**. (4) Structural changes of **36** and **38** in genin moiety from 16β-acetoxy-14-hydroxy-5β,14β-card-20(22)-enolide to 8,14-epoxy-5β, 14β-card-20(22)-enolide such as **40** and **41** or 8,14-epoxy-5β,14β-card-16,20(22)-dienolide such as **42** induced a large decrease of the activity. (5) The change of the 5 β,14β-card-20(22)-enolide structure of **36** and **38** to the corresponding 5α,14β-card-20(22)-enolide structure of **44** and **45** led to a large decrease in activity. (6) Compounds **36, 37, 39, 41–45** showed inhibitory activities on the induction of ICAM-1 induced by IL-1α and TNF-α at the same level.

Table 1.14: Effect of cardenolide diglycosides **35-45** on induction of ICAM-1 and on cell viability

Compound	*ICAM-1[a] [IC_{50} (μM)][b]*		*Cell Viability by MTT Assay[c]*
	IL-1[d]	*TNF-α[d]*	*[IC_{50} (μM)]*
35	>320	>320	>320
36	0.63	0.62	>320
37	0.34	0.25	>320
38	0.65	NT[e]	>320
39	0.72	0.60	>320
40	>320	300	>320
41	28	16	>320
42	35	21	>320
43	34	28	>320
44	29	22	>320
45	28	19	>320
odoroside A[f]	0.20	0.48	>320

a: A549 cells were pretreated with various concentrations of the compound for 1 h and then incubated in the presence of IL-1α or TNF-α for 6 h. Absorbance of 415 nm was assayed after treatment of the cells with primary and secondary antibodies and addition of the enzyme substrate. b: The experiment were carried out in triplicate cultures. c: A549 cells were incubated with serial dilutions of the compounds for 24 h. Cell viability (per cent) was measured by MTT assay and used for determination of IC_{50}. The experiments were carried out in triplicate cultures. d: IC_{50} represent the means of two independent experiment except for **38**. e: Not tested. f: 3β-*O*-(β-D-diginopyranosyl)-14-hydroxy-5β,14β-card-20(22)-enolide (**14**).

Inhibitory Activity of Cardenolide Triglycosides 46–61 on the Expression of ICAM-1 Induced by IL-1α and TNF-α

The *in vitro* anti-inflammatory activity of isolated cardenolide triglycosides **46–61** was estimated by inhibition of the induction of ICAM-1 in the presence of IL-1α and TNF-α using human cultured cell line A549 cells. Cell viability was measured by MTT assay (Table 1.15). The assay results of **46–61** are summarized as follows: (1) The 14-hydroxy-5β,14β-card-20(22)-enolide structure in genin moiety is important for the inhibitory activity on the induction of ICAM-1 as that shown for **46–50**. (2) In them, 3β-*O*-(4-*O*-Gentiobiosyl-L-oleandrosyl)-16-β-acetoxy-14-hydroxy-5β,14β-card-20(22)-enolide (**50**) is the most effective compound. Since **50** showed very weak cytotoxic activity (IC_{50} > 316 μM), it is a desirable compound as an antiinflammatory agent. (3) The structural change at C-3 of **50** from 3β-*O*-(4-*O*-gentiobiosyl-L-oleandrosyl) to 3β-*O*-(4-*O*-gentiobiosyl-D-diginosyl) or 3β-O-(4-*O*-gentiobiosyl-D-digitalosyl) did not show as great a change in the activity as that shown for **48** and **49**. (4) Elimination of an acetoxy group at C-16 in **48** and **49** did not induce as great a change in the activities as that shown in the corresponding compounds **46** and **47**.

(5) Introduction of an additional hydroxyl group at C-8 in **46** to **58** or a change of the 14-hydroxy group of **46** and **47** to the 8,14-epoxide ring of **53** and **54** led to a large decrease in activity. (6) The change of the 5β,14β-card-20(22)-enolide structure of **46** and **47** to the corresponding 5α,14β-card-20(22)-enolide structure of **51** and **52** led to a large decrease in activity. (7) Introduction of an epoxide ring at 7,8-position of **46** led to a large decrease in activity as that shown for **61**. In conclusion, 14-hydroxy-5β,14β-card-20(22)-enolide is the essential structure for the inhibitory activity of induction of ICAM-1. Introduction of one more hydroxy group at C-8 or C-16 and change of 14-hydroxy group to 8,14-epoxy group led to a large decrease of activity. Introduction of a new epoxide ring in 7β,8β-position of **46** also led to a large decrease of activity in **61**. Compounds **46–61** showed inhibitory activity on the induction of ICAM-1 induced by IL-1α and TNF-α at the same level.

Cardenolides and cardenolide glycosides which are indicated in Tables 1.12–1.15 showed inhibitory activity on the induction of ICAM-1 induced by IL-1α and TNF-α at nearly the same level. The results suggest that these compounds block the common signaling NF-kB activation downstream of IkB kinase activation. Consistent with this, we have recently shown that odoroside A and ouabain inhibit Na^+/K^+-ATPase and prevent NF-kB-inducible protein expression by blocking Na^+-dependent amino acid transport (Takada *et al.*, 2009).

Cell Growth Inhibitory Activities of Compounds to Three Cell Lines, WI-38 Fibroblast Cell, VA-13 Marignant Tumor Cell, and HepG2 Human Liver Tumor Cell In vitro

Cell Growth Inhibitory Activities of of Pregnanes 1–8 to WI-38, VA-13, and HepG2

The cytotoxic activities of compounds **1–8** were evaluated against three human cell lines, WI-38, VA-13, and HepG2. Compound **4** exhibited significant growth inhibition of VA-13 and HepG2 cells. It is interesting to note that the cytotoxicity of **4** to the parental normal WI-38 cells (14.3 μM) was less than that to VA-13 (Table 1.16).

Table 1.15: Effect of cardenolide triglycosides **46-61** on induction of ICAM-1 and on cell viability.

Assay	***46***	***47***	***48***	***49***	***50***	***51***	***52***	***53***	***54***	***55***	***56***	***57***	***58***	***59***	***60***	***61***
							IC_{50} (μM)[a]									
ICAM-1[b]																
IL-1α	5.31	3.16	4.71	6.54	1.69	65.4	34.3	>316	67.8	>316	78.1	36.2	66.6	53.6	>316	150
TNF-α	3.40	2.01	2.48	3.29	1.20	46.0	25.2	>316	44.5	203	62.2	25.7	49.0	36.5	149	66.2
							IC_{50} (μM)[c]									
Cell viability by MTT assay[d]	>316	>316	>316	>316	>316	>316	>316	>316	>316	>316	>316	>316	>316	>316	>316	>316

a: IC_{50} was calculated using the following equation. Expression of ICAM-1 (per cent of control) = [(absorbance with sample and IL-1α/TNFα treatment – absorbance without IL-1α/TNF-α treatment)/(absorbance with IL-1α/TNF-α treatment – absorbance without IL-1α/TNF-α treatment)] x 100. IC_{50} represents the means of two independent experiment except for **61**. b: A549 cells (2 x 10^4 cells/well) were pretreated with various concentrations of the compounds for 1 h and then incubated in the presence of IL-1α or TNF-α for 6 h. Absorbance of 415 nm was assayed after treatment of the cells with primary and secondary antibodies and addition of the enzyme substrate as described in Experimental Section. The experiments were carried out in triplicate cultures. c: IC_{50} was determined using the following equation. Cell viability (per cent) = [(experimental absorbance – background absorbance)/(control absorbance – background absorbance)] x 100. The representative IC_{50} of two independent experiments are shown except for **16**. [d]A549 cells were incubated with serial dilutions of the compounds for 24 h. Cell viability (per cent) was measured by MTT assay. The experiments were carried out in triplicate cultures.

Table 1.16: Cell growth inhibitory activities of pregnanes **1**–**8** against WI-38, VA-13 and HepG2 cells.

Compound	IC_{50} (μM)[a]		
	WI-38	*VA-13*	*HepG2*
1	140	256	277
2	202	175	150
3	149	213	181
4	14.3	1.97	7.20
5	213	>290	>290
6	>290	>290	>290
7	>200	>200	>200
8	66.9	125	98.3
paclitaxel	0.04	0.005	8.1
adriamycin	0.70	0.40	1.3

a: IC_{50} represents the mean of duplicate determination.

Cell Growth Inhibitory Activities of of Less Polar Cardenolide Monoglycosides 9–21 to WI-38, VA-13, and HepG2

Cytotoxic activities of **9–21** were evaluated against three cell lines, WI-38, VA-13, and HepG2 cells (Table 1.17). The results of **9–21** are summarized as follows: (1) The 5β,14β-card-20(22)-enolide structure is important for the cell growth inhibitory activity of cardenolides. Thus, compounds **14** and **21** with 5 β,14β-card-20(22)-enolide functionalities showed stronger activity toward VA-13 and HepG2 cells than those of the corresponding compounds **15** and **12** with 5 α,14β-card-20(22)-enolide functions. (2) Cardenolide N-1 (**9**) is the most effective compound toward HepG2 cells. Its 3 β-*O*-(ᴅ-diginosyl)-derivative (**14**) also showed strong activity toward VA-13 cells. Their IC_{50} values were less than 0.18 μM. Compound **21**, the C-16 acetoxy derivative of **14**, and its aglycone (**20**) showed strong activity toward VA-13. Their IC_{50} values were also less than 0.2 μM. (3) Compound **19**, the 3β-*O*-(ᴅ-sarmentosyl)-derivative of **21**, also showed effective cytotoxic activity toward VA-13 and HepG2 cells at IC_{50} values of less than 1 μM. In conclusion, the compounds possessing the 3 β-*O*-(ᴅ-sarmentosyl)- or 3β-*O*-(ᴅ-diginosyl)-14-hydroxy-5β,14β-card-20(22)-enolide structure with or without an acetoxy group at C-16 are effective for expression of cytotoxicity toward VA-13 and HepG2 cells. (4) Change of the functional group of **14** from the 14-hydroxy group to the 8,14-epoxy or 8,14-dihydroxy groups led to a 10 to 100 fold decrease in the activity as shown by the increase in the IC_{50} values of **17** and **18**. (5) Introduction of a double bond or an α-epoxide ring into C-16,17 position of **17** induced a further decrease in the activity as shown by the ca. 10 fold increase in the IC_{50} values of compounds **16** and **11**. Thus, the 14-hydroxy group in **9**, **14**, **19**, **20**, and **21** is the essential functional group for expression of strong cytotoxic activities toward VA-13, and HepG2 cells. (6) IC_{50} values of compounds **12**, **13**, **17**, **18**, and **20** toward WI-38 cells are 2–10 fold higher concentrations than those toward VA-13. The assay results indicated that compounds **12**, **13**, **17**, **18**, and **20** showed stronger cytotoxicity toward

VA-13 malignant tumor cells than those toward parental WI-38 normal cells. Thus, they are desirable compounds as antitumor agents toward VA-13 because the side reaction toward WI-38 normal cells is expected to be low *in vivo*. Compound **20** is especially interesting because it exhibited significant cytotoxicity with an IC_{50} value of less than 0.2 μM and more than 10 fold lower cytotoxic activity toward the parental WI-38 cells. Although compounds**9, 14,19,** and **21** also exhibited significant cytotoxic activity toward VA-13 cells with IC_{50} values of less than 1 μM, they also exhibited 2–40 fold stronger cytotoxic activity toward WI-38 cells. Thus, compounds **9, 14, 19,** and **21** are undesirable compounds as antitumor agents toward VA-13, because their citotoxicity toward parental WI-38 normal cells are stronger than those toward VA-13 malignant tumor cells.

Table 1.17: Cell growth inhibitory activities of less polar cardenolide monoglycosides **9**–**21** against WI-38, VA-13 and HepG2 cells.

Compound	*IC_{50} (μM)*[a]		
	WI-38	*VA-13*	*HepG2*
9	<0.02	0.80	0.14
10	16.3	85.7	81.4
11	40.9	178	74.1
12	20.1	8.63	16.5
13	11.8	1.9	18
14	0.07	0.18	1.5
15	0.37	1.3	10.2
16	102	161	151
17	33.1	13.4	76.4
18	9.4	1.6	4.7
19	0.08	0.24	0.82
20	1.7	0.16	0.20
21	0.09	0.17	1.5
paclitaxel	0.04	0.005	8.1
adriamycin	0.70	0.40	1.3

a: IC_{50} represents the mean of duplicate determination.

Cell Growth Inhibitory Activities of More Polar Cardenolide Monoglycosides 22–34 against WI-38, VA-13, and HepG2 Cells

Cytotoxic activities of compounds **22**–**34** were evaluated against three cell lines, WI-38 (normal human fibroblast cells), VA-13 (malignant tumor cells induced from WI-38), and HepG2 (human liver tumor cells) (Table 1.18). The assay results of **22**–**34** are summarized as follows: (1) 5 β,14β-Card-20(22)-enolide structure is important for cell growth inhibitory activity of cardenolides. Thus, compound **25** with 5β,14β-card-20(22)-enolide structure showed stronger activity than the corresponding 5α,14β-card-20(22)-enolide **30** as shown by the increase of IC_{50} values of **30** in the range from 30 to 1000 times. (2) The skeletal rearrangement of the 3β-*O*-(glycosyl)-5β,14β-cardenolide structure of **25** to the corresponding 3β-*O*-(glycosyl)-15(14→8)*abeo*-cardenolide **33** and 3β-*O*-(glycosyl)-8,14-seco-cardenolide **34** also induced decrease of cytotoxic activities of the compounds as shown by the increase of IC_{50} values of **33** and **34** in the range from 40 to 100 times and 80 to 800 times, respectively. (3) 3β-*O*-(Glycosyl)-16β-acetoxy-14-hydroxy-5β,14β-cardenolides **27** and **28** are the most effective compounds toward HepG2 cells. The change of 3 β-*O*-(glycosyl) moiety of L-oleandrosyl in **27** to D-glucosyl in **28** has no influence toward the activity. Their IC_{50} value was less than 0.14 μM. (3) 3β-*O*-(glycosyl)-14-hydroxy-5β,14β-cardenolide **25** and its 16-acetoxy derivatives **26, 27** and **28** showed strong activity toward VA-13 at the IC_{50} values of less than 0.7 μM. (4) Thus, 3β-*O*-(glycosy)-14-hydroxy-5β,14β-card-20(22)-enolide structures with or without an acetoxyl group at C-16 are effective for expression of cytotoxic activity toward VA-13 and HepG2 cells. (5) Introduction of a new epoxide ring at 7,8-position of **25** induced decrease of the activity as shown by the increase of IC_{50} values of **23** in the range from 20 to 700 times. Change of the functional group of **25** from 14-hydroxyl group to 8,14-epoxy ring such as **22** induced further decrease of the activity as shown by the increase of IC_{50} values of **22** in the range from 400 to 8000 times. Introduction of a double bond at C-16 of 14-hydroxy-5β,14β-card-20(22)-enolide structure induced significant decrease of activity as shown in that of **31**. Thus, the 14β-hydroxy and 17β-α,β-unsaturated γ-lactone groups in **25–28** are the essential functional groups for expression of their strong cytotoxic activities toward VA-13, and HepG2 cells.

Table 1.18: Cell growth inhibitory activities of more polar cardenolide monoglycosides **22–34** against WI-38, VA-13, and HepG2 cells.

Compound	*IC_{50} (μM)*[a]		
	WI-38	*VA-13*	*HepG2*
22	125	>188	171
23	10.8	14.2	6.48
24	184	224	165
25	0.016	0.123	0.41
26	0.013	0.121	1.35
27	0.019	0.128	0.09
28	0.11	0.68	0.14
29	1.50	1.53	1.50
30	18.1	149	11.0
31	128	131	73.9
32	34.6	79.5	90.2
33	1.85	10.9	18.2
34	13.1	9.5	78.2
paclitaxel	0.04	0.005	8.1
adriamycin	0.70	0.40	1.3

a: IC_{50} represents the mean of duplicate determination.

Cell Growth inhibitory Activities of Cardenolide Diglycosides 35–45 against WI-38, VA-13, and HepG2 Cells

Cytotoxic activities of **35–45** were evaluated against three cell lines, WI-38, VA-13, and HepG2 cells (Table 1.19). The results of **35–45** are summarized as follows: (1) 16β-Acetoxy-14-hydroxy-5β,14β-card-20(22)-enolide structure is important for the cell growth inhibitory activity of cardenolide diglycosides. Thus, compounds **36** and **38** with 16β-acetoxy-14-hydroxy-5β,14β-card-20(22)-enolide structure showed stronger activity toward WI-38, VA-13 and, HepG2 cells than those of the corresponding compounds **44** and **45** with 16β-acetoxy-14-hydroxy-5α,14β-card-20(22)-enolide structure. (2) 3β-*O*-(β-D-glucopyranosyl-(1→4)-α-L-oleandropyranosyl)-16β-acetoxy-14-hydroxy-5β,14β-card-20(22)-enolide (**37**) is the most effective compound toward WI-38, VA-13, and HepG2 cells. Its 3β-*O*-[β-D-glucopyranosyl-(1→4)-β-D-diginopyranosyl]-, 3β-*O*-[β-D-glucopyranosyl-(1→4)-β-D-digitalopyranosyl], or 3β-*O*-[β-D-glucopyranosyl-(1→4)-β -D-sarmentopyranosyl]]-derivatives (**36**, **38**, and **39**) also showed strong activity toward WI-38 and HepG2 cells. Their IC_{50} values were less than 1.3 μM. (3) Structural changes of **36** and **38** in genin moiety from 16β-acetoxy-14-hydroxy-5β,14β-card-20(22)-enolide to 8,14-epoxy-5β,14β-card-20(22)-enolide such as **41** or 8,14-epoxy-5β,14β-card-16,20(22)-dienolide such as **42** led to a 10 to 100 fold decrease in the activity as shown by the increase in the IC_{50} values of **41** and **42**. Thus, the 14β-hydroxy group in **36–39** is the essential functional group for expression of strong cytotoxic activities.

Table 1.19: Cell growth inhibitory activities of cardenolide diglycosides **35**–**45** against WI-38, VA-13, and HepG2 cells.

Compound	*IC_{50} (μM)[a]*		
	WI-38	*VA-13*	*HepG2*
35	117.0	>143	130.0
36	0.95	9.2	0.80
37	0.37	2.32	0.83
38	0.94	8.05	1.29
39	0.39	3.08	0.79
40	>147	>147	>147
41	57.7	114	24.8
42	46.6	87.3	87.9
43	22.0	125	17.9
44	36.9	71.2	9.25
45	23.2	88.5	12.8
Paclitaxel	0.04	0.005	8.1
Adriamycin	0.70	0.40	1.3

a: IC_{50} represents the mean of duplicate determination.

Cell Growth Inhibitory Activities of Cardenolide Triglycosides 46–61 Against WI-38, VA-13, and HepG2 Cells

Cytotoxic activities of cardenolide triglycosides **46–61** were evaluated against three cell lines, WI-38, VA-13, and HepG2 (Table 1.20). The results of **46–61** are summarized as follows: (1) The 14-hydroxy-5β,14β-card-20(22)-enolide structure is important for the cell growth inhibitory activity of cardenolides. Thus compounds**46** and **47**, with 14-hydroxy-5β,14β-card-20(22)-enolide functionalities, showed stronger activity toward WI-38, VA-13, and HepG2 cells than those of the corresponding compounds **51** and **52** with 14-hydroxy-5α,14β-card-20(22)-enolide functions. (2) 3β-*O*-(4-*O*-Gentiobiosyl-L-oleandrosyl)-16-β-acetoxy-14-hydroxy-5β,14β-card-20(22)-enolide (**50**) is the most effective compound toward WI-38, VA-13, and HepG2 cells. Its 3β-*O*-(4-*O*-gentiobiosyl-D-diginosyl) derivative (**48**) and 3 β-*O*-(4-*O*-gentiobiosyl-D-digitalosyl) derivative (**49**) also showed strong activity toward HepG2. (3) Change of the functional group of **46** and **47** from the 14-hydroxy group to the 8,14-epoxy group led to a large decrease in the activity as shown by the increase in the IC_{50} values of **53** and **54**. (4) Introduction of an additional hydroxyl group at C-8 in **46** led to a large decrease in the activity as shown by the increase in the IC_{50} values of **58**. (5) Introduction

Table 1.20: Cell growth inhibitory activities of cardenolide triglycosides against WI-38, VA-13, and HepG2 cells.

Compound	*IC_{50} (μM)^a*		
	WI-38	*VA-13*	*HepG2*
46	3.93	8.38	3.63
47	4.58	12.6	4.66
48	7.99	10.90	5.43
49	3.44	15.0	6.54
50	0.62	6.53	3.01
51	92.9	116	78.8
52	79.7	115.0	46.5
53	>119	>119	>119
54	101	>117	80.9
55	>119	>119	>119
56	99.2	>117	73.8
57	16.6	88.4	30.0
58	56.1	110	43.1
59	10.7	95.9	51.5
60	92.1	>119	115
61	75.6	103	76.9
Paclitaxel	0.04	0.005	8.1
Adriamycin	0.70	0.40	1.3

a: IC_{50} represents the mean of duplicate determination.

of a new epoxide ring in 7β,8β-position of **46** also led to a large decrease of activity as shown by the increase in the IC_{50} values of **61**. (6) Change of the functional group at C-16 of **50** from 16-acetoxy group to 16-hydroxy group led to a large decrease in the activity as shown by the increase in the IC_{50} values of **57**. In conclusion, 14-hydroxy-5β,14β-card-20(22)-enolide is the essential structure for expression of cytotoxic activity toward WI-38, VA-13, and HepG2. Introduction of one more hydroxy group at C-8 or C-16, a new epoxide ring at 7β,8β-position, and the change of 14-hydroxy group to 8,14-epoxy group led to a large decrease of activity.

MDR Reversal Activity

In cancer chemotherapy, occurrence of multidrug resistance (MDR) of cancer cells caused by repeated administration of anticancer agents is a serious problem. One mechanism underlying multidrug resistance (MDR) in mammalian tumor cells has been ascribed to enhanced removal of drugs due to overexpression of efflux transporter proteins, such as P-glycoprotein (Pgp), a multidrug resistance protein (MRP) (Wortelboer *et al.*, 2005). Thus, agents that inhibit the function of this protein could overcome the MDR effect. Calcein derived from calcein AM by endogenous esterase is used as an easily operated functional fluorescent probe for this drug efflux protein (Eneroth *et al.*, 2001; Tsuruo *et al.*, 1986; Jonsson *et al.*, 1996).

MDR Reversal Activity of Pregnanes 1–8

The effects of pregnane derivatives, **1**–**8** on the cellular accumulation of calcein in MDR human ovarian cancer 2780AD cells were examined. Compounds **1**, **2**, and **5** showed significant and **4**, **6**, and **7** showed moderate MDR reversal activity toward these cells by comparison with a control (Table 1.21). It is interesting to note that the

Table 1.21: Effects of compounds **1**–**8** on the accumulation of calcein in MDR 2780 AD cells and cytotoxic activities of compounds against WI-38, VA-13, and HepG2 cells.

Compound	*Calcein Accumulation (% of control)*[a,b]			*Cytotoxicity IC_{50} (μg/ml)*[c]		
	0.25 μg/ml	*2.5 μg/ml*	*25 μg/ml*	*WI-38*	*VA-13*	*HepG2*
1	110	105	140	48.1	87.7	94.9
2 (1)	100	122	136	66.4	57.4	49.2
2 (2)	116	127	138			
3	103	108	99	51.1	73.1	62.1
4	109	92	107	4.9	0.68	2.5
5	110	154	148	73.5	>100	>100
6	102	114	112	>100	>100	>100
7	98	109	109	>100	>100	>100
8	93	110	98	53.7	>100	78.9

a: The amount of calcein accumulated in multidrug-resistant human ovarian cancer 2780 AD cells was determined relative to a control in the presence of 0.25, 2.5, and 25 μg/mL of each test compound. b: Values are the relative amount of calcein accumulated in the cell compared with the control experiment and represent the means of triplicate determinations. [c]IC_{50} values represent the means of duplicate determinations.

Table 1.22: Effect of compounds 2 and 5 on the accumulation of calcein in multidrug-resistant 2780 AD cells.

Compound	*Calcein Accumulation*[a]					*Evaluation Max. Verapamil % Concentration*
	Concentration (µg/mL)	*Average*[b] *(Count/well)*	*Per cent of Control*[c]	*Activity*[d]	*Verapamil (per cent)*[e]	
2(2)	0.25	3937	116	+	120	P[f]
	2.5	4327	127	+	117	120
	25	4679	138	++	93	0.25 µg/mL
5	0.25	3743	110	±	113	P[f]
	2.5	5240	154	++	141	141
	25	5019	148	++	100	2.5 µg/mL
Verapamil	0 (control)	3395	100			
	0.25	3298	97	±	100	
	2.5	3701	109	±	100	
	25	5034	148	++	100	

a: The amount of calcein that accumulated in multi drug-resistant human ovarian cancer 2780 AD cells was determined relative the control in the presence of 0.25, 2.5, and 25 µg/mL of the pregnanes. b: Values represent the means of triplicate determinations. c: Values are the relative amount of calcein accumulated in the cell compared with the control experiment. d: Indices are expressed on a scales of four by the range of the relative amount of calcein accumluation as compared with a control experiment (per cent): +++. >151; ++, 131-150 per cent; +, 111-130 per cent; ±, 91-110 per cent; -, <90 per cent. e: Values are expressed as the relative amount of calcein accumulation in the cell as compared with that of verapamil. [f]P, positive; the activity was more potent than that of verapamil (verapamil per cent > 100 per cent).

cytotoxic activity of compounds **1–3** and **5–8** toward WI-38, VA-13, and HepG2 cells is weak in addition to significant to moderate effects on the accumulation of calcein in MDR A2789AD, because cytotoxicity is not a desirable feature of MDR cancer reversal agents. Pregnanes **2** and **5** showed stronger activities than those of verapamil and maximum verapamil per cent is 120 per cent and 141 per cent, respectively (Table 1.22).

MDR Reversal Activity of Less Polar Cardenolide Monoglycosides 9–21

The effects of cardenolide derivatives, **9–21** on the cellular accumulation of calcein in MDR human ovarian cancer 2780AD cells were examined. Compounds **12**, **17**, and **18** showed effects on the accumulation of calcein in MDR A2780AD cells by comparison with a control (Table 1.23). It is interesting to note that the cytotoxic activity of compound **17** toward WI-38, VA-13, and HepG2 cells is relatively weak in addition to the significant effect on the accumulation of calcein in MDR A2789AD, because cytotoxicity is unnecessary for MDR cancer reversal agents. On the contrary, compounds **12** and **18** showed significant to moderate cytotoxicity toward VA-13 or VA-13 and HepG2. Thus, compound **17** is a possible lead compound for an MDR cancer reversal agent and compounds **12** and **18** are expected to be lead compounds in development of anti-MDR cancer agents. Compound **12** exhibited 128 maximum verapamil per cent, at 2.5 μg/ml using verapamil as a positive control (Table 1.24).

Table 1.23: Effect of compounds **9–21** on the accumulation of calcein in MDR 2780 AD cells.

Compounds	*Calcein Accumulation (per cent of control)*[a,b]		
	0.25 μg/ml	*2.5 μg/ml*	*25 μg/ml*
9	89	83	86
10	99	100	102
11	104	96	97
12	105	126	109
13	86	74	66
14	93	89	96
15	78	67	58
16	88	89	99
17	92	102	112
18	112	107	112
19	90	81	91
20	92	100	99
21	67	77	75

a: The amount of calcein accumulated in multidrug-resistant human ovarian cancer 2780 AD cells was determined relative to a control in the presence of 0.25, 2.5 and 25 μg/ml of test compounds. b: Values are the relative amount of calcein accumulated in the cell compared with the control experiment and represent the means of triplicate determinations.

Table 1.24: Effect of compounds **12** on the accumulation of calcein in multi drug-resistant 2780 AD cells

Compound	*Calcein Accumulation*[a]					*Evaluation Max. Verapamil % Concentration*
	Concentration (μg/mL)	*Average*[b] *(Count/well)*	*Per cent of Control*[c]	*Activities*[d]	*Verapamil (per cent)*[e]	
12	0.25	2559	105	±	113	P[f]
	2.5	3081	126	+	128	128
	25	2665	109	±	82	2.5 μg/ml
Verapamil	0 (control)	2445				
	0.25	2268	93	±	100	
	2.5	2407	98	±	100	
	25	3249	133	++	100	

a: The amount of calcein that accumulated in multi drug-resistant human ovarian cancer 2780 AD cells was determined relative the control in the presence of 0.25, 2.5, and 25 μg/mL of the pregnanes. b: Values represent the means of triplicate determinations. c: Values are the relative amount of calcein accumulated in the cell compared with the control experiment. d: Indices are expressed on a scales of four by the range of the relative amount of calcein accumluation as compared with a control experiment (per cent): +++. >151; ++, 131-150 per cent; +, 111-130 per cent; ±, 91-110 per cent; -, <90 per cent. e: Values are expressed as the relative amount of calcein accumulation in the cell as compared with that of verapamil. [f]P, positive; the activity was more potent than that of verapamil (verapamil per cent > 100 per cent).

MDR Reversal Activity of More Polar Cardenolide Monoglycosides 22–34

The effect of thirteen kinds of cardenolide derivatives **22–34** on the cellular accumulation in MDR human ovarian cancer 2780AD cells was examined. Compounds **22, 27, 33,** and **34** showed MDR reversal activity by the comparison with a control (Table 1.25). Since compounds **22** showed very weak cytotoxic activity, it is a potential lead compound as a MDR cancer-reversal agent.

Table 1.25: Effect of compounds **22**–**34** on the accumulation of calcein in MDR 2780AD cells.

Compounds	*Calcein Accumulation (per cent of control)*[a,b]		
	0.25 μg/ml	*2.5 μg/ml*	*25 μg/ml*
22	109[c]	110[c]	130[c]
23	108	81	86
24	91	95	92
25	96	83	91
26	94[c]	85[c]	85[c]
27	97	87	111
28	79	79	75
30	99	84	82
31	101[c]	105[c]	99[c]
32	97	99	98
33	112	126	117
34	108	96	106

a: The amount of calcein accumulated in multidrug-resistant human ovarian cancer 2780 AD cells was determined relative to a control in the presence of 0.25, 2.5 and 25 μg/ml of test compounds. b: Values are the relative amount of calcein accumulated in the cell compared with the control experiment and represent the means of triplicate determinations. c: Values represent the means of duplicate determinations.

MDR Reversal Activity of Cardenolides Diglycosides 35–45

The effects of cardenolide diglycosides, **35–45** on the cellular accumulation of calcein in MDR human ovarian cancer 2780AD cells were examined. Compounds**35** and **42** showed effects on the accumulation of calcein in MDR 2780AD cells by comparison with a control (Table 1.26). It is interesting to note that the cytotoxic activity of compounds **35** and **42** toward WI-38, VA-13, and HepG2 cells is relatively weak in addition to the significant effect on the accumulation of calcein in MDR 2789AD, because cytotoxicity is unnecessary for MDR cancer reversal agents. Thus, compounds **35** and **42** are possible lead compounds for an MDR cancer reversal agent.

Table 1.26: Effect of cardenolides diglycosides **35**–**45** on the accumulation of calcein in MDR 2780AD cells.

Compounds	*Calcein Accumulation (per cent of control)*[a,b]		
	0.25 µg/ml	*2.5 µg/ml*	*25 µg/ml*
35	103	93	118
36	87	88	76
37	97	93	92
38	95	70	83
39	98	93	96
40	90	93	95
41	104	110	86
42	126	110	111
43	105	94	84
44	95	83	88
45	92	91	64

a: The amount of calcein accumulated in multidrug-resistant human ovarian cancer 2780 AD cells was determined relative to a control in the presence of 0.25, 2.5 and 25 µg/ml of test compounds. b: Values are the relative amount of calcein accumulated in the cell compared with the control experiment and represent the means of triplicate determinations.

Table 1.27: Effect of cardenolide triglycosides **46**–**61** on the accumulation of calcein in MDR 2780AD cells.

Compounds	*Calcein Accumulation (per cent of control)*[a,b]		
	0.25 µg/ml	*2.5 µg/ml*	*25 µg/ml*
46	113	98	81
47	98	92	79
48	86	88	75
49	112	103	94
50	105	90	82
51	98	99	90
52	107	102	86
53	99	95	93
54	114	102	104
55	108	100	106
56	95	96	106
57	93	101	66
58	104	101	117
59	111	109	117
60	108	106	103
61	93	91	97

a: The amount of calcein accumulated in multidrug-resistant human ovarian cancer 2780 AD cells was determined relative to a control in the presence of 0.25, 2.5 and 25 µg/ml of test compounds. b: Values are the relative amount of calcein accumulated in the cell compared with the control experiment and represent the means of triplicate determinations.

MDR Revrsal Activity of Cardenolides Triglycosides 46–61

The effects of cardenolide triglycoside derivatives **46–61** on the cellular accumulation of calcein in MDR human ovarian cancer 2780AD cells were examined. Compounds **54–56** and **58–60** showed moderate to significant effects on the accumulation of calcein in MDR 2780AD cells by comparison with a control (Table 1.27). It is interesting to note that the cytotoxic activities of compounds **58** and **59** toward HepG2 are moderate activity in addition to the significant effect on the accumulation of calcein in MDR 2780AD. On the contrary, compounds**54–56** and **60** showed very week cytotoxic activity toward VA-13 and HepG2. Thus, compounds **54–56** and **60** are possible lead compounds for MDR cancer reversal agent and compounds **58** and **59** are expected to be lead compounds in development of anti-MDR cancer agent.

Acknowledgements

This work was supported by Young Academic Backbone Program of Heilongjiang Province, China (No. 1153G051). We thank our colleagues in the Niigata Research Laboratory of Mitsubishi Gas Chemical Company, Inc.: Dr. Sinyo Gayama and Ryuichiro Harada for their considerable cooperation and Ms. Sachiko Shimizu for her technical assistance in biological evaluation. We thank Mss Seiko Oka and Hiroko Tsushima of Center for Instrmental Analysis, Hokkaido University for HR FAB-MS

References

Abe, F. and Yamauchi, T. (1976). Pregnanes in the root bark of *Nerium odorum*. *Phytochemistry*, **15**: 1745-1748.

Abe, F. and Yamauchi, T. (1978). Digitoxigenin oleandroside and 5α-adynerin in the leaves of *Nerium odorum* (*Nerium* 9). *Chemical & Pharmaceutical Bulletin*, **26**: 3023-3027

Abe, F. and Yamauchi, T. (1979). Oleaside; Novel cardenolides with an unusual framework in *Nerium odorum* (*Nerium* 10). *Chemical & Pharmaceutical Bulletin*. **27**: 1604-1610.

Abe, F. and Yamauchi, T. (1992). Cardenolide triosides of oleander leaves. *Phytochemistry*, **31**: 2459-2463.

Abe, F. and Yamauchi, T. (1992). Two pregnanes from oleander leaves. *Phytochemistry*, **31**: 2819-2820.

Abe, F., Yamauchi, T., and Minato, K. (1996). Presence of cardenolides and ursolic acid from oleander leaves in larvae and frass of *Daphnis nerii*. *Phytochemistry*, **42**: 45-49.

Aebi, A. and Reichstein, T. (1950). Über die glycoside der blätter von Cryptostegia grandiflora (*Roxb.*) *R. Br.* (Asclepiadaceae). *Helvetica Chimica Acta*, **33**: 1013-1034.

Ahmed, A.F., Hsieh, Y.T., Wen, Z.H., Wu, Y.C., and Sheu, J.H. (2006). Polyoxygenated sterols from the Formosan soft coral *Sinularia gibberosa*. *Journal of Natural Products*, **69**: 1275-1279.

Ando, M., Akahane, A., Yamaoka, H. and Takase, K. (1982). Syntheses of arborescin, 1,10-epiarborescin, and (11*S*)-guaia-3,10(14)-dieno-13,6α-lactone, the key intermediate in Greene and Grabbé's estafiatin synthesis, and the stereochemical assighment of arborescin. *The Journal of Organic Chemistry*, **47**: 3909-3916.

Ando, M. and Yoshimura, H. (1993). Syntheses of four possible diastereoisomers of Bohlmann's Structure of isoepoxyestafiatin. The stereochemical assignment of isoepoxyestafiatin. *The Journal of Organic Chemistry*, **58**: 4127-4131.

Ando, M., Arai, K., Kikuchi, K. and Isogai, K. (1994) Synthetic studies of sesquiterpenes with a cis-fused decalin system, 4. Synthesis of (+)-5βH-eudesma-3,11-diene, (–) -5βH-eudesmane-4β,11-diol, and (+)-5βH-eudesmane-4α,11-diol, and structure revision of a natural eudesmane-4,11-diol isolated from *Pluchea arguta*. *Journal of Natural Products*, **57**: 1189-1199.

Bauer, P. and Franz, G. (1985). Untersuchungen zur biosynthese von 2,6-didsoxy-3-*O*-methylhexosen in *Nerium oleander*. *Planta Medica*, **3**: 202-205.

Begum, S., Siddiqui, B.S., Sultana, R., Zia, A. and Suria, A. (1999). Bio-active cardenolides from the leaves of *Nerium oleander*. *Phytochemistry*, **50**: 435-438.

Cabrera, G.M., Deluca, M.E., Seldes, A.M., Gros, E.G., Oberti, J., Crockett, J. and Gross, M. L. (1993). Cardenolide glycosides from the roots of *Mandevilla pentlandiana*. *Phytochemistry*, **32**: 1253-1259.

Chao, M., Zhang, S., Fu, L., Li, N., Bai, J., Sakai, J., Wang, L., Tang, W., Hasegawa, T., Ogura, H., Kataoka T., Oka, S., Kiuchi, M., Hirose, K. and Ando, M. (2006). Taraxasterane- and ursane-type triterpenes from *Nerium oleander* and their biological activities. *Journal of Natural Products*, **69**: 1164-1167.

Chopra, R.N., Nayara, S.L. and Chopra, I.C. (1956). Glossary of Indian Medicinal Plants. Council of Scientific Research, New Delhi, pp 175-177.

Eneroth, A., Åström, E., Hoogstraate, J., Schrenk, D., Conrad, S., Kauffmann, H.M., Gjellan, K. (2001). Evaluation of a vincristine resistant Caco-2 cell line for use in a calcein/AM extrusion screening assaay for P-glycoprotein interactio. *European Journal of Pharmaceutical Sciences*, **12**: 205–214.

Fieser, L. F. and Fieser, M. (1959). *Steroids*; Reinhold Publishing Corporation: New York, 1959; pp 727-809.

Fu, L., Zhang, S., Li, N., Wang, J., Zhao, M., Sakai, J., Hasegawa, T., Mitsui, T., Kataoka, T., Oka, S., Kiuchi, M., Hirose, K. and Ando, M. (2005). Three new triterpenes from *Nerium oleander* and biological activity of the isolated compounds. *Journal of Natural Products*, **68**: 198-206.

Hanada, R., Abe, F. and Yamauchi, T. (1992). Steroid glycoside from the roots of *Nerium odorum*. *Phytochemistry*, **31**: 3183-3187.

Higuchi, Y., Shimoma, F., Koyanagi, R., Suda, K., Mitui, T., Kataoka, T., Nagai, K. and Ando, M. (2003). Synthetic approach to exo-endo cross-conjugated cyclohexadienones and its application to the syntheses of dehydrobrachylaenolide, isodehydrochamaecynone, and *trans*-isodehydrochamaecynone. *Journal of Natural Products*, **66**: 588-594.

Hill, R.A., Kirk, D.N., Makin, H.L.J. and Murphy, G.M. (1991). Dictionary of Steroids; Chapman & Hall: London, New York, Tokyo, Melbourne, Madras. p 237 [gentiobiosylodoroside A (**46**), odoroside G (**47**)] and p 939 [odoroside K **51**)].

Hong, B.C., Kim, S., Kim, T.S., and Corey, E. J. (2006). Synthesis and properties of several isomers of the cardioactive steroid ouabain.*Tetrahedron Letters*, **47**: 2711-2715.

Huq, M.M., Jabbar, A., Rashid, M.A., Hasan, C.M., Ito, C., and Furukawa, H. (1999). Steroids from the roots of *Nerium oleander*. *Journal of Natural Products*, **62**: 1065-1067.

Jäger, H., Schindler, O. and Reichstein, T. (1959). Die glycoside der samen von*Nerium oleander* L. *Helvetica Chimica Acta*., **42**: 977-1013.

Janiak, P.S., Weiss, E., Euw, J. v. and Reichstein, T. (1963). Die konstitution von adynerin. *Helvetica Chimica Acta.*, **46**: 374-391.

Jolad, S.D., Hoffmann, J.J., Cole, J.R., Tempesta, M.S. and Bates R.B. (1981). 3'-*O*-methylevomonoside: A new cytotoxic cardiac glycoside from *Thevetia ahoubia* A. DC (Apocynaceae). The *Journal of Organic Chemistry*, **46**: 1946-1947.

Jonsson, B., Liminga, G., Csoka, K., Fridborg, H., Dhar, S., Nygren, P., Larsson, R. and Oka, S. (**1996**). Cytotoxic activity of calcein acetoxymethyl ester (calcein/AM) on primary cultures of human haematological and solid tumours. *Europian Journal of Cancer*, **32A**: 883–887.

Kawai, K., Kataoka, T., Sugimoto, H., Nakamura, A., Kobayashi, T., Arao, K., Higuchi, Y., Ando, M. and Nagai, K. (2000). Santonin-related compound 2 inhibits the expression of ICAM-1 in response to IL-1 stimulation by blocking the signaling pathway upstream of I*k*B degradation. *Immunopharmacology*, **48**: 129-135.

Kesselmans, R.P.W., Wijnberg, J.B.P.A., Minnaard, A.J., Walinga, R.E. and de Groot, A. (1991). Synthesis of all stereoisomers of eudesm-11-en-4-ol. 2. Total synthesis of Selin-11-en-4α-ol, intermedeol, neointermedeol, and paradisiol. First total synthesis of amiteol. *The Journal of Organic Chemistry*, **56**: 7237-7244.

López-Lázaro, M.; Postor, N., Azrak, S.S., Ayuso, M. J., Austin, C.A. and Cortés, F. (2005). Digoxin Inhibits the growth of cancer cell lines at concentrations commonly found in cardiac patients. *Journal of Natural Products*, **68**: 1642-1645.

Miyatake, K., Okano, A., Hoji, K., Miki, T. and Sakashita, A. (1959). *Chemical & Pharmaceutical Bulletin*, **7**: 634-640.

Paper, D. and Franz, G. (1989). Glycosylation of cardenolide aglycones in the leaves of *Nerium oleander*. *Planta Medica*, **55**: 30-34.

Paquette, L.A., Fristad, W.E., Schuman, C.A., Beno, M.A. and Cristoph, G.G. (1979). Reappraisal of the Stereochemistry of electrophilic additions to 3-norcarenes. X-ray and ^{1}H NMR analysis of norcarene epoxide conformation. The role of magnetic anisotropic contributions of epoxide rings *Journal of American Society*, **101**: 4645-4655.

Rangaswami, V.S. and Reichstein, T. (1949). Die glycoside von *Nerium odorum* Sol. I. *Pharmaceutica Acta Helvetiae*, **24**: 159-183.

Rittel, W. and Reichstein, T. (1954). Odoroside K and odorobioside K. Die glycoside von *Nerium odorum* Sol. *Helvetica Chimica Acta*., **37**: 1361-1373.

Roy, M.C., Chang, F.R., Huang, H.C., Chiang, M.Y.N. and Wu, Y.C. (2005). Cytotoxic Principles from the formosan milkweed, *Asclepias curassavica*. *Journal of Natural Products*, **68**: 1494-1499.

Siddiiqui, B. S., Sultana, R., Begum, S., Zai, A., and Suria, A. (1997). Cardenolide from the methanolide extract of *Nerium oleander* leaves possessing central nervous system depressant in mice. *Chemical & Pharmaceutical Bulletin*, **60**: 540-544.

Sugimoto, H., Kataoka, T., Igarashi, M., Hamada, M., Takeuchi, T. and Nagai, K. (2000). E-73, acetoxy analogue of cycloheximide, blocks the tumor necrosis factor-induced NF-kB signaling pathway. *Biochemical Biophysical Reserch Communications*, **277**: 330–333.

Tori, K., Ishii, H., Wolkowski, Z.W., Chachaty, C., Sangaré, M. and Lukacs G. (1973). Carbon-13 nuclear magnetic resonance spectra of cardenolide. *Tetrahedron Letters*, **13**: 1077-1080.

Tsuruo, T., Iida-Saito, H., Kawabata, H., Oh-hara, T., Hamada, H. and Utakoji, T. (1986). Characteristics of resistance to adriamycin in human myelogenouse leukemia K562 resistant to adryammycin and in isolated clones. *Jpnanese Journal Cancer Reserch (Gann)*, **77**: 682–692.

Ueda, K. and Komano, T. (1988). The multidrug-resistance gene MDR1. *Japanese Journal of Cancer and Chemotherapy (Gan To Kagaku Ryoho)*, **15**: 2858-2862.

Ueda, K., Pastan, I. and Gottesman, M.M. (1987). Isolation and sequence of the promoter region of human multidrug-resistance (P-glycoprotein) gene. *Journal of Biological Chemistry*, **262**: 17432-17436.

Wang, S.K., Dai, C.F. and Duh, C.Y. (2006). Cytotoxic pregnane steroids from the Formosan soft coral *Stereonephythya crystalliana*. *Journal of Natural Products*, **69**: 103-106.

Wortelboer, H.M., Usta, M., van Zanden, J.J., van Bladeren, P.J., Rietjens, I.M.C.M. and Cnubben, N.H.P. (2005). Inhibition of multidrug resistance proteins MRP1 and MRP2 by a series of α,β-unsaturated carbonyl compounds. *Biochemical. Pharmacolgy*, **69**: 1879–1890.

Yamauchi, T., Hara, M. and Mihashi K. (1972). Pregnenolone glucosides of *Nerium odorum*. *Phytochemistry*, **11**: 3345-3347.

Yamauchi, T., Mõri, Y. and Ogata, Y. (1973). D[16]-Dehydroadynerigenin glycosides of *Nerium odorum*. *Phytochemistry*, **12**: 2737-2739.

Yamauchi, T., Takata, N. and Mimura, T. (1975). Cardiac glycosides of the leaves of *Nerium odorum*. *Phytochemistry*, **14**: 1379-1382.

Yamauchi, T., Abe, F. and Takahashi, M. (1976). Neriumosides, cardenolide pigments in the root bark of *Nerium odorum*. *Tetrahedron Letters*, 1115-1116.

Yamauchi, T., Takahashi, M., and Abe, F. (1976). Cardiac glycosides of the root bark of *Nerium odorum. Phytochemistry*, **15**: 1275-1278.

Yamauchi, T. and Abe, F. (1978). Neriaside, a 8,14-*seco*-cardenolide in*Nerium odorum. Tetrahedron Letters,* 1825-1828.

Yamauchi, T., Abe, F. and Tachibana Y., Atal, C. (1983). Quantitative variations in the cardiac glycosides of oleander. *Phytochemistry*, **22**: 2211-2214.

Yamauchi, T. and Abe, F. (1990). Cardiac glycosides and pregnanes from *Adenium obesum* (Studies of the constituents of *Adenium*. I). *Chemical & Pharmaceutical Bulletin,* **38**: 669-672.

Yuuya, S., Hagiwara, H., Suzuki, T., Ando M., Yamada, A., Suda, K., Kataoka, T. and Nagai, K. (1999). Guaianolides as immunomodulators. Synthesis and biological activities of dehydrocostus lactone, mokko lactone, eremanthin, and their derivatives. *Journal of Natural Prodducts*. **62**: 22-30.

Zhao, M., Bai, L., Wang, L., Toki, A, Hasegaw, T., Kikuchi, M., Abe, M., Sakai, J., Hasegawa, R., Bai, Y., Mitsui, T., Ogura, H., Kataoka, T., Oka, S., Tsushima, H., Kiuchi, M., Hirose, K.,Tomida, A., Tsuruo, T. and Ando, M. (2007). Bioactive cardenolides from the stems and twigs of *Nerium oleander*. *Journal of Natural Products,* **70**: 1098-1103.

Bioactive Phytochemicals: Perspectives for Modern Medicine Vol. 1 (2012) *Pages* **79–106**
Editor: **V.K. Gupta**
Published by: **DAYA PUBLISHING HOUSE, NEW DELHI**

2

Flavonoids and their Anti-Diabetic Potentials

A.O. Ayeleso[1], O.O. Oguntibeju[1*] and N. Brooks[2]

ABSTRACT

Diabetes mellitus is a major health problem not only in urban, but also in the rural areas. It is a syndrome that is characterized by abnormal insulin action, resulting into high level of glucose in the body. Diabetes is diagnosed by the presence of hyperglycaemia and its prevalence is rapidly increasing in every part of the world. Oxidative stress is known to be actively involved in developmental diabetic-mediated disorders. Continuous uses of synthetic anti-diabetic drugs have been reported to have side effects and produce numerous complications affecting various vascular and metabolic functions. As a result, research studies on the use of phytochemicals from plants are on the increase as they are known to be very effective and safer in the management of diabetes and its complications. Flavonoids are a group of naturally-occurring compounds widely distributed as secondary metabolites in the plant kingdom. They are phenolic compounds known for very high antioxidant potentials. Many studies have demonstrated the hypoglycemic effects of flavonoids using different experimental models and treatments. The review covers the chemical characteristics and health promoting potentials of flavonoids in the management of diabetes.

Keywords: Flavonoids, Diabetes, Phenolic compounds, Plant kingdom, Hyperglycaemia.

1 Oxidative Stress Research Centre, Department of Biomedical Sciences, Faculty of Health and Wellness Sciences, Cape Peninsula University of Technology, Bellville, South Africa.

2 Department of Wellness Sciences, Faculty of Health and Wellness Sciences, Cape Peninsula University of Technology, Cape Town, South Africa.

* *Corresponding author*: E-mail: oguntibejuo@cput.ac.za; bejufemi@yahoo.co.uk, Tel: +27 21 9538495; Fax: +27 21 9538490

Introduction

Diabetes mellitus (DM) is a complex, progressive disease, which is accompanied by multiple complications. It is a metabolic disorder of the endocrine system (Li *et al.*, 2004) and among the most common disorders in developed and developing countries (Mukund *et al.*, 2008; Zhou *et al.*, 2009). The number of people affected by diabetes is estimated to rise by 50 per cent by 2010, and will almost be doubled by 2025 (Zimmet *et al.*, 2001; Bethel *et al.*, 2007). Increase in the estimated number of diabetic people from the present 150 to 230 million in 2025 has been reported (Iraj *et al.*, 2009; Abu-Zaiton, 2010). Oxidative stress has been suggested to be a common pathway linking diverse mechanisms for the pathogenesis of complications in diabetes (Mehrotra *et al*, 2001; Shih *et al.*, 2002). Prolonged hyperglycaemia results in the formation of advanced glycation end-products (AGEs) in body tissues of these patients (Deepralard *et al.*, 2009). It has been reported that diabetes is a risk factor for cardiovascular disease (Oguntibeju *et al.*, 2009b; Laakso, 1999; 2010) and more than 70 per cent of patients with type 2 diabetes die of cardiovascular diseases (Laakso, 2001).

Many drugs are available for use in the treatment of diabetes but their long-term use may cause adverse side effects and hence, the search for natural remedies is in progress to find effective remedies for diabetes (Nabeel *et al.*, 2010). Dietary factors play a key role in the prevention and management of various human diseases such as cardiovascular diseases (Menlanson, 2007, Oguntibeju *et al.*, 2009b), hypertension (Appel *et al.*, 2006), HIV/AIDS and tuberculosis (Oguntibeju *et al.*, 2010), diabetes (Ble-Castillo *et al.*, 2005) and cancer (Williams and Hord, 2005, Oguntibeju *et al.*, 2009a). Flavonoids are biologically active, polyphenolic constituents of plant foods which are found in various fruits, vegetables, legumes and beverages such as tea and wine (Nettleton *et al.*, 2006) and have the ability to scavenge free radicals and chelate metals (Saija *et al.*, 1995; Wilcox *et al.*, 2000; Geckil *et al.*, 2005). Some bioflavonoids have been reported to help in the improvement of hyperglycemia by affecting glucose transport (Ong and Khoo, 1996; Hsu *et al.*, 2003; Lee *et al.*, 2010), insulin receptor function (Shisheva and Shechter, 1992) and insulin-like properties (Choi *et al.*, 1991). Jung *et al.* (2004) reported that flavonoids play vital roles in preventing the progression of hyperglycaemia partly by increasing hepatic glycolysis and glycogen concentration and/or by lowering hepatic gluconeogenesis.

Overview of Diabetes as an Endocrine Disorder

Diabetes mellitus is a complex metabolic disorder in the endocrine system characterized by abnormalities in insulin secretion and/or insulin action that leads to the progressive deterioration of glucose tolerance which causes hyperglycemia. The immediate symptoms of the endocrine disorder include glucosuria, ketoacidosis, hypertriglyceridemia and hypercholesterolemia with weight loss and caloric deficits (Granner, 2000). There are two main categories of the disease. Type 1 diabetes mellitus also called juvenile onset or insulin-dependent diabetes mellitus (IDDM) and type 2, the non-insulin dependent diabetes mellitus (NIDDM) (Gale, 2001). The most prevalent form of diabetes mellitus is type 2 diabetes and it typically makes its appearance at the later stage of life (Grundy *et al.*, 1999). Type 2 diabetes may be caused by the combined effects of impairment in the insulin-mediated glucose disposal and defective secretion of insulin by the β-cells of the pancreas and is more common (Grundy *et al.*, 1999).

Hyperglycemia has tissue-damaging effects on a subset of cell types such as capillary endothelial cells of the retina, mesangial cells in the renal glomerulus, and neurons in the peripheral nerves (Brownlee, 2005). Great efforts have been made in the management of diabetes but serious problems such as diabetic retinopathy (Ferris *et al.*, 1999), diabetic nephropathy (Ritz and Orth, 1999), diabetic neuropathy (Androne *et al.*, 2000; Chistyakov *et al.*, 2001), lower extremity amputation (Reiber *et al.*, 1995) and accelerated coronary artery disease (Skyrme-Jones *et al.*, 2000; Mackness *et al.*, 2002) are still confronting diabetic patients.

Chronic hyperglycemia leads to many long-term complications in the eyes, kidneys, nerves, heart, and blood vessels (Laakso, 2010). In diabetic patients, the interaction of autoantibodies with AGEs is capable of forming AGE-immune complexes which may play a role in atherogenesis (Turk *et al*, 2001). Atherogenesis involves endothelial dysfunction, activation and injury, inflammation, and smooth muscle cell migration and proliferation (Mehta *et al.*, 2006). There is increasing

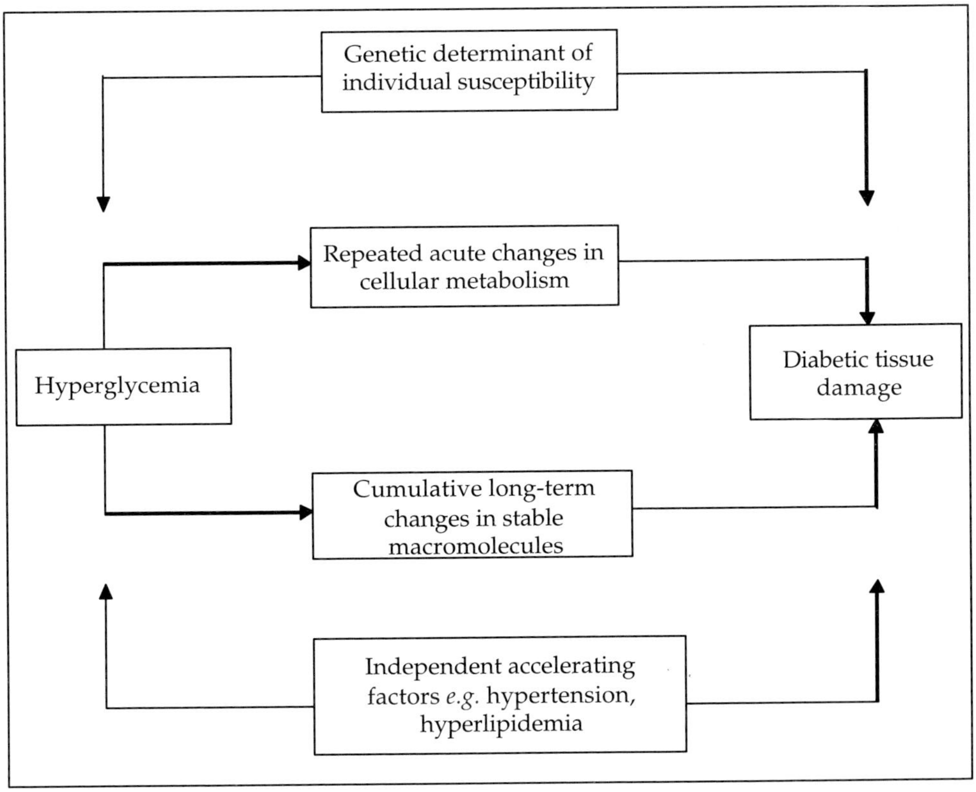

Figure 2.1: General features of hyperglycemia-induced tissue damage (modified by genetic determinant of individual susceptibility and independent accelerating factors such as hypertension and hyperlipidemia) (Brownlee, 2005).

evidence for the role of genetic factors inseveral diabetic complications, particularly diabetic nephropathy and cardiovascularcomplications of diabetes (Bowden, 2002).

Oxidative Stress in Diabetes

Oxidative stress, an imbalance between the generation of reactive oxygen species/ reactive nitrogen species and antioxidant defence capacity of the body, is actively involved in the pathogenesis of diabetes and its complications (Ha and Lee, 2000; Bonnefont-Rousselot, 2002; Johansen *et al.*, 2005; Oguntibeju *et al.*, 2010). Reactive oxygen species/reactive nitrogen species include free radicals such as superoxide ($^{\bullet}O_2^-$), hydroxyl ($^{\bullet}OH$), peroxyl ($^{\bullet}RO_2$), hydroperoxyl ($^{\bullet}HRO_2^-$), nitric oxide (NO) and nitrogen dioxide ($\bullet NO_2$-) and non-free radicals such as hydrogen peroxide (H_2O_2), hydrochlorous acid (HOCl), peroxynitrite (ONOO-), nitrous oxide (HNO2) and alkyl peroxynitrates (RONOO) (Johansen *et al.*,2005; Higashi *et al.*, 2006; Oguntibeju *et al.*, 2010). Diabetes has been associated with increased oxidative stress, which may contribute to microvascular and macrovascular complications (Giugliano and Ceriello, 1996). Hyperglycemia is mediated to some extent, by a state of enhanced oxidative stress which results in excessive production of reactive oxygen species and cause adverse structural and functional changes in tissues (Mehta *et al.*, 2006; Robertson and Harmon, 2006).

Several mechanisms appear to be involved in hyperglycemia such as glucose autoxidation, stimulation of the polyol pathway, activation of the reduced form of nicotinamide adenine dinucleotide phosphate oxidase, and production of advanced glycation end-products which leads to increased generation of reactive oxygen species (Bonnefont-Rousselot *et al.*, 2000; Bonnefont-Rousselot, 2002). Glycation is a major source of reactive oxygen species and reactive carbonyl species that are caused by both oxidative (glycoxidative) and non-oxidative pathways (Rahbar and Figarola, 2003). Elevated non-enzymatic glycation of proteins, lipids and nucleic acids due to the formation of advanced glycation end-products (AGE's) is accompanied by oxidative, radical-generating reactions and therefore represents a major source for oxygen free radicals under hyperglycemic conditions (Mohamed *et al.*, 1999).Studies have reported that glycation may result in production of superoxide (Jones *et al.*, 1987; Sakurai and Tsuchiya, 1988).

Protein glycation alters protein and cellular function, and binding of advanced glycated end-products (AGEs) to their receptors can result to modification in cell signalling and further production of free radicals (Penckofer *et al.*,2002). In an*in vitro* study on HIT-T15 cells, induced glycation suppressed insulin gene promoter activity and its mRNA levels by provoking oxidative stress through the glycation reaction (Matsuoka *et al.*, 1997). Glucose can oxidize *in vitro* (catalyzed by trace amounts of transition metal), generating hydrogen peroxide, highly reactive oxidants, and protein-reactive ketoaldehyde compounds (Wolff *et al.*, 1991). Reactive oxygen species, particularly superoxide anions could inactivate endothelium-derived nitric oxide (NO) to form potent oxidant peroxynitrite which contributes to the development of endothelial dysfunction in diabetes (Kodja and Harrison, 1999; Laight *et al.*, 2000; Johansen *et al.*, 2005). Superoxide anions ($^{\bullet}O_2^-$) can also activate several damaging pathways in diabetes including accelerated formation of advanced glycation end-products (AGE), polyol pathway, hexosamine pathway and protein kinase C, all of which have been proven to be involved in micro and macro vascular complications (Johansen *et al.*, 2005).

Oxidative stress can alter insulin action through a change in the physical state of the plasma membrane of target cells, increase in intracellular calcium content and reduction in nitric oxide (NO) availability (Paolisso and Giugliano, 1996). Mitochondrial overproduction of free radicals is possibly a potential mechanism causing impaired first phase of glucose-induced insulin secretion (Knight, 1998; Sakai *et al.*, 2003) and this process has been associated with the onset of type 1 diabetes via apoptosis of pancreatic beta-cells, and the onset of type 2 diabetes via insulin resistance (Bonnefont-Rousselot *et al.*, 2000). Oxidative stress caused by short

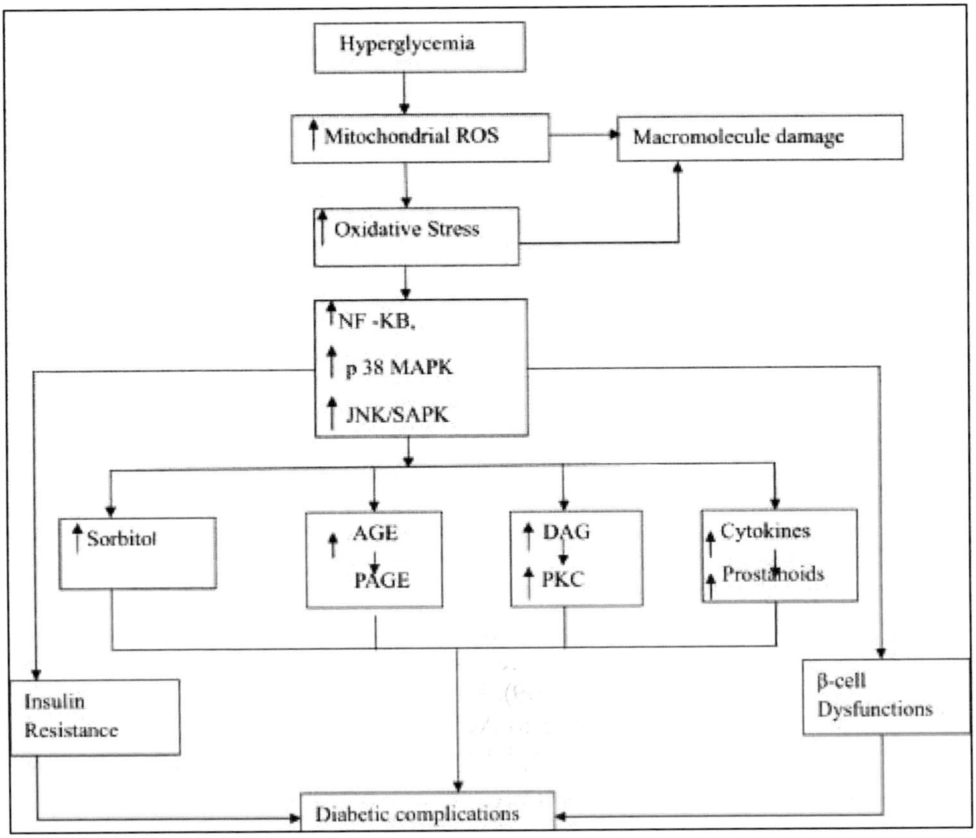

Figure 2.2: The diagram describes the link between hyperglycaemia, mitochondrial ROS generation, oxidative stress, activation of stress-sensitive pathways (NF-kB, p38 MAPK, JNK/SAPK, and others), insulin resistance, B-cell dysfunction, and diabetic complications. Increased production of sorbitol (formed as a consequence of the hyperglycemia-mediated increase in aldose reductase activity), AGE, cytokines, prostanoids, along with PKC activation could function as positive regulatory feedback loops to chronically stimulate stress-sensitive pathways. ROS (and RNS) can also cause oxidative damage directly upon cellular macromolecules and result in oxidative stress (Evans *et al.*, 2002).

exposure of β-cell preparations to H_2O_2 has been shown to increase the production of p21 and decreases insulin mRNA, cytosolic ATP, and calcium flux in cytosol and mitochondria (Maechler *et al.,* 1999). B-Cells are particularly sensitive to reactive oxygen species due to their low free-radical quenching (antioxidant) enzymes such as catalase, glutathione peroxidase, and superoxide dismutase (Tiedge *et al.,* 1997).

Signal transduction pathways such as c-Jun N-terminal kinase (JNK) (also known as stress-activated protein kinase), p38 mitogen-activated protein kinase (p38 MAPK), and protein kinase C (PKC) are activated by oxidative stress in several cell types including pancreatic β-cells. Kaneto *et al.* (2002) reported that that activation of the JNK pathway is involved in reduction of insulin gene expression by oxidative stress and that suppression of the JNK pathway protects β-cells from oxidative stress. The JNK pathway is reported to be activated under diabetic conditions and is possibly involved in the progression of insulin resistance (Evans *et al.,* 2002). The modulation of the JNK pathway in the liver on insulin resistance and glucose tolerance showed that, suppression of the JNK pathway in the liver produced highly beneficial effects on insulin resistance status and glucose tolerance in both genetic and dietary models of diabetes (Nakatani *et al.,* 2004).

One primary intracellular target of hyperglycaemia, ROS and oxidative stress is the transcription factor NF-kB (Barnes and Karin, 1997; Mohamed *et al.,* 1999; Bierhaus *et al.,* 2001; Evans *et al.,* 2002). NF-κB belongs to the Rel-family of pluriprotein transcription activators. It is a regulatory protein that controls the expression of numerous inducible and tissue- specific NF-κB responsible genes (Ghosh *et al.,* 1998). NF-κB is generally considered a central regulator of stress responses, because it can be activated by hundreds of different stimuli, such as lipopolysaccharide (LPS), tumor necrosis factor α (TNFα), and other proinflammatory cytokines, as well as environmental stress (Wu *et al.,* 2009). Kabe *et al.* (2005) reported that reactive oxygen species could enhance the signal transduction pathways for NF-kB activation in the cytoplasm and translocation into the nucleus. Reactive oxygen species appeared to serve as common secondary messengers of many different stimuli that activate NF-κB (Shreck *et al.,* 1991). AGE's can influence cellular function by binding to several binding sites including the receptor for AGE's (RAGE). It has been shown that binding of AGE's (and other ligands) to RAGE results in generation of intra-cellular oxidative stress and subsequent activation of the redox-sensitive transcription factor NF-kB *in vitro* and *in vivo* (Mohamed *et al.,* 1999). Modification of plasma proteins by AGE precursors creates ligands that bind to AGE receptors, inducing changes in gene expression in endothelial cells, mesangial cells and macrophages (Brownlee, 2001).

Activation of protein kinase C (PKC) occurs in response to increase in diacylglycerol (DAG) in various tissues in diabetes and hence, it is involved in the pathological events that cause diabetes complications (Tomkin, 2001). DAG can be generated from the hydrolysis of phosphatidylinositides or the metabolism of phosphatidylcholine (PC) by phospholipase C or phospholipase D and also, by *de novo* synthesis from glycolytic intermediates (Park *et al.,* 1999). High glucose appears to stimulate messengial cell proliferation through PKC/NF-kB pathways (Park *et al.,* 2000). The activation of PKC by intracellular hyperglycemia has a variety of effects on gene expression (Brownlee, 2005).

In the polyol pathway, high concentration of glucose in the cell is reduced to sorbitol by aldose reductase which is later oxidized to fructose. In the process of reducing high intracellular glucose to sorbitol, the aldose reductase consumes the cofactor NADPH, an essential cofactor for regenerating a critical intracellular antioxidant, reduced glutathione. By reduction in the amount of reduced glutathione, the polyol pathway increases susceptibility to intracellular oxidative stress (Brownlee, 2005). Glucose metabolism through the hexosamine pathway has been implicated in many of the adverse effects of chronic hyperglycemia. In the hexosamine pathway, fructose-6-phosphate is converted to N-acetylglucosamine-6-phosphate by glutamine:fructose-6-phosphate amidotransferase (GFAT). N-Acetylglucosamine-6-phosphate is then converted to N-acetylglucosamine-1,6-phosphate and to Uridine diphosphate *N*-acetyl Glucosamine (UDP-GlcNAc) (Kaneto *et al.,* 2001; Brownlee *et al.,* 2005). UDP-Glc- NAc is a substrate for *O*-linked glycosylation, which is catalyzed by *O*-GlcNAc transferase. The *O*-linked glycosylation is reversed by *O*-GlcNAc -*N*-acetylglucosaminidase (*O*-GlcNAcase) (Kaneto *et al.,* 2001). The elevated intracellular *O*-GlcNAc-mediated modification of certain kinds of proteins may suppress the process of glucose transport, thus causing insulin resistance (Akimoto *et al.,* 2005). Streptozotocin, a diabetogenic agent, elevated *O*-GlcNAc levels in pancreatic islets and contributed to the destruction of β-cells (Liu *et al.,* 2000).

Flavonoids and their Chemical Characteristics

Rusznyak and Szent- Györgi in the 1930s identified a substance called vitamin P from lemon peels that reduced capillary permeability which was effective in the treatment of purpura patients who were resistant to vitamin C (Rusznyak and Szent-Györgyi, 1936). It later became clear that the substance was actually a flavonoid (Bruckner and Szent-Gyorgyi, 1936; Ranaud and de Lorgeril, 1992). However, the term vitamin P was abandoned because these flavonoids ultimately did not meet the definition of a vitamin (Hollman *et al.,* 1996). Flavonoids are a class of secondary plant phenolic compounds that are well distributed in the plant kingdom. Flavonoids are characterized by two or more aromatic rings, each bearing at least one aromatic hydroxyl and connected with a carbon bridge (Clifford, 2001; Beecher, 2003). The basic flavonoid structure is the flavan nucleus, which consists of 15 carbon atoms arranged in three rings (C_6–C_3–C_6) (Pietta, 2000).

The various classes of flavonoids differ in the level of oxidation and pattern of substitution of the C ring, while individual compounds within a class vary in the pattern of substitution of the A and B rings (Pietta, 2000). Multiple combinations of hydroxyl groups, sugars, oxygen and methyl groups attached to the common structural components of flavonoids (two benzene on either side of a 3-carbon ring) create the various classes of flavonoids (Alan and Miller, 1996). Several classes of flavonoids such as anthocyanins, flavones, flavonols, flavanones, dihydroflavonols, chalcones, aurones, flavan and proanthocyanidins, isoflavonoids, bioflavonoids have been reported ((Alan and Miller, 1996; Iwashina, 2000). More than 8000 flavonoids are known and they are the most important and the largest group of polyphenolic compounds in plants (Lukaèínová *et al.,* 2008).

They generally occur in plants as glycosylated derivatives, and they contribute to the brilliant shades of blue, scarlet, and orange, in leaves, flowers, and fruits (Brouillard and Cheminat, 1988). Flavonoids take part in light phase photosynthesis by acting as catalyst and or as regulators of iron channels involved in phosphorylation (Pietta and Simonetti, 1999). Flavones, flavonols and anthocyanidins could act as visual signals in plants for pollinating insects due to their attractive colours (Pietta, 2000). They are broadly distributed in many frequently consumed beverages and food products of a plant origin, such as fruit, vegetables, wine, tea, and cocoa (Ross and Kasum, 2002). The flavonoids are frequently components of the human diet, and intake can be between 50 to 800 mg/day (Pietta, 2000; Yang *et al.*, 2001).

Table 2.1: Classes of flavonoids and the names of prominent food flavonoids and typical food sources (Beecher, 2003).

Flavonoids	*B Ring Connection to C Ring (Position on C-ring)*	*C Ring Unsatu-ration*	*C Ring Functional*	*Prominent Food Flavonoids*	*Typical Rich Food Sources*
Flavanol	2	None	3-hydroxyl	(+)-Catechin (+)-Gallocatechin (-)-Epicatechin (-)-Epigallocatechin	Teas, red grapes, red wines
			3-O-gallate	(-)-Epicatechin-3-gallate (-)-Epigallocatechin-3-gallate	
Flavonones	2	None	4-Oxo	Eriodictyol Hesperetin Naringenin	Citrus foods
Flavones	2	2-3 Double bond	4-Oxo	Apigenin Luteolin	Green leafy spices *e.g.*, Parsley
Isoflavones	2	2-3 Double bond	4-Oxo	Daidzein Genistein Glycitein Biochanin A Formononentin	Soyabeans, soy foods and legumes
Flavonols	2	2-3 Double bond	3-hydroxy, 4-Oxo	Isorhamnetin Kaemferol Myricetin Quercetin	Nearly ubiquitos in foods *e.g.*, Quercetin
Anthocyanidins	2	1-2, 3-4 Double	3-hydroxy	Cyanidin Dephinidin Petunidin Malvidin Pelargonidin	Red, purple, blue berries

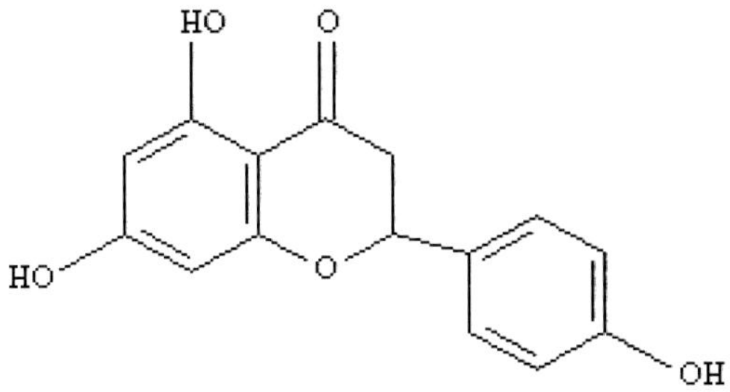

Flavonone

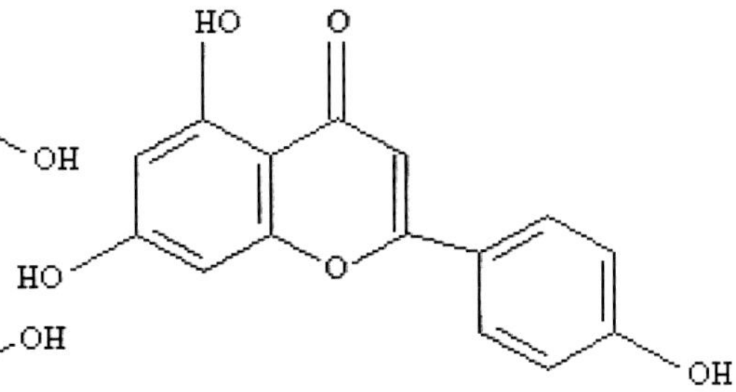

Flavones

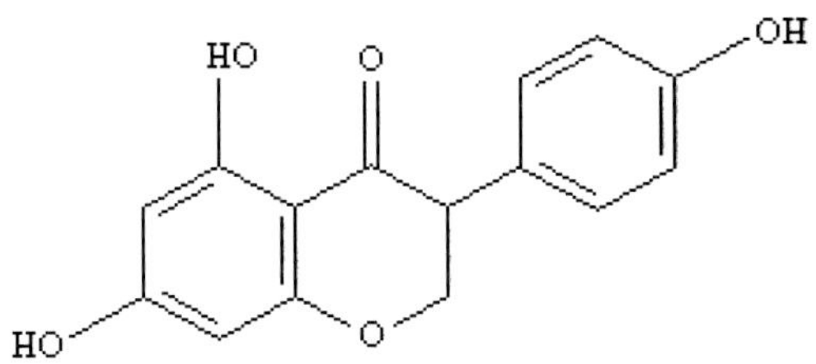

Isoflavones

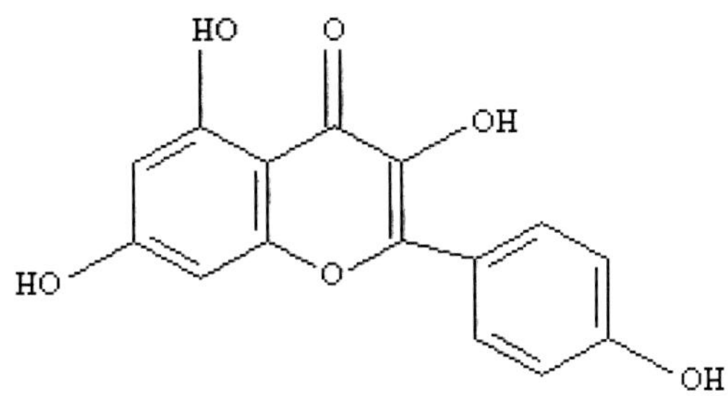

Flavonols

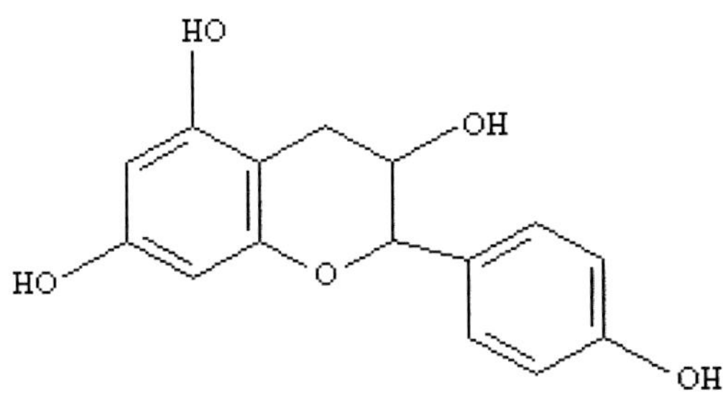

Anthocyanin

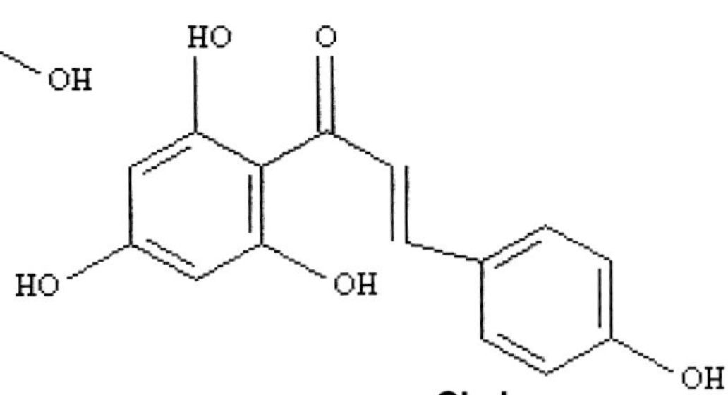

Chalcones

Figure 2.3: Structures of the different classes of flavonoids.

Potentials Roles of Flavonoids on Diabetes and its Complications

Polyphenolic compounds are known to play vital roles in protecting the body against various chronic diseases, such as cardiovascular diseases (Vita, 2005; Manach *et al.*, 2005; Stangl *et al.*, 2007), diabetes mellitus (Knekt *et al.*, 2002; Jung *et al.*, 2006; Pinent *et al.*, 2008; Lukacínová *et al.*, 2008), cancer (Carroll *et al.*, 1998; Mukhtar and Ahmad, 2000; Le Marchand, 2002; Knekt *et al.*, 2002; Surh, 2003; Manson, 2003) and asthma (Knekt *et al.*, 2002). Bonnefont-Rousselot (2004) reported that some antioxidants micronutrients can indirectly participate in the decrease of oxidative stress in diabetic patients by improving glycemic control and/or are able to exert antioxidant activity. Flavonoids can exert their antioxidant activity by various mechanisms, *e.g.*, by scavenging or quenching free radicals, by chelating metal ions, or by inhibiting enzymatic systems responsible for free radical generation (Pietta, 2000; Nijveldt *et al.*, 2001).

Flavonoids are soluble chain-breaking inhibitors of the peroxidation process, scavenging intermediate peroxyl and alkoxyl radicals (Saija *et al.*, 1995; Jovanovic *et al.*, 1998). Flavonoids inhibit the enzymes responsible for superoxide anion production, such as xanthine oxidase (Hanasaki *et al.*, 1994) and protein kinase C (Ursini *et al.*, 1994). The scavenging ability of flavonoids has been reported to be in the order: Myrcetin > quercetin > rhamnetin > morin > diosmetin > naringenin > apigenin > catechin > 5,7-dihydroxy-3′,4′,5′-trimethoxyflavone > robinin > kaempferol > flavones (Ratty and Das, 1988). The ability of quercetin to protect against oxidative stress-induced cellular damage is commonly associated with its anti-oxidative action as well as its metal chelatory properties (Mira *et al.*, 2002; Anjaneyulu and Chopra, 2004).

Lukacínová *et al.* (2008) studied the hypoglycaemic and antioxidant effects of quercetin and chrysin in alloxan-induced diabetic rats and found that serum glucose elevation was prevented but the effect of chrysin was weaker, particularly at the higher dose. Furusawa *et al.* (2005) had earlier reported that chrysin has only moderate antioxidant effect and almost no metal chelatory properties. It was suggested that the protective effect of quercetin and chrysin to a certain extent is due to their antioxidative/chelatory properties and partly to the alteration of renal glucose absorption (Lukacínová *et al.*, 2008).

Quercetin significantly attenuated renal dysfunction and oxidative stress in diabetic rats and the neuropathic pain that accompanies the disease (Anjaneyulu *et al.*, 2003; Anjaneyulu and Chopra, 2004). Machha (2007) also showed that the administration of quercetin to diabetic rats was able to restore vascular function, probably through enhancement in the bioavailability of endothelium-derived nitric oxide coupled to reduced blood glucose level and oxidative stress. Through an *in vitro* study, kaempferol was shown to protect HIT-T15 pancreatic beta cells from 2-deoxy-D-ribose-induced oxidative damage and it was suggested that kaempferol could be viewed as a possible means of preventing beta cell apoptosis under hyperglycaemic conditions (Lee *et al.*, 2010). Rutin was shown to decrease plasma glucose levels and prevent STZ-induced oxidative stress (Kamalakkannan and Prince,

2006b). In another study, Torres-Piedra *et al.* (2010) showed that the sub-acute administration of chrysin, 3-hydroxyflavone and quercetin produced significant lowered levels of blood glucose in STZ- nicotinamide diabetic rats.

Flavonoids may have the ability to reduce the occurrence of diabetes by preventing the progressive impairment of pancreatic beta-cells function (Coskun *et al.*, 2005; Song *et al.*, 2005), and thereby regenerate the damaged pancreatic cells or stimulate the secretion of insulin by β–cells of the pancreas (Seetharam *et al.*, 2002). Genistein (Lee, 2006) and epigallocatechin gallate (Wolfram, 2006) were reported to increase plasma insulin in diabetic animals. Liu *et al.* (2006) showed that genistein could increase rapid glucose-stimulated insulin secretion (GSIS) in both insulin-secreting cell lines (INS-1 and MIN6) and mouse pancreatic islets.

Geinstein acted directly on pancreatic β-cells, leading to the activation of cAMP/PKA signalling cascade to exert an insulinotropic effect, thereby providing a novel role of soy isoflavones in the regulation of insulin secretion (Liu *et al.*, 2006). In another study, geinsten was reported to promote beta-cell survival, insulin secretory function and ameliorate hyperglycaemia in streptozotocin-induced diabetes in mice (Fu and Liu, 2007). The protective effect of genistein in diabetes and its late secondary complications has been attributed to its antioxidant properties (Exner *et al.*, 2001; Mizushige *et al.*, 2007; Wu and Chan, 2007).

Hif *et al.* (1985) reported that quercetin was able to stimulate insulin release and enhanced Ca^{2+} uptake from isolated islets cell and suggested the involvement of flavonoids in non-insulin dependent diabetes. Quercetin could regenerate pancreatic islets and probably increases insulin release in streptozotocin-induced diabetic rats (Vessal *et al.*, 2003). Kobori *et al.* (2009) suggested that quercetin increased pancreatic insulin production by promoting cell proliferation through suppression of Cyclin-dependent kinase inhibitor 1A (Cdkn1a) expression induced by STZ. Rutin, in a long-term treatment of diabetic rats was found to significantly increase plasma insulin and the histopathological observations revealed the protective role of rutin in streptozotocin-induced diabetes mellitus (Kamalakkannan and Prince, 2006a). Fernandes *et al.* (2009) suggested that the serum glucose lowering effect of naringerin in the absence of a significant change in serum insulin concentration could involve an insulin-independent-mechanism. Intraperitoneal injection of prunin (Naringenin-7-O-glucoside), a glycoside from naringenin, also produced a significant hypoglycemic effect in diabetic rats (Choi *et al.*, 1991).

Diosmin was shown to significantly restore plasma glucose, insulin, glycosylated haemoglobin and therefore, it possesses antihyperglycemic activity by stimulating insulin production from the existing β-cells of the pancreas (Pari and Srinivasan, 2010). Similarly, Kawano *et al.* (2009) showed that aspalathin significantly suppressed the rise in fasting blood glucose levels and improved the impaired glucose tolerance in db/db mice. The *in vitro* study revealed that aspalathin, a rooibos tea component from *Aspalathus linearis* was able to increase both glucose uptake by muscle cells and insulin secretion from pancreatic β-cells in type 2 diabetic model db/db mice (Kawano *et al.*, 2009). Waltner-Law *et al.* (2002) showed that epigallocatechin gallate had an insulin-like effect on hepatocytes mediated by changes in the redox state that affected the functional states of some intracellular mediators of insulin signalling. Similarly, the administration of epigallocatechin gallate to rats was found to lower blood glucose and insulin levels (Kao *et al.*, 2000). Cazarolli *et al.* (2009b) reported that apigenin-6-C-β-L-fucopyranoside has anti-hyperglycemic (insulin secretion) as well as insulinomimetic (glycogen synthesis) effects.

Zorzano *et al.* (1989) reported that GLUT4 which is the predominant glucose transporter isoform in muscles and adipose tissue, is the major carrier involved in insulin-stimulated glucose transport. Insulin stimulates glucose transport in adipocytes through a mechanism involving the translocation of GLUT4, in which tyrosine phosphorylation plays a key role in the signal-transduction cascade (Watanabe *et al.*, 1991). Insulin has been reported to stimulate GLUT4 activation through p38 MAPK signalling (Michelle Furtado *et al.*, 2003). Lee *et al.* (2010) showed that nobiletin, a polymethoxylated flavone could improve hyperglycemia and insulin resistance in obese diabetic ob/ob mice by regulating the expression of GLUT1 and GLUT4 in white adipose tissue (WAT) and muscle, and the expression of adipokines in WAT.

Like the action of insulin, Pinent *et al.* (2004) showed that the extract of grape seed procyanidins was able to stimulate glucose uptake in adipocytes and myotubes through some of the main intracellular mediators described for the insulin signalling pathway (PI3K and p38 MAPK) and also increase the amount of insulin-sensitive glucose transporter, GLUT4, in the plasma membrane. Kaempferol 3-neohesperidoside exhibited its stimulatory effect on glucose uptake in the rat soleus muscle through the PI3K and PKC pathways and is, at least in part, independent of the MEK pathway and the synthesis of the new glucose transporter (Zannata *et al.*, 2008). Similarly, the stimulatory effects of kaempferol 3-neohesperidoside and apigenin-6-C-β-L-fucopyranoside on glycogen synthesis in rat soleus muscle have also been shown to involve PI3K – GSK3 and MAPK – PP1 pathways (Cazarolli *et al.*, 2009a, 2009b). In contrast, naringenin, but not its glucoside naringin was reported to suppress hepatic glucose production and the inhibition of hepatic glucose production by naringenin was independent of PI3-kinase signalling (Purushotham *et al.*, 2009).

Naik *et al.* (1991) had also earlier reported that flavonoids exerted their effects by either promoting the entry of glucose into cells, stimulation of glycolytic enzymes and glycogenic enzymes, depression of gluconeogenic enzymes or inhibiting the glucose- 6-phosphatase in the liver and subsequently reducing the release of glucose in the blood. Hepatic glucokinase is the most sensitive indicator of the glycolytic pathway in diabetes and its increase can enhance the utilization of blood glucose for glycogen storage in the liver (Iynedjian *et al.*, 1988). Quercetin was found to increase hexokinase and glucokinase activity in diabetic rats (Vessal *et al.*, 2003). Jung *et al.* (2004) showed that hesperidin and narigenin increased glycogen concentration and the activity of glucokinase in db/db mice. Narigenin had a significant regulatory effect on gluconeogenesis of glucose-6-phosphatase and phosphoenolpyruvate carboxykinase (PEPCK) by lowering their activities (Jung *et al.*, 2004).

In another study, Jung *et al.* (2006) investigated the effect of hesperidin and naringin on glucose and lipid regulation and it was suggested that they altered the expression of the genes encoding the regulatory enzymes of glycolysis and gluconeogenesis and significantly up-regulated the mRNA level of hepatic glucokinase in the liver of the db/db mice. Hesperidin and naringin both significantly increased the glucokinase mRNA, while naringin also lowered the mRNA expression of phosphoenol pyruvate carboxykinase and G-6-Pase in the liver (Jung *et al.*, 2006). Koyama *et al.* (2004) showed that epigallocatechin 3- gallate could mimic the effects of insulin on the gene expression/reduction of phosphoenol pyruvate carboxykinase and glucose-6-phosphatase in mouse liver.

Epigallocatechin 3-gallate has also been shown to up-regulate glucokinase mRNA expression in the liver of db/db mice in a dose-dependent manner and decreased the mRNA expression of phosphoenolpyruvate carboxykinase in H4IIE cells as well as in the liver and adipose tissue of db/db mice (Wolfram *et al.*, 2006). Epigallocatechin 3- gallate could potentially improve glucose tolerance in humans with type 2 diabetes (Wolfram *et al.*, 2006). Pari and Scrinivasan (2010) showed that hepatic hexokinase and glucose-6-phosphate dehydrogenase were significantly increased whereas, glucose-6-phosphatase and fructose-1, 6-bisphosphatase were significantly decreased in diosmin-treated diabetic rats.

Glucose/glycogen homeostasis is mainly regulated by two enzymes: glycogen phosphorylase and glycogen synthase (Jakobs *et al.*, 2006). Quercetin, cyanidin and delphinidin were reported to have potent inhibitory effects on both glycogen phosphorylase *a* (phosphorylated, active) and *b* (unphosphorylated, inactive) in isolated muscle (Jakobs *et al.*, 2006). Myricetin was also shown to increase the levels of hepatic glycogen, glucose-6- phosphate and hepatic glycogen synthase I activity without having any effect on either total glycogen synthase or hepatic phosphorylase *a* activity in diabetic rats and on the other hand, decreased phosphorylase *a* activity in the muscle (Ong and Khoo, 2000).

It was suggested that the hypoglycemic effect of myricetin is likely to be due to its effect on glycogen metabolism (Ong and Khoo, 2000). Catechin was found to increase hepatic glycogen and glycogen synthase activity significantly whereas there was a decrease in glycogen phosphorylase, showing that the hypoglycemic effect of catechin is due to increased glycogenesis and decreased glycogenolysis (Valsa *et al.*, 1997). Similarly, dietary supplementation of gallated catechins or the green tea extract containing catechins was reported to inhibit both α-glucosidases and glycogen phosphorylase *in vitro* and in cell culture and could be helpful in the management of type 2 diabetes (Kamiyama *et al.*, 2010).

Glucocorticoids (GC) are potent functional antagonists of insulin action, and promote gluconeogenesis in the liver, potentially leading to raised blood glucose concentrations in diabetes (Albert *et al.*, 2003). The access of active glucocorticoids to its receptors is governed by 11β-hydroxysteroid dehydrogenase type 1 (11β-HSD1) at the tissue level (Albert *et al.*, 2002; Webster and Pallin, 2007). The selective inhibition of 11β-HSD1 may proffer a means of treating diabetes and other metabolic syndrome because 11b-HSD1 mediates glucocorticoid hormone action in target tissues for insulin action and has been suggested to play a regulatory role in glucose homeostasis (Albert, *et al.*, 2002; Webster and Pallin, 2007).

Quercetin, tangeretin, morin and naringenin have been reported to be inhibitors of 11b-HSD (Wang *et al.*, 2002). Ortiz-Andrade *et al.* (2008) showed that naringenin was able to exert its antidiabetic effect by inhibiting 11b-HSD1 activity. Through an *in vitro* study, the inhibitory effects of six structurally related flavonoids (flavones, 3-hydroxyflavone, 6-hydroxyflavone, 7-hydroxyflavone, chrysin and quercetin) on 11β-HSD1 were investigated and only flavones and quercetin were reported to be active analogues of flavonoids showing inhibition of 11β-HSD1 (Torres-Piedra *et al.*, 2010).

Diabetes mellitus affects several lipid metabolism mechanisms and hyperlipidemia is a common finding among diabetic patients (Mengesha, 2006). The increase in the levels of triacylglycerols, cholesterol and lipoprotein (LDL and VLDL-cholesterol) in the serum of the diabetic rats has been shown (Fernandes *et al.*, 2010). Naringenin has been reported to penetrate lipid membranes and protected LDL from oxidation (Wilcox *et al.*, 2000). Hesperidin, marsupin, pterosupin, liquiritigenin, biochanin A, formononetin, and pratensein have also been reported to cause significant reductions in serum total cholesterol and triglyceride (Wilcox *et al.*, 2000). Similarly, flavones, 3-hydroxyflavone, 6-hydroxyflavone, 7-hydroxyflavone, chrysin and quercetin were also reported to significantly lowered triglycerides and LDL (Torres-Piedra *et al.*, 2010).

3-hydroxy-3-methyl-glutaryl-CoA (HMG-CoA) reductase is the rate-controlling enzyme of the mevalonate pathway, the metabolic pathway that produces cholesterol and other isoprenoids. Acyl CoA: cholesterol *O*-acyltransferase (ACAT) is another key cholesterol-regulating enzyme involved in the esterification and absorption of cholesterol, secretion of hepatic LDL-cholesterol, and cholesterol accumulation in the arterial wall (Suckling and Stange, 1985). Naringerin and hesperidin are reported to be potent inhibitors of HMG-CoA reductase and ACAT activities and hence, helpful in lowering serum cholesterol levels (Bok *et al.*, 1999; Jung *et al.*, 2006). Rutin has also been associated with marked decreased hepatic and cardiac levels of triacylglycerols in streptozotocin-induced diabetic rats (Fernandes *et al.*, 2010).

Glycation and advanced glycated end-product (AGE) formation are also accompanied by increased oxidation of LDL and an increase in this atherogenic oxidized LDL occurs in diabetes (Bucala, 1997). The non-enzymatic glycation of hemoglobin has been established and shown to be significantly increased in diabetes (Goldstein, 1995). Glycoxidation of collagens contributes to development of vascular complications in diabetes (Urios *et al.*, 2007). Measurement of glycated hemoglobin has proven to be particularly useful in monitoring the effectiveness of therapy in diabetes (Goldstein, 1995). Attention has been focused on preventing protein glycation by antioxidants (Bonnefont-Rousselot, 2002; Rahbar and Figarola, 2003). Flavonoids have been reported to inhibit protein glycation (Wu and Yen, 2005; Urios *et al.*, 2007). The inhibitory mechanism of flavonoids against glycation was, at least partly, due to their antioxidant properties (Wu and Yen, 2005).

Asgary *et al.* (1999) through an *in vitro* study showed that flavonoids such as quercetin, rutin and kaempferol were able to inhibit glycation possibly due to the relation between structure activity of flavonoids and the preventive effect on haemoglobin glycosylation. The inhibitory effect of the flavonoids on glycation was in this pattern: Quercetin> Rutin> Kaempferol (Asgary *et al.*, 1999). Similarly, Urios *et al*. (2007) showed the decreasing order of the inhibitory activity of flavonoids on the formation of a cross-linking advanced glycation end product, pentosidine, in collagens in this pattern: myricetin ? quercetin > rutin > (+)catechin > kaempferol. The characteristic of AGEs was earlier shown to decrease in streptozotocin-diabetic rats orally treated with rutin (Odetti *et al.,* 1990) and diosmin (Vertommen *et al.,* 1994). Isoquercitrin and astragalin isolated from the leaves of *Eucommia ulmoides,* a plant traditionally used in Korea to treat diabetes, have also been reported to inhibit protein glycation (Kim *et al.,* 2004). Epigallocatechin gallate (EGCG) has been shown to have a protective effect on hyperglycaemic induction of intracellular AGEs (Wu *et al.,* 2009). Wu *et al.* (2010) suggested that plasma loaded with EGCG is an efficient way to increase the content of EGCG in LDL, which may produce a favourable *in vivo* activity in diabetes. Pelargonidin has been shown to offset hyperglycaemia and reduced oxidative stress including Hb-induced iron-mediated oxidative reactions by lowering the glycation level and free iron of Hb (Roy *et al.,* 2008).

Diabetes has been linked with reproductive impairment in both men and women (Baccetti *et al.,* 2002). Oxidative stress is increased in diabetes resulting in impaired sexual dysfunction and impotence in the modern world. (Thakur and Dixit, 2008). Decrease in reproductive functions has been reported in both alloxan and streptozotocin-induced diabetic rats. Streptozotocin caused testicular dysfunction and degeneration under situations of experimentally induced diabetes in animal models (Shrilatha and Muralidhara, 2007) and alloxan- induced diabetes in male rats was reported to reduce semen parameters and impairs distinct phases of spermatogenesis (Arikawe *et al.,* 2006). Quercetin significantly increased sperm viability, motility and total serum testosterone levels as well as degeneration and inflammation in testes cells associated with diabetes were improved when compared with control groups (Khaki *et al.,* 2009, 2010).

Conclusion

The effect of hyperglycemia is mediated to a significant extent through increased production of reactive oxygen species (ROS) which subsequently leads to oxidative stress and various diabetic complications. Flavonoids, generally found in the plant kingdom, display a remarkable array of biochemical and pharmacological actions and significantly affect the functions of various mammalian cellular systems in diabetic conditions. Flavonoids exhibit their anti-diabetic properties through various mechanisms. The dietary intake of fruits, vegetables, onion, teas, red wine and other polyphenolic-rich foods are strongly recommended as they could help to prevent or reduce the scourge of diabetes. Presently, in our research group, we are trying to investigate the anti-diabetic potentials of dietary intake rooibos, a herbal tea known to be very rich in different flavonoids. However, more research studies need to be done to explore more possibilities on the anti-diabetic properties of plants containing flavonoids and other several individual flavonoids on diabetes, its complications as well as their mechanism of actions.

References

Abu-Zaiton, A.S. (2010). Anti-diabetic activity of *Ferula assafoetida* extract in normal and alloxan-induced diabetic rats. *Pakistan Journal of Biological Sciences*, **13**: 97-100.

Akimoto, Y., Hart, G.W., Hirano, H. and Kawakami, H. (2005). O-GlcNAc modification of nucleocytoplasmic proteins and diabetes. *Medical Molecular Morphology*, **38**: 84-91.

Appel, L.J., Brands, M.W., Daniels, S.R., Karanja, N., Elmer, P.J. and Sacks, F.M. (2006). Dietary Approaches to Prevent and Treat Hypertension: A Scientific Statement from the American Heart Association. *Hypertension*, **47**: 296-308.

Alan, L. and Miller, N.D. (1996). Antioxidant flavonoids: Structure, function and clinical usage. *Alternative Medicine Review*, **1(2)**: 103-111.

Alberts, P., Engblom, L., Edling, N., Forsgren, M., Klingström, G., Larsson, C., Rönquist-Nii Y., Öhman, B and Abrahmsén, L. (2002). Selective inhibition of 11β-hydroxysteroid dehydrogenase type 1 decreases blood glucose concentrations in hyperglycemic mice. *Diabetologia*, **45**: 1528 -1532.

Alberts, P., Nilsson, C., Selén, G., Engblom, L.O.M., Edling, N.H.M., Norling, S., Klingström, G., Larsson, C., Forsgren, M., Ashkzari, M., Nilsson, C.E., Fiedler, M., Bergqvist, E., Öhman, B., Björkstrand, E. and Abrahmsén L. (2003). Selective inhibition of 11β-hydroxysteroid dehydrogenase type 1 improves hepatic insulin sensitivity in hyperglycemic mice strains. *Endocrinology*, **144**: 4755 - 4762.

Androne, L., Gavan, N.A., Veresiu, I.A. and Orasan, R. (2000). *In vivo* effect of lipoic acid on lipid peroxidation in patients with diabetic neuropathy. *In Vivo*, **14**: 327-330.

Anjaneyulu, M., Chopra, K. and Kaur, I. (2003). Antidepressant activity of quercetin, a bioflavonoid, in streptozotocin-induced diabetic mice. *Journal of Medicinal Food*, **6(4)**: 391-395.

Anjaneyulu, M. and Chopra, K. (2004). Quercetin, an anti-oxidant bioflavonoid, attenuates diabetic nephropathy in rats. *Clinical and Experimental Pharmacology and Physiology*, **31(4)**: 244-248.

Arikawe, A.P., Daramola, A.O., Odofin, A.O. and Obika, L.F.O. (2006). Alloxan-induced and Insulin-resistant diabetes mellitus affect semen parameters and impair spermatogenesis in male rats. *African Journal of Reproductive Health*, **10(3)**: 106-113.

Asgary, S. Naderi, G., Sarrafzadegan, N., Ghassemi, N., Boshtam, M., Rafie, M. and Arefia, A. (1999). Anti-oxidant effect of flavonoids on haemoglobin glycosylation. *Pharmaceutica Acta Helvetiae*, **73**: 223-226.

Baccetti, B., La Marca, A., Piomboni, P., Capitani, S., Bruni, E., Petraglia, F. and De Leo, V. (2002). Insulin-dependent diabetes in men is associated with hypothalamo-pituitary derangement and with impairment in semen quality. *Human Reproduction*, **17**: 2673-2677.

Barnes, P.J. and Karin, M. (1997). Nuclear factor-kappa B: a pivotal transcription factor in chronic inflammatory diseases. *New England Journal of Medicine*, **336**: 1066 -1071.

Beecher, G.R. (2003). Overview of dietary flavonoids: Nomenclature, occurrence and intake. *Journal of Nutrition*, **133**: 3248-3254.

Bethel, M.A., Sloan, F.A, Belsky, D. and Feinglos, M.N. (2007). Longitudinal incidence and prevalence of adverse outcomes of diabetes mellitus in elderly patients, *Archives of Internal Medicine*, **167(9)**: 921-927.

Bierhaus, A., Schiekofer, S., Schwaninger, M., Andrassy, M., Humpert, P.M., Chen, J., Hong, M., Luther, T., Henle, T., Kloting, I., Morcos, M., Hofmann, M., Tritschler, H., Weigle, B., Kasper, M., Smith, M, Perry, G., Schmidt, A.M., Stern, D.M., Haring, H.U., Schleicher, E. and Nawroth, P.P. (2001). Diabetes-associated sustained activation of the transcription factor nuclear factor-kappaB. *Diabetes*, **50**: 2792 - 2808.

Ble-Castillo, J.L., Carmona-Diaz, E., Mendez, J.D., Larios-Medina, F.J., Medina-Santillan, R., Cleva-Villanueva, G. and Diaz-Zagoya, J.C. (2005). Effect of alpha-tocopherol on the metabolic control and oxidative stress in female type 2 diabetics. *Biomedicine Pharmacotherapy*, **59**: 290-295.

Bok, S.H., Lee, S.H. and Park, Y.B. (1999). Plasma and hepatic cholesterol and hepatic activities of 3-hydroxy-3-methyl-glutaryl-CoA reductase and acyl CoA: cholesterol transferase are lower in rats fed citrus peel extractor a mixture of citrus bioflavonoids. *Journal Nutrition*, **129**: 1182-1185.

Bonnefont-Rousselot, D. (2002). Glucose and reactive oxygen species. *Current Opinion in Clinical Nutrition and Metabolic Care*, **5**: 561-568.

Bonnefont-Rousselot, D. (2004). The role of antioxidant micronutrients in the prevention of diabetic complications. *Treatments in Endocrinology*, **3**: 41-52.

Bonnefont-Rousselot, D., Bastard, J.P., Jaudon, M.C. and Delattre, J. (2000). Consequences of the diabetic status on the oxidant/antioxidant balance. *Diabetes Metabolism*, **26(3)**: 163-176.

Bowden, D.W. (2002). Genetics of diabetes complications. *Current Diabetes Report*, **2**: 191-200.

Brouillard, R. and Cheminat, A. (1988). Flavonoids and plant color. *Progress in Clinical and Biological Research*, **280**: 93-106.

Brownlee, M. (2001). Review article biochemistry and molecular cell biology of diabetic complications. *Nature*, **414**: 813-820.

Brownlee, M. (2005). The pathobiology of diabetic complications: A unifying mechanism *Diabetes*. **54**: 1615-1625.

Bruckner, V. and Szent-Gyorgyi, A. (1936), Chemical nature of citrin. *Nature*, **138**: 1057.

Bucala, R. (1997). Lipid and lipoprotein modification by AGEs: role in atherosclerosis. *Experimental Physiology*, **82**: 327-337.

Carroll, K.K., Guthrie, N., So, F.V. and Chambers, A.F. (1998). Anticancer properties of flavonoids with emphasis on Citrus flavonoids. In: Flavonoids in health and disease, Rice-Evans CA, Parker L, eds., Marcel Dekker Inc, NY, ISBN 0-824700961.

Cazarolli, L.H. Folador, P. Pizzolatti, M.G. and Barreto Silva, F.R.M. (2009a). Signalling pathways of kaempferol-3-neohesperidoside in glycogen synthesis in rat soleus muscle. *Biochimie,* **91**: 843-849.

Cazarolli, L.H., Folador, P., Moresco, H.H., Brighente, I.M.C., Pizzolatti, M.G. and Barreto Silva F.R.M. (2009b). Stimulatory effect of apigenin-6-C-b-L-fucopyranoside on insulin secretion and glycogen synthesis. *European Journal of Medicinal Chemistry,* **44**: 4668-4673.

Chistyakov, D.A., Savost'anov, K.V., Zotova, E.V. and Nosikov, V.V. (2001). Polymorphisms in the Mn-SOD and EC-SOD genes and their relationship to diabetic neuropathy in type 1 diabetes mellitus. *BMC Medical Genetics,* **2**: 4.

Choi, J.S., Yokozawa, T. and Oura, H. (1991). Improvement of hyperglycemia and hyperlipidemia in streptozotocin-diabetic rats by a methanolic extract of *Prunus davidiana* stems and its main component, pruning. *Planta Medica,* **57(3)**: 208-211.

Clifford, M. (2001). A nomenclature for phenols with special reference to tea. *Critical Reviews in Food Science and Nutrition,* **41(5)**: 393-397.

Coskun, O., Kanter, M., Korkmaz, A. and Oter, S. (2005). Quercetin, a flavonoid antioxidant, prevents and protects streptozotocin induced oxidative stress and beta-cell damage in rat pancreas. *Pharmacology Research,* **51(2)**: 117-123.

Deepralard, K., Kawanishi, K., Moriyasu, M., Pengsuparp, T. and Suttisri, R. (2009). Flavonoid glycosides from the leaves of *Uvaria rufa* with advanced glycation end-products inhibitory activity. *Thai Journal of Pharmaceutical Sciences,* **33**: 84-90.

Evans, J.L, Goldfine, I.D., Maddux, B.A and Grosdky, G.M. (2002). Oxidative stress and stress–activated signalling pathways: A unifying hypothesis of type 2 diabetes. *Endocrine Reviews,* **23(5)**: 599-622.

Exner, M., Hermann, M., Hofbauer, R., Kapiotis, S., Quehenberger, P., Speiser, W., Held, I. and Gmeiner, B.M.K. (2001). Genistein prevents the glucose autoxidation mediated atherogenic modification of low density lipoprotein. *Free Radical Research,* **34**(1): 101-112.

Fernandes, A.A.H., Novelli, E.L.B., Junior, A.F. and Galhardi, C.M. (2009). Effect of naringerin on biochemical parameters in the streptozotocin-induced diabetic rats. *Brazillian achieves of Biology and Technology,* **52**(1): 51-59.

Fernandes, A.A.H., Novelli, E.L.B., Okoshi, K., Okoshi, M.P., Muzio, B.P.D., Guimaraes J.F.C. and Junior, A.F. (2010). Influence of rutin treatment on biochemical alterations in experimental diabetes. *Biomedicine and Pharmacotherapy,* 64: 214-219.

Ferris, F.L. III, Davis, M.D. and Aiello, L.M. (1999). Treatment of diabetic retinopathy. *The New England Journal of Medicine,* **341**: 667-678.

Fu, Z. and Liu, D.M. (2007). Phytochemical genistein promotes beta cell survival, insulin secretory function and ameliorates hyperglycemia in streptozotocin-induced diabetic mice. *Diabetes, 56*: A415.

Furusawa, M., Tanaka, T., Ito, T., Nishikawa, A., Yamazaki, N., Nakaya, K., Matsuura, N., Tsuchyi, H., Nagayama, M. and Iinuma, M. (2005). Antioxidant activity of hydroxyflavonoids. *Journal of health Sciences,* **51**: 376-378.

Gale, A.M. (2001). The discovery of type I diabetes. *Diabetes.* **50**: 217-226.

Geckil, H., Ates, B., Durmaz, G., Erdogan, S. and Yilmaz, I. (2005). Antioxidant, free radical scavenging and metal chelating characteristics of propolis. *American Journal of Biochemistry and Biotechnology,* **1(1)**: 27?31.

Ghosh, S., May, M. and Kopp, E. (1998). NF-kB and Rel proteins: evolutionaril conserved mediators of immune responses. *Annual Review Immunology,* **16**: 225-260.

Giugliano, D. and Ceriello, A. (1996). Oxidative stress and diabetic vascular complications. *Diabetes care,* **19(3)**: 257–267.

Goldstein, D.E. (1995). How much do you know about glycated haemoglobin testing. *Clinical diabetes,* 60–63.

Granner, D.K. (2000). Hormones of the Pancrease and Gastrointestinal Tract. In: Harpers Biochemistry, Meyes, P.A. (Ed.). McGraw Hill, New York, pp: 610-626.

Grundy, M.S., Benjamin. J.I., Burke, L.G., Chait. A., Eckel, H.R., Howard, V.B., Mitch, M., Smith, C.S and Sowers, R.J (1999). Diabetes and cardiovascular disease: A statement for health care professionals from the America Heart Association. *Circulation,* **100**: 1134-1146.

Ha, H. and Lee, H.B. (2000). Reactive oxygen species as glucose signaling molecules in mesangial cells cultured under high glucose. *Kidney International Supplement,* **77**: S19-25.

Hanasaki, Y., Ogawa, S. and Fukui, S. (1994). The correlation between active oxygen's scavenging and anti-oxidative effects of flavonoids. In: *Free Radical Biology and Medicine,* **16**: 845-850

Hif, C.S. and Howell, S.L. (1985). Effects of flavonoids on insulin secretion and 45Ca+2 handling in rat islets of langerhans. *Journal of Endocrinology,* **107**: 1-8.

Higashi, Y., Jitsuiki, D., Chayama, K. and Yoshizumi, M. (2006). Edaravone (3- methyl-1-phenyl-2-pyrazolin-5-one), a novel free radical scavenger, for treatment of cardiovascular diseases. *Recent Patents on Cardiovascular Drug Discovery* 1(1): 85-93.

Hollman, P.C.H., Hertog, M.G.L and Katan, M.B. (1996). Analysis and health effects of flavonoids. *Food Chemistry,* **51(1)**: 43-46.

Hsu, F.L., Liu, I.M., Kuo, D.H., Chen, W.C., Su, H.C. and Cheng, J.T. (2003). Antihyperglycemic effect of puerarin in streptozotocin-induced diabetic rats. *Journal of Natural Products,* **66**: 788-792.

Iraj, H., Vida, R., Sara, R. and Afsaneh, A. (2009). Chronic complications of diabetes mellitus in newly diagnosed patients. *International Journal of diabetes Mellitus,* **4**: 34-37.

Iynedjidan, P.B., Gjinovci, A. and Renold, A.E. (1988). Stimulation by insulin of glucokinase gene transcription in liver of diabetic rats. *Journal of Biological Chemistry*, **263**: 740-744.

Iwashina, T. (2000). The structure and distribution of the flavonoids in plants. *Journal of Plants Research*, **113**: 287-299.

Jakobs, S., Fridrich, D., Hofem, S., Pahlke, G. and Eisenbrand, G. (2006). Natural flavonoids are potent inhibitors of glycogen phosphorylase. *Molecular Nutrition and Food Research*, **50**: 52-57.

Johansen, J.S., Harris, A.K., Rychly, D.J. and Ergul, A. (2005). Oxidative stress and the use of antioxidants in diabetes: linking basic science to clinical practice. *Cardiovascular Diabetology*, **4**(1): 5.

Jones, A.F., Winkles, J.W., Thornalley, P.J., Lunec, J., Jennings, P.E., and Barnett, A.H. (1987). Inhibitory effect of superoxide dismutase on fructosamine assay. *Clinical Chemistry* **33**: 147-149.

Jovanovic, S.V., Steenken, S., Simic, M.G, and Hara, Y.(1998). Antioxidant properties of flavonoids: reduction potentials and electron transfer reactions of flavonoid radicals. *In* Flavonoids in Health and Disease. C Rice Evans, L Packer (eds). NewYork; Marcel Dekker, pp 137-161.

Jung, U.J., Lee, M.K., Jeong, K.S. and Choi, M.S. (2004), The hypoglycemic effects of hesperidin and naringin are partly mediated by hepatic glucose regulating enzymes in C57BL/KsJ-db/db mice. *Journal of Nutrition*, **134**: 2499-2503.

Jung U.J., Lee, M.K., Park, Y.B., Kang, M.A. and Choi, M.S. (2006). Effect of citrus flavonoids on lipid metabolism and glucose-regulating enzyme mRNA levels in type-2 diabetic mice. *The International Journal of Biochemistry and Cell Biology*, **38**: 1134–1145.

Kabe, Y., Ando, K., Hirao, S., Yoshida, M. and Handa, H. (2005). Redox regulation of NF-kappaB activation: distinct redox regulation between the cytoplasm and the nucleus. *Antioxidants and Redox Signaling*, **7**: 395-403.

Kamalakkannan, N. and Prince, P.S. (2006a). Rutin improves the antioxidant status in streptozotocin-induced diabetic rat tissues. *Molecular and Cellular Biochemistry*, **293**: 211-219.

Kamalakkannan, N. and Prince, P.S. (2006b). The antihyperglycemic and antioxidant effect of rutin, a polyphenolic flavonoid, in streptozotocin-induced diabetic Wistar rats. *Basic and Clinical Pharmacology and Toxicology*, **98**: 97-103.

Kamiyama, O., Sanae, F., Ikeda, K., Higashi, Y. Minami, Y. Asano, N., Adachi, I. and Kato, A. (2010). *In vitro* inhibition of α-glucosidases and glycogen phosphorylase by catechin gallates in green tea. *Food Chemistry*, **122**: 1061-1066.

Kaneto H, Xu G, Song KH, Suzuma K, Bonner-Weir S, Sharma A, and Weir GC (2001). Activation of the hexosamine pathway leads to deterioration of pancreatic β-cell function through the induction of oxidative stress. *Journal of Biological Chemistry*, **276**: 31099-31104.

Kaneto, H., Xu, G., Fujii, N., Kim, S., Bonner-Weir, S. and Weir, G.C. (2002). Involvement of c-Jun N-terminal kinase in oxidative stressmediated suppression of insulin gene expression. *Journal of Biological Chemistry*, **277**: 30010-30018.

Kao, Y.H., Hiipakka. R.A. and Liao, S. (2000). Modulation of endocrine systems and food intake by green tea epigallocatechin gallate. *Endocrinology*, **141**: 980-987.

Kawano, A., Nakamura, H., Hata, S., Minakawa, M., Miura, Y. and Yagasaki, K. (2009). Hypoglycaemic effect of aspalathin, a rooibos tea component from *Aspalathus linearis*, in type 2 diabetic model db/db mice. *Phytomedicine*, **16**: 437-443.

Khaki, A., Nouri, M., Fathiazad, F., Ahmadi-Ashtiani, H.R., Rastgar, H. and Rezazadeh, Sh. (2009). Protective effects of quercetin on spermatogenesis in streptozotocin-induced diabetic rat. *Journal of Medicinal Plants*, **8 supplement 5**: 57-64

Khaki, A., Fathiazad, F., Nouri, M. Khaki, A., Maleke, N.A, Khamnei, H.J. and Ahmadi P. (2010). Beneficial effects of quercetin on sperm parameters in streptozotocin-induced diabetic male rats. *Phytotherapy research.* Published online in Wiley InterScience. DOI: 10.1002/ptr.3100.

Kim,H.Y, Moon,B.H., Lee, H.J., and Choi, D.H.(2004). Flavonol glycosides from the leaves of *Eucommia ulmoides* O. with glycation inhibitory activity. *Journal of Ethnopharmacology*, **93**: 227-230.

Knekt, P., Kumpulainen, J., Jarvinen, R., Rissanen, H., Heliovaara, M, Reunanena, A., Hakulinent, T. and Aromaa, A. (2002). Flavonoid intake and risk of chronic diseases. *American Journal of Clinical Nutrition*, **76**: 560-568.

Knight, J.A. (1998). Free radicals: their history and current status in aging and disease. *Annals of Clinical and Laboratory Science*, **28**: 331-346.

Kobori, M., Masumoto, S., Akimoto, Y. and Takahashi, Y. (2009). Dietary quercetin alleviates diabetic symptoms and reduces streptozotocin-induced disturbance of hepatic gene expression in mice. *Molecular Nutrition and Food Research*, **53**: 859-868.

Kodja, G. and Harrison, D. (1999). Interactions between NO and reactive oxygen species: pathophysiological importance in atherosclerosis, hypertension, diabetes and heart failure, *Cardiovascular Research*, **43**: 552-557.

Koyama, Y., Abe, K., Sano, Y., Ishizaki, Y., Njelekela, M., Shoji,Y., Hara, Y. and Isemura, M. (2004). Effects of green tea on gene expression of hepatic gluconeogenic enzymes in vivo. *Planta Medica*, **70**(11): 1100-1102.

Laakso, M. (1999). Hyperglycaemia and cardiovascular disease in type 2 diabetes. *Diabetes* **48(5)**: 937-942.

Laakso M. (2001). Cardiovascular disease in type 2 diabetes: challenge for treatment and prevention. *Journal of Internal Medicine*, **249**: 225-235.

Laakso M. (2010). Cardiovascular disease in type 2 diabetes from population to man to mechanisms. *Diabetes Care*, **33(2)**: 442-449.

Laight, D.W., Carrier, M.J., and Anggard, E.E. (2000). Antioxidants, diabetes and endothelial dysfunction. *Cardiovascular Research*, **47**: 457-464.

Le Marchand, L. (2002). Cancer preventive effects of flavonoids-a review. *Biomedical Pharmacotherapy*, **56**: 296–301.

Lee, J.S. (2006). Effects of soy protein and genistein on blood glucose, antioxidant enzyme. *Life Sciences*, **79**: 1578-1584.

Lee, Y.J., Suh, K.S., Choi, M.C., Chon, S. Oh, S. Woo, J.T., Kim, S.W., Kim, J.W. and Kim,Y.S. (2010). Kaempferol protects HIT-T15 pancreatic beta cells from 2-deoxy-D-ribose-induced oxidative damage. *Phytotherapy Research*, **24**: 419-423.

Li, W.L., Zheng, H.C., Bukuru, J. and De Kimpe, N. (2004). Natural medicines used in the traditional Chinese medical system for therapy of diabetes mellitus. *Journal of Ethnopharmacology*, **92**: 1-21.

Liu, K, Paterson, A.J., Chin, E. and Kudlow, J.E. (2000). Glucose stimulates protein modification by O-linked GlcNAc in pancreatic beta cells: linkage of O-linked GlcNAc to beta cell death. *Proceeding of national Academic of Sciences, USA*, **97**: 2820-2825.

Liu, D., Zhen, W., Yang, Z., Carter, J.D., Si, H. and Reynolds, K.A. (2006). Genistein acutely stimulates insulin secretion in pancreatic β-cells through a cAMP-dependent protein kinase pathway. *Diabetes*, **55**: 1043-1050.

Lukacínová, A. Mojžiš, J. Beòaèka, R. Rácz, O. and Ništiar, F. (2008). Structure-activity relationships of preventive effects of flavonoids in alloxan-induced diabetes mellitus in rats. *Journal of Animal and Feed Sciences*, **17**: 411-421.

Machha, A., Achike, F.I., Mustafa, A.L. and Mustafa, M.R. (2007). Quercetin, a flavonoid antioxidant, modulates endothelium-derived nitric oxide bioavailability in diabetic rat aortas. *Nitric Oxide*, **16**: 442-447.

Mackness, B., Durrington, P.N., Boulton, A.J., Hine, D. and Mackness, M.I. (2002). Serum paraoxonase activity in patients with type 1 diabetes compared to healthy controls. *European Journal Clinical Investigation*, **32**: 259-64.

Maechler, P., Jornot, L. And Wolheim, C.B. (1999). Hydrogen peroxide alters mitochondrial activation and insulin secretion in pancreatic beta cells. *Journal of Biological Chemistry*, **274**: 27905–27913.

Manach, C., Mazur, A. and Scalbert, A. (2005). Polyphenols and prevention of cardiovascular diseases. *Current Opinions in Lipidology*, **16**: 77-84.

Manson, M. (2003). Cancer prevention-the potential for diet to modulate molecular signaling. *Trends in Molecular Medicine*, **9**: 11-18.

Matsuoka, T., Kajimoto, Y. and Watada, H. (1997). Glycation-dependent, reactive oxygen species-mediated suppression of the insulin gene promoter activity in HIT cells. *Journal of Clinical Investigation*, **99**: 144-150.

Mehrotra, S, Ling, K.L., Bekele, Y., Gerbino, E., Earle, K.A. (2001). Lipid hydroperoxide and markers of renal disease susceptibility in African–Caribbean and Caucasian patients with Type 2 diabetes mellitus. *Diabetic Medicine*, **18**: 109–115.

Mehta, J.L., Rasouli, N., Sinha, A.K., and Molavi, B. (2006). Oxidative stress in diabetes: a mechanistic overview of its effects on atherogenesis and myocardial dysfunction. *International Journal of Biochemistry and Cell Biology,* **38**: 794-803.

Melanson, K.J. (2007). Dietary Factors in Reducing Risk of Cardiovascular Diseases. *American Journal of Lifestyle Medicine,* **1(1)**: 24-28.

Mengesha, A.Y. (2006). Lipid profile among diabetes patients in Gaborone, Botswana. *South African Medical Journal,* 2006; **96**: 147-148.

Michelle Furtado, L., Poon, V. and Klip, A. (2003). GLUT4 activation: thoughts on possible mechanisms. *Acta Physiologica Scandinavica,* **178**: 287-296.

Mira, L., Fernandez, M.T., Santos, M., Rocha, R., Florencio, M.H. and Jennings, K.R. (2002). Interactions of flavonoids with iron and copper ions: a mechanism for their antioxidant activity. *Free Radical Research,* **36**: 1199-1208.

Mizushige, T., Mizushige, K., Miyatake, A., Kishida, T. and Ebihara, K. (2007). Inhibitory effects of soy isoflavones on cardiovascular collagen accumulation in rats. *Journal of Nutritional Science and Vitaminology,* **53(1)**: 48-52.

Mohamed, A.K, Bierhaus, A., Schiekofer, S., Tritschler, H., Ziegler, R. and Nawroth, P.P. (1999). The role of oxidative stress and NF-kB activation in late diabetic complications. *Biofactors,* **10**: 157-167.

Mukund, H., Rao, C.M., Srinivasan, K.K., Mamathadevi, D.S. and Satish, H. (2008). Hypoglycaemic and hypolipidemic effect of strobilanthes heyneanus in alloxan-induced diabetic rats. *Pharmacognosy Magazine,* **15**: 819- 824.

Mukhtar, H. and Ahmad, N. (2000).Tea polyphenols: prevention of cancer and optimizing health. *American Journal of Clinical Nutrition,* **71(6)**: 1698S-1702S.

Nabeel, M.A., Kathiresan, K. and Manivannan, S. (2010). Antidiabetic activity of the mangrove species *Ceriops decandra* in alloxan-induced diabetic rats. *Journal of Diabetes,* **2**: 97-103.

Naik, S.R., Dhuley, J.N. and Deshmukh, A. (1991), Probable mechanism of hypoglycaemic activity of basic acid, a natural product isolated from *Bumelia sartorum. Journal of Ethnopharmacology,* **33**: 37-44.

Nakatani, Y., Kaneto, H., Kawamori, D., Hatazaki, M., Miyatsuka, T., Matsuoka, T.A., Kajimoto, Y., Matsuhisa, M., Yamasaki, Y. and Hori, M. (2004). Modulation of the JNK pathway in liver affects insulin resistance status. *Journal of Biological Chemistry,* **279**: 45803–45809.

Nettleton, J.A., Harnack, L.J., Scrafford, C.G., Mink, P.J., Barra,j L.M., Jacobs,Jr D.R. (2006). Dietary flavonoids and flavonoid-rich foods are not associated with risk of type 2 diabetes in postmenopausal women. *Journal of Nutrition,* **136**: 3039-3045.

Nijveldt, R.J., van Nood, E., van Hoorn, D.E., Boelens, P.G., van Norren, K. and van Leeuwen, P.A. (2001). Flavonoids: a review of probable mechanisms of action and potential applications. *American Journal of Clinical Nutrition,* **74**: 418-425.

Odetti, P.R., Borgoglio, A., De Pascale, A., Rolandi, R. and Adezati, L. (1990). Prevention of diabetes-increased aging effect on rat collagen-linked fluorescence by aminoguanidine and rutin. *Diabetes*, **39**: 796–801.

Oguntibeju, O.O., Esterhuyse, A.J. and Truter, E.J. (2009a). Red palm oil: nutritional, physiological and therapeutic roles in improving human wellbeing and quality of life. *British Journal of Biomedical Science*, **66(4)**: 216-222.

Oguntibeju, O.O., Esterhuyse, A.J. and Truter, E.J. (2009b). Cardiovascular disease and the potential protective role of antioxidants. *African Journal of Biotechnology*, **8(14)**: 3107-3117.

Oguntibeju, O.O., Esterhuyse, A.J. and Truter, E.J. (2010). Possible role of red palm oil supplementation in reducing oxidative stress in HIV / AIDS and TB patients: A Review. *Journal of Medicinal Plants Research*, **4(3)**: 188-196.

Ong, K.C. and Khoo, H.E. (1996). Insulinomimetic effects of myricetin on lipogenesis and glucose transport in rat adipocytes but not glucose transporter translocation. *Biochemical Pharmacology*, **51**: 423-429.

Ong, K.E. and Khoo, H.E. (2000). Effects of myricetin on glycemia and glycogen metabolism. *Life Sciences*, **67**: 1695-1705.

Ortiz-Andrade, R.R., Sánchez-Salgado, J.C., Navarrete-Vázquez, G., Webster, S.P., Binnie, M., Garcia-Jimenez, S., León-Rivera, I., Cigarroa-Vázquez, P., Villalobos-Molina, R. and Estrada-Soto, S. (2008). Antidiabetic and toxicological evaluations of naringenin in normoglycaemic and NIDDM rat models and its implications on extra-pancreatic glucose regulation. *Diabetes, Obesity and Metabolism*, **10**: 1097-1104.

Paolisso, G. and Giugliano, D. (1996). Oxidative Stress and insulin action. Is there a relationship? *Diabetologia*, **39**: 357-363.

Pari, L. and Srinivasan, S. (2010). Antihyperglycemic effect of diosmin on hepatic key enzymes of carbohydrate metabolism in streptozotocin-nicotinamide-induced diabetic rats. *Biomedicine and Pharmacotherapy* (Article in press).

Park, J.Y., Ha, S.W. and King, G.L. (1999). The role of protein kinase C activation in the pathogenesis of diabetic vascular complications. Proceedings of *the* ISPD '98 - The VIIIth Congress of the ISPD. *Peritoneal Dialysis International*, **19 Supplement 2.**

Park, CW., Kim, J.H, Lee, J.H., Kim, Y.S., Ahn, H.J., Shin, Y.S., Kim, S.Y., Choi, E.J., Chang, Y.S. and Bang, B.K. (2000). High glucose-induced intercellular adhesion molecule-1 (ICAM)-1 expression through osmotic effect in rat mesangial cells is PKC-NF-kappa B-dependent. *Diabetologia*, **43**: 1544-1553.

Penckofer, S., Schwertz, D. and Florczak, K. (2002). Oxidative stress and cardiovascular disease in type 2 diabetes: the role of antioxidants and prooxidants. *Journals Cardiovascular Nursing*, **16(2)**: 68-85.

Pietta, P.G. and Simonetti, P. (1999). Dietary flavonoids and interaction with physiologic antioxidants. In: Packer, L., Hiramatsu, M. and Yoshikawa, T.,

Editors, *Antioxidant food supplements in human health*, Academic Press, San Diego, California, pp. 283-308.

Pietta, P.G. (2000). Flavonoids as antioxidants. *Journal of natural Products*, **63**: 1035-1042.

Pinent, M., Blay, M., Bladé, M.C., Salvadó, M.J. and Arola, L. (2004). Grape seed-derived procyanidins have an antihyperglycemic effect in streptozotocin induced diabetic rats and insulinomimetic activity in insulin-sensitive cell lines. *Endocrinology*, **145(11)**: 4985-4990.

Pinent, M., Castell, A., Baiges, I., Montagut, G., Arola, L. and Ardévol, A. (2008). Bioactivity of flavonoids on insulin-secreting cells. *Comprehensive Reviews of Food Science and Food Safety*, **7**: 299-308.

Purushotham, A., Tian, M. and Belury, M.A. (2009). The citrus fruit flavonoid naringenin suppresses hepatic glucose production from Fao hepatoma cells. *Molecular Nutrition and Food Research*, **53**: 303-307.

Rahbar, S. and Figarola, J.L. (2003). Novel inhibitors of advanced glycation endproducts. *Archives of Biochemistry and Biophysics*, **419**: 63-79.

Ranaud, S., and de Lorgeril, M. (1992). Wine, alcohol, platelets, and the french paradox for coronary heart disease. *Lancet*, **339**: 1523-1526.

Ratty, A.K. and Das, N.P. (1988). Effects of flavonoids on nonenzymatic lipid peroxidation: structure activity relationship. *Biochemical Medicine and Metabolic Biology*, **39(1)**: 69-79.

Reiber, G.E., Boyko, E.J. and Smith, D.G.(1995). Lower extremity foot ulcers and amputations in diabetes. In Diabetes in America. 2nd ed. Harris, M.I., Cowie, C.C., Stern M.P., Boyko, E.J., Reiber, G.E. and Bennett, P.H., Eds. Washington, D.C., U.S. Govt. Printing Office (NIH publ. no. 95-1468), pp 409-428.

Ritz, E. and Orth, S. R. (1999). Nephropathy in patients with type 2 diabetes mellitus. *New England Journal of Medicine*, **341(15)**: 1127-1133

Robertson, R.P. and Harmon, J.S. (2006). Diabetes, glucose toxicity, and oxidative stress: a case of double jeopardy for the pancreatic islet beta-cell. *Free Radical Biology of Medicine*, **41**: 177-184.

Ross, J.A. and Kasum, C.M. (2002). Dietary flavonoids: bioavailability, metabolic effects, and safety. *Annual Review of Nutrition*, **22**: 19-34.

Roy, M., Sen, S. and Chakraborti, A.S. (2008). Action of pelargonidin on hyperglycemia and oxidative damage in diabetic rats: Implication for glycation-induced hemoglobin modification. *Life Sciences*, **82**: 1102-1110.

Rusznyak, S. and Szent-Gyorgyi, A. (1936). Vitamin P: flavonols as vitamins. *Nature*, **138**: 27.

Saija, A., Scalese, M., Marzullo, D., Bonina, F. and Castelli, F. (1995). Flavonoids as antioxidant agents: Impotance of their interaction with biomembranes. *Free Radical Biology of Medicine*, **19**: 481-486.

Sakai, K., Matsumoto, K., Nishikawa, T., Suefuji, M., Nakamaru, K., Hirashima, Y., awashima, J., Shirotani, T., Ichinose, K., Brownlee, M. and Araki, E. (2003). Mitochondrial reactive oxygen species reduce insulin secretion by pancreatic beta-cells. *Biochemical Biophysical Research Communications,* **300**: 216–222.

Sakurai, T. and Tsuchiya, S. (1988). Superoxide production from non-enzymatically glycated protein. *FEBS Letters,* **236**: 406-410.

Schreck, R., Rieber, P. and Baeuerle, P.A. (1991). Reactive oxygen intermediates as apparently widely used messengers in the activation of the NF-kappa B transcription factor and HIV-1. *EMBO Journal,* **10**: 2247–2258.

Seetharam, Y.N., Chalageri, G., Setty, S.R. and Bheemachar, (2002). Hypoglycaemic activity of *Abutilon indicum* leaf extracts in rats. *Fitoterapia,* **73**: 156-159.

Shih, C.C., Wu, Y.W. and Lin, W.C. (2002). Antihyperglycemic and antioxidant properties of Anoectochilus Formosanus in diabetic rats. *Clinical and Experiment pharmacology and physiology,* **29**: 684-688.

Shisheva, A. and Schechter, Y. (1992). Quercetin selectively inhibits insulin receptor function in vitro and the bioresponses of insulin and insulinomimetic agents in rat adipocytes. *Biochemistry,* **31**: 8059-8063.

Shrilatha, B. and Muralidhara, (2007). Early oxidative stress in testis and epididymal sperm in streptozotocin-induced diabetic mice: its progression and genotoxic consequences. *Journal* of *Reproductive Toxicology,* **23 (4)**: 578-587.

Skyrme-Jones, R.A., O'Brien, R.C., Luo, M. and Meredith, I.T. (2000). Endothelial vasodilator function is related to low-density lipoprotein particle size and low-density lipoprotein vitamin E content in type 1 diabetes. *Journal of American College of Cardiology,* **35**: 292- 299.

Song, Y.Q., Manson, J.E., Buring, J.E., Sesso, H.D., and Liu, S.M. (2005). Associations of dietary flavonoids with risk of type 2 diabetes and markers of insulin resistance and systemic inflammation in women: A prospective study and cross-sectional analysis. *Journal of American College of Nutrition,* **24(5)**: 376-384.

Stangl, V., Dreger, H., Stangle, K. and Lorenz, M. (2007). Molecular targets of tea polyphenols in the cardiovascular system. *Cardiovascular Research,* **73**: 348-358.

Suckling, K.E. and Strange, E.F. (1985). Role of acyl-CoA,Cholesterol acyl-transferase in cellular cholesterol metabolism. *Journal of Lipid research*, **26**: 647-647.

Surh, Y.J. (2003). Cancer chemoprevention with dietary phytochemicals. *Nature Review Cancer,* **3**: 768-780.

Thakur, M. and Dixit, V.K. (2008). Ameliorative effect of fructo-oligosaccharide rich extract of *Orchis latifolia* Linn. on sexual dysfunction in hyperglycaemic male rats. *Sexuality and Disability,* **26**: 37-46.

Tiedge, M., Lortz, S., Drinkgern, J., and Lenzen, S. (1997). Relation between antioxidant enzyme gene expression and antioxidative defense status of insulin producing cells. *Diabetes,* **46**: 1733-1742.

Tomkin, G.H. (2001). Diabetic vascular disease and the rising star of Protein Kinase C. *Diabetologia*, **44**: 657-658.

Turk, Z., Ljubic, S., Turk, N. and Benko, B. (2001). Detection of autoantibodies against advanced glycation end products and AGE immune complexes in serum of patients with diabetes mellitus. *Clinical Chimica Acta*, **303**: 105-115.

Torres-Piedra, M. Ortiz-Andrade, R.R., Villalobos-Molina, R., Singh, N., Medina-Franco, J.L., Webster, S.P., Binnie, M., Navarrete-Vázquez, G. and Estrada-Soto, S. (2010). Comparative Study of Flavonoid analogues on Streptozotocin-nicotinamide induced diabetic rats: Quercetin as Potential Antidiabetic Agent acting via 11β-Hydroxysteroid Dehydrogenase Type 1 Inhibition. *European Journal of Medicinal Chemistry*, **45**: 2606-2612.

Urios, P., Grigorova-Borsos, A.M. and Sternberg, M. (2007). Flavonoids inhibit the formation of the cross-linking AGE pentosidine in collagen incubated with glucose, according to their structure. *European Journal of Nutrition*, **46**: 139-146.

Ursini, F., Maiorino, M., Morazzoni, P., Roveri, A. and Pifferi, G. (1994). A novel antioxidant flavonoid (IdB 1031) affecting molecular mechanisms of cellular activation. *Free Radical Biology and Medicine*, **16**: 547-553.

Valsa, A.K., Sudheesh, S. and Vijayalakshmi, N.R. (1997). Effect of catechin on carbohydrate metabolism. *Indian Journal of Biochemistry and Biophysics*, **34**: 406-408.

Vertommen, J., Van den Enden, M., Simoens, L. and De Leew, I. (1994). Flavonoid treatment reduces glycation and lipid peroxidation in experimental diabetic rats. *Phytotherapy Research*, **8**: 430-432.

Vessal, M., Hemmati, M. and Vasei, M. (2003). Antidiabetic effects of quercetin in streptozocin induced diabetic rats. *Comparative Biochemistry Physiology C*, **135**: 357-364.

Vita, J.A. (2005). Polyphenols and cardiovascular disease: effects on endothelial and platelet function. *American Journal of Clinical Nutrition*, **81(1)**: 292S-297S.

Waltner-Law, M.E., Wang, X.L., Law, B.K., Hall, R.K., Nawano, M. and Granner, D.K. (2002). Epigallocatechin gallate, a constituent of green tea, represses hepatic glucose production. *Journal of Biological Chemistry*, **277**: 34933–34940.

Wang, M.S., Shi, H., Wang, K.S., Reidenberg, M.M. (2002). Inhibition of 11b-hydroxysteroid dehydrogenase in guinea pig kidney by three bioflavonoids and their interactions with gossypol. *Acta Pharmacologica Sinica*, **23**: 92-96.

Watanabe, T., Kondo, K. and Oishi, M. (1991). Induction of in vitro differentiation of mouse erythroleukemia cells by genistein, an inhibitor of tyrosine protein kinases. *Cancer Research*, **51**: 764-768.

Webster, S.P. and Pallin, T.D. (2007). 11b-hydroxysteroid dehydrogenase type 1 inhibitors as therapeutic agents. *Expert Opinion on Therapeutic Patents*, **17**: 1407-1422.

Wilcox, L.J., Borradaile, M.N. and Huff, M.W. (2000). Antiatherogenic properties of naringerin, a citrus flavonoids. *Cardiovascular Drug Reviews*, **17**: 160- 178.

Williams M.T. and Hord, N.G. (2005). The role of dietary factors in cancer prevention: Beyond fruits and vegetables. *Nutrition in Clinical Practice*, **20(4)**: 451-459.

Wolfram, S., Raederstorff, D., Preller, M., Wang, Y., Teixeira, S.R., Riegger, C. and Weber, P. (2006). Epigallocatechin gallate supplementation alleviates diabetes in rodents. *Journal of Nutrition*, **136(10)**: 2512-2518.

Wolff, S. P., Jiang, Z. Y. and Hunt, J. V. (1991). Protein glycation and oxidative stress in diabetes mellitus and aging. *Free Radical Biology and Medicine*, **10**: 339-352.

Wu, H. and Yen, G.C. (2005). Inhibitory effect of naturally occurring flavonoids on the formation of advanced glycation end products. *Journal of Agricultural and Food Chemistry*, **53**: 3167-3173.

Wu, H.J. and Chan, W.H. (2007). Genistein protects methylglyoxal induced oxidative DNA damage and cell injury in human mononuclear cells. *Toxicology in Vitro*, **21(3)**: 335-342.

Wu, C.H., Wu, C.F., Huang, H.W., Jao, R.C. and Yen, G.C. (2009). Naturally occurring flavonoids attenuate high glucose-induced expression of proinflammatory cytokines in human monocytic THP-1 cells. *Molecular Nutrition and Food Research*, **53(8)**: 984–995.

Wu, M., Bian, Q., Liu, Y. Fernandes, A.F., Taylor, A., Pereira, P. and Shang, F. (2009). Sustained oxidative stress inhibits NF-κB activation partially via inactivating the proteasome. *Free Radical Biology and Medicine*, **46**: 62-69.

Wu, C.H., Yeh, C.T. and Yen, G.C. (2010). Epigallocatechin gallate (EGCG) binds to low-density lipoproteins (LDL) and protects them from oxidation and glycation under high-glucose conditions mimicking diabetes. *Food Chemistry*, **121(3)**: 639-644.

Yang, B., Kotani, A., Arai, K. and Kusu, F. (2001). Estimation of the antioxidant activities of flavonoids from their oxidation potentials. *Analytical Sciences*, **17**: 599-604.

Zanatta, L., Rosso, A., Folador, P., Figueiredo, M.B.S.R., Pizzolatti, M.G., Leite, L.D. and Silva, F.R. (2008). Insulinomimetic effect of kaempferol 3-neohesperidoside on the rat soleus muscle. *Journal of Natural Products*, **71**: 532-535.

Zhou, T.Y., Luo, D.H., Li, X.Y. and Luo, Y.B. (2009). Hypoglycemic and hypolipidemic effects of flavonoids from lotus (*Nelumbo nuficera* Gaertn) leaf in diabetic mice. *Journal of Medicinal Plants Research*, **3**: 290-293.

Zimmet, P., Alberti, K.G. and Shaw, J. (2001). Global and societal implications of the diabetes epidemic. *Nature*, **414**: 782-787.

Zorzano, A., Wilkinson, W., Kotliar, N., Thoidis, G., Wadzinkski, B.E., Ruoho, A.E. and Pilch, P.F. (1989). Insulin-regulated glucose uptake in rat adipocytes is mediated by two transporter isoforms present in at least two vesicle populations. *Journal of Biological Chemstry*, **264**: 12358-12363.

Bioactive Phytochemicals: Perspectives for Modern Medicine Vol. 1 (2012) *Pages* **107–125**
Editor: **V.K. Gupta**
Published by: **DAYA PUBLISHING HOUSE, NEW DELHI**

3

Limonene: A Systematic Overview for its Chemistry and Bioactivity

P. Koul[1*], G. D. Singh[1], R. Sharma[1], V. K. Gupta[1] and S. Singh[1]

ABSTRACT

Pure limonene, a monoterpene, is a colourless liquid, made up of two isoprene units and occurs in two optically active forms i.e., l-limonene and d-limonen. Both isomers having different odours such as l-limonene smells piney and turpentine like whereas d-limonene has a pleasing orange scent with molecular weigh 136.23 and molecular formula $C_{10}H_{16}$. It is often used as an additive in food products and fragrances, and is classified by the U.S. Food and Drug Administration (FDA) as Generally Recognized as Safe (GRAS). It has also been approved by the U.S. Environmental Protection Agency (EPA) for usage as a natural pesticide and insect repellent. Limonene occurs naturally in certain trees and bushes. It is also released in large amounts along with other monoterpenes mainly to the atmosphere, from both biogenic and anthropogenic sources. The major impurities in limonene are other monoterpenes, such as myrcene, alpha-pinene, sabinene and Gamma3-carene. It is a skin irritant in both experimental animals and humans. The critical organ in animals (except for male rats), following per oral or intraperitoneal administration, is the liver. In male rats, exposure to d-limonene causes damage to the kidneys and renal tumours. d-Limonene has been studied in a battery of short-term in vitro tests and found to be non-genotoxic. There is no evidence that limonene has teratogenic or embryotoxic effects in the absence of maternal toxicity. In general, d-limonene could be considered to be a lead molecule for exploring new drugs with fairly low toxicity.

Keywords: Limonene, Isomers, Fragrance, Monoterpenes, Nephropathy, Carcinogenic, Toxicity.

1 Indian Institute of Integrative Medicine (CSIR), Canal Road, Jammu – 180 001, J&K State, India.

* *Corresponding author*: E-mail: pkoul@iiim.ac.in

Introduction

Limonene is a hydrocarbon, chiral molecule, classified as a cyclic terpene (monoterpene) made up of two isoprene units. It is a colorless liquid at room temperature with a strong smell of oranges. Its name is derived from lemon, as the rind of the lemon, like other citrus fruits, contains considerable amounts of this chemical compound, which is responsible for much of their odor. Limonene exists in two isomeric forms (compounds with the same molecular formula-in this case, $C_{10}H_{16}$- but with different structures), namely *l*-limonene, the isomer that rotates the plane of polarized light counterclockwise, and *d*-limonene, the isomer that causes rotation in the opposite direction. Both isomers have different odors: *l*-limonene smells piney and turpentine like and *d*-limonene has a pleasing orange scent. D-Limonene is a common naturally occurring compound with a citrus scent. D-limonene [(+)-limonene], which is the (*R*)-enantiomer is also known as dipentene (Simonsen, 1947). It is often used as an additive in food products and fragrances, and is classified by the U.S. Food and Drug Administration (FDA) as Generally Recognized as Safe (GRAS). It has also been approved by the U.S. Environmental Protection Agency (EPA) for usage as a natural pesticide and insect repellent because it is a contact poison which intensifies sensory nerve activity in insects.

Limonene occurs naturally in certain trees and bushes. The two enantiomers of limonene are the most abundant monocyclic monoterpenes in nature; *l*-limonene is mainly found in a variety of trees and herbs such as*Mentha* spp., while*d*-limonene is the major component of peel oil from oranges and lemons. Limonene and other monoterpenes are released in large amounts mainly to the atmosphere, from both biogenic and anthropogenic sources. Limonene is used as a solvent in degreasing metals prior to industrial painting, for cleaning in the electronic and printing industries, and in paint as a solvent. Limonene is also used as a flavour and fragrance additive in food, household cleaning products, and perfumes.

Limonene is a skin irritant in both experimental animals and humans. In rabbits, *d*-limonene was found to be an eye irritant. Studies in guinea-pigs revealed that air-oxidized *d*-limonene, but not *d*-limonene itself, induced contact allergy. Because *d*- and *l*-limonene are enantiomers, this could also be true for *l*-limonene and dipentene (the mixture). Handling and purity of the chemical, and possibly addition of antioxidants, may thus be crucial for the allergenic capacity of limonene. The critical organ in animals (except for male rats), following per oral or intraperitoneal administration, is the liver. Studies in which experimental animals were exposed by inhalation to limonene have not been identified. Exposure to limonene affects the amount and activity of different liver enzymes, liver weight, cholesterol levels, and bile flow. These changes have been observed in mice, rats, and dogs. Available data are insufficient to determine the critical organ in humans. In male rats, exposure to*d*-limonene causes damage to the kidneys and renal tumors. The male rat specific protein alpha2µ-globulin is considered to play a crucial role in the development of neoplastic as well as non-neoplastic kidney lesions. Thus, these kidney lesions are considered not relevant for human risk assessment. *d*-Limonene has been studied in a battery of short-term *in vitro* tests and found to be non-genotoxic. There is no evidence that limonene has teratogenic or embryo-toxic effects in the absence of maternal toxicity.

In general, *d*-limonene could be considered (with the exception of its irritative and sensitizing properties) to be a chemical with fairly low toxicity.

Food is the principal source of exposure to limonene, based on available data. A guidance value for the ingestion of limonene was calculated to be 0.1 mg/kg body weight per day. At current estimated levels of exposure, limonene in foodstuffs does not appear to represent a significant risk to human health. In the atmosphere, limonene and other terpenes react rapidly with photo- chemically produced hydroxyl and nitrate radicals and ozone. The oxidation of terpenes such as limonene contributes to aerosol and photochemical smog formation. In soil, limonene is expected to have low mobility; in the aquatic environment, it is expected to bind strongly to sediment. Limonene is resistant to hydrolysis. Biodegradation occurs under aerobic, but not anaerobic, conditions.

Natural Sources of Limonene

Limonene and other monoterpenes are released in large amounts mainly to the atmosphere, from both biogenic and anthropogenic sources. Limonene occurs naturally in certain trees and bushes especially in the peels of oranges and lemons, pine stumps and caraway seeds. The two enantiomers of limonene are the most abundant monocyclic monoterpenes in nature; *l*-limonene is mainly found in a variety of trees and herbs such as *Mentha* spp., while *d*-limonene is the major component of peel oil from oranges and lemons.

Chemistry

Limonene is a colorless liquid at room temperature. It is miscible with alcohol and ether whereas in water upto 7.57mg/L at 25°C it is soluble. The structural formula for limonene is given below in the Table 3.1. Chemically it exists as two optical isomers, *d*- and *l*-limonene (Figure 3.1), and the racemic mixture dipentene. The 3D structure and ball and socket model of *d*-limonine are given in Figures 3.2 and 3.3. The purity of commercial *d*-limonene is about 90-98 per cent.

Table 3.1: Physico-chemical constants of limonene.

	d-Limonene	*l-Limonene*
Chemical name	(R)-1-methyl-4-(1-methylethenyl) cyclohexene	(S)-1-methyl-4-(1-methylethenyl) cyclohexene
Empirical formula	$C_{10}H_{16}$	$C_{10}H_{16}$
Molecular weight	136.23	136.23
Melting point (°C)	–74.35	–74.35
Boiling point (°C)	175.5-176.0	175.5-176.0
Density (g/cm^3 at 20°C)	0.8411	0.8422
Vapour pressure (Pa at 20°C)	190	190
Water solubility (mg/litre at 25°C)	13.8	–
Henry's law constant (kPa m^3/mol at 25°C)	34.8	–
Log K_{ow}	4.23	–

The impurities in Limonene are mainly other monoterpenes, such as myrcene (7-methyl-3-methylene-1,6-octadiene), alpha-pinene (2,6,6-trimethyl-bicyclo[3.1.1]hept-2-ene), alpha-pinene (6,6-dimethyl-2-methylene-bicyclo[3.1.1]heptane), sabinene (2-methyl-5-(1-methylethyl)-bicyclo[3.1.0]hexan-2-ol), and Gamma3-carene ((1S-cis)-3,7,7-trimethyl-bicyclo[4.1.0]hept-2-ene). The vapour pressure of limonene is high and its solubility in water is low, giving a high value of the Henry's law constant, which predicts a high rate of vaporization of limonene.

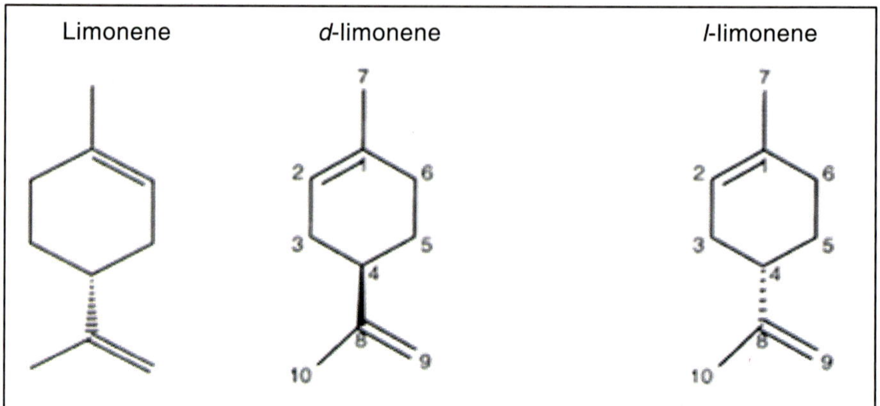

Molecular Structure of *d* and *l*-limonene

It is relatively a stable terpene, which can be distilled without decomposition, although at elevated temperatures it cracks to form isoprene (Pakdela *et al.*, 2001). It oxidizes easily in moist air to produce carveol and carvone. Dehydration with sulfur gives *p*-cymene, hydrogen sulfide, and some other sulfides. In nature it occurs as the (*R*)-enantiomer, but racemizes to dipentene at 300 °C. When warmed with mineral acid, limonene isomerizes to the conjugated diene α-terpinene, which can itself easily be oxidized to *p*-cymene, an aromatic hydrocarbon. Evidence for this isomerization includes the formation of Diels-Alder α-terpinene adducts when limonene is heated with maleic anhydride.

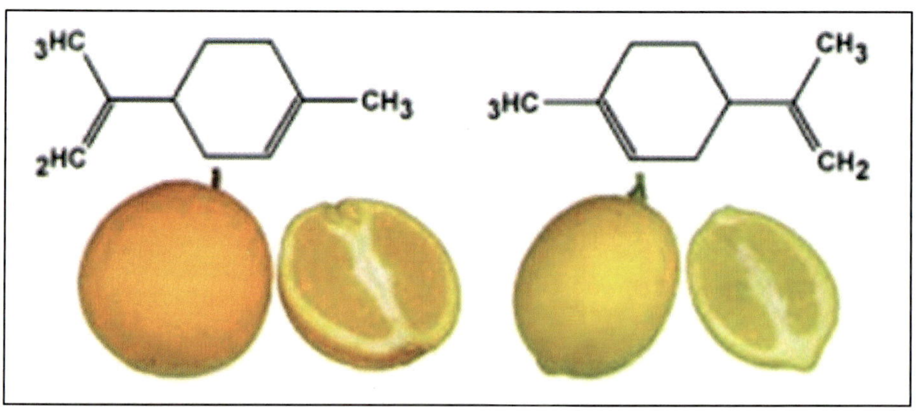

Figure 3.1: *d*- and *l*-Limonene, the two enantiomers of Limonene.

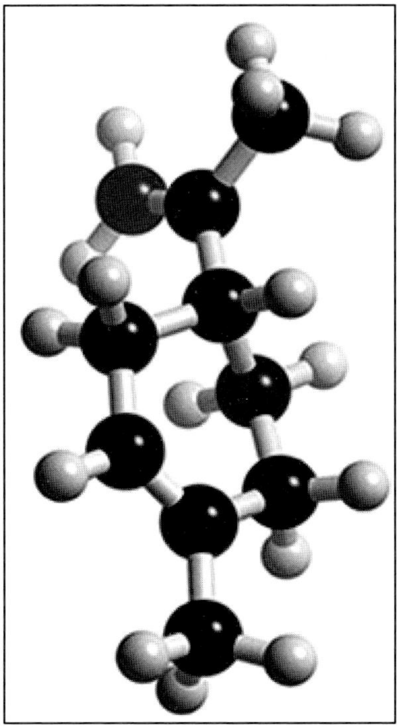

Figure 3.2: 3D model of the Limonene structure.

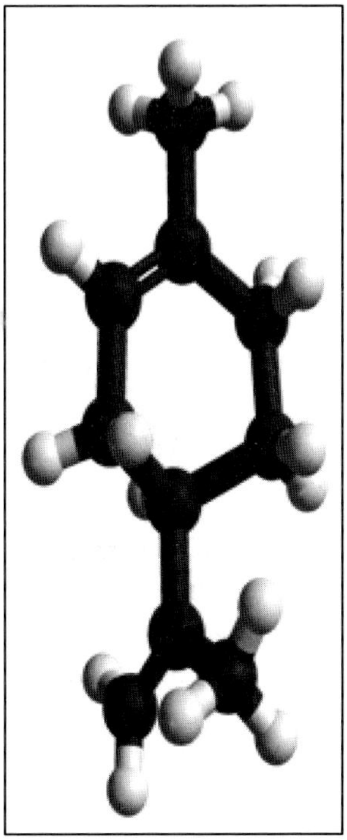

Figure 3.3: Ball and stick model of *d*-limonene.

It is possible to effect reaction at one of the double bonds selectively. Anhydrous hydrogen chloride reacts preferentially at the disubstituted alkene, whereas epoxidation with MCPBA occurs at the trisubstituted alkene. In both cases the second C=C double bond can then be made to react if desired. In another synthetic method Markovnikov addition of trifluoroacetic acid followed by hydrolysis of the acetate gives terpinol.

The most widely practiced conversion of limonene is to carvone. The three step reaction begins with the regioselective addition of nitrosyl chloride across the trisubstituted double bond. This species is then converted to the oxime with base, and the hydroxylamine is removed to give the ketone-containing carvone (Karl-Georg *et al.*, 2002). Limonene, a candidate for renewable volatile bioresource, allowed for the successful production of optically active polymers having weak intermolecular forces, such as π/π, van der Waals and CH/π interactions. The protocol used for this may provide an environmentally friendly, safe and mild process to rapidly produce ambidextrous light-emitting polymers with a minimal loss of starting polymers at ambient temperature, from CD-silent polymers without any specific chiral substituents or chiral catalyst (Kawagoe *et al.*, 2010).

In the past 10 years, trends in analytical chemistry have turned toward the green chemistry which endeavours to develop new techniques that reduce the influence of chemicals on the environment. The challenge of the green analytical chemistry is to develop techniques that meet the request for information output while reducing the environmental impact of the analyses. For this purpose petroleum-based solvents have to be avoided. Therefore, increasing interest was given to new green solvents such as limonene and their potential as alternative solvents in analytical chemistry. In this work limonene was used instead of toluene in the Dean-Stark procedure. Moisture determination on wide range of food matrices were performed either using toluene or limonene. Both solvents gave similar water percentages in food materials, *i.e.* 89.3+/-0.5 and 89.5+/-0.7 for carrot, 68.0+/-0.7 and 68.6+/-1.9 for garlic, 64.1+/-0.5 and 64.0+/-0.3 for minced meat with toluene and limonene, respectively. Consequently limonene could be used as a good alternative solvent in the Dean-Stark procedure (Veillet *et al.*, 2010).

Biosynthesis

Limonene is formed from geranyl pyrophosphate, via cyclization of a neryl carbocation or its equivalent. The final step involves loss of a proton from the cation to form the alkene (Figure 3.4).

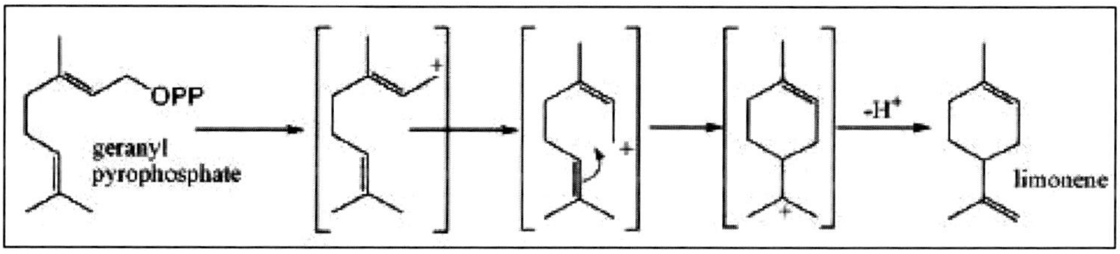

Figure 3.4: Biosynthesis of Limonene from geranyl pyrophosphate.

Methods of Manufacturing

Limonene is manufactured for the commercial by the following different methods such as:

1. Extraction from Southeastern pine stumps, and citrus fruits (especially from the peels of oranges and lemons); from pyrolysis of alpha-pinene.
2. Isolation of *d*-limonene from Mandarin peel oil (*Citrus reticulata* Blanco) (O'Neil, 2001).
3. As a by-product in the manufacture of terpineol and in various synthetic products made from alpha-pinene or turpentine oil (Opdyke, 1979).
4. Derivation: Lemon, bergamot, caraway, orange, and other oils./Also/ peppermint and spearmint oils (Lewis, 2001).

Significant Uses

Limonene is a natural organic chemical compound which is used for number of activities/purposes. As it occurs in two different forms (*d*- and *l*-limonene) and both the forms have different utilities. Although both the forms of Limonene are useful but *d*-limonene is more in use because of its peculiar odor. The major use of *d*-limonene is as a precursor for the synthesis of carvone (Karl-Georg Fahlbusch, 2002). Limonene can be used as an alternative to mineral oils. Obviously mineral oils are a non-renewable source and they are not biodegradable. Because it is from a natural source, limonene does not release anything that would not occur naturally anyway. Therefore it is an environmentally preferred product. It is biodegradable, but it must be treated as hazardous waste.

It is commonly used in cosmetic products and perfumery. As the main odor constituent of citrus, *d*-limonene is used in the manufacturing of food items as a flavor and fragrance additive and in some medicines, *e.g.* bitter alkaloids, as a flavoring; it is also used as botanical insecticide and antimicrobial, antiviral, antifungal, antilarval, and insect attractant and repellent properties. In Japan, it has been used to dissolve gallstones and in wound healing. It is added to cleaning products such as hand cleansers to give a lemon-orange fragrance. In contrast, *l*-limonene has a piney, turpentine-like odor. Polylimonene is used as a flavor fixative (Bingham *et al.*, 2001)

Limonene is increasingly being used as a solvent for cleaning purposes, such as the removal of oil from machine parts, as it is produced from a renewable source (citrus oil, as a byproduct of orange juice manufacture). Furthermore, limonene is used as a substitute for chlorinated hydrocarbons, chlorofluorocarbons, and other solvents. It also serves as a paint stripper when applied to painted wood. Limonene is also used as a solvent in some model airplane glues. As it is combustible, limonene has also been considered as a bio-fuel (SAE Event, 2007).

Biological Effects

Limonene is a biologically active molecule. A number of biological studies have been carried out with it. Limonene is a skin irritant in experimental animals and humans. *d*-Limonene is an eye irritant in rabbits. Studies in guinea-pigs have revealed that air-oxidized *d*-limonene, but not *d*-limonene itself, induced contact allergy. Similar results are likely with *l*-limonene and dipentene. The critical organ in animals (except for male rats) following peroral or intraperitoneal administration is the liver. Exposure to limonene affects the amount and activity of different liver enzymes, liver weight, cholesterol levels, and bile flow, with effects having been observed in mice, rats, and dogs. In male rats, exposure to *d*-limonene results in damage to the kidneys and an increased incidence of renal tumours. As the male rat specific protein alpha2µ-globulin is considered to play a crucial role in the development of the neoplastic and non-neoplastic kidney lesions, they are considered not relevant for human risk assessment.

A dose-related nephropathy was observed in the kidneys of male rats after oral administration of *d*-limonene. This lesion, consisting of degeneration of epithelial cells in the convoluted tubules, granular casts in the outer stripe of the outer medulla, and epithelial regeneration, is characteristic of hyaline droplet nephropathy associated with the accumulation of alpha2µ-globulin in the cytoplasm of tubular cells (Alden *et al.*, 1984; Halder *et al.*, 1985) in response to a variety of hydrocarbon compounds (Swenberg *et al.*, 1992). Some compounds fit deeply into a hydrophobic pocket of alpha2µ-globulin. When hydrogen bonding between the chemical and protein occurs, the digestibility of alpha2µ-globulin by proteases is inhibited, leading to accumulation of the male rat specific protein in lysosomes of the P2 segment of the nephron (Lehman-McKeeman *et al.*, 1990). Although such chemicals fall into rather diverse classes, molecular modelling studies have demonstrated a strong structure-activity relationship with respect to alpha2μ-globulin binding (Borghoff *et al.*, 1991). The accumulation of alpha2μ-globulin is cytotoxic, resulting in single-cell necrosis (Dietrich and Swenberg, 1991). The exfoliated renal epithelium is restored by compensatory cell proliferation. The increase in cell proliferation associated with alpha2μ-globulin is reversible. Damage of this type has not been observed in female rats, male rats that do not produce alpha2μ-globulin, or other mammals, such as mice, hamsters, guinea-pigs, dogs, and monkeys (Dietrich and Swenberg, 1991). The processes leading to nephropathy and the development of renal cancer by such compounds are among the best understood for non-genotoxic chemicals and strongly indicate that it is a male rat specific process. Acute and chronic renal effects induced in male rats by limonene will be unlikely to occur in any species not producing alpha2μ-globulin or a very closely related protein in the large quantities typically seen in the male rat (US EPA, 1991; Swenberg, 1993). *d*-Limonene has been studied in a variety of short-term *in vitro* tests and has been found to be non-genotoxic. There is no evidence that limonene has teratogenic or embryotoxic effects in the absence of maternal toxicity.

Preclinical and Clinical Safety Studies

D-limonene is one of the most common terpenes in nature. It is a major constituent in several citrus oils (orange, lemon, mandarin, lime, and grapefruit). *D*-limonene is listed in the Code of Federal Regulations as generally recognized as safe (GRAS) for a flavoring agent and is used in common food items such as fruit juices, soft drinks, baked goods, ice cream, and pudding.

It is considered to have fairly low toxicity. It has been tested for carcinogenicity in mice and rats. Although initial results showed *d*-limonene increased the incidence of renal tubular tumors in male rats, female rats and mice in both genders showed no evidence of any tumor. Subsequent it has been established that *d*-limonene does not pose a mutagenic, carcinogenic, or nephrotoxic risk to humans. In humans, d-limonene has demonstrated low toxicity after single and repeated dosing for up to one year.

D-limonene is considered as an excellent solvent of cholesterol, it has been used clinically to dissolve cholesterol-containing gallstones. Because of its gastric acid neutralizing effect and its support of normal peristalsis, it has also been used for relief of heartburn. *D*-limonene has well-established chemopreventive activity against many types of cancers. Evidence from a phase I clinical trial shows a partial response in a patient with breast cancer and stable disease for more than six months in three patients with colorectal cancer (Jidong, 2007).

D-limonene (1-methyl-4-(1-methylethenyl) cyclohexane) is a monocyclic monoterpene with a lemon-like odor and is a major constituent in several citrus oils (orange, lemon, mandarin, lime, and grapefruit). Because of its pleasant citrus fragrance, *d*-limonene is widely used as a flavor and fragrance additive in perfumes, soaps, foods, chewing gum, and beverages. *D*-limonene is listed in the Code of Federal Regulation as generally recognized as safe (GRAS) for a flavoring agent. The typical concentration of *d*-limonene in orange juice, ice cream, candy, and chewing gum is 100 ppm, 68 ppm, 49 ppm, and 2,300 ppm, respectively.

Acute and Sub-acute Toxicity Study

The oral LD_{50} of *d*-limonene in male and female mice is reported to be 5.6 and 6.6 g/kg body weight, respectively, while LD_{50} in male and female rats is reported to be 4.4 and 5.1 g/kg body weight, respectively. No histological abnormality was found 30 minutes after infusion of 10 mL *d*-limonene into the duodenum of rats. (Igimi *et al.*, 1992). In pigs, 20 mL d-limonene was infused into the gallbladder once daily for two days. Twenty-four hours after the last infusion, histological examination found no abnormality in the mucosa of the gallbladder, common bile duct, or duodenum, which were directly in contacted with *d*-limonene. (Igimi *et al.*, 1976) In dogs, 10 mL d-limonene was infused daily for seven days via a cholecystostomy tube. On the day following the last infusion, no major abnormality was found except slight inflammatory cell infiltration and fibrosis in the duodenal papilla. (Igimi *et al.*, 1992).

Three weeks toxicity of *d*-limonene (>99 per cent pure) at doses ranging from 413-6,600 mg/kg daily administered to rats and mice five days/week revealed no signs of compound-related toxicity at doses < 1,650 mg/kg daily (National Toxicology Program, 2007; Whysner and Williams, 1996). Another study observed decreased weight gain and even death in male rats starting at a dose of 600 mg/kg daily. As doses reached 1,200-2,400 mg/kg/day, surviving male rats developed rough hair coats, lethargy, and excessive lacrimation. Nephropathy was noted in all male rats at the end of the study. In the case of mice, decreased body weight gain, lethargy, and rough hair coats were observed in male mice given the two highest doses of d-limonene (1,000 and 2,000 mg/kg daily). No other compound-related signs of toxicity or lesions were observed (National Toxicology Program, 2007; Whysner and Williams 1996).

Chronic Toxicity Studies

The results of the chronic toxicity study revealed that although male rats experienced an increased incidence of tubular cell hyperplasia, adenomas, and adenocarcinomas of the kidney, no evidence of carcinogenic activity was observed in female rats or male or female mice at any dose (National Toxicology Program, 2007).

Human Safety Studies

In the limited clinical early study, five healthy males received a single dose of 20 g *d*-limonene. Although subjects complained about increased bowel movements (2-3 times daily) and tenesmus, blood tests showed no abnormalities in liver (total protein, bilirubin, cholesterol, AST, ALT, and alkaline phosphatase), kidney (BUN), or pancreatic (amylase) functions (Igimi *et al.*, 1992).

D-limonene has also been found to be safe, without gradable toxicity, when 100 mg/kg (equivalent to about 7 g for an average adult male) was ingested. Only mild eructation for 1-4 hours post-ingestion, mild satiety for 10 hours post-ingestion, and slight fatigue for four hours post-ingestion were reported (Crowell, 1994).

In an escalated dose study of 32 patients with refractory solid tumors, *d*-limonene was given orally at 0.5-12 g/[m.sup.2]/day (1-24 g/day, considering an average area per person is 1.9 [m.sup.2]). Patients initially received d-limonene for 21 days. The maximum tolerated oral dose was 8 g/[m.sup.2]/day (15 g/day). Nausea, vomiting, and diarrhea were the only side effects observed and were dose dependent. One breast cancer patient was on the dose of 8 g/[m.sup.2]/day (15 g/day) for 11 months. The authors concluded that *d*-limonene had low toxicity after single and repeated dosing for up to one year (Vigushin, 1998).

Nephropathy seen in rats after high-dose limonene does not appear to be possible in humans, since neither the quantity nor type of protein that binds *d*-limonene or *d*-limonene-l,2-oxide is present. The protein content of human urine is very different from rat urine, as humans excrete very little protein if any (1 per cent or less of the concentration found in urine of male rats). There is also no protein in human plasma or urine identical to [{alpha}.sub.2u]-globulin and no [{alpha}.sub.2u]-g-like protein has been detected in human kidney tissue. Although *d*-limonene-1,2-oxide binds to [{alpha}.sub.2u]-g, no other proteins, particularly those synthesized by humans, bind d-limonene-1,2-oxide. Finally, there is no evidence that any human protein can contribute to a renal syndrome similar to [{alpha}.sub.2u]-globulin nephropathy (Igimi *et al.*, 1999; Whysner and Williams, 1996)

A study with 200 patients reported a direct infusion of 20-30 mL d-limonene (97 per cent solution) completely or partially dissolved gallstones in 141 patients. Stones completely dissolved in 96 cases (48 per cent); partial dissolution was observed in 29 cases (14.5 per cent); and in 16 cases (8 per cent) complete dissolution was achieved with the inclusion of hexamethaphosphate (HMP), a chelating agent that can dissolve bilirubin calcium stones. All the stones were between 0.5 and 1.5 cm with an average diameter of 1.0 cm. The duration of the treatment ranged from three weeks to four months (Igimi, 1991).

Gastroesophageal Reflux

D-limonene has been shown to be effective in relieving occasional heartburn and gastroesophageal reflux disorder (GERD). In a clinical setting, 19 adults suffering from chronic heartburn or GERD were invited to use d-limonene to relieve their symptoms. All participants had a history of chronic heartburn or GERD, with symptoms ranging from mild/moderate to severe for at least five years. Before taking *d*-limonene, each participant was asked to rate the frequency and severity of symptoms on a scale of 1-10, with 1 corresponding to complete relief and 10 corresponding to severe and/or painful symptoms that occur every day. Most participants had an initial severity and frequency rating of 5 or greater. Participants were asked to discontinue current treatments (OTC and/or prescription medications), take one capsule containing 1,000 mg d-limonene every day or every other day, and rate symptoms daily using the frequency/severity index described above. On the second day of taking *d*-limonene, 32 per cent of participants experienced a significant relief of symptoms (severity rating=1-2); this relief rate improved gradually during the regimen. By day 14, 89 per cent of participants achieved complete relief of symptoms (Wilkins, 2002).

In a double-blind, placebo-controlled study, 13 participants suffering from mild/ moderate to severe heartburn/GERD was randomized to *d*-limonene or placebo.

Seven participants in the d-limonene group received 1,000 mg *d*-limonene once daily or every other day, while six participants received an identical capsule containing soybean oil (placebo). Each participant was asked to rate the frequency and severity of symptoms on a scale of 1-10 described above. On day four, 29 per cent of participants in the d-limonene group experienced significant relief of symptoms (severity rating=1-2), compared to no relief of symptoms in the placebo group. By day 14, 86 percent of participants achieved complete relief of symptoms, compared to 29 percent of participants in the placebo group (Wilkins, 2002).

Anticancer Activity

Animal studies of d-limonene for chemoprotective activity on several types of cancers have shown inhibitory activity. Several experiments demonstrated inhibition of chemically-induced mammary cancer in rodents administered with different doses of d-limonene (Maltzman, 1989). Inhibition occurs in either the initiation or promotion phases, depending on the chemically-induced medium used (Crowell, 1999; Uedo *et al.*, 1999; Yano *et al.*, 1999). Other animal trials demonstrated *d*-limonene inhibited development of liver cancer, pulmonary adenoma, and forestomach tumors (Dietrich and Swenberg, 1991; Wattenberg *et al.*, 1989; Wattenberg and Coccia, 1991).

Mechanistic studies revealed that limonene inhibits the posttranslational isoprenylation of 21-26 kDa cellular proteins implicated in cell growth and proliferation. It is also presumed that the mechanism through which d-limonene influences its effect is by inducing phase I and phase II carcinogen-metabolizing enzymes (cytochrome p450), which metabolize carcinogens to less toxic forms and prevent the interaction of chemical carcinogens with DNA. D-limonene has been shown to enhance gastrointestinal UDP-glucuronosyltransferase (UGT) activity in rats (Van der Logt *et al.*, 2004). It also inhibits tumor cell proliferation, acceleration of the rate of tumor cell death and/or induction of tumor cell differentiation. Furthermore, d-limonene inhibits protein isoprenylation. Many prenylated proteins regulate cell growth and/or transformation. Impairment of prenylation of one or more of these proteins might account for the antitumor activity of d-limonene. It was found that *d*-limonene attenuates gastric cancer through increasing apoptosis, while decreasing DNA synthesis and ornithine decarboxylase activity of cancer cells. D-limonene inhibits hepatocarcinogenesis via inhibition of cell proliferation, enhancement of apoptosis, and blockage of oncogene expression (Girl *et al.*, 1999; Karl *et al.*, 2001).

D-limonene may also exhibit immune-modulating properties. In one of the animal study, results observed increased survival in lymphoma-bearing mice placed on a high d-limonene diet. These mice also demonstrated increased phagocytosis, microbicidal activity, and nitric oxide production (Del Toro-Arreola *et al.*, 2005).

In a phase I pharmacokinetics study of d-limonene in patients with advanced cancer, a female breast cancer patient demonstrated partial beneficial response to d-limonene at a dose of 8 g/[m.sup.2]/day. Axillary and supraclavicular lymph nodes containing metastatic infiltrating ductal carcinoma remained stable during the first five treatment cycles. At the beginning of the sixth cycle, supraclavicular lymphadenopathy was reduced by >50 per cent, and by the 14th course axillary lymph nodes were no longer palpable; bone pain decreased as well. Response was maintained for 11 months before progression of cancer in the bone forced the patient to withdraw from the study.

Three individuals with colorectal carcinoma, while on *d*-limonene, were able to suspend progression of the disease for over six months. Similarly, *d*-limonene at a dosage of 0.5 g/[m.sup.2]/day was able to halt progression of cancer for nine months in a patient diagnosed with locally advanced mucinous cystadenocarcinoma of the appendix. A patient with presacral recurrence of an adenocarcinoma in the sigmoid colon experienced a minor reduction (<50 per cent) in tumor size at a dose of 0.5 g/[m.sup.2]/day for 12 months. Another patient with local retrovesical recurrence of colorectal adenocarcinoma remained stabilized on 1 g/[m.sup.2]/day (2 g/day) for 7.5 months (Vigushin *et al.*, 1998).

One epidemiological study reported that people without epithelial cell carcinomas consumed significantly more citrus peel, rich in *d*-limonene, than those having epithelial cell carcinomas. Moreover, a dose-response relationship was observed between higher citrus peel in the diet and reduced risk of skin cell carcinoma. The authors concluded that citrus peel consumption, the major source of dietary d-limonene, might have a potential preventive effect on squamous cell carcinoma (Hakim, 2000).

While these case and epidemiological reports are of interest, larger, more comprehensive studies are necessary to confirm d-limonene's effectiveness as a potential chemopreventive and treatment agent. An early phase clinical study with limonene conducted in University of Arizona in January 2010 evaluate the distribution of limonene to the breast tissue and its associated biological activities after 2 to 6 weeks of limonene dosing in women with a recent diagnosis of early stage breast cancer. This study will help evaluate the potentials of developing limonene as a breast cancer preventive agent.

The results of the clinical trials on docetaxel in combined with other novel agents revealed that the combination can improve the survival of androgen-independent prostate cancer patients. *d* -Limonene, a non-nutrient dietary component, has been found to inhibit various cancer cell growths without toxicity. Results of *d* -limonene in combination with docetaxel enhanced the antitumor effect against prostate cancer cells without being toxic to normal prostate epithelial cells. The combined beneficial effect could be through the modulation of proteins involved in mitochondrial pathway of apoptosis. *d* -Limonene could be used as a potent non-toxic agent to improve the treatment outcome of hormone-refractory prostate cancer with docetaxel (Thangaiyan and Anupam, 2009).

Kinetics and Metabolism

D-Limonene has a high partition coefficient between blood and air (lambda$_{blood/air}$ = 42) and is easily taken up in the blood at the alveolus (Falk *et al.*, 1990). The net uptake of *d*-limonene in volunteers exposed to the chemical at concentrations of 450, 225, and 10 mg/m^3 for 2 hours during light physical exercise averaged 65 per cent (Falk *et al.*, 1993). Orally administered *d*-limonene is rapidly and almost completely taken up from the gastrointestinal tract in humans as well as in animals (Igimi *et al.*,

1974; Kodama *et al.*, 1976). Infusion of labeled *d*-limonene into the common bile duct of volunteers revealed that the chemical was very poorly absorbed from the biliary system (Igimi *et al.*, 1991). In shaved mice, the dermal absorption of [^{3}H] *d/l*-limonene from bathing water was rapid, reaching the maximum level in 10 minutes (von Schäfer and Schäfer, 1982). In one study (one hand exposed to 98 per cent *d*-limonene for 2 hours), the dermal uptake of *d*-limonene in humans was reported to be low compared with that by inhalation (Falk *et al.*, 1991), however, quantitative data were not provided.

D-Limonene is rapidly distributed to different tissues in the body and is readily metabolized. Clearance from the blood was 1.1 litre/kg body weight per hour in males exposed for 2 hours to *d*-limonene at 450 mg/m^3 (Falk *et al.*, 1993). A high oil/blood partition coefficient and a long half-life during the slow elimination phase suggest high affinity to adipose tissues (Falk *et al.*, 1990; Falk *et al.*, 1993). In rats, the tissue distribution of radioactivity was initially high in the liver, kidneys, and blood after the oral administration of [^{14}C] *d*-limonene (Igimi *et al.*, 1974); however, negligible amounts of radioactivity were found after 48 hours. Differences between species regarding the renal disposition and protein binding of *d*-limonene have been observed. For rats, there is also a sex-related variation (Lehman-McKeeman *et al.*, 1989; Webb *et al.*, 1989). The concentration of *d*-limonene equivalents was about 3 times higher in male rats than in females, and about 40 per cent was reversibly bound to the male rat specific protein, alpha2μ-globulin (Lehman-McKeeman *et al.*, 1989; Lehman-McKeeman and Caudill, 1992).

The biotransformation of *d*-limonene has been studied in many species, with several possible pathways of metabolism. Metabolic differences between species have been observed with respect to the metabolites present in both plasma and urine. About 25-30 per cent of an oral dose of *d*-limonene in humans was found in urine as *d*-limonene-8,9-diol and its glucuronide; about 7-11 per cent was eliminated as perillic acid (4-(1-methylethenyl)-1-cyclohexene-1-carboxylic acid) and its metabolites (Smith *et al.*, 1969; Kodama *et al.*, 1976). *d*-Limonene-8,9-diol is probably formed via *d*-limonene-8,9-epoxide (Kodama *et al.*, 1976; Watabe *et al.*, 1981). In another study, perillic acid was reported to be the principal metabolite in plasma in both rats and humans (Crowell *et al.*, 1992). Other reported pathways of limonene metabolism involve ring hydroxylation and oxidation of the methyl group (Kodama *et al.*, 1976). Following the inhalation exposure of volunteers to *d*-limonene at 450 mg/m^3 for 2 hours, three phases of elimination were observed in the blood, with half-lives of about 3, 33, and 750 minutes, respectively (Falk *et al.*, 1993). About 1 per cent of the amount taken up was eliminated unchanged in exhaled air, whereas about 0.003 per cent was eliminated unchanged in the urine. When male volunteers were administered (per os) 1.6 g [^{14}C] *d*-limonene, 50-80 per cent of the radioactivity was eliminated in the urine within 2 days (Kodama *et al.*, 1976). Limonene has been detected, but not quantified, in breast milk of non-occupationally exposed mothers (Pellizzari *et al.*, 1982).

Mechanism of Action

Being a biologically active molecule limonene has been studied for number of activities. Its mechanism has been worked with reference to the anti-carcinogenic

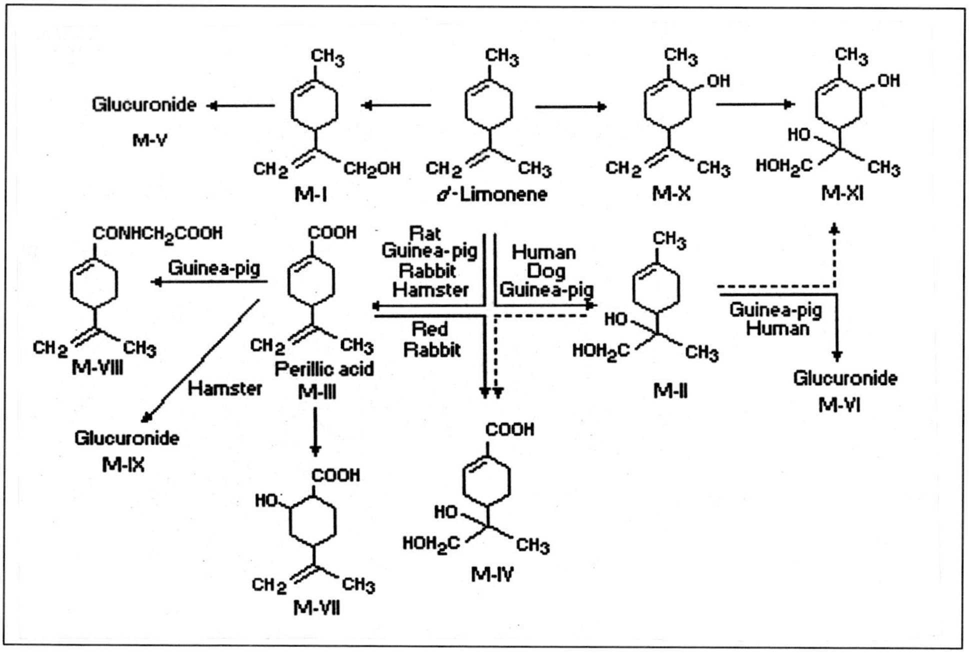

Figure 3.5: Possible metabolic pathways of *d*-Limonene.

(M-1, *p*-Mentha-1,8-dien-10-ol; M-II, *p*-Mentha-1-ene-8,3-diol; M-III, Perillic acid; M-IV, Perillic acid-8,3-diol; M-V, *p*-mentha-1,8- dien-10-yl-β-D-glycopyrosiduronic acid; M-VI, 8-hydroxy-p-mentha-1-on-3-yl- β-D-glycopyrosiduronic acid; M-VII, 2-hydroxy-p-methyl-8-on-7-oic acid; M-VIII, perillyiglycine; M-IX, perillyl- β-D-glycopyrosiduronic acid; M-X, *p*-mentha-1,8-dien-6-ol; M-XI, *p*-mentha-1-ene-6,8,9- triol).

effects. The anti-carcinogenic effects of monocyclic monoterpenes such as limonene were demonstrated when given during the initiation phase of 7,12-dimethylbenz[a]anthracene induced mammary cancer in Wistar-Furth rats. The possible mechanisms for this chemoprevention activity including limonene's effects on 7,12-dimethylbenz(a)anthracene-DNA adduct formation and hepatic metabolism of 7,12-dimethylbenz[a]anthracene were investigated. Twenty four hours after carcinogen administration, there were approx 50 per cent decreases in 7,12-dimethylbenz(a)anthracene-DNA adducts found in control animals formed in the liver, spleen, kidney and lung of limonene fed animals. While circulating levels of 7,12-dimethylbenz(a)anthracene and/or its metabolites were not different in control and limonene fed rats, there was a 2.3 fold increase in 7,12-dimethylbenz(a)anthracene and/or 7,12-dimethylbenz(a)anthracene derived metabolites in the urine of the limonene fed animals. Limonene and sobrerol, a hydroxylated monocyclic monoterpenoid with increased chemoprevention activity, modulated cytochrome p450 and epoxide hydrolyase activity. The 5 per cent limonene diet increased total cytochrome p450 to the same extent as phenobarbital treatment, while 1 per cent sobrerol (isoeffective in chemoprevention to 5 per cent limonene) did not. However, both 5 per cent limonene and 1 per cent sobrerol diets greatly increased the levels of microsomal epoxide hydrolyase protein and associated hydrating activities towards benzo[a]pyrene 4,5-oxide when compared to control and phenobarbital treatment. These changes also modified the rate and regioselectivity of *in vitro* microsomal 7,12-dimethylbenz(a)anthracene metabolism when compared to phenobarbital treatment or control. Identification of the specific isoforms of cytochrome p450 induced by these terpenoids was performed with antibodies to cytochrome p450 isozymes in Western blot analysis and inhibition studies of microsomal 7,12-dimethylbenz(a)anthracene metabolism. Five per cent limonene was more effective than 1 per cent sobrerol at increasing the levels of members of the cytochrome p450 2B and 2C families but was equally effective at increasing epoxide hydrolyase. Furthermore, both terpenoid diets caused increased formation of the proximate carcinogen, 7,12-dimethylbenz (a)anthracene 3,4-dihydrodiol.

The monocyclic monoterpenoid compounds limonene and sobrerol have anticarcinogenic activity when fed during the initiation stage of dimethylbenz(a)anthracene induced rat mammary carcinogenesis. The potential roles of hepatic glutathione-S-transferase and uridine diphosphoglucuronosyl transferase were studied in monoterpene-mediated chemoprevention. Diets containing the isoeffective anticarcinogenic terpenes, 5 per cent limonene or 1 per cent sobrerol, elevated hepatic glutathione-S-transferase activity > 2 fold when measured using the general substrate 1-chloro-2,4-dinitrobenzene and 3,4-dichloronitrobenzene for the glutathione-S-transferase dimer 3-3. However, there were no significant changes in hepatic glutathione-S-transferase activity when 1,2-epoxy-3-(*p*-nitrophenoxy)propane was used. Liver glutathione-S-transferase subunit 3 had the greatest increase followed by 1 and 4 with no change in subunit 2. Both terpene diets significantly increased the activity of the methylcholanthrene inducible and the phenobarbital inducible uridine diphosphoglucuronosyl transferase isozymes. It was proposed that much of the anticarcinogenic activity of these monocyclic monoterpenes during the initiation phase of dimethylbenz[a]anthracene carcinogenesis is mediated through the induction of the hepatic detoxification enzymes glutathione-S-transferase and uridine diphosphoglucuronosyl transferase.

Conclusions

Limonene is considered a molecule with highly significant values from household to medicine and industry with fairly low toxicity, which is one among primary requirements of new drug applications and the utilization of any chemical towards human beings. Although it is found in two isoforms but *d*-limonene has the much more significant importance in comparison to the *l*- limonene. It is often used as an additive in food products and fragrances, and is classified by the U.S. FDA as GRAS. It has also been approved by the U.S. EPA for usage as a natural pesticide and insect repellent. Limonene can be used as an alternative to mineral oils. The well-established chemo-preventive activity of *d*-limonene against many types of cancers has led this molecule for phase-I clinical trials and showed partial anticancer response in patients against different types of cancers. Although, it is biodegradable but it must be treated as hazardous waste. Keeping all the significant activities and utilities into consideration and its low toxicity effects, limonene can be considered as a lead molecule for new drug development in the near future.

References

Alden, C.L., Kanerva, R.L., Ridder, G., and Stone, L.C. (1984). Pathogenesis of the nephrotoxicity of volatile hydrocarbons in the male rat. *In*: *Advances in modern environmental toxicology. Vol. VII.* Princeton, NJ, Princeton Scientific Publ., pp. 107-120.

Bingham, E., Cohrssen, B., and Powell, C.H. (2001). *In*: Patty's Toxicology Volumes 1-9, 5th ed. John Wiley and Sons. New York, N.Y. pp. 185.

Borghoff, S.J., Miller, A.B., Bowen, P., and Swenberg, J.A. (1991). Characteristics of chemical binding to alpha2μ-globulin *in vitro* – evaluating structure-activity relationships. *Toxicology and applied pharmacology,* **107**: 228-238.

Crowell, P.L., Elegbede, J.A., Elson, C.E., Lin, S., Vedejs, E., Cunningham, D., Bailey, H.H., and Gould, M.N. (1992). Human metabolism of orally administered *d*-limonene. *Proceedings of the American Association for Cancer Research,* **33**: 524.

Crowell, P.L., Elson, C.E., Bailey, H.H, *et al.* (1994). Human metabolism of the experimental cancer therapeutic agent d-limonene. *Cancer Chemother Pharmaco,* **35**: 31-37.

Crowell, P.L. (1999). Prevention and therapy of cancer by dietary monoterpenes. *J Nutr.,* 1**29**: 775S-778S.

Del Toro-Arreola, S., Flores-Torales, E., Torres-Lozano, C., *et al.* (2005). Effect of d-limonene on immune response in BALB/c mice with lymphoma. *Int Immunopharmacol.,* **5**: 829-838.

Dietrich, D.R., and Swenberg, J.A. (1991). The presence of alpha2μ-globulin is necessary for *d*-Limonene promotion of male rat kidney tumors. *Cancer research,* **51**: 3512-3521.

Elegbede, J.A., Maltzman, T.H., Elson, C.E., and Gould, M.N. (1993). Effects of anticarcinogenic monoterpenes on phase II hepatic metabolizing enzymes. *Carcinogenesis.* **14(6)**: 1221-1223

Falk, A., Fischer, T.,and Hagberg, M. (1991). Purpuric rash caused by dermal exposure to *d*-limonene. *Contact dermatitis,* **25**: 198-199.

Falk, Filipsson, A., Löf, A., Hagberg, M., Wigaeus, Hjelm, E., and Wang, Z. (1993). *d*-Limonene exposure to humans by inhalation: Uptake, distribution,elimination, and effects on the pulmonary function. *Journal of toxicology and environmental health,* **38**: 77-88.

Girl, R.K., Parija, T., and Das, B.R. (1999). D-limonene chemoprevention of hepatocarcinogenesis in AKR mice: inhibition of c-jun and c-myc. *Oncol Rep.,* **6**: 1123-1127.

Pakdela, H., Panteaa, D. and Roy C. (2001). Production of dl-limonene by vacuum pyrolysis of used tires. *J. Anal. Appl. Pyrolysis.,* **57 (1)**: 91–107.

Hakim, I.A., Harris, R.B., and Ritenbaugh, C. (2000). Citrus peel use is associated with reduced risk of squamous cell carcinoma of the skin. *Nutr Cancer.,* **37**: 161-168.

Halder, C.A., Holdsworth, C.E., Cockrell, B.Y., and Piccirillo, V.J. (1985). Hydrocarbon nephropathy in male rats: Identification of the nephrotoxic components of unleaded gasoline. *Toxicology and industrial health,* **1**: 67-87.

Igimi, H., Hisatsugu, T., and Nishimura, M. (1976). The use of d-limonene preparation as a dissolving agent of gallstones. *Am J Dig Dis.,* **21**: 926-939.

Igimi, H., Nishimura, M., Kodama, R., and Ide, H. (1974). Studies on the metabolism of *d*-limonene (*p*-mentha-1,8-diene). I. The absorption, distribution and excretion of *d*-limonene in rats. *Xenobiotica,* **4**: 77-84.

Igimi, H., Tamura, R., Toraishi, K., *et al.* (1991). Medical dissolution of gallstones. Clinical experience of d-limonene as a simple, safe, and effective solvent. *Dig Dis Sci.,* **36**: 200-208.

Igimi, H., Watanabe, D., Yamamoto, F., *et al.* (1992). A useful cholesterol solvent for medical dissolution of gallstones. *Gastroenterol Jpn.,* **27**: 536-545.

Igimi, H., Watanabe, D., Yamamoto, F., *et al.* (1999). d-limonene a useful cholesterol solvent for medical dissolution. *IARC Monogr Eval Carcinog Risk Chem Hum.,***73**: 307-327.

Simonsen, J. L. (1947). *The Terpenes.* **1** (2nd ed.). Cambridge University Press.

Jidong Sun (2007). D-limonene: safety and clinical applications. *Altern Med Rev.,* **12(3)**: 259-264.

Karl, I., Tatsuta, M., Iishi, H., *et al.* (2001). Inhibition by *d*-limonene of experimental hepatocarcinogenesis in Sprague-Dawley rats does not involve p21(ras) plasma membrane association. *Int J Cancer,* **93**: 441-444.

Karl-Georg, F., Franz-Josef, H., Johannes, P., Wilhelm, P., Dietmar, S., Kurt, B., Dorothea G., and Horst, S. (2002). "Flavors and Fragrances" *In*: Ullmann's Encyclopedia of Industrial Chemistry, Wiley-VCH, Weinheim.

Kawagoe, Y., Fujiki, M., and Nakano, Y. (2010). Limonene magic: noncovalent molecular chirality transfer leading to ambidextrous circularly polarised luminescent-conjugated polymers. *New J. Che.,* **34**: 637 – 647.

Kodama, R., Yano, T., Furukawa, K., Noda, K., and Ide, H. (1976). Studies on the metabolism of *d*-limonene (*p*-mentha-1,8-diene). IV. Isolation and characterization of new metabolites and species differences in metabolism. *Xenobiotica,* **6**: 377-389.

Lehman-McKeeman, L.D., and Caudill, D. (1992). Biochemical basis for mouse resistance to hyaline droplet nephropathy: lack of relevance of the alpha2µ-globulin protein superfamily in this male rat specific syndrome. *Toxicology and applied pharmacology,* **112**: 214-221.

Lehman-McKeeman, L.D., Rodriguez, M.I., and Caudill, D. (1990). Lysosomal degradation of alpha2µ-globulin and alpha2µ-globulin-xenobiotic conjugates. *Toxicology and applied pharmacology,* **103**: 539-548.

Lehman-McKeeman, L.D., Rodriguez, P.A., Takigiku, R., Caudill, D., and Fey. M.L. (1989). *d*-Limonene induced male rat specific nephrotoxicity: Evaluation of the association between *d*-limonene and alpha2μ-globulin. *Toxicology and applied pharmacology,* **99**: 250-259.

Lewis, R.J. (2001). Hawley's Condensed Chemical Dictionary 14th Edition. John Wiley and Sons, Inc. New York, NY. p. 669

Maltzman, T.H., Cristou, M., Gould, M.N., and Jefcoate, C.R. (1991). Effects on monoterpenoids on *in vivo* DMBA-DNA adduct formation and on phase I hepatic metabolizing enzymes. *Carcinogenesis,* **12**: 2081-2087.

Maltzman, T.H., Hurt, L.M., Elson. C.E., *et al.* (1989). The prevention of nitrosomethylurea-induced mammary tumors by d-limonene and orange oil. *Carcinogenesis,***10**: 781-783.

National Toxicology Program (2007). Toxicology and Carcinogenesis Studies of d-Limonene (CAS No. 5989-27-5) in F344/N Rats and B6C3F1 Mice.http: //ntp. niehs.nih.gov/index. cfm? objectid=07086449-9787-5414-556E052773467BE9. [Accessed July 11],

O'Neil, M.J. (2001). *Ed* : The Merck Index - An Encyclopedia of Chemicals, Drugs, and Biologicals. 13th Edition, Whitehouse Station, NJ: Merck and Co., Inc. p. 984.

Opdyke, D.L.J.(1979). *Ed* : Monographs on Fragrance Raw Materials. New York: Pergamon Press, p. 333

Pellizzari, E.D., Hartwell, T.D., Harris, B.S.H. III., Wadell, R.D., Whitaker, D.A., and Erickson, M.D. (1982). Purgeable organic compounds in mother's milk. *Bulletin of environmental contamination and toxicology,* **28**: 322-328.

Smith, O.W., Wade, A.P. and Dean,F.M. (1969). Uroterpenol, a pettenkofer chromogen of dietary origin and a common constituent of human urine. *Journal of endocrinology,* **45**: 17-28.

Swenberg, J.A. (1993). alpha2μ-globulin nephropathy: Review of the cellular and molecular mechanisms involved and their implications for human risk assessment. *Environmental health perspectives,* **101(Suppl. 6)**: 39-44.

Swenberg, J.A., Dietrich, D.R., McClain, R.M., and Cohen, S.M. (1992). Species-specific mechanisms of carcinogenesis. *In*: Vaino, H., Magee, P.N., McGregor, D.B., and McMichael, A.J. Eds. *Mechanisms of carcinogenesis in risk identification.* Lyon, International Agency for Research on Cancer, pp. 477-500 (IARC Monograph No. 116).

Thangaiyan, R., and Anupam, B. (2009). *d* -Limonene sensitizes docetaxel-induced cytotoxicity in human prostate cancer cells: Generation of reactive oxygen species and induction of apoptosis. *J. Carcinog.,* **8**: 9.

Uedo, N., Tatsuta, M., Iishi, H., *et al.* (1999).Inhibition by d-limonene of gastric carcinogenesis induced by N-methyl-N'-nitro-N-nitrosoguanidine in Wistar rats. *Cancer Lett,* **137**: 131-136.

US EPA (1991). *Alpha-2μ-globulin: Association with chemically induced renal toxicity and neoplasia in the male rat.* Washington,DC, US Environmental Protection Agency, Risk Assessment Forum (EPA-625-3-91-019F).

Van der Logt, E.M., Roelofs, H.M., van Lieshout, E.M., *et al.* (2004). Effects of dietary anticarcinogens and non-steroidal anti-inflammatory drugs on rat gastrointestinal UDP-glucuronosyltransferases. *Anticancer Res.*, **24**: 843-849.

Veillet, S., Tomao, V., Ruiz, K., and Chemat. F. (2010).Green procedure using limonene in the Dean-Stark apparatus for moisture determination in food products. *Anal Chim Acta.*, **674(1)**: 49-52.

Vigushin, D.M., Poon, G.K., Boddy, A., *et al.* (1998).Phase I and pharmacokinetic study of *d*-limonene in patients with advanced cancer. Cancer Research Campaign Phase I/II Clinical Trials Committee. *Cancer Chemother Pharmacol.*, **42**: 111-117.

Von Schäfer, R., and Schäfer, W. (1982). Die perkutane Resorption verschiedener Terpene-Menthol, Campher, Limonen, Isobornylacetat, alpha-pinen-ausbadezusätzen. *Drug research*, **32**: 56-58.

Watabe, T., Hiratsuka, A., Osawa, N., and Isobe, M. (1981). A comparative study on the metabolism of *d*-limonene and 4-vinylcyclohex-1-ene by hepatic microsomes. *Xenobiotica*, **11**: 333-344.

Wattenberg, L.W., and Coccia, J.B. (1991). Inhibition of 4-(methylnitrosamino)-1-(3-pyridyl)-1-butanone carcinogenesis in mice by *d*-limonene and citrus fruit oils. *Carcinogenesis*, **12**: 115-117.

Wattenberg, L.W., Sparnins, V.L., and Barany, G. (1989). Inhibition of N-nitrosodiethylamine carcinogenesis in mice by naturally occurring organosulfur compounds and monoterpenes. *Cancer Res.*, **49**: 2689-2692.

Webb, D.R., Ridder, G.M., and Alden, C.L. (1989). Acute and subchronic nephrotoxicity of *d*-limonene in Fischer 344 rats. *Food and chemical toxicology*, **27**: 639-649.

Whysner, J., and Williams, G.M. (1996). D-limonene mechanistic data and risk assessment: absolute species-specific cytotoxicity, enhanced cell proliferation, and tumor promotion. *Pharmacol Ther.*,**71**: 127-136.

Yano, H., Tatsuta, M., and Iishi, H., *et al.* (1999). Attenuation by *d*-limonene of sodium chloride-enhanced gastric carcinogenesis induced by N-methyl-N′-nitro-N-nitrosoguanidine in Wistar rats. *Int J Cancer*, **82**: 665-668.

Bioactive Phytochemicals: Perspectives for Modern Medicine Vol. 1 (2012) *Pages* **127–175**
Editor: **V.K. Gupta**
Published by: **DAYA PUBLISHING HOUSE, NEW DELHI**

4

Phytochemicals Against Liver Disease I: Recent Progress in the Treatment of NAFLD and AFLD by Natural Drug Products and their Active Chemical Entities, in China and other Countries

Fang Peng[1], Shawn Spencer[2], Xiumei Wu[1], Yan Xu[3], Su Zeng[3], Guangming Liu[1], Chenggui Zhang[1], Pengfei Gao[1], Yu Zhao[1*] and Xiaojiang Hao[4]

ABSTRACT

This chapter presents an up-to-date review of natural drug products and active chemical entities showing promise in the treatment of Non-Alcoholic and Alcoholic Fatty Liver Disease (NAFLD and AFLD). This Review covers 134 natural products, both whole herbal/natural preparations and isolated chemicals utilized mostly in China, however includes natural products used in other countries. The treatments have been categorized according to the basic structure of their active component(s) where possible, as a potential framework for future structure-based activity relationships in designing improved therapies against NAFLD and

1 Key Laboratory of Insects and Antiviral Drugs of Yunnan Province, College of Pharmacy, Dali University, Dali 671000, China.

2 College of Pharmacy and Pharmaceutical Sciences, Florida A&M University, Tallahassee, Florida 32307, USA.

3 College of Pharmaceutical Sciences, Zhejiang University, Hangzhou 310058, China.

4 Key Laboratory of Natural Products Chemistry of Guizhou Province and Chinese Academy of Sciences, Guiyang 550002, China.

* *Corresponding author*: E-mail: dryuzhao@126.com; dryuzhao@hotmail.com.

AFLD. Perspectives on current trends in the field are also discussed, with some suggestions for future research and development in NAFLD and AFLD.

Keywords: Natural drugs, Natural products, TCM, Homeopathic medicine, Complementary and alternative medicine, NAFLD, AFLD, Anti-fatty liver disease.

Introduction

Fatty liver disease (FLD) is recognized as the most common form of liver disease affecting at least 10-20 per cent of the population in western countries (Bellentani *et al.*, 2004; Angulo *et al.*, 2007) Presently, there are about 80 million people with fatty liver, and 70 million people in the USA. The incidence of FLD in developing economies (particularly in parts of Asia, South America and Africa) is growing, and has been linked to dietary lifestyle changes trending towards the western world. Fatty liver can be either alcoholic or non-alcoholic (AFLD or NAFLD), and is known to cause liver-related morbidity and/or mortality in a subset of individuals characterized by fibrosis, cirrhosis, and the eventual development of hepatocellular carcinoma (Reddy and Rao, 2006). As such, FLD, when untreated, presents as a serious threat to the majority people's health. It is generally difficult to distinguish between NAFLD and AFLD morphologically, as the histological feature of macro-vesicular hepatic steatosis is predominant in FLD, despite differences in etiology (Hubscher, 2006). The classification of FLD cases remains a broad spectrum of pathologic disease states (*e.g.*, steatohepatitis and steatonecrosis), however is gradually being accepted into the family of metabolic syndromes, such as obesity and diabetes. The shaping issues regarding FLD begin with a discussion of the etiology and pathogenesis of fatty liver.

The Etiology and Pathogenesis of Fatty Liver Disease

Definition and Diagnosis of Fatty Liver

Fatty Liver Disease refers to lipid accumulation in hepatocytes of more than 5 per cent of liver wet weight, or histologically, 1/3 of the cells have steatosis per unit area throughout the liver. The diagnosis of FLD is usually suspected in persons with elevated aminotransferase levels, radiologic findings of fatty liver, or unexplained persistent hepatomegaly (Brunt, 2010), however a definitive diagnosis is made on a liver biopsy. The clinical presentation is often asymptomatic, and may include general fatigue, and upper right-quadrant discomfort, and laboratory findings of excessive accumulation of triglycerides in liver cells and diffuse fatty degeneration of liver cells (Petta *et al.*, 2009).

Pathogenesis and Differentiation of Fatty Liver States in Traditional Chinese Medicine (TCM)

In Traditional Chinese Medicine (TCM), discussions and concerns of a Fatty Liver corresponds to records of "hepatic fullness", "hepatic distention" or "costalgia" etc. in the book of *Neijing, Canon of Medicine* (*Huangdi's Internal Classic*). Based on the records of *Jin Kui Yao Lue* (*Synopsis of the Golden Chamber*), *Jing Yue Quan Shu* (*Complete Works of Jingyue*) and *Zhu Bing Yuan Hou Lun* (*General Treatise on Causes and*

Manifestations of all Diseases), it is also described as a problem of abdominal mass, liver stuffiness, jaundice, fullness retention, gynecologic abdominal lumps, etc. The pathogenesis has been hypothesized as imbalances with phlegm, sputum, stagnation, blockages, retention, dampness, blood stasis, heat and liver-qi stagnation, and so on. As such, the basic syndromes of fatty liver include insufficiency of liver and kidney, flaring fire/heat due to yin deficiency, liver-qi stagnation and spleen deficiency, spleen deficiency, spleen deficiency and dampness stagnation, mild syndrome of internal accumulation of damp-heat, blood stasis, severe syndrome of internal accumulation of damp-heat, and internal stagnation of phlegm-dampness (Wei *et al.*, 2009; Hu, 2007).

The etiology of FLD according to TCM considers "seven emotions depression", "internal damage caused by diet", "overwork", "improper diet and drink", "moodiness", "improper oily food", "pathogenic qi" etc. This leads to the liver being stifled from functioning as "wood failing to regulate earth", "qi depression and blood stasis", "blockages in spleen function", " turbid phlegm", "dysfunction of kidney in qi transformation", "blood failing to produce", "poor elimination of pathogens" and such conditions accumulating in the liver and the disease occurs (Qiang and Wang, 2008; Ye, 2004).

Pathogenesis and Differentiation of Fatty Liver Disease in Western Medicine

Although FLD is generally currently classified as either alcoholic or nonalcoholic, NAFLD comprises a wider spectrum of diseases including simple steatosis (fatty liver), the more serious non-alcoholic steatohepatitis (NASH), and fibrosis, and cirrhosis. The exact pathogenesis of fatty liver has not been fully elucidated in western medicine, however a number of factors have been implicated. The primary theory of FLD pathogenesis is based on altered fat homeostasis, and the role that free fatty acids (FFA) play in promoting hepatic injury. In cases of increased FFA transport to the liver (seen in obesity and insulin resistance), these FFA either undergo β-oxidation or are esterified with glycerol to form triglycerides, leading to hepatic fat accumulation (Dowman *et al.*, 2010). The FFA themselves may cause toxicity by increasing oxidative stress, and via activation of inflammatory pathways (Feldstein *et al.*, 2004). Oxidative stress inhibits the replication of mature hepatocytes, which is indirectly correlated with the development of fibrosis/cirrhosis and hepatocellular carcinogenesis (Roskams *et al.*, 2003). Triglycerides may be exported as very low density lipoproteins, and decreased transport away from the liver has been proposed as a mechanism underlying the pathogenesis of FLD (Namikawa *et al.*, 2004; Charlton *et al.*, 2002).

Insulin resistance has become a hallmark of FLD, and is thus thought to play a critical role in the mechanism involved in developing FLD. Insulin resistance is known to be a key factor in the promotion of liver fat accumulation, and in stimulating lipogenesis (Basaranoglu and Neuschwander-Tetri, 2006). Likewise, obesity and visceral body fat are well established risk factors in developing FLD. Research outlining biochemical pathways implicated in FLD are the subject of numerous reviews (Han *et al.*, 2008; Méndez-Sánchez *et al.*, 2007), and describe the potential influence of hormones such as glucocorticoids, oxidative stress, mitochondrial dysfunction, adipokine and inflammatory cytokine abnormalities, small-intestinal bacterial overgrowth, and other genetic, and/or environmental factors.

Treatment of Fatty Liver Disease

Pharmacotherapy

The treatment of FLD patients does not change materially whether they are classified as AFLD or NAFLD, as both groups are recommended for nutritional support, and abstention from alcohol. NAFLD patients in particular are strongly recommended to reduce excess body fat through exercise and diet control (Ding and Fan, 2009). NAFLD patients with moderate to severe progression of the disease cannot effectively remove the deposition of liver fat through exercise and diet alone (Clark, 2006), and is not known to materially improve liver function or reduce the risk of cirrhosis and hepatocellular carcinomar. Consequently, pharmacologic treatment is the only data-supported option in the management of moderate to severe patients with NAFLD and AFLD (Moscatiello *et al.*, 2008). Pharmacotherapy strategies include a) improving insulin resistance to address the metabolic syndrome, and b) using hepato-protective agents such as antioxidants to protect the liver (Adams and Angulo, 2006). The main therapies reported are metformin (Schwimmer *et al.*, 2005) and thiazolidinediones (Belfort *et al.*, 2006) as insulin sensitizers, orlistat (Zelber-Sagi, 2006), and sibutramine (Sabuncu *et al.*, 2003) as anti-obesity drugs; losartan, an angiotensin II receptor antagonist (Yokohama *et al.*, 2004); lipid-lowering agents such as the fibrates (Basaranoglu *et al.*, 1999) or statins (Antonopoulos *et al.*, 2006), anti-oxidants (Harrison *et al.*, 2003); and ursodiol as a liver protectants/choleretics (Dufour *et al.*, 2006). The choice of pharmacologic agent should be selected based on whether patients present with hyperlipidemia, or marked liver injury. Most lipid-lowering drugs only show limited effects on reducing liver fat while a number of lipid-lowering drugs can cause liver damage. As such, the role and status of lipid-lowering drugs in the treatment of fatty liver is still controversial (Kaser *et al.*, 2010; Ahmed and Byrne, 2009; Quercioli *et al.*, 2009; Trappoliere *et al.*, 2005).

Natural Products and Traditional Chinese Medicine

Comprehensive reviews describing Chinese medicine treatment of NAFLD and AFLD in the literature is limited (Ding *et al.*, 2007; Hu, 2004; Zhang, 1992). Generally speaking, the approach to treating FLD in Traditional Chinese Medicine is 1) soothing the liver, strengthening the spleen and resolving phlegm; 2) tonifying the liver and kidney, resolving phlegm and dispelling stasis; 3) soothing the liver and promoting blood circulation, strengthening the spleen and alleviating dampness; 4) soothing the depressed liver to regulate the circulation of qi, softening hardness and promoting blood circulation; and 5) strengthening the spleen and excreting dampness and soothing the depressed liver to regulate the circulation of qi (Zhao, 2004). Chinese medicine traditionally uses a combination of natural products expected to work together to achieve the intended clinical outcome. As such, descriptions of the individual herbs or natural components are rare. It is of interest for researchers designing targeted evidence-based therapies, to become abreast of individual phytochemicals showing potential in the treatment of emerging diseases. Only Mei *et al.* reviewed more than twenty kinds of herbs for the treatment of NAFLD and AFLD from 1985 to 2006 (Mei *et al.*, 2006), however, the active components have not been mentioned in this review. Furthermore, no other comprehensive report of an individual natural products or their active components for treatment of NAFLD and AFLD has been available in recent years (circa 2005-2009) (Zhang *et al.*, 2009). This chapter reviews these types of substances in the treatment of NAFLD and AFLD from the beginning of this century, particularly in the last five years. Following, are descriptions and studies delineating the pharmacological effects and clinical observations of natural medicines for the treatment of FLD. The active components of natural products are classified by their basic structure or type.

Profiles of Natural Products Used to Treat NAFLD and AFLD

Alkaloids

Berberine (Berberidaceae/Berberis)

Bai (Bai *et al.*, 2009) and Luo (Luo *et al.*, 2006) respectively treated 47 cases and 34 cases of patients with NAFLD and dyslipidemia with Berberine (BBR) for 8 weeks. The TC, TG, LDL-C and BMI values were all significantly lower after treatment, and the serum ALT, FBG, PBG, HbA1c decreased remarkably compared to pre-treatment levels. No significant change in HDL-C, AST, TBiL, serum creatinine or BUN was found. B-mode ultrasonography examination revealed markedly improved degrees of steatosis without adverse effects. This implies that BBR treatment in NAFLD can improve the clinical state of lipid dysregulation while lowering the activity of liver enzymes, as well as offering a hypoglycemic effect. Kim *et al.* (2009) administered orally BBR to the db/db fatty liver model of obese mice and found that BBR ameliorates fatty liver by improving blood lipid regulation barriers, enhancing peripheral tissue AMPK activity and fatty acid oxidation capacity, and improving liver metabolism related genes. Following oral administration of BBR, the liver weight, TG and cholesterol of the db/db and ob/ob mice were all reduced. Wei *et al.* (2004) used BBR on 30 cases of type-II diabetic patients with fatty liver for eight weeks. Their ALT, AST, GGT values were reduced to normal levels, while TC, TG, LDL-C and BMI values were significantly lower than pre-treatment levels. Furthermore, the FPG and HbA1c levels were decreased compared to pre-treatment levels, whereas HOMA-IR and HOMA-IAI values were significantly differentpost-treatment which suggested that BBR can improve insulin resistance and insulin sensitivity, reduce enzyme activity of ALT and AST while lowering glucose and cholesterol. Additional similar findings with Berberine are also reported in the literature (Chang *et al.*, 2010; Yi and Wang, 2008; Wang *et al.*, 2007).

Aconine (Ranunculaceae/Aconitum)

Shou and Fan (2008) administered aconine (2 mg/kg/d) in the non-alcoholic fatty liver rat model of leptin and insulin resistance for 4 weeks. The serum TC, TG, LP, and insulin levels of treatment groups were significantly lower compared with controls. The degree of fat degeneration was reduced, and suggested that aconine may attenuate hepatic fat degeneration, lower serum leptin and reduce insulin resistance in rats.

Oxymatrine (Leguminosae/Cassia genus)

Yu *et al.* (2007) investigated 24 cases of non-alcoholic fatty liver patients taking combined treatment of oxymatrine and metformin for six months. Their serum ALT, insulin resistance index, serum TNF-α compared with controls were significantly decreased; while their liver/spleen computerized tomography (CT) density ratios (a marker of liver fat content) were significantly higher than the control group. This suggests that oxymatrine combined with metformin may have remarkable curative effects and favorable safety profile in NAFLD patients.

Betaine (Chenopodiaceae/Beta L.)

The benign effects of betaine in fatty liver have been reported for years (Savel and Leroi, 1964; Brignon and Wolff, 1956). More recently, Xu *et al.* (2006) applied 0.2-0.8 g/kg/d dose of betaine in the treatment of AFLD rats for 6 weeks. The indexes of TC, TG, LDL-C, cholesterol, free fatty acids of the treated group were all decreased. The liver weight index, liver lipid and decreased malondialdehyde (MDA) content, fatty degeneration of liver cells of the treated rats were also reduced significantly, while the HDL-C was increased. The result demonstrated that betaine has a satisfactory therapeutic effect on AFLD. Potential mechanisms of action for betaine in AFLD have been reported (Kharbanda *et al.*, 2007; Cheng *et al.*, 2004; Barak *et al.*, 1997; Barak *et al.*, 1993). Conversely, effects of betaine in NAFLD are also encouraging for the potential use of betaine against FLD (Kathirvel *et al.*, 2010; Wang *et al.*, 2010; Abdelmalek *et al.*, 2009; Song *et al.*, 2007; Liu *et al.*, 2006).

Pentoxifylline (Sterculiaceae/Theobroma L)

Fan *et al.* (2006) fed pentoxifylline (100 mg/kg/d) to 24 of NASH Sprague Dawley rats for 20 weeks, the NF-kB and TNF-α values of drug group were significantly decreased and the IRS-2 expression was apparently reduced. Additionally, the IkBα levels showed an increase whereas liver IRS-1 and GLUT2 expression differences between the three groups were not statistically significant. These results and other reports (Lee *et al.*, 2008; Satapathy *et al.*, 2007; Adams *et al.*, 2004) show that pentoxifylline helps to improve insulin resistance in rats, important in NASH.

Melatonin

Pan *et al.* (2006) treated fatty liver rats by intraperitoneal injection of melatonin (2.5, 5.0, 10 mg/kg/d) for 12 weeks. Melatonin (5.0 or 10 mg/kg) was effective in reducing hepatic steatosis and inflammation, lowers serum ALT, and AST, and reduces TC and TG in high-fat diet rats. Additionally, the study shows that melatonin at 10 mg/kg reduces MDA levels, indicative of potential antioxidant actions (Ferraro and López-Ortega, 2008). The results show that melatonin has a dose-dependent effect in potentially ameliorating some biochemical components of FLD.

Total Flavonoid and Phenolic Extracts

Litsea coreana flavonoids (Lauraceae/Litsea)

Liu *et al.* (2009) administered total flavonoids on AFLD rats orally for 6 weeks and found that *Litsea coreana* flavonoids can reduce ALT, AST, MDA, and TNF-α levels in rats, the expression of hepatic TNF-α mRNA was decreased, whereas SOD an GSH-PX increased. Pathologic investigation revealed a reduction in hepatic steatosis and inflammation status. The studies revealed that *Litsea coreana* flavonoids can significantly reduce the degree of liver pathological damage in AFLD, and potentially NAFLD (Wang *et al.*, 2009).

Hawthorn Leaf Flavonoids (Rosaceae/Crataegus)

Ye *et al.* (2009) performed oral administration (20, 40, and 80 mg/kg/d) of hawthorn leaves flavonoids to 60 quail for 61 months. They discovered that the TC, TG, LDL-C, MDA, AST, ALT, etc. were all significantly decreased in the serum and liver homogenate of the test groups, while the contents of HDL-C, GSH, SOD were significantly higher. This suggested that hawthorn leaves flavonoids reduce serum lipids, which may play a significant role in prevention and treatment of hyperlipidemia and fatty liver. Additional recent studies have shed light on potential mechanisms (Chen *et al.*, 2009; Yan *et al.*, 2009; Liu *et al.*, 2008).

Gingko biloba Flavonoids (Ginkgoaceae/Ginkgo L.)

Tang *et al.* (2009) fed (150 mg/kg/d) total flavonoids in *Gingko biloba* to insulin resistant rats for 12 weeks. The blood glucose level together with their HOMA-IR, IAI, TC, TG, MDA, ALT and AST were all significantly decreased, whereas the HDL-C, T-AOC and SOD of the treatment group were significantly increased. Lipid droplets in liver cells of the treatment group were small and lesser in number than controls. The results show that total flavonoids in *G. biloba* can effectively regulate blood sugar and lipids, increase insulin sensitivity and reduce hepatic steatosis.

Phenolic Acids of Oenanthe javanica (Umbelliferae/Oenanthe sp.)

Hu *et al.* (2009) fed NAFLD rats induced by high-sugar and high-fat diets with total phenolic acids of *Oenanthe javanic* (300, 150, 75 mg/kg/d) for 4 weeks. The TG and serum ALT activity in the treatment group were significantly lowered, TC, MDA, and FFA content in liver tissue were decreased whereas SOD activity increased. Additionally, steatosis and necrosis in liver cells were significantly attenuated. The results suggest that total phenolic acids of *O. javanic* can reduce blood and liver TG content thus having potential benign effects against NAFLD.

Green Tea, Black Tea and Green Tea Polyphenols (Theaceae/Camellia spp)

Pan *et al.* (2005) fed NAFLD Sprague Dawley rats with green tea, black tea (165 mg/kg/d) and green tea polyphenols (25 mg/kg/d). The weights of the testicular fat pad of test groups were reduced compared to control groups, and liver TG and TC were significantly lower than controls. Only Yunnan black tea exhibited similar indexes with the control group. The result implied that green tea and their polyphenols markedly inhibit the formation of fatty liver in rats; but not Yunnan black tea. Bruno *et al.* (2008) also administered 0, 1, and 2 per cent green tea extract to ob/ob obese mice for 6 weeks. The mice were observed to lose weight by 23-25 per cent while their symptoms of fatty liver were significantly reduced. Serum ALT and AST were reduced by 30-41 per cent and 22-33 per cent, along with a reduction in liver content of the very lipophilic α-tocopherol. This suggests that green tea extract can inhibit the intestinal absorption of fat and regulate liver lipid accumulation, thus showing potential in controlling NAFLD (Park *et al.*, 2010; DiNatale *et al.*, 2009; Hamdaoui *et al.*, 2008).

Silymarin (Asteraceae/Silibum)

Du and Li (2007) treated 23 cases of fatty liver patients with silymarin (total flavonoids) at 450 mg/d. After treatment, 13 cases displayed a significant effect (TC decreased > 20 per cent, TG decreased > 30 per cent or B-mode ultrasonophy indicated fatty liver reduction), 7 cases displayed a moderate effect, and was non-effective in 3 cases, for a total effective rate of 87 per cent. This confirmed that silymarin is likely an effective treatment in FLD. The benefits of silymarin in liver disease has been the subject of numerous studies and review articles (Fehér *et al.*, 2009; Berger and Kowdley, 2003; Saller *et al.*, 2001; Kropácová *et al.*, 1998; Ulicná *et al.*, 1985). In a recent trial of 50 NASH patients treated with 280 mg of silymarin, AST and ALT levels in the treatment group saw significant decreases compared to controls (Hashemi *et al.*, 2009). Such studies and reports indicate that silymarin may be one of the more effective treatments in AFLD and NAFLD.

Citrus Flavonoids (Hesperidin and Diosmin) (Rutaceae/Citrus)

Rapavi *et al.* (2007) fed Wistar albino rats with a combination containing 450 mg diosmin and 50 mg hesperidin (60 mg/kg/d orally) for 9 days. After treatment, both the free sulfhydryl concentration in rat liver and hydrogen-donating ability were elevated while the amount of MDA decreased. This suggests these two kinds of citrus flavonoids may be of use as antioxidant agents for prevention of fatty liver.

Phenolic Compounds

Epigallocatechin Gallate (EGCG) (Theaceae/Camellia)

Ge *et al.* (2009) administered (10, 20, 40 mg/kg/d), a green tea component, to NAFLD rats for 6 weeks. The liver weight, liver index, TC, TG, LDL-C, FFA, ALT, AST levels, as well as TC, TG, MDA concentrations in liver tissue were all significantly decreased. The HDL-C and SOD activity in liver tissue were significantly increased whereas liver lipid levels and liver cell degeneration were reduced. This suggests the EGCG may effectively treat NAFLD in animal models (Fiorini *et al.*, 2005). Kaviarasan *et al.* (2008) fed chronic alcoholic fatty liver rats with (-)EGCG for 60 days (6.0 g/kg/d), and the level of blood lipids, liver collagen and collagen cross-linking in the test rats were significantly reduced whereas collagen solubility characteristics were increased. This indicated that consumption of (-)EGCG can reduce AFLD damage. Bose *et al.* (2008) administered oral (-)EGCG to NAFLD mice (3.2 g/kg/d) for 16 weeks. Their body weight, body fat percentage, visceral fat weight, serum cholesterol, and monocyte chemoattractant protein levels were all significantly decreased. Also, insulin resistance, mesenteric fat weight, blood glucose, liver fat accumulation, TG, ALT activity were all decreased. The results implied long-term use of (-)EGCG can attenuate obesity and fatty liver, while short-term administration may reverse metabolic syndrome disorder in mice.

Puerarin (Leguminosae/Pueraria)

Zheng *et al.* (2008) treated NAFLD Sprague Dawley rats with puerarin (0.8 g/kg/d) for 4 weeks. The TG, TC, and liver inflammation were noticeably reduced, whereas liver steatosis was improved. Compared with simvastatin, puerarin can more effectively reduce lipid accumulation in the liver, reduce inflammation, and protect liver cells. The results suggest puerarin may be an effective option in the treatment of NAFLD and inflammation in rats. Additional studies reveal that the effect may be achieved through improvement of leptin signal transduction via JAK2/STAT3 pathways (Zheng *et al.*, 2009).

Rhein (Polygonaceae/Rheum)

Ying *et al.* (2007) fed NAFLD rats rhein orally (20, 40, 80 mg/kg/d) for 8 weeks. The results show an improvement in liver indices of steatosis.

Emodin (Polygonaceae/Rheum)

Zhou *et al.* (2006) fed emodin to male Japanese quails (20, 40, 80 mg/kg/d) for 8 weeks. The results show a dose-dependent effect of emodin on fatty liver, and blood lipids.

Curcumin (Zingiberaceae/Curcuma)

Ren *et al.* (2008) administered NAFLD ducks with oral curcumin at two, four, and eight times an equivalent adult dose (20, 40, 80 mg/kg/d), respectively. Curcumin dose-dependently reduces the liver index, liver TG, serum TG, serum FFA, and increases HL activity. Parameters of liver and kidney function were also significantly improved. The results suggest that curcumin has a strong anti-fatty liver effect in the optimal dose range of 80-160 mg. Zhang *et al.* (2008) administered curcumin (100, 200, 300 mg/kg/d) to NAFLD mice, and found that the liver weight and liver index decreased, and the serum TG and TC were significantly lowered, whereas the serum LDL-C were decreased in a dose-dependent manner. Similar results were seen in another study (Tan *et al.*, 2007). The authors suggest curcumin may operate via blood lipid modulation and anti-lipid peroxidation as possible mechanisms (Ren *et al.*, 2008), although other biochemical effects have been reported (Li *et al.*, 2010).

Resveratrol (Polygonum/Polygonum)

Xiao *et al.* (2008) fed NAFLD model Wistar rats by resveratrol (100 mg/kg/d) for 16 weeks and found that GIR and liver steatosis improved and serum TNF-α decreased by 31.5 per cent. The results suggest that resveratrol may reduce fatty liver by lowering serum levels of TNF-α and improving insulin resistance. Bujanda*et al.* (2008) studied oral administration of resveratrol in Wistar rats at 10 mg/kg/d for 4 weeks, and found that fat deposition, MDA and glucose levels decreased, while SOD, GSH-PX and catalase were significantly increased, suggestive of an improvement in NAFLD pathology. In another experiment, Xiao *et al.* (2008) fed resveratrol to NASH mice (400 mg/kg/d) for 16 weeks. Liver steatosis was significantly attenuated whereas COX-2 mRNA and protein expression were also reduced indicating that resveratrol may improve NASH at least in part by reducing hepatic expression of COX-2. Additional studies reported also show promising results with links to AMP-activated kinase as a factor in the mechanism (Ajmo *et al.*, 2008; Shang *et al.*, 2008a; Shang *et al.*, 2008b).

Danshensu (Lamiaceae/Salvia)

Ding *et al.* (2005) co-cultured Danshensu with NAFLD rat liver cells for 1 week adding polysaccharides and insulin. The discovered the sugar content after 2 and 24 hours were both lower than the controls. The 24-hour insulin concentration was also significantly lower than the control group. These results suggest that Danshensu treatment may enhance hepatocyte capacity of glucose metabolism and insulin uptake and binding.

Silibinin (Asteraceae/Silybum)

Lu *et al.* (2008) reported 33 cases of NAFLD patients treated with silibinin capsules (70 mg, 3 times a day). The serum TG and blood lipids of the treatment group were significantly decreased whereas the degree of fatty liver on CT was remarkably improved. These results demonstrated that silibinin treatment of fatty liver has both efficacy and safety. Zhu *et al.* (2008) investigated 46 cases of NAFLD patients taking silibinin (210 mg/d) for 2 months and reported an efficiency ratio is 80.7 per cent. After treatment, the ALT, AST, GGT, TG, CHO, LDL-C values of the patients were decreased while HDL-C was elevated. This confirmed that the combination of diet, weight loss and oral administration of silibinin may be a viable treatment option for NAFLD (Liu *et al.*, 2007).

Quercetin

Zhang *et al.* (2007) gave intraperitoneal injections of quercetin to AFLD model Wistar rats (0.5 mg/kg) for 4 weeks, and found that the blood AST, ALT, TNF-α and liver expression of NF-κB were significantly decreased. The authors suggest that quercetin may control AFLD via inhibiting expressions of NF-κB and TNF-α.

Raspberry Ketone (Rosaceae/Rubus)

Zhou *et al.* (2008) fed 1 per cent raspberry ketone to NAFLD Sprague Dawley rats for 8 weeks, the insulin sensitivity index of the raspberry ketone group was significantly decreased, while the serum TNF-α was apparently elevated, as well as the PPARγ positively expression cells were remarkably increased. The results suggest that raspberry ketone may effectively influence NAFLD by comprehensive effects.

Honokiol (Magnolia/Magnolia)

Yin *et al.* (2009) investigated AFLD Wistar rats administered oral honokiol (10 mg/kg/d) for 2 weeks. They reported that the TG, liver GSH, TNF-α and other indicators attributable to liver toxicity was markedly improved. The SREBP-1c protein maturation, the expression of Srebf1c and its target genes for hepatic lipogenesis were inhibited *in vivo*. The authors suggest that honokiol has the ability to ameliorate alcoholic steatosis by blocking fatty acid synthesis regulated by SREBP-1c.

α-Tocopherol/Vitamin-E

Botella-carretero *et al.* (2010) treated morbidly obese NAFLD patients with α-tocopherol. Serum α-tocopherol concentrations showed a negative correlation with the body mass index. The results suggested that oral administration of a-tocopherol can improve body weight in patients with NAFLD. Cankurtaran *et al.* (2006) studied the effects of vitamin-E in 52 patients with NAFLD. A correlation was found between low vitamin-E levels and high triglyceride levels as well as sonographic findings. Patients with low vitamin-E levels did not respond to a classical diet for FLD. Based on the data, the authors suggest that vitamin-E supplementation be added to lifestyle regimens for FLD.

Rhaponitin (Polygonaceae/Rheum)

Chen *et al.* (2009) investigated oral administration of rhaponitin (from rhubarb) (125 mg/kg/d) to the KK/Ay II diabetic mice. The blood glucose levels, TG, LDL, CHO, non-esterified free fatty acid, insulin levels of the treated group were significantly decreased after administration. Glucose tolerance improved, serum enzymes LDH, CK, AST, ALT were increased and the hepatic fibrosis and steatosis both decreased. This indicated that rhaponitin can significantly lower blood sugar, and serve as treatment against type-II diabetes and complicated fatty liver diseases.

Baicalin (Labiatae/Scutellaria L.)

Guo *et al.* (2009) fed NAFLD rats with baicalin (80 mg/kg/d) for 16 weeks. The body weight of the test animals were significantly decreased along with a reduction in visceral fat. The serum cholesterol, FFA, liver lipid accumulation, and insulin levels were also significantly decreased. Additionally, TNF-α was lowered while phosphorylations of AMPK and ACC were increased. The result suggests that baicalin can improve fatty liver and obesity-induced diseases through modulation of liver AMPK.

Terpene Derivatives and Steroidal Compounds

Cucurbitacin (Cucurbitaceae/Lagenaria sp)

Fu *et al.* (2005) gave pediatric obesity patients oral cucurbitacin (0.1 mg, 3 times a day) for one month, the ALT, AST of the patients decreased but ultrasound examinations did not exhibit differences compared to the control group. ALT values of the patients returned to normal after 3 months of treatment, while AST values returned to nearly normal. Cucurbitacin may improve liver function in children suffering from high GPT, and protect liver cells. The results suggest that cucurbitacin is a sound option in the treatment of children with NASH, and without obvious side effects.

Andrographolide (AGH, diterpenoic lactones) (Acanthaceae/Andrographis)

Ye *et al.* (2008) gave intraperitoneal injections of andrographolide to NASH Sprague Dawley rats (100 mg/kg/d) for 3 weeks. The TG, MDA, and TNF-a in both serum and liver of the treated animals were significantly lower whereas liver SOD activity reduced. The hepatic steatosis and inflammation of the treated rats were reduced remarkably. These results indicated that andrographolide may alleviate NASH in rats.

Retinol/Vitamin-A

Botella-Carretero *et al.* (2010) treated morbidly obese patients with retinol, and found that serum retinol concentration was not only negatively correlated with body mass index, but also negatively correlated with concentrations of serum AST, ALT.

This implied that orally administered retinol can improve body weight and symptoms in patients with NAFLD.

Ursodeoxycholic Acid (UDCA) (Ursidae/Ursus)

Uzun *et al.* (2009) fed NAFLD rats having a two-thirds liver resection with UDCA, and found that the MI values and proliferating-cell nuclear antigen levels of the control group were significantly lower than both the UDCA treated and normal rats. Additionally, GSH values after hepatectomy in the control group was far lower than normal and treated rats. The results suggest administration of UDCA may prompt liver regeneration in NAFLD rats. Santos*et al.* (2003) studied 15 patients with 10 mg/kg/day of UDCA and observed a significant reduction in serum levels of ALT, AST and gamma-glutamyltransferase, but the effects were not related to modifications in liver fat content.

9-cis β-carotene (Powder of the Alga Dunaliella bardawil) (Polyblepharidaceae/Dunaliella genus)

Harari *et al.* (2008) treated high-fat-diet fed LDL receptor knockout mice with 50 per cent 9-cis and 50 per cent all-trans beta-carotene in the diet. The authors observed a 40-63 per cent inhibition of serum cholesterol and lowered VLDL and LDL values. Atherosclerotic lesions in the mice were reduced by 60-83 per cent, while both fat accumulation in the liver and liver inflammation were reduced. The results suggest that 9-cis β-carotene can dose-dependently inhibit atherosclerosis and fatty liver symptoms.

Corosolic Acid (CRA, Lagerstroemia Specious Leaf) (Lythraceae/Lagerstroemia)

Yamada *et al.* (2008) fed 0.023 per cent CRA to KK-Ay obese mice for 9 weeks. The weight loss of the animals were ca. 10 per cent while total fat reduced 15 per cent, the fasting blood glucose reduced 23 per cent, the plasma insulin decreased 41 per cent, TG decreased 22 per cent and insulin sensitivity improved. Additionally, there was an increase in plasma adiponectin receptors and white adipose tissue adiponectin receptors. This means corosolic acid can reduce the weight and symptoms of fatty liver which may be related to high expressions of PPAR-a in liver and white adipose tissue.

Lycopene (Tomato Fruit) (Solanaceae/Lycopersicon)

Ma *et al.* (2007) reported oral administration of lycopene to fatty liver quails (10, 20 mg/kg/d) for 4 weeks. They found that the TC and TG in plasma were significantly decreased, and after 8 weeks treatment, the TC, TG, MDA levels and fatty liver pathology in quail livers were markedly reduced, whereas SOD activity was increased in a dose-dependent manner. The authors believe that lycopene has the capability to control experimental fatty liver of quails. The results are supported by a more recent study showing the positive effects of lycopene in NAFLD rats (Wei and Zhao, 2010).

Capsaicin (Solanaceae/Capsicum)

Kang *et al.* (2009) fed capsaicin 0.015 per cent to C57BL/6 model NAFLD obese mice for 10 weeks. The fasting blood glucose, insulin, leptin, and TG levels of the treated mice were all decreased whereas the glucose tolerance of the obese mice was improved. The TNF-a, MCP-1, and expression of interleukin IL-6 mRNA TRPV-1 were significantly reduced, while the adiponectin mRNA/protein, PPAR-a/PGC-1 a mRNA were increased. The results indicated that capsaicin may interact with PPAR-a to reduce glucose tolerance, and can not only inhibit inflammation but also promote fatty acid oxidation. As such, capsaicin may have the ability to reduce insulin resistance and treat fatty liver diseases. Capsaicin also shows the ability to reduce the formation of liver TG in rats fed orotic acid (Cha *et al.*, 2004).

Saponin Extracts

Saponins from Panax ginseng (ginsenosides GSL, total saponins) (Araliaceae/ Panax)

Hu *et al.* (2009) fed NAFLD mice with high and low dose GSL (50, 100 mg/kg/ d) for 2 weeks. The high-dose group significantly reduced blood lipids, liver lipids, MDA, and the liver index, and increased SOD activity and liver pathology. Additionally, the level of PPAR-α mRNA in liver tissue increased but decreased the level of CYP2E1 mRNA in liver tissue. The results suggest that GSL can reduce blood and liver fat, and inhibit lipid peroxidation.

Panax Notoginsenosides (PNS, Total Saponins) (Araliaceae/Panax)

Na *et al.* (2008) fed PNS on NAFLD Sprague Dawley rats (200 mg/kg/d) for 20 weeks. The fat-based degeneration of liver cells in the PNS group was significantly attenuated, the lipid droplets reduced, CYP 2E1 expression, MDA and FFA were all markedly decreased, whereas liver SOD activity increased. The results demonstrate that PNS may significantly inhibit expression of CYP 2E1 in rat liver and plays a role in the prevention and treatment of fatty liver.

Passepartout (Araliaceae/Panax)

Cao (2005) treated 34 cases of NAFLD patients daily with Passepartout (500 mg in 500 mL of 10 per cent glucose solution) via intravenous infusion. After 4 weeks treatment, 17 cases were classified as significantly effective, 7 cases effective and 10 cases ineffective. As such, passepartout demonstrates potential as an efficacious agent in NAFLD.

Tripterygium Glycosides (TWP, Total Saponins) (Celastraceae/Tripterygium)

He *et al.* (2007) investigated oral administration of TWP to 22 hyperlipidemic NAFLD New Zealand white rabbits (1.5 mg/kg/d). After 16 weeks treatment, the serum TC and TG levels in the liver were significantly reduced. The results implied that TWP has a hypolipidemic effect and may inhibit high-fat diet-induced fatty liver.

Fenugreek Saponins (TFGs, total saponins) (Leguminosae/Trigonella L.)

Zhang *et al.* (2006) administered TFGs orally to AFLD Wistar rats (60, 90, 120 mg/kg/d) for 4 weeks. The TC, TG and fat in rat hepatocytes were significantly decreased. The TC, LDL-C, activity of AST and ALT, and TBil in serum were significantly reduced, and liver morphology improved. These results suggest that

TFGs have a hypolipidemic and inhibiting effect on ALT and AST, while significantly reducing liver lipid depositions.

Saponins of Litchi (Total Saponins) (Sapindaceae/Litchi L.)

Guo *et al.* (2005) administered litchi saponins orally to hyperlipidemic fatty liver insulin resistant (IR) Sprague Dawley rats (50, 100 mg/kg/d) for 4 weeks. At 2 hours after administration, the FSG, TC, TG, insulin levels and TNF-α of the treated rats were found to be decreased significantly while the HDL-C was significantly increased. The insulin sensitivity and hyperinsulinemia of the treated rats also improved. The authors suggest that litchi saponins may modulate glucose and lipid metabolism disorders, and may improve hyperlipidemia in rats via a similar mechanism of rosiglitazone.

Platycodin (Total Saponins) (Campanulaceae/Platycodon L.)

Khanal *et al.* (2009) fed the alcoholic liver injury Sprague Dawley rats with platycodins for 2 weeks. The ALT, AST and albumin levels in serum were significantly decreased. The expression of cytochrome P450 2E1 and the accumulation of TG were reduced, while the AMP-activated protein kinase-α (AMPK-a) phosphorylation was restored. The results indicate that platycodin may be effective in the treatment and prevention of AFLD.

Amino Acids, Peptides and Simple Organic Compounds

Taurine

Yang *et al.* (2007) recorded of 80 patients with NAFLD taking taurine (2.0 g, 3 times a day) for 12 weeks. The TBil, AST, ALT, GGT, TC, TG, GLU indices of the treated patients were all significantly decreased compared to controls. The study supports an analeptic role of taurine in FLD (Chen *et al.*, 2005; Chen *et al.*, 2006). Chen *et al.* (2009) reported that rats fed taurine can prevent ethanol-induced oxidative stress, whereas the expression of inflammatory cytokines in the adipose tissue is increased. Taurine can also prevent decreases in CCAAT/enhancer binding protein-α and peroxisome proliferator-activated receptor-α, and can improve the concentration of serum adiponectin. The results suggest taking taurine can prevent ethanol-induced expression of adiponectin and oxidative stress.

Glutamine

Li *et al.* (2008) found that NAFLD rats administered glutamine for 4 weeks results in their serum ALT, AST, and liver inflammation scores to be significantly decreased, and supports an earlier finding on the effects of glutamine in preventing fatty liver (Helton *et al.*, 1990). The portal plasma endotoxin, D-xylose concentrations in plasma of the abdominal aorta as well as the MDA content in intestinal tissue of the treated rats were significantly reduced. Meanwhile, the SIgA levels in intestinal mucus SOD levels in small intestine were apparently higher compared with controls. The authors indicate that glutamine may reduce the inflammation of liver tissue injuries in NAFLD rats, but cannot completely stop the progress of inflammation.

L-arginine

The role of arginine in the development of fatty liver has been reported for some time (Milner and Hassan, 1981; Milner *et al.*, 1979). Ijaz *et al.* (2009) found that intravenous injection of L-arginine to fatty liver Sprague Dawley rats (50, 100, 300, 500 mg/kg/d) may significantly improve their hepatic artery, portal vein, and hepatic microcirculation while reducing liver tissue oxidation. The authors conclude that continuous use of large doses of L-arginine may improve both liver microcirculation and liver blood flow in fatty liver, while relieving symptoms of liver tissue degeneration.

Fructus Lycii Glucopeptide

Xing *et al.* (2008) treated 82 NAFLD patients with oral administration of Fructus lycii glucopeptide (30 mg 2 times a day) for 6 months and the effectiveness rate was 70.7 per cent. The ALT, AST, GGT levels of treated patients decreased significantly, with positive results in blood fat indices. The authors suggest that long-term treatment of Fructus lycii glucopeptide on NAFLD patients is safe and efficacious.

Soybean Peptide (Leguminosae/Glycine L.)

Lv *et al.* (2008) fed NAFLD rats with 500 mg/kg soy peptide for 10 weeks. They found that soy peptides could significantly lower TG and TC in serum and liver of high-fat diet rats whereas the steatosis and FFA content in rat livers were also significantly reduced. The findings suggest that aerobic exercise and soy peptide administration can improve fat metabolism in rats with high fat diet, and is potentially capable of preventing fatty liver.

Ligustrazine (Apiaceae/Ligusticum)

Sun *et al.* (2007) studied an acute liver injury model of fatty liver in mice by intraperitoneal injections of ligustrazine (50, 25, and12.5 mg/kg/d). After 7 days treatment, the ALT and AST activity in mice serum were decreased, in addition to FFA, TG, and MDA levels in liver. Conversely, hepatic lipase and SOD in rat liver were increased whereas hepatic steatosis was reduced.

Allicin (Alliaceae/Allium)

Shao *et al.* (2006) administered NAFLD rats with allicin (the active component in garlic) at high, medium and low doses (30, 20, and 10 mg/kg/d) for 12 weeks. Results showed that all doses of allicin can significantly decrease lipids and endotoxin levels in rat plasma, whereas differences in SOD activity, MDA, FFA, MDA, and GSH contents between the treated groups and controls were statistically significant. The authors suggest that allicin has a positive effect against NAFLD in rats, in a dose-dependent manner.

Osthol [Mature Fruit of Cnidium monnieri (L) Cuss] (Apiaceae/Cnidium)

Song *et al.* (2008) administered osthol to AFLD Sprague Dawley rats at three doses (5, 10, 25 mg/kg/d) orally for 6 weeks. The osthol treatment significantly decreased the TC and TG contents in serum and can dose-dependently raise the expression of CYP7AmRNA and PPARct mRNA in AFLD rat liver tissue. Meanwhile the expression of DGAT mRNA was lowered in the treatment groups. The results suggest that osthol may exhibit a therapeutic effect on lipid accumulation in AFLD, potentially by regulating PPAR alpha mediated lipogenic gene expression (Sun *et al.*, 2010), thereby reducing alcohol induced injury on the liver.

Polysaccharides

Chicory Polysaccharide (Asteraceae/Cichorium Genus)

Zheng *et al.* (2008) administered Chicory polysaccharide to NAFLD Wistar rats (10, 20 g/kg/d) for 19 days. The TC, TG and liver index were significantly decreased in addition to plasma TC, TG and glucose. Liver ALP decreased, but levels of total lipase, LPL and HL were increased. The results indicate that Chicory polysaccharide significantly reduces liver fat in NAFLD rats.

Lycium Barbarum Polysaccharides (LBP) (Solanaceae/Lycium)

Gu *et al.* (2007a; 2007b; 2007c) fed AFLD Wistar rats with LBP (250, 500 mg/kg/d) for 5-10 weeks. The authors found that the CYP2E1 gene and protein expression of the rats were inhibited, while ALT, AST, γ-GT and MDA were reduced however the activities of GSH-PX, SOD, and GSH were increased. LBP causes a significant improvement in liver pathological changes of AFLD and the authors suggest that LBP can effectively prevent AFLD through reduction of lipid peroxidation. Similar effects were observed in NAFLD rat models (Song *et al.*, 2007).

Chondroitin Sulfate

Wu *et al.* (Wu 2006) reported that intraperitoneal administration of AFLD rats with chondroitin sulfate (25 mg/kg•/d) for 4 weeks may significantly reduce the values of serum ALT, AST, MDA, TG, TC, and alleviate liver inflammation and fat content of AFLD rats. The results suggest that chondroitin sulfate, a common drug too many, may have a potential therapeutic benefit in AFLD.

Sweet Potato Vines (Total Polysaccharides) (Convolvulaceae/Ipomoea)

According to a study by Gao *et al.* (2005), hyperlipidemic Sprague Dawley rats fed sweet potato vines polysaccharide (100, 200, 400 mg/kg/d) for 8weeks, showed a reduction in TC, TG, LDL-C levels and AI in the serum of the treated rats. As such, sweet potato vines polysaccharides possess efficacy in reduction of blood lipids and possible prevention of NAFLD.

Polydextrose (Konjac Glucomannan) (Araceae/Amorphophallus)

According to a study by Deng *et al.* (2003), NAFLD model Wistar rats fed konjac glucomannan (20 mg/d) for 4weeks and ALT, TG, TC and the degree of liver steatosis remarkably decreased whereas AST did not show an improvement. The author concludes that polydextrose may show efficacy in prevention and treatment of experimental fatty liver steatohepatitis.

Unsaturated Fatty Acids

Conjugated Linoleic Acid (CLA)

According to the report of Noto *et al.* (2006) feeding fa/fa and lean Zucker rats with 1.5 per cent CLA for 8 weeks can reduce 62 per cent of liver fat accumulation in insulin resistance fa/fa rats, while the liver function and serum lipoproteins were all improved. The data shows that CLA can actively improve lipid metabolism of fa/fa Zucker rats and may be unrelated to an improvement in overall body fat content (Purushotham *et al.*, 2007).

Dietary ω-3 and ω-6 Polyunsaturated Fatty Acids

Yeh *et al.* (2009) fed laying hens with soybean oil or flaxseed oil supplements in a cross-breeding experiment. The hens fed with a large number of ω-6polyunsaturated fatty acids in soybean oil diets exhibited elevated activities of blood coagulation factor V, VII and X when compared with flax seed oil. The authors found relationships between liver hemorrhage score and liver weight, and between liver weight percentage and severity of histological haemorrhagic and fatty changes. The authors hypothesized that the clotting activity of fatty liver haemorrhagic syndrome in laying hens can be improved by feeding diets rich in ω-3 and ω-6 fatty acids.

Seal Oil ω-3 Polyunsaturated Fatty Acids (Otariidae/Callorhimus L.)

Li *et al.* (2004) found that NAFLD Wistar rats fed with seal oil (0.5, 1.6, 4.8 g/kg/d) for 8 weeks results in significant loss of TG, TC, MDA, FFA while the liver weight of the treated rats were decreased. Conversely, their SOD activity and 6-keto-PGF1α/TxB2 increased while steatosis and the expression of CYP2E1 were reduced. The authors conclude that the seal oil may prevent and treat NAFLD via inhibition of lipid formation and modulation of lipid metabolism.

n-3 Polyunsaturated Gatty Acids

Spadaro *et al.* (2008) studied 40 NAFLD patients given 2.0 g/d doses of n-3 polyunsaturated fatty acids for 6 months. The ALT level, TG, NGF-a and HOMA (IR) values of the treated patients were decreased whereas complete fatty liver regression was observed in 33.4 per cent of the patients, and an overall reduction in 50 per cent. The result indicated that n-3 polyunsaturated fatty acids may lower liver fat production, and reduce liver inflammation.

γ-Linolenic Acid

Nakanishi *et al.* (2004) reported on conjugated linoleic acid-induced fatty liver mice given linoleic acid (LA) or γ-linolenic acid (GLA) for 4 weeks. A single administration of CLA significantly increased PGE-2 levels in the liver 12 h after administration, however, long-term administration of CLA significantly decreased the liver PGE-2 level and induced fatty liver. GLA increased PGE-2 levels, and coadministration with GLA, but not with LA, prevented the CLA-induced fatty liver. The results suggest that fatty liver associated with PGE-2 reduction by CLA ingestion can be attenuated by GLA in mice.

Eicosapentaenoic Acid (EPA)

Kurihara *et al.* (1997) reported on fatty liver Sprague Dawley rats simultaneously given EPA (1.0 g/kg/d) and a choline deficient diet for 4 weeks. The microchannel passage time of the EPA treated group were significantly shorter than the choline deficient diet group, which indicated that platelet aggregation changes of leukocyte adhesion of platelet aggregation are less in the EPA treated group. The authors conclude that EPA may amend blood flow changes of fatty liver rats caused by inadequate choline.

Eicosapentaenoic Acid Ethyl Ester (EPA-E)

Kajikawa *et al.* (2009) fed NAFLD mice induced by a high-fat and high-sucrose diet with EPA-E. The hepatic TG value, mRNA, and SREBP-1c expression and contents of monounsaturated fatty acids C16: 1 and C18: 1 were decreased, while n-3 PUFA content (including EPA and DHA) increased. The authors conclude that oral administration of EPA-E can reduce the deposition of fat in the liver via inhibition of TG synthesis enzymes and via reduction of MUFA accumulation.

Docosahexaenoic Acid (DHA)

Yanagita *et al.* (2005) fed C57BL/6N mice with a combination diet of CLA with 0.5 per cent DHA for 4 weeks, which alleviated fatty liver without decreasing the antiobesity effect of CLA, significantly attenuated the increase in enzyme activity induced by CLA and reduced hepatic fatty acid synthesis without affecting adipocytokine production in C57BL/6N mice.

Arachidonic Acid (ARA)

Oikawa *et al.* (2008) fed NAFLD mice with 3 per cent CLA +1-2 per cent ARA for four weeks. The concentration of serum TAG as well as liver weight of the mice decreased, whereas cholesterol and NEFA concentrations were unaffected and liver fat accumulation was suppressed. Furthermore, liver PGE-2 increased while PGE-1 did not exhibit significant changes in treated mice. Consequently, the symptoms of fatty liver caused by CLA can be alleviated via co-administration with ARA without influencing the anti-obesity effect of CLA.

Roots and Stems

Polygonum cuspidatum (Root Aqueous Extract) (Polygonaceae/Polygonum Genus)

Jiang *et al.* (2009) reported the continuous administration of polygonum (11 g/kg/d) to NAFLD Wistar rats for 4 weeks. They noticed declines in adipose tissue leptin mRNA and adiponectin mRNA compared with the control group and the relative levels of TNF-α mRNA in adipose tissue of the treatment group were significantly lower than controls. Uncoupling protein 2mRNA were detected in all samples of the control group, while only a rather low level of uncoupling protein 2mRNA could be detected in a few samples of the intervention group. Resistin mRNA was not found in both treatment and control groups. These results indicated that *P. cuspidatum*, as an inhibitor of TNF-α, can improve liver conditions from steatosis and inflammation (Jiang *et al.*, 2007).

Rhubarb (Root Alcoholic Extract) (Polygonaceae/Rhubarb L.)

Xu *et al.* (2007) studied experimental rabbits of hyperlipidemia and fatty liver with successive administration of ethanolic extract of rhubarb (1.4, 4.2, 12.6 g/d, i.g.) for 10 weeks. The authors found that extract of rhubarb can increase HDL-C, reduce

TG and LDL-C, and hepatic steatosis in a dose-dependent manner. The results suggest that ethanolic extract of rhubarb can reduce lipid levels of atherosclerotic rabbits to reduce the development of fatty liver.

Panax notoginseng (Root Powder) (Araliaceae/Panax L.)

Cai *et al.* (2007) reported on fatty liver Sprague Dawley rats continuously administered *Panax notoginseng* (0.6, 1.2 g/kg/d, i.g.) for 14 weeks. Liver steatosis of the animals was significantly reduced in treatment groups with large and small doses of *P. notoginseng* compared with controls. Additionally, COX-2 expression was significantly reduced, while plasma TXB2, 6-Keto-PGF1 α, and TXB2/6-Keto-PGF1 α values were also markedly decreased. These indicated that *P. notoginseng* can improve the microcirculation in fatty liver rats and inhibit COX-2 expression in liver tissue.

Danshen (Root Aqueous Extract) (Lamiaceae/Salvia L.)

Sun *et al.* (2007) reported the TC and TG contents in serum and liver tissue of NAFLD rats could be reduced by treatment with Danshen intraperitoneal injection (1.65, 3.3 mL/kg/d) for 8 weeks. Levels of serum and liver tissue MDA were reduced while levels of serum SOD were increased. It was concluded that Danshen injection inhibits lipid peroxidation and adipopexis.

Sophora Tonkinensis (Root Vinegar Extract) (Leguminosae/Sophora L.)

Dai *et al.* (2007) (Infectious Disease Dept. of Shanghai Huadong Hospital) reported that tonkinensis liquid treatment of fatty liver patients demonstrated a preliminary effect in lowering ALT and cholesterol. Compared with Traditional Chinese Medicine decoctions, vinegar extract can avoid losses of active components caused by the heat and evaporation.

Radix Polygoni Multiflori (Root Aqueous Extract of Polygonum multiflorum Thuna.) (Polygonaceae/Polygonum)

Wang *et al.* (2006) administered *Polygonum multiflorum* (5 g/kg/d, i.g.) to NAFLD Sprague Dawley rats for 26 days. Their TC and TG levels exhibited significant differences compared to controls, and hepatic steatosis significantly lower than controls. The results suggest *P. multiflorum* possesses inhibitory effects on fatty liver.

Zedoary (Aqueous Extract of Curcuma root) (Zingiberaceae/Curcuma L.)

According to Li *et al.* (2006) the MDA, TC, and TG levels in the liver homogenate of NAFLD Sprague Dawley rats fed with Zedoary (2.0, 4.0 g/d) for 12 weeks, were significantly reduced, while the indexes of ALT and AST were also lowered. The aqueous extract of Curcuma root clears the accumulation of TG and reduces MDA in the liver. The results show that Zedoary has a lipid-lowering and liver protective effect in NAFLD rats.

Red Peony Root (Radix Concentrate of Paeonia lactiflora) (Ranunculaceae/Paeonia L.)

Zhao *et al.* (2005) administered NAFLD Sprague Dawley rats with red peony root (10, 20g/kg/d, i.g.) for 7 weeks. They found that the body weights and liver index of all treated groups were lower than controls, while leptin levels and insulin resistance decreased significantly compared to controls. The results indicate that Red Peony Root has the effect of improving leptin and insulin resistance.

Platycodon grandiflorum (Campanulaceae/Platycodon)

Kim *et al.* (2007) investigated prophylactic administration with Platycodon radix (PR) extracts to rats. PR can not only prevent development of AFLD, but also decrease the lipid formation in liver and serum. PR can also normalize the expression of the L-FABP gene and the activity of cytochrome P450 2E1 (CYP2E1).

Alisma (Rhizome Aqueous Extract) (Alismataceae/Alisma L.)

Li and Feng (2006), also reported that fatty liver Sprague Dawley rats administered with an aqueous extract of *Alisma orientalis* (2.0, 4.0 g/d) for 12 weeks can significantly reduce liver homogenate MDA, TC, TG, ALT and AST. TG accumulated in liver was cleared while the MDA content was reduced. Hong et *al.* (2006) also studied NAFLD rats fed with methanol extracts of *A. orientalis* (150, 300, 600 mg/kgd) for 6 weeks. Serum and liver fat were significantly reduced, fasting blood glucose lowered, insulin resistance increased, anti-lipid peroxidation capacity and antioxidant enzyme activities and transaminases improved. It was concluded that methanol extracts of *A. orientalis* have good effect a in NAFLD.

Leaves

Perilla Leaf Extract (Labiatae/Perilla)

Xu *et al.* (2009) fed NAFLD New Zealand rabbits with *Perilla* leaf extract (0.17, 0.5, 1.5 g/kg/d) for 8 weeks, and the TC, TG, LDL levels of three treatment groups were significantly lower than a hyperlipidemic control group. HDL levels were significantly higher than controls, and only the high dose group demonstrated a significant reduction in the liver index when compared to the hyperlipidemic control. The degree of liver steatosis in treatment groups were all attenuated compared to controls, in a dose-dependent manner. The authors indicated that *Perilla* leaf extract is effective against high-fat high-cholesterol diet induced NAFLD rabbits, and its mechanism of action may be related to lipid regulation.

Crataegus pinnatifida Bge. var. major (Ethanol Extract) (Rosaceae/Crataegus L.)

In the study of Zhang *et al.* (2008) NAFLD model Wistar rats administered with the leaves of *Crataegus pinnatifida* (0.12, 0.72 g/kg/d) for 16 days, saw significant differences in hepatosomatic ratios among the model group, normal group, and treatment group ($P < 0.05$). Levels of serum TC and TG were higher than the normal group ($P< 0.05$), while a significant improvement could be found in liver pathological examination for the treatment groups. The results indicated that the butanol partition of the 70 per cent ethanol extract of the leaves of *C. pinnatifida* can significantly reduce hepatosomatic ratios, and therefore may be effective against fatty liver.

Gingko biloba Leaf Extract (Ginkgoaceae/Ginkgo L.)

According to the study of Liu *et al.* (2008), NAFLD Sprague Dawley rats were administered Ginkgo leaf extract (10 mg/kg/d, i.g.) for 6 weeks. Differences were observed for the liver tissues and levels of cholesterol, TG, HDL, ALT, and AST in treatment and NAFLD control groups ($P < 0.05$), while no difference could be observed between the treatment group and normal animals. Gu *et al.* (Gu *et al.*, 2009) reported the effect of *G. biloba* leaf extract GBE50 on NAFLD rats (i.g., 19 weeks), and found that the development of high fat-induced fatty liver was reduced while the levels of serum cholesterol and lactate dehydrogenase were suppressed. Some genes related to lipid metabolism, glucose metabolism, vascular contraction, ion transportation and drug metabolism may be regulated by GBE50. The results indicated that GBE50 can inhibit the synthesis of fatty acids, and promote the metabolism of fatty acids.

Green Tea (Aqueous Extract) (Theaceae/Camellia)

Wang *et al.* (2006) found that after administration of green tea water extract (5 g/kg/d, i.g.) for 26 days, the TC, TG of NAFLD Sprague Dawley rats were significantly different compared to controls and liver fat infiltration was significantly lower than untreated animals. The results showed that green tea extracts may inhibit the formation of fatty liver in rats.

Olive Leaf Extract (Burseraceae/Canarium L.)

Omagari *et al.* (2010) investigated the preventive effects of olive leaf extract on hepatic fat accumulation in a rat model of NASH. In the study, the spontaneously hypertensive/NIH-corpulent rats were administered olive leaf extract (0.5, 1.0, 2.0 g/kg/d, i.g.) for 23 weeks, and the high and medium doses of olive leaf extract prevented the emergence of NASH. Thioredoxin-1 expression was more evident in the liver, while the expression of 4-hydroxy nonene in the liver was less evident. The results show that olive leaf extract may prevent NAFLD through an antioxidant mechanism.

Rosemary Leaf (RE, Extract of Rosamarinus officinalis L.) (Labiatae/Rosemarinus)

The study of Harach *et al.* (2010) explored fatty liver mice fed with rosemary leaf extract (50, 200 mg/kg/d, i.g.) for 50 days. The body weights of the high dose group reduced by 64 per cent, while a measure of fat mass decreased by 57 per cent. *In vitro* experiments showed that rosemary leaf extract inhibited pancreatic lipase and hepatic TG decreased 39 per cent, while no significant effect was found for a low dose group (20 mg/kg/d). The results showed that 200 mg/kg rosemary leaf extract can inhibit high-fat diet induced obesity and prevent obesity-related liver steatosis.

Fruits and Seeds

Raw Hawthorn (Aqueous Extract) (Rosaceae/Crataegus L.)

Li and Feng (2006), reported on NAFLD Sprague Dawley rats administered raw hawthorn fruit aqueous extract (5 g/kg/d, i.g.) for 26 days. Their TC and TG values were significantly different compared to untreated animals, and fat infiltration of the liver was also significantly lower than controls. The results suggest that raw hawthorn fruit aqueous extract may inhibit the development of fatty liver.

Zhijuzi (Granules of Semen Hoveniae orHovenia acerba Seeds) (Rhamnaceae/ Hovenia L.)

Zhu *et al.* (2007) found that after the AFLD rats were continuously administered with Zhijuzi (1, 2 g/rat/d, i.g.) for 45 days, the serum AST and ALT of high and low dose groups decreased significantly. Conditions related to liver steatosis and inflammations were also improved significantly. The results showed that early intervention by Zhijuzi can prevent AFLD in rats.

Fructus Lycii (Fruit Extract of Lycium barbarum L.) (Solanaceae/Lycium L.)

According to the study of Sun *et al.* (2006) Wistar rats with fatty liver were administered Chinese wolfberry fruit liquid (2,0, 4.0 g/kg/d) for 5 weeks and the serum TC of the high-dose group was significantly decreased. Pathologic slices revealed less liver steatosis and infiltration of inflammatory cells than in untreated animals. The results suggest that Chinese wolfberry fruit solution can reduce TC levels of serum and liver tissue and reduce the degree of liver steatosis.

Soy Protein Concentrate (Papilionaceae/Glycine sp.)

Gudbrandesen *et al.* (2007) fed obese Zucker rats with soy protein preparations enriched with isoflavones for 6 weeks. It was found that the serum ALT and AST of the high dose group were reduced, and the incidence of fatty liver was also reduced. Meanwhile, the activities of mitochondrial and peroxisomal β-oxidation, acetyl coenzyme A carboxylase, fatty acid synthase and glycerol 3-phosphate transferase in the liver increased. The authors suggest that both soy protein preparations with fruitful isoflavone and soy protein may be used as supplemental therapy against NAFLD. These results are supported by data on the prevention of hepatic steatosis using soy isoflavones (Brackett *et al.*, 2006).

Fenugreek (FEN, Seeds of Trigonella foenum graecum) (Leguminosae/ Trigonella L.)

Raju and Bird (2006), fed both fat and lean female Zucker rats with 5 per cent FEN diet for 8 weeks. The liver weight, TG, and TNF-a protein (soluble and bound forms) in obese animals were significantly reduced (lean animals showed no effect), and TNF-II receptor proteins in the obese animals were significantly increased. The results indicate that FEN seed supplementation reduces triglyceride accumulation in the liver and that TNF-alpha may play an important role in this process.

Barks

Ash Bark (Extract of Cortex fraxini) (Oleaceae/Fraxinus L.)

Yang *et al.* (2007) reported that fatty liver Wistar rats administered with Cortex fraxini (0.2, 0.4, 0.8 g/kg/d, i.g) for 21 days. The liver secretary TG and ApoB levels were significantly lower than untreated animals in a dose-dependent manner. The TG and ApoB levels in the microsomal lumen, and the VLDL of rat liver cells were significantly lower than untreated animals, in a dose-dependent manner. These results show that ash bark extract has a therapeutic effect on experimental fatty liver rats, which may be related to the inhibition of the generation and transport of TG and ApoB.

Magnolia officinalis (MO, Bark Extract) (Magnoliaceae/Magnolia L.)

Yin *et al.* (2009) found that Magnolia extract (MO) can protect RAW 264.7 cells from attack by reactive oxygen species, superoxide anions and TNF-α caused by ethanol, and can prevent cell death induced by activation of NADPH oxidase. The authors also studied administration of MO to AFLD model Lieber-DeCarli ethanol diet-fed rats for the last two weeks, and found that the indicators liver function and fatty liver was completely reversed, while increased mutation of binding protein-1c was blocked. The authors suggest that MO extracts have the potential to be developed as a drug in the treatment of AFLD.

Cinnamon (Ethanol Extract of Cinnamomum cassia bark) (Lauraceae/ Cinnamomum)

In the experiments of Kanuri *et al.* (2009), acute alcohol-induced steatosis in mice was prevented by administration of cinnamon extract, which significantly reduced hepatic lipid accumulation in the treated animals. *In vitro* studied showed that cinnamon extract could suppress the expression of LPS-induced MyD88, iNOS and TNF-a in RAW 264.7 macrophages (a model of Kupffer cells), and could control the degradation of kappaB inhibitor. The authors suggested that the ethanol extract of cinnamon bark can treat acute AFLD, and its mechanism of action may include inhibiting the expression of proteins such as MyD88.

Flowers

Safflower (Iridaceae/Crocus L.)

Zuo (2004) reported intravenous safflower (16 g/d) for 14 days, led to gastrointestinal symptoms of patients disappearing more quickly with earlier recovery of function. The treated cases saw a lowering of ALT and lipid levels and suggest that injection of safflower may have an effect in the treatment of fatty liver complicated with hyperlipidemia.

Pomegranate Flower (PGF) (Punicaceae/Punica)

Xu *et al.* (2009) investigated obese diabetic ZDF rats administered PGF (0.5 g/kg/d) for 6 weeks. The ratio of liver weight/tibia length, TG, and lipid droplets were decreased whereas peroxisome proliferator-activated receptor PPAR-α, ACO, and gene expression of stearoyl coenzyme A dehydrogenase-1 were increased, while stearoyl coenzyme A dehydrogenase-1 activity decreased. Moreover, the gene expression for synthesis, hydrolysis and absorption of fatty acids and TG were minimized by PGF treatment. PGF treatment also increased PPAR and ACO mRNA levels in HepG2 cells. The authors suggest that PGF extract can alleviate diabetes and obesity-related fatty liver, at least in part by activating gene expression for oxidation of fatty acids in the liver.

Algae

Sargassum fusiforme (Sargassum Decoction of Whole Plant) (Sargassaceae/ Sargassum)

Zhang *et al.* (2006) investigated fatty liver Sprague Dawley rats administered Sargassum decoction (1, 5, 10, 20, 40 g/kg/d, i.g.) for 4 weeks. Their body weights, liver index, steatosis, and serum TG in the high dose group were all decreased. The results show large doses of Sargassum decoction possess therapeutic effects on experimental fatty liver of rats.

Arthrospira maxima (Oscillatoriaceae/Arthrospira)

Torres-Durán and Paredes-Carbajal (2006), reported Wistar rats fed with 5 per cent *Arthrospira maxima* were injected a single sublethal, intraperitoneal dose of CCl_4. At 48 hours post-administration, the reduction of serum AST, and liver TG values were 2.2 and 1.4 times the control group, respectively. Free saturated fatty acids in the liver increased significantly in the treatment group and the amount of unsaturated fatty acids reduced by 50 per cent. The results show that *A. maxima* may protect CCl_4-induced liver injury by anti-oxidation mechanisms, or increase of the synthesis and release of nitric oxide.

Spirulina platensis (Oscillatoriaceae/Spirulina)

Liu *et al.* (2007) reported 98 patients treated with *Spirulina platensis* and 52 control cases using a lipid-lowering drug for 3 months. The authors found that the total effective rate for treatment of fatty liver with *Spirulina platensis* was 89.9 per cent, while the control group was 65.38 per cent, which was a statistically significant difference ($P < 0.05$). This suggests that *S. platensis* is more efficacious in the treatment of fatty liver in lowering blood lipids and improving liver function.

Whole Plants

Chinese Allium fistulosum Linn. (Liliaceae/Allium)

Zhang *et al.* (2007) fed fatty liver Sprague Dawley rats with a preparation of Chinese *Allium fistulosum* Linn (0.06, 0.12, 0.24 g/kg/d) for 8 weeks, and found that the TC, TG, NO, NOS, VEGFmRNA, and ICAM-1 values of untreated animals were significantly higher than healthy animals. The levels of TC, TG, NO, NOS, VEGFmRNA, and ICAM-1 values in the low, medium and high doses of Chinese *A. fistulosum* Linn groups and methionine choline treated groups were significantly lower than untreated animals. The results show that the preparation of Chinese *A. fistulosum* Linn has preventive and curative effect on fatty liver in rats, and its mechanism of action might be related to lipid-lowering and preventing body injury from the activity of nitrogen and cytokines.

Evening Primrose (Onagraceae/Oenothera L.)

Mao (2008) treated NAFLD patients with aerobic and Evening Primrose for 12 weeks. The serum LDL-C, TC, and TG concentrations of the treated group were significantly reduced, the HDL-C level was increased, and liver morphology was also improved. The results indicated that aerobic exercise combined with evening primrose can effectively regulate lipid metabolism and improve liver morphology in NAFLD patients.

Gynostemma pentaphyllum (Cucurbitaceae/Gynostemma)

Tan (2006) reported fatty liver Japanese white rabbits were fed with Gynostemma (5 g/d) for 8 and 12 weeks. Histological observations showed that 2/3 of the treated liver improved significantly as gynostemma has a preventive effect on hyperlipidemia in controlling TG, HDL-C, LDL-C compared to simvastatin. The authors speculated that alterations in lipid metabolism and blood rheology may be the mechanism of *G. pentaphyllum* in fatty liver prevention. The anti-hyperlipidemic effect of *G. gypenosides* has been reported elsewhere (Megalli *et al.*, 2005; Megalli *et al.*, 2006).

Artemisia capillaries (Whole Plant Extract) (Asteraceae/Artemisia spp.)

Shen *et al.* (2008) continuously administered fatty liver and insulin resistance rats with *Artemisia capillaries* (6.9, 2.3 g/kg/d) for 4 weeks. The fasting blood glucose and serum insulin levels of the high dose group were significantly lower than untreated animals, the insulin sensitivity index returned to normal ($P < 0.05$) and the SOD activity was significantly increased while the MDA content was decreased. Moreover, the TC, TG, FFA, and LDL-C levels were decreased while the HDL-C level was increased, and the activities of AST and ALT as well as the TGF-β1 levels were significantly reduced, and liver steatosis was alleviated. The results indicated *A. capillaries* extract has the effect of blood lipid regulation and liver protection in cases of insulin resistance and fatty liver. The mechanism of action may be related to increased antioxidant capacity, restoration of insulin sensitivity and reduction of TGF-β1.

Peristrophe roxburghiana [Schult.] Brem (HSX, Aqueous Extract) (Acanthaceae/Peristrophe spp.)

Liu and Lv (2006) preventively administered insulin resistance fatty liver rats with HSX (0.38, 1.14 g/kg/d i.g.) for 8 weeks. The fasting serum insulin, plasma FFA and TG levels almost returned to normal in both high and low dose groups. Additionally, HDL-C levels in plasma were increased, while ALT and AST activities, the liver index and degree of steatosis of liver tissue was decreased. Low doses of HSX increased insulin sensitivity and improved glucose tolerance.

Erigeron breviscapus [Vant.] Hand.-Mazz. (Asteraceae/Erigeron spp)

Zhan (2006) reported 83 hepatitis B patients with fatty liver disease treated with *Erigeron breviscapus* (30-40 mL i.v., daily). The results show that *E. breviscapus* can effectively reduce blood TC and TG, and improve liver function. The authors conclude that *E. breviscapus* is effective for the treatment of experimental chronic hepatitis B complicated with fatty liver.

Herba Anoectochili mxburghii [Wall.] lindl (Whole Plant Juice) (Orchidaceae/Anoectochilus spp.)

Huang and Zhu (2005) found that alcoholic liver injury ICR mice with continuous administration of Herba Anoectochili (1.0, 5.0 g/kg, 2 times a day) for 10 days saw no significant differences in ALT and AST levels among treatment group, normal group, and untreated animals. The TG level of untreated and treated animals were significantly lower than that of the normal group ($P < 0.01$), but between the two groups showed no significant difference. The extent of cell necrosis and inflammatory cell infiltration of two Herba Anoectochili treated groups were markedly less than untreated animals. The results showed that the whole plant Herba Anoectochili juice can reduce cell necrosis and inflammation in alcoholic liver injury mice.

Phyllanthus urinaria L. (Euphorbiaceae/Phyllanthus)

Zheng *et al.* (2005) treated fatty liver patients consecutively with tablet preparations of *Phyllanthus urinaria* L. (6 tabs, 3 times a day) for 30 days. 63 cases were strongly effective and 33 cases were classified as effective for a total effective rate of 94.11 per cent. The results show that *P. urinaria* L. can both improve liver function and regulate lipid metabolism in the body.

Sedum sarmentosum Bunge (SSB) (Crassulaceae/Sedum spp.)

Dai *et al.* (2004) reported on NAFLD patients with continuous administration with SSB granules (20 g orally, 3 times a day) for 2 months. The normalization rate of ALT was 57.13 per cent and for TG was 33.29 per cent and AST was decreased to (12.31 + 7.17) U/L. The results showed that SSB granules can improve liver function and reduce serum TG.

Pleurotus serotinus (Aqueous Extract of Mukitake Mushroom) (Pleurotaceae/ Pleurotus spp.)

The study of Nagao *et al.* (2010) reported that after db/db mice were administered aqueous extracts of *Pleurotus serotinus* (i.g.) for 4 weeks, the hepatomegaly, hepatic TG accumulation, and the serum markers of liver injury of the treated mice were all significantly reduced. Additionally, the insulin dependency of the mice and production of inflammatory cytokines MCP1 were significantly lowered, and *P. serotinus* appeared to be a kappaB kinase (IkappaB, IKK) inhibitor. The authors concluded that aqueous extracts of *P. serotinus* can inhibit NFkappaB-mediated inflammatory response and other symptoms of NAFLD.

Cucumis Melo Extract (Extramel®) (Cucurbitaceae/Cucumis L.)

The investigation of Dédordé *et al.* (2010) observed hamsters administered Cucumis melo extract Extramel® (0.7, 2.8, 5.6 mg/d, i.g.) for 12 weeks. Their plasma cholesterol lowered, and SOD activity in blood and liver was induced to increase. The liver lipid profiles of the aorta and heart were significantly decreased and the development of hepatic steatosis was attenuated. The results suggested that long-term consumption Cucumis melo extract can prevent atherosclerosis and fatty liver.

Picroliv (PIC) (Indian Picrorhiza kurroa extract) (Scrophulariaceae/Picrorhiza spp)

Vivikanandan *et al.* (2007) reported that the administration of Indian PIC (50 mg/kg, i.g.) can significantly reduce TG, CHO, FFA, TL, PL of the hydrazine-induced hyperlipidemia in rats and increase the mobility of adipose tissue.

Bulbus Allii Caespitosi Extract (Liliaceae/Allium)

Shi *et al.* (2009) investigated the influence of extract of Bulbus Allii Caespitosi on NAFLD Sprague Dawley rats. Administration with dose equivalent of 41.6 g/kg crude drugs for 4 weeks, revealed that the TC, TG, ALT, AST values in the plasma of the treated rats were significantly decreased, while their PPAR-γ values were significantly increased. These indicated that extract of Bulbus Allii Caespitosi can reduce fatty liver, and prevent NAFLD in rats.

Oils

Flaxseed Oil (Linaceae/Linum spp)

Yang *et al.* (2009) found that after the hyperlipidemic-induced NAFLD hamsters were administered flaxseed oil (i.g.), the GPT, GOT and other indicators of liver damage for the treatment group were lower than those of CO and the BU groups. Liver stromal MMP-9 gene expression and activity were decreased in treatment group, but the expression and activity of MMP-2 had no significant change. The results suggested that the symptoms of hyperlipidemia-induced NAFLD can be alleviated by feeding linseed oil to hamsters, and may be more effective than soy (Bhathena *et al.*, 2003).

Garlic Oil (Liliaceae/Allium)

The study of Zeng *et al.* (2008) discovered that when fatty liver mice were fed with garlic oil (50, 100, 200 mg/kg/d, i.g.), their MDA levels were reduced in a dose-dependent manner, GSH levels were restored and the activities of SOD, GR and GST were enhanced. The authors theorize that garlic oil can prevent and treat acute AFLD, if taken prophylactically, and the mechanism of action is associated with antioxidant activity. Wang *et al.* (2007) examined the protective effect of garlic oil in carbon tetrachloride induced NAFLD rats, and the garlic oil significantly reduced markers of fatty liver. Similar results have been reported using garlic mash diet (Bao and Wu, 2007).

Pine Nut Oil (Pinaceae/Pinus spp.)

Ferramosca *et al.* (2008) fed mice with 7.5 per cent of supplemental pine nut oil (i.g.) for 8 weeks. The CLA induces weight loss whereas the CLA side effects of fatty liver and hyperinsulinemia was avoided with concomitant administration of pine nut oil. These results showed that pine nut oil may aid controlling fatty liver.

Olive Oil (Oleaceae/Olea)

Hussein *et al.* (2007) studied 32 Sprague Dawley rats on a methionine choline-deficient diet (MCDD) enriched with olive oil. After 2 months, the increase in hepatic TG levels was blunted by 30 per cent in MCDD with olive oil group compared with controls. The authors concluded that olive oil decreases the accumulation of triglyceride in the liver of rats with NAFLD. Hernández *et al.* (2005) examined the effects of an olive oil enriched diet (14 per cent versus a normal 5 per cent enriched diet) on recovery from hepatic steatosis, and observed that fatty infiltration in steatotic livers decreased. The potential effects of olive oil in NAFLD has been reviewed by Assy *et al.* (2009).

Dietary Fish Oil

The experiments of Wada *et al.* (2008) discovered that feeding mice with fish oil, can reduce 73 per cent of the incidence of ethanol-induced fatty liver and reduce SREBP-1c activity while increasing PPAR-a activity of the treated mice. The levels of DGAT1, DGAT2, ChREBP, LPK, and PPAR-γ mRNAs were all elevated. The authors suggest that preventively feeding fish oil can reduce the activity of SREBP-1c, which may control the occurrence of AFLD.

Animal and Fungal Preparations

Silkworm Chrysalis Oil (Pupa Microwave Extract) (Saturniidae/Bombyx L.)

He *et al.* (2007) reported oral administration of Chrysalis oil to Sprague Dawley rats in various doses (for prevention and treatment) for 5 to 9 weeks. The liver weight index, liver TG, TC and MDA of the prevention group, of the treatment group and of the positive control (evening primrose oil) group were significantly lower than those of the control group ($P<0.05$) in a dose-dependent manner. The results suggest that silkworm chrysalis oil has a preventive and treatment effect on NAFLD, which is more effective than evening primrose oil.

China Oak Silkworm Liquid (Male Tussah Moth Extract of Whole Insects) (Saturniidae/Antheraea Genus)

Jia *et al.* (2007) gave NAFLD mice oral China oak silkworm liquid (0.12 mL/10g) for 4 weeks. The hepatic steatosis of treated mice was milder compared with untreated mice, while the low dose group treatment was more effective. The MDA concentration in liver mitochondria and the ALT and AST activities in the low-dose group were decreased whereas the SOD activity increased, but those in the high-dose group and untreated animals showed no significant difference.

Bovine Fetal Liver Extract (Bovidae/Bos. L.)

Li *et al.* (2007) administered NAFLD Sprague Dawley rats with Bovine fetal liver (15, 24, 40 mg/kg/d) orally for 16 weeks. They found that the body weight of the high-dose group was significantly decreased, and liver weights of each dose group were reduced, liver index (liver weight/body weight × 100 per cent) in the large and medium dose groups were decreased, and the TG, TC contents were also lowered. The authors concluded that bovine fetal liver extract has a positive effect on NAFLD.

Lecithin

Liu *et al.* (2005) studied lecithin treatment (lecithin 0.1 g, 4 tablets 3 times a day) on 75 NAFLD patients. Three months after treatment, the efficiency rate was 89.3 per cent, while all of the TG, TC, ALT and γ - serum glutamine glutamyl (γ-GT) were lowered. The results implied that lecithin can improve liver function, blood lipid, B-mode ultrasonic images and the clinical symptoms, and no obvious adverse reactions were observed. Lecithin is also known to decrease hepatic steatosis in long-term total parenteral nutrition (Buchman *et al.*, 1992). Consequently, lecithin has potential as a clinical treatment of choice in NAFLD.

Seal Oil (Otariidae/Arctocephalus)

Zhu *et al.* (2008) found that after the NAFLD patients were administered seal oil (2 g, 3 times a day) for 24 weeks, their body weight, fasting blood glucose (FBG), renal function, blood cells were all unchanged. However, their ALT, TG values and total symptom scores were decreased, while the AST, GGT, HDL, TCHO values of the tested patients having treatment or placebo were improved. The LDL content was only improved in the seal oil treated patients. About 20 per cent of patients were cured, while 53.0 per cent of them responders were classified as effective, and no serious side effects were found during the treatment. The author noted that seal oil rich in n-3 polyunsaturated fatty acids is safe and proved to be an effective treatment of patients with NAFLD.

Mortierella isabellina (Lipid Extract of Mildew Fungus Mortierella) (Mortierellaceae/Mortierella Genus)

Zhang *et al.* (2004) administered NAFLD Wistar rats with *Mortierella isabellina* extract orally for 12 weeks. The levels of blood lipids, liver lipids, superoxide dismutase (SOD) were increased in the treatment group compared with untreated animals, while the transaminases, and malondialdehyde (MDA) decreased significantly in the treatment group. The authors suggested that *M. isabellina* extract can prevent both high blood cholesterol and fat deposition in the liver.

Cordyceps sinensis (Clavicipitaceae/Cordyceps spp)

Wang and Wang (2008) fed AFLD Sprague Dawley rats with *Cordyceps sinensis*, and the AST, ALT, TC, TG levels in the serum of the treatment mice were significantly reduced compared to controls. The authors theorized that *C. sinensis* is effective in the treatment of AFLD.

Leptin

Canbakan *et al.* (2008) studied 52 NAFLD patients to investigate whether serum leptin levels correlate with insulin resistance, oxidative stress parameters and the severity of histological changes in NAFLD. The results showed that there was no apparent association among serum leptin, fasting insulin levels, and oxidative stress parameters. No association between the severity of histological changes and serum leptin levels could be found either. A 6-month follow-up research showed ALT and AST were significantly decreased in the NASH group with elevated leptin levels. The authors suggest that leptin can prevent progressive liver injury in NAFLD.

Interleukin-10 (IL-10)

den Boer *et al.* (2006) investigated the protective role of endogenous IL-10 in the development of diet-induced insulin resistance. IL-10 (-/-) mice and wild-type (WT) mice were fed high-fat food for 6 weeks and the plasma free fatty acid content of the IL-10 (-/-) group of mice after overnight fasting increased by 75 per cent compared with WT group and the TG by 54 per cent in IL-10 (-/-) group mice. However, no differences could be observed in whole-body or hepatic insulin sensitivity between IL-10 (-/-) and WT groups during a hyperinsulinemic euglycemic clamp. These results suggest that during high-fat feeding, basal IL-10 production may prevent the hepatic steatosis but does not improve liver pathology and insulin sensitivity.

Krill Oil (KO) (Euphausiidae/Euphausia)

Tandy *et al.* (2009) investigated the effects of dietary KO on cardiometabolic risk factors in male C57BL/6 mice fed a high-fat diet. The mice were fed a 1.25 wt per cent, 2.5 wt per cent, 5.0 wt per cent krill oil diet and the results showed that their liver weight and liver fat were significantly reduced due to a dose-dependent decrease in hepatic TG. Serum cholesterol and blood glucose were also reduced while serum adiponectin was markedly elevated in treated mice. The results indicated that krill oil dietary supplements can effectively reduce blood sugar, high fat and improve metabolic parameters, and may be effective in the metabolic syndrome of NAFLD.

Summary and Future Directions

The previous pages describe recent progress in the treatment of Fatty Liver Disease using phytochemicals and natural products. To date, tremendous progress has been made by researchers particularly in China, but also in many other countries. However, it should be mentioned that the review was not intended to be exhaustive, as not all phytochemicals used to treat FLD were covered in this review (*e.g.*, *Gymnema sylvestre* and *Gymnema montanum* (gurmar) herb, *Vaccinium ashei* (Asian Rabbiteye blueberry) leaves, *Schisandra chinensis* (five flavor berry) fruit, *Glycyrrhiza glabra* (licorice) root, *Vitis coignetiae* (crimson glory vine) leaves, *Teuerium polium* and *Teucrium chamaedrys* (germander) root (Yarnell *et al.,* 2010). The approach to treating Fatty Liver Disease in Traditional Chinese Medicine versus Western medicine although different, need not be viewed separately. An integrated approach combining the best of both Western and Eastern medicine seems to be the best course of action for clinical practitioners. The basic principles in the etiology and pathogenesis of Fatty Liver Disease is an unfavorable diet, but may also include emotional mood based disorders manifesting in asthenia and eventual hepatic injury. Therefore, although the disease is expressed by the liver, tight relationships are believed to exist between all the major organs such as the spleen and kidney (Liu *et al.,* 2004). Based on this, TCM physicians treat FLD using complex prescriptions of multiple components directed at rebalancing various "energy blockages" impeding normal physiologic function. As such the focus in TCM is not on the individual active entities involved, but rather the overall clinical and pharmacodynamic response to a combination of natural products (Jiang, 2005).

From the natural products reviewed here, it becomes apparent that crude preparations of single herbs (active chemical species unknown) still represent the majority of investigative research into natural product activity in FLD, especially in China. Many other countries are still biased towards western medicine, or at best, an integrative approach (Yu and Zhao, 2007). As such, there remains much enthusiasm on identifying the active chemical species in herbal decoctions, and delineating the biochemical mechanism(s) involved. Despite these differences in philosophy, the abundance of research supports clinical utilization of natural medicines against FLD. Bringing together the natural products currently showing promise into a comprehensive review as in this chapter, draws attention to a number of viewpoints worth mentioning. Natural medicines utilized in TCM have a unique advantage of a long history of use and clinical outcomes. In the future, evidence-based research on classical "folk medicines" could bring such natural medicines into a competitive marketplace, improving worldwide treatment of FLD patients, and overall health-care. Some crude preparation are appropriate for development into their 'active' chemical entities, as this could potentially reduce adverse side effects, and improve patient compliance due to unfavorable organoleptic (*e.g.*, taste and smell) properties of many phytochemicals. However readers are reminded that there is often synergism between diverse chemical species in herbal extracts (Yuan and Lin, 2000), and attempts to isolate the most effective chemical structures is not always successful. Nonetheless, the separation and characterization of individual chemicals, remains an important aspect in the current modernization of Traditional Chinese Medicine, and controlling the quality of products from multiple manufacturers. Using chemometric methods (such as principle component analysis) researchers are able to evaluate complex preparations on multiple molecular targets due to advances in separation science (Liang *et al.*, 2008; Zhang *et al.*, 2008). Such technologies fail to bridge the gap between the holistic approach of TCM and single target indications, such as ALD, AFLD, NAFLD, and NASH in western therapeutics (Chan *et al.*, 2010).

It is suggested that researchers take full advantage of the well-developed FLD animal models currently in use, to cross-screen active fractions or single natural products. Most of the new anti-FLD drug applications in China are still on the complex preparations (Class XI New TCM Drug) in lieu of active single compounds (Class I New TCM Drug). This may be in part due to a higher burden in proving to the Chinese SDFA (State Food and Drug Administration) whether the safety, efficacy and quality control of the single chemical entities is/are favorable compared to crude extracts. Moreover, scientists and practitioners are encouraged to invest in preclinical studies on the pathologic and histologic observations of liver tissue, which is expected to reduce risk of toxicity during clinical trials. The Chinese SFDA also recommends investigators observe the current monographed anti-FLD drugs (and those in clinical trials) for their toxicological status during the course of long-term treatment in FLD cases.

Although there are natural products that show promise against FLD, currently, no drugs have been proven safe and efficacious in the treatment of FLD. This is likely due in part to the complex syndrome of insulin resistance confounding symptoms of fatty liver. As such, concerted interventions with liver-protective agents, lipid-lowering drugs, and drugs with promote glucose tolerance is the trend in FLD therapy. The successful development of drugs to prevent and treat FLD may depend on an ongoing commitment to designing novel compounds based on phytochemicals which show potential in the fight against fatty liver.

Acknowledgements

The authors thank Yunnan Province Project (Lead high-level personnel training project No. 2009CI121), Key Industries Innovation Project of Yunnan Science and Technology Department (Modernization of Chinese Technology Industry Base Construction in Yunnan Province No. 2008IF012) and Program for Innovative Research Team (in Science and Technology) in University of Yunnan Province (IRTSTYN, 2010-11) and Program for Yunnan Innovative Research Team.

References

Abdelmalek, M.F., Sanderson, S.O., Angulo, P., Soldevila-Pico, C., Liu, C., Peter, J., Keach, J., Cave, M., Chen, T., McClain, C.J., and Lindor, K.D. (2009). Betaine for nonalcoholic fatty liver disease: results of a randomized placebo-controlled trial. *Hepatology*, **50**(6): 1818-1826.

Adams, L.A., and Angulo, P. (2006). Treatment of non-alcoholic fatty liver disease. *British Medical Journal*, **82**(967): 315-322.

Adams, L.A., Zein, C.O., Angulo, P., and Lindor, K.D. (2004). A pilot trial of pentoxifylline in non-alcoholic steatohepatitis. *The American Journal of Gastroenterology*, **99**(12): 2365-2368.

Ahmed, M.H., and Byrne, C.D. (2009). Current treatment of non-alcoholic fatty liver disease. *Diabetes, Obesity and Metabolism*, **11**(3): 188-195.

Ajmo, J.M., Liang, X., Rogers, C.Q., Pennock, B., and You, M. (2008). Resveratrol alleviates alcoholic fatty liver in mice. *American Journal of Physiology-Gastrointestinal and Liver Physiology*, **295**(4): G833-G842.

Angulo, P. (2007). GI epidemiology: nonalcoholic fatty liver disease. *Alimentary Pharmacology and Therapeutics*, **25**(8): 883-889.

Antonopoulos, S., Mikros, S., Mylonopoulou, M., Kokkoris, S., and Giannoulis, G. (2006). Rosuvastatin as a novel treatment of non-alcoholic fatty liver disease in hyperlipidemic patients. *Atherosclerosis*, **184**(1): 233-234.

Assy, N., Nassar, F., Nasser, G., and Grosovski, M. (2009). Olive oil consumption and non-alcoholic fatty liver disease. *World Journal of Gastroenterology*, **15**(15): 1809-1815.

Bai, M., Ren, M., and Liu, Z. (2009). Clinical observation on berberine treating non-alcoholic fatty liver disease. *ChongQing Medical Journal*, **38**(10): 1215-1216, and 1218.

Bao, B., and Wu, W.-H. (2007). Prevention of non-alcoholic fatty liver by garlic diet in rats. *Food Science*, **28**(9): 505-509.

Barak, A.J, Beckenhauer, H.C., Badakhsh, S., and Tuma, D.J. (1997). The effect of betaine in reversing alcoholic steatosis. *Alcoholism: Clinical and Experimental Research*, **21**(6): 1100-1102.

Barak, A.J, Beckenhauer, H.C., Badakhsh, S., and Tuma, D.J. (1993). Dietary betaine promotes generation of hepatic S-adenosylmethionine and protects the liver from ethanol-induced fatty infiltration. *Alcoholism: Clinical and Experimental Research*, **17**(3): 552-555.

Basaranoglu, M., and Neuschwander-Tetri, B. (2006). Non-alcoholic fatty liver disease: clinical features and pathogenesis. *Gastroenterology and Hepatology*, **2**(4): 282-291.

Basaranoglu, M., Acbay, O., and Sonsuz, A. (1999). A controlled trial of gemfibrozil in the treatment of patients with nonalcoholic steatohepatitis. *Journal of Hepatology*, **31**(2): 384.

Belfort, R., Harrison, S.A., Brown, K., Darland, C., Finch, J., Hardies, J., Balas, B., Gastaldelli, A., Tio, F., Pulcini, J., Berria, R., Ma, J.Z., Dwivedi, S., Havranek, R., Fincke, C., DeFronzo, R., Bannayan, G.A., Schenker, S., and Cusi, K. (2006). A placebo-controlled trial of pioglitazone in subjects with non-alcoholic steatohepatitis. *New England Journal of Medicine*, **355**(22): 2297-2307.

Bellentani, S., Bedogn, G., Miglioli, L., and Tiribelli, C. (2004). The epidemiology of fatty liver. *European Journal of Gastroenterology*, **16**(11): 1087-1093.

Berger, J., and Kowdley, K. (2003). Is silymarin hepatoprotective in alcoholic liver disease? *Journal of Clinical Gastroenterology*, **37**(4): 278-279.

Bhathena, S.J., Ali, A.A., Haudenschild, C., Latham, P., Ranich, T., Mohamed, A.I., Hansen, C.T., and Velasquez, M.T. (2003). Dietary flaxseed meal is more protective than soy protein concentrate against hypertriglyceridemia and steatosis of the liver in an animal model of obesity. *Journal of American College of Nutrition*. **22**(2): 157-164.

Bose, M., Lambert, J.D., Ju, J., Reuhl, K.R., Shapses, S.A., and Yang, C.S. (2008). The major green tea polyphenol,(-)-epigallocatechin-3-gallate, inhibits obesity, metabolic syndrome, and fatty liver disease in high-fat-fed mice. *Journal of Nutrition*, **138**(9): 1677-1683.

Botella-Carretero, J.I., Balsa, J.A., Vázquez, C., Peromingo, R., Díaz-Enriquez, M., and Escobar-Morreale, H.F. (2010). Retinol and alpha-tocopherol in morbid obesity and nonalcoholic fatty liver disease. *Obesity Surgery*, **20**(1): 69-76.

Brackett, D., Droke, E., Lerner, M., Gusev, Y., Lightfoot, S., Postier, R., Bronze, M., and Smith, B. (2006). Gene expression profile alterations and hepatic steatosis induced by chronic inflammation are prevented by soy isoflavones. *Shock*, **25**(6): 43-44.

Brignon, J., and Wolff, R. (1956). Effect of betaine on hepatic steatosis of dietary origin in the rat. *Comptes Rendus des Séances de la Société de Biologie et de Ses Filiales*, **150**(5): 1001-1004.

Bruno, R., Dugan, C.E., Smyth, J.A., DiNatale, D.A., and Koo, S.I. (2008). Green tea extract protects leptin-deficient, spontaneously obese mice from hepatic steatosis and injury. *Journal of Nutrition*, **138**(2): 323-331.

Brunt, E.M. (2010). Pathology of nonalcoholic fatty liver disease. *Nature Reviews Gastroenterology and Hepatology*. **7**(4): 195-203.

Buchman, A.L., Dubin, M., Jenden, D., Moukarzel, A., Roch, M.H., Rice, K., Gornbein, J., Ament, M.E., and Eckhert, C.D. (1992). Lecithin increases plasma free choline and decreases hepatic steatosis in long-term total parenteral nutrition patients. *Gastroenterology*, **102**: 1363-1370.

Bujanda, L., Hijona, E., Larzabal, M., Beraza, M., Aldazabal, P., García-Urkia, N., Sarasqueta, C., Cosme, A., Irastorza, B., González, A., and Arenas, J.I. Jr. (2008). Resveratrol inhibits nonalcoholic fatty liver disease in rats. *BMC Gastroenterology*. **8**: 40.

Cai, D., Chen, Z., Yan, M., He, B., and Xiang, B. (2007). Effect of *Panax Notogenseng* on the COX-2 expression in liver of rats with alcoholic fatty liver. *Chinese Archives of Traditional Chinese Medicine*, **25**: 1391-1393.

Canbakan, B., Tahan, V., Balci, H., Hatemi, I., Erer, B., Ozbay, G., Sut, N., Hacibekiroglu, M., Imeryuz, N., and Senturk, H. (2008). Leptin in nonalcoholic fatty liver disease. *Annals of Hepatology*, **7**(3): 249-254.

Cankurtaran, M., Kav, T., Yavuz, B., Shorbagi, A., Halil, M., Coskun, T., and Arslan, S. (2006). Serum vitamin-E levels and its relation to clinical features in nonalcoholic fatty liver disease with elevated ALT levels. *Acta Gastro-Enterologica Belgica*, **69**(1): 5-11.

Cao, Y. (2005). The investigation of the effect of Passepartout injection on fatty liver patients. *Journal of Liaoning College of TCM*, **7**: 245.

Cha, J., Jun, B., and Cho, Y. (2004). Prevention of orotic acid-induced fatty liver in rats by capsaicin. *Food Science and Biotechnology*, **13**(5): 597-602.

Chan, E., Tan, M., Xin, J., Sudarsanam, S., and Johnson, D.E. (2010). Interactions between traditional Chinese medicines and Western therapeutics. *Current Opinion in Drug Discovery and Development*, **13**(1): 50-65.

Chang, X.,Yan, H., Fei, J., Jiang, M., Zhu, H., Lu, D., and Gao, X. (2010). Berberine reduces methylation of the MTTP promoter and alleviates fatty liver induced by a high-fat diet in rats. *The Journal of Lipid Research*, **51**(9): 2504-2515.

Charlton, M., Sreekumar, R., Rasmussen, D., Lindor, K., and Nair, K.S. (2002). Apolipoprotein synthesis in nonalcoholic steatohepatitis. *Hepatology*, **35**(4): 898-904.

Clark, J.M. (2006). Weight loss as a treatment for nonalcoholic fatty liver disease. *Journal of Clinical Gastroenterology*, **40**: S39-S43.

Chen, J., Ma, M., Lu, Y., Wang, L., Wu, C., and Duan, H. (2009). Rhaponticin from rhubarb rhizomes alleviates liver steatosis and improves blood glucose and lipid profiles in KK/Ay diabetic mice. *Planta Medica*, **75**(5): 472-477.

Chen, S.-W., Chen, Y.-X., Zhang, X.-R., Zeng, X., Liu, S., and Xie, W.-F. (2006). The prevention and therapeutic effect of taurine on experimental rat nonalcoholic fatty livers. *Zhonghua ganzangbing zazhi = Chinese Journal of Hepatology*, **14**(3): 226-227.

Chen, X., Sebastian, B.M., Tang, H., McMullen, M.M., Axhemi, A., Jacobsen, D.W., and Nagy, L.E. (2009). Taurine supplementation prevents ethanol-induced decrease in serum adiponectin and reduces hepatic steatosis in rats. *Hepatology*, **49**(5): 1554-1562.

Chen, Y., Liu, S., Zeng, X., and Xie, W. (2005). A pilot study of the effect of taurine on patients with nonalcoholic fatty liver. *Chinese Journal of Practical Internal Medicine*, **25**(3): 249-250.

Chen, Z., Wen, X.,Yan M., and He, B. (2009). Effect of total flavones of hawthorn leafon (TFHL) on expression of UCP2 in liver of NASH rats. *China Journal of Chinese Materia Medica*, **34**(24): 3272-3276.

Cheng, R., Ye, X., Zhang, L., Ren, Y., and Wang, Y. (2004). Study on preventive effect of betaine on experimental hyperlipidemia and fatty liver in mice. *China Pharmacist*, **6**: 411-413.

Dai. (2007). *Tonkinensis liquid treatment of fatty liver.* Popular Medicine, **4**: 58.

Dai, Z., Gu, X., and Wu, Y. (2004). Therapeutic effects of sarmentosum and glycyrrhiza decoction and sarmentosum medicinal granule for non-alcohol steatosis hepatitis. *World Journal of Infection*, **3**: 403-404.

Décordé, K., Ventura, E., Lacan, D., Ramos, J., Cristol, J.P., and Rouanet, J.M. (2010). An SOD rich melon extract Extramel® prevents aortic lipids and liver steatosis in diet-induced model of atherosclerosis. *Nutrition, Metabolism and Cardiovascular Diseases*, **20**: 301-307.

den Boer, M.A.M., Voshol, P.J., Schröder-van der Elst, J.P., Korsheninnikova, E., Ouwens, D.M., Kuipers, F., Havekes, L.M., and Romijn, J.A. (2006). Endogenous interleukin-10 protects against hepatic steatosis but does not improve insulin sensitivity during high-fat feeding in mice. *Endocrinology*, **147**(10): 4553-4558.

Deng, C., He, X., Sheng, X.Y., Li, X., Long, H., Wang, M., and Chen, F. (2003). The investigation of the effect of polydextrose on steatohepatitis induced by high fat diet and carbon tetrachloride in Wistar rats. *Chinese Journal of Clinical Medicine Practice*, **2**: 615-616.

Ding, G., Wang, B., and Chen, L. (2005). The influence of adding Danshensu and ursodeoxycholic acid on glucose metabolism in liver cells of fatty liver. *World Chinese Journal of Digestology*, **13**: 1907-1909.

Ding, K., Wu, Y., and Pu, Z. (2007). Recent research on fatty liver by Traditional Chinese Medicine. *Lishizhen Medicine and Materia Medica Research*, **18**: 1776-1778.

Ding, W., and Fan, J. (2009). Current pharmacologic treatment of nonalcoholic fatty liver disease. *Chinese Journal of Gastroenterology*, **14**(007): 442-445.

DiNatale, D., DiNatale, D.A., Park, H.J., Chung, M.-Y., Koo, S., and Bruno, R. (2009). Green tea extract (GTE) protects against nonalcoholic fatty liver disease (NAFLD) in obese mice by decreasing liver injury and improving enzymatic antioxidant defenses. The *FASEB Journal*, **23**(1_MeetingAbstracts): 718.5.

Dowman, J.K., Tomlinson, J.W., and Newsome, P.N. (2010). Pathogenesis of non-alcoholic fatty liver disease. *QJM: An International Journal of Medicine*, **103**(2): 71-83.

Du, X., and Li, X. (2007). Clinical studies of silymarin treatment of fatty liver disease. *Journal of Shandong University of TCM*, **31**: 135-136.

Dufour, J.F., Oneta, C.M, Gonvers, J.J., Bihl, F., Cerny, A., Cereda, J.M., Zala, J.F., Helbling, B., Steuerwald, M., and Zimmermann, A. (2006). Randomized placebo-controlled trial of ursodeoxycholic acid with vitamin e in nonalcoholic steatohepatitis. *Clinical Gastroenterology and Hepatology*, **4**(12): 1537-1543.

Fan, J., Qian, Y., Zheng, X., Cai, X., and Lu, Y. (2006). Effects of pentoxifylline on hepatic nuclear factor-kappa B signaling pathway and insulin resistance in nonalcoholic steatohepatitis rats induced by fat-rich diet. Chinese Journal of Hepatology = *Zhonghua Gan Zang Bing Za Zhi*, **14**(10): 762-766.

Feldstein, A.E., Werneburg, N.W., Canbay, A., Guicciardi, M.E., Bronk, S.F., Rydzewski, R., Burgart, L.J., and Gores, G.J. (2004). Free fatty acids promote hepatic lipotoxicity by stimulating TNF-alpha expression via a lysosomal pathway. *Hepatology*, **40**(1): 185-194.

Fehér, J., and Lengyel, G. (2009). Silymarin in the treatment of chronic liver diseases: past and future. *Clinical and Experimental Medical Journal*, **3**(3): 403-413.

Ferraro, S., and López-Ortega, A. (2008). Antioxidant activity of melatonin on fatty liver induced by ethionine in mice. *Archivos de Medicina Veterinaria*, **40**: 51-57.

Ferramosca, A., Savy, V., Conte, L., and Zara, V. (2008). Dietary combination of conjugated linoleic acid (CLA) and pine nut oil prevents CLA-induced fatty liver in mice. *Journal of Agricutural and Food Chemistry*, **56**(17): 8148-8158.

Fiorini, R.N., Donovan, J.L., Rodwell, D., Evans, Z., Cheng, G., May, H.D., Milliken, C.E., Markowitz, J.S., Campbell, C., Haines, J.K., Schmidt, M.G., and Chavin, K.D. (2005). Short-term administration of (-)-epigallocatechin gallate reduces hepatic steatosis and protects against warm hepatic ischemia / reperfusion injury in steatotic mice. *Liver Transplantation*, **11**(3): 298-308.

Fu, J., Liang, L., and Wang, C. (2005). Intervention effects of cucurbitacin and vitamin E on fatty liver in obese children. *Zhejiang Journal of Preventive Medicine*, **17**: 46–48.

Gao, Y., Luo, L., Wang, Y., Xia, D., and Hong, X. (2005). Antilipidemic effect of polysaccharides extracted from sweet potato vines. *Food Science*, **26**: 197-201.

Ge, B., Xie, M., Gu, Z., Qian, P., Zhou, W., and Guo, C. (2009). Therapeutic effect of epigallocatechin gallate on hyperlipidemic fatty liver in rats. *Chinese Pharmacological Bulletin*, **25**: 510-514.

Gudbrandsen, O.A., Wergedahl, H., Mørk, S., Liaset, B., Espe, M., and Berge, R.K. (2007). Dietary soya protein concentrate enriched with isoflavones reduced fatty liver, increased hepatic fatty acid oxidation and decreased the hepatic mRNA level of VLDL receptor in obese Zucker rats. *British Journal of Nutrition*, **96**(02): 249-257.

Guo, H.-X., Liu, D.-H., Ma, Y., Liu, J.-F., Wang, Y., Du, Z.-Y., Wang, X., Shen, J.-K., and Peng, H.-L. (2009). Long-term baicalin administration ameliorates metabolic disorders and hepatic steatosis in rats given a high-fat diet. *Acta Pharmacologica Sinica*, **30**(11): 1505-1512.

Guo, J., Liao, H., Pan, J., Ye, B., Jian, X., Wei, D., and Dai. L. (2005). Study on the mechanism of mitchi saponin in improving action of insulin resistance in rats with hyper-lipemia-hepar adiposum. *China Pharmacy*, **16**: 732-734.

Gu, S. and Jiang, H.-L. (2007a). Effect and mechanism of *Lycium barbarum* polysaccharide on rat of alcoholic fatty liver. *Chongqing Medicine*, **36**(1): 60-62.

Gu, S., and Jiang, R. (2007b). Action mechanism of *Lycium barbarum* polysaccharide in the prevention and treatment of alcoholic fatty liver in rats. *China Pharmacy*, **18**(21): 1606-1610.

Gu, S., Wang, P.L., and Jiang, R. (2007c). A study on the preventive effect of *Lycium barbarum* polysaccharide on the development of alcoholic fatty liver in rats and its possible mechanisms. *Zhonghua Gan Zang Bing Za Zhi = Chinese Journal of Hepatology*, **15**(3): 204-208.

Gu, X., Xie, Z., Wang, Q., Liu, G., Qu, Y., Zhang, L., Pan, J., Zhao, G., and Zhang, Q. (2009). Transcriptome profiling analysis reveals multiple modulatory effects of *Ginkgo biloba* extract in the liver of rats on a high-fat diet. *FEBS Journal*, **276**(5): 1450-1458.

Hamdaoui, M., Abid, Z. B., Akrem, J., and Jaafoura, H. (2008). Influence of long-term treatment with a green tea (*Camellia sinensis*) decoction with or without citrus juice on liver steatosis and some plasma variables in the elderly rat. *Proceedings of the Nutrition Society*, **67**(OCE5), E195.

Han, T., Jing, Y., Wu, J., and Dong Y. (2008). Advanced and recent research of alcoholic fatty liver. *Chinese Journal of Gastroenterology and Hepatology*, **17**(10): 862-866.

Harach, T., Aprikian, O., Monnard, I., Moulin, J., Membrez, M., Béolor, J.C., Raab, T., Macé, K., and Darimont, C. (2010). Rosemary (*Rosmarinus officinalis* L.) leaf extract limits weight gain and liver steatosis in mice fed a high-fat diet. *Planta Medica*, **76**(6): 566-571.

Harari, A., Harats, D., Marko, D., Cohen, H., Barshack, I., Kamari, Y., Gonen, A., Gerber, Y., Ben-Amotz, A., and Shaish, A. (2008). A 9-cis {beta}-carotene-enriched diet inhibits atherogenesis and fatty liver formation in LDL receptor knockout mice. *Journal of Nutrition*, **138**(10): 1923-1930.

Harrison, S.A., Torgerson, S., Hayashi, P., Ward, J., and Schenker, S. (2003). Vitamins E and C treatment improves fibrosis in patients with nonalcoholic steatohepatitis. *American Journal of Gastroenterology*, **98**(11): 2485-2490.

Hashemi, S.J., Hajiani, E., Haidari S.E., and Eskandar H. (2009). A placebo-controlled trial of Silymarin in patients with nonalcoholic fatty liver disease. *Hepatitis Monthly*, **9**(4): 265-270.

He, F., Xia, Y., Li, F., Sun, H., Xu, Z., Peng, Q., Peng, K., and Yang, Y. (2007). Investigation of tripterygium glycosides inhibits the formation of fatty liver in hyperlipidemic NAFLD male New Zealand white rabbit. *Chinese Journal of Arteriosclerosis*, **15**: 561-562.

He, Z.L., Chen, W.P., and Shan, W. (2007). The effects of chrysalis oil on the formation of nonalcoholic steatohepatitis. *Chinese Journal of Microecology*, **19**(6): 483-485.

Helton, W.S., Smith, R.J., Rounds, J., and Wilmore, D.W. (1990). Glutamine prevents pancreatic atrophy and fatty liver during elemental feeding. *Journal of Surgical Research*, **48**(4): 297-303.

Hernández, R., Martínez-Lara, E., Cañuelo, A., Del Moral, M.L., Blanco, S., Siles, E., Jiménez, A., Pedrosa, J.A., and Peinado, M.A. (2005). Steatosis recovery after treatment with a balanced sunflower or olive oil-based diet: involvement of perisinusoidal stellate cells. *World Journal of Gastroenterology*, **11**(47): 7480-7485.

Hong, X., Tang, H., Wu, L., and Li, L. (2006). Protective effects of the *Alisma orientalis* extract on the experimental non-alcoholic fatty liver disease. *Journal of Pharmacy and Pharmacology*, **58**(10): 1391-1398.

Hu, C., Lu, D., Sun, L., and Qin. L. (2009). The effect of ginsenosides of stem and leaf on mouse fatty liver and its mechanism. *Chinese Pharmacological Bulletin*, **25**: 663-667.

Hu, K., Nian, G., Yang, K., and Huang, Z. (2009). The study of therapeutical effect of total phenolic acid extracted from Oenanthe Javanica (Bl) DC on non-alcoholic fatty liver in rats. *Pharmaceutical Journal of Chinese People's Liberation*, **25**(1): 29-33.

Hu, Y.Y. (2007). Strengthening research of traditional Chinese medicine on fatty liver. *Zhongguo Zhong Xi Yi Jie He Za Zhi = Chinese Journal of Integrated Traditional and Western Medicine*, **27**(4): 293-294.

Hu, Y.Y (2004). To promote further study on treatment of lipoidal liver diseases with traditional Chinese medicine. *Chinese Journal of Integrated Traditional and Western Medicine = Zhongguo Zhong Xi Yi Jie He Za Zhi*, **24**(1): 12.

Huang, L., and Zhu, Q. (2005). The protection effect of Herba Anoectochilus against alcoholic liver injured ICR mice. *Journal of Fuzhou General Hospital*, **12**: 279-280.

Hubscher, S.G. (2006). Histological assessment of non-alcoholic fatty liver disease. *Histopathology*, **49**(5): 450-465.

Hussein, O., Grosovski, M., Lasri, E., Svalb, S., Ravid, U., and Assy, N. (2007). Monounsaturated fat decreases hepatic lipid content in non-alcoholic fatty liver disease in rats. *World Journal of Gastroenterology*, **13**(3): 361-368.

Ijaz, S., Winslet, M., and Seifalian, A. (2009). The effect of consecutively larger doses of L-arginine on hepatic microcirculation and tissue oxygenation in hepatic steatosis. *Microvascular Research*, **78**(2): 206-211.

Jia, Q., Zhang, W.D., Wang, C.X., and Zhang, Y.Y. (2007). The experiment of male China oak silkworm liquid's obviating function on alcoholic fatty liver in rats. *Modern Journal of Integrated Traditional Chinese and Western Medicine*, **16**(22): 3151-3153.

Jiang, Q., Ma, J., Pan, J., Li, Y., and Lian, J. (2009). Gene expressions in the adipose tissue of NAFLD rats intervened with the extracts of *Polygonum cuspidatum*. *Journal of Medical Research*, **38**(005): 54-57.

Jiang, Q.L., Pan, J.Y., Ma, J., Li, Y.Y., and Xu, B.L. (2007). Variances of leptin mRNA in the adipose tissue of NAFLD rats Intervened with the extracts of Polygonum cuspidatum compound. *Zhong Yao Cai = Journal of Chinese Medicinal*

Jiang, W. (2005). Therapeutic wisdom in traditional Chinese medicine: a perspective from modern science. *Trends in Pharmacological Sciences*, **26**(11): 558-563.

Kajikawa, S., Harada, T., Kawashima, A., Imada, K., and Mizuguchi, K. (2009). Highly purified eicosapentaenoic acid prevents the progression of hepatic steatosis by repressing monounsaturated fatty acid synthesis in high-fat/high-sucrose diet-fed mice. *Prostaglandins, Leukotrienes and Essential Fatty Acids*, **80**(4): 229-238.

Kang, J.-H., Tsuyoshi, G., Han, I.-S., Kawada, T., Kim, Y.M., and Yu, R. (2009). Dietary capsaicin reduces obesity-induced insulin resistance and hepatic steatosis in obese mice fed a high-fat diet. *Obesity*, **18**(4): 780-787.

Kanuri, G., Weber, S., Volynets, V., Spruss, A., Bischoff, S.C., and Bergheim, I. (2009). Cinnamon extract protects against acute alcohol-induced liver steatosis in mice. *Journal of Nutrition*, **139**(3): 482-487.

Kaser, S., Ebenbichler, C.F. and Tilg, H. (2010). Pharmacological and non-pharmacological treatment of non-alcoholic fatty liver disease. *International Journal of Clinical Practice*, **64**(7): 968-983.

Kathirvel, E., Morgan, K., Nandgiri, G., Sandoval, B.C., Caudill, M., Bottiglieri, T., French, S.W., and Morgan, T.R. (2010). Betaine improves non alcoholic fatty liver and associated hepatic insulin resistance: a potential mechanism for hepatoprotection by betaine. *American Journal of Physiology-Gastrointestinal and Liver Physiology*, (Doi: 10.1152/ajpgi.00249.2010)

Kaviarasan, S., Viswanathan, P., Ravichandran, M.K., and Anuradha, C.V. (2008). (-) Epigallocatechin gallate (EGCG) prevents lipid changes and collagen abnormalities in chronic ethanol-fed rats. *Toxicology Mechanisms and Methods*, **18**(5): 425-432.

Khanal, T., Choi, J.H., Hwang, Y.P., Chung, Y.C., and Jeong, H.G. (2009). Protective effects of saponins from the root of *Platycodon grandiflorum* against fatty liver in chronic ethanol feeding via the activation of AMP-dependent protein kinase. *Food and Chemical Toxicology*, **47**(11): 2749-2754.

Kim, W.S., Lee, Y.S., Cha, S.H., Jeong, H.W., Choe, S.S., Lee, M.R., Oh, G.T., Park, H.S., Lee, K.U., Lane, M.D., and Kim, J.B. (2009). Berberine improves lipid dysregulation in obesity by controlling central and peripheral AMPK activity. *American Journal of Physiology-Endocrinology And Metabolism*, **296**(4): E812-E819.

Lee, Y.-M., Sutedja, D.S., Wai, C.-T., Dan, Y.-Y., Aung, M.-O., Zhou, L., Cheng, C.-L., Wee, A., and Lim, S.-G. (2008). A randomized controlled pilot study of pentoxifylline in patients with non-alcoholic steatohepatitis (NASH). *Hepatology International*, **2**(2): 196-201.

Li, H.Z., Xu, L., Xu, G.Y., Shi, Q.J., and Yu, C.H. (2007). Intervention study of the effect of bovine fetal liver extract on non-alcoholic fatty liver rats. *Zhejiang Journal of Preventive Medicine*, **19**(3): 75-76, 80.

Li, J., and Feng, W. (2006). Experimental study into the effect of raw hawthorn fruit, alisma and zedoary in treating fatty liver and the interaction for the three herbs. *Shanxi Journal of Traditional Chinese Medicine*, **22**: 57-59.

Li, J.-M., Li, Y.-C., Kong, L.-D., and Hu, Q.-H. (2010). Curcumin inhibits hepatic protein-tyrosine phosphatase 1B and prevents hypertriglyceridemia and hepatic steatosis in fructose-fed rats. *Hepatology*, **51**(5): 1555-1566.

Li, S., Wu, W., He, C., Han, Z., and Jin, D. (2008). The protective effect of glutamine on the intestinal mucosa barrier function in non-alcoholic steatohepatitis rats. *Chinese Journal of Clinical Gastroenterology*, **20**: 241-244.

Li, Z., Deng, L., Le, J., Yan, A., and Xu, K. (2004). Therapeutic effect of ω-3 polyunsaturated fatty acids from seal oil on rat fatty liver. *Chinese Journal of Biochemical Pharmaceutics*, **25**: 324-327.

Liang, Y.Z., Yi, L.Z., and Xu. Q.S. (2008). Chemometrics and modernization of traditional Chinese medicine. *Science in China Series B: Chemistry*, **51**(8): 718-728.

Liu, F., Xie, X., Ji, Z., Duan, X., Zhao, X., and Han, D. (2007). Experimental research of the therapeutic effect of Silibinin capsule on fatty liver in rats. *The Journal of Medical Theory and Practice*, **20**(3): 251-253.

Liu, H., Li, J., Hu, C., and Wang, Y. (2009). Effect of total flavonoids of litsea coreana on lipid peroxidation and TNF-α in rats with alcoholic fatty liver. *Acta Universitatis Medicinalis Anhui*, **44**(2): 236-240.

Liu, J., Tong, Z., Zhang, Z., Wong, Y., and Ye, X. (2008). Empirical study of flavone from hawthorn biloba in preventing and treating insulin resistance and fatty liver in rats. *Journal of East China Normal University (Natural Science)*, (**6**): 127-132.

Liu, Q.-Q, Liu, X.-L., and Ma, X. (2007). Clinical effect observation of Spirulina in treatment of fatty livers. *Journal of Dali University*, **6**: 17-18.

Liu, R., Chen, L., and McClain, C. (2006). Betaine modulates high carbohydrate diet-induced fatty liver in mice. *The FASEB Journal*, **20**(4): A183.

Liu, T.H. (2004). The treatment of 34 cases of fatty liver with spleen and kidney strengthening and stasis removing. *Hebei Journal of Traditional Chinese Medicine*, **26**(11): 818.

Liu, W., Wang, Y., Duan, F., Kou, S., Sun, X., and Ma, Y. (2008). *Experimental observation of* Ginkgo leaf extract on the rats with hyperlipidemia fatty liver. *Lishizhen Medicine and Materia Medica Research*, **19**: 428-429.

Liu, Y., and Lv, J. (2006). Clinical analysis of *Erigeron breviscapus* treating patients with cerebral hemorrhage on rehabilitation phase. *Journal of Liaoning College of Traditional Chinese Medicine*, **8**: 4-6.

Liu, Y., Zhang, X.D., and Liu, J.H. (2005). Clinical effect observation of lecithin treatment of 142 NAFLD patients. *Medical Journal of National Defending Forces in North China*, **17**: 358-359.

Lu, X., Dong, L., Zhang, K., Wang, J., Gong, J., Zhang, J., and Yan, H. (2008). Observation on the therapeutic efficacy of silibinin capsules for patients with fatty liver disease. *Journal of Clinical Hepatology*, **11**: 398-400.

Luo, C., Liu, L., Wu, X., and Zhang, S. (2006). Berberine treatment of non-alcoholic fatty liver. *Medical Forum of Grass Roots = Ji Ceng Xi Xue Lun Tan (B edition)*, **10**: 533-535.

Lv, H., Deng, Y., Niu, M., and Jin, Q. (2008). Effect of long-term swimming and supplementation of soybean polypeptide on lipids metabolism during the formation of fatty liver in high-fat-diet rats. *Chinese Journal of Sports Medicine*, **27**: 575-578.

Kharbanda, K.K., Mailliard, M.E., Baldwin, C.R., Beckenhauer, H.C., Sorrell, M.F., and Tuma, D.J. (2007). Betaine attenuates alcoholic steatosis by restoring phosphatidylcholine generation via the phosphatidylethanolamine methyltransferase pathway. *Journal of Hepatology*, **46**(2): 314-321.

Kim, H., Kim, D., and Cho, H. (2007). Protective effects of Platycodi radix on alcohol-induced fatty liver. *Bioscience, Biotechnology, and Biochemistry*, **71**(6): 1550-1552.

Kim, W.S., Lee, Y.S., Cha, S.H., Jeong, H.W., Choe, S.S., Lee, M.R., Oh, G.T., Park, H.S., Lee, K.U., Lane, M.D., and Kim, J.B. (2009). Berberine improves lipid dysregulation in obesity by controlling central and peripheral AMPK activity. *American Journal of Physiology-Endocrinology And Metabolism*, **296**(4): E812-E819.

Kropácová, K., Misúrová, E., and Haková, H. (1998). Protective and therapeutic effect of silymarin on the development of latent liver damage. *Radiatsionnaia Biologiia, Radioecologiia*, **38**(3): 411-415.

Kurihara, T., Akimoto, M., Tsuchiya, M., Hashimoto, H., Ishiguro, H., Niimi, A., Maeda, A., Shigemoto, M., Yamashita, K., Yokoyama, I., Kashima, S., and Kikuchi, Y. (1997). Effects of eicosapentaenoic acid on blood rheology in rats with fatty liver. *Current Therapeutic Research*, **58**(8): 525-532.

Ma, J.-H., Zheng, X.-Z., and Liu, H.-H. (2007). The effect of lycopene on the fatty liver of hyperlipidemic quail. *Chinese Journal of Gerontology*, **27**: 730-731.

Mao, Z.-H. (2008). Effect of *Oenothera erythrosepala* Borb with aerobic exercise on serum lipid metabolism and liver histolomorph of non-alcoholic fatty liver patients. *Journal of Beijing Sport University*, **31**: 1087-1089.

Megalli, S., Davies, N.M., and Roufogalis, B.D. (2006). Anti-hyperlipidemic and hypoglycemic effects of *Gynostemma pentaphyllum* in the Zucker fatty rat. *Journal of Pharmacy and Pharmaceutical Sciences*, **9**(3): 281-291.

Megalli, S., Aktan, F., Davies, N.M., and Roufogalis, B.D. (2005). Phytopreventative anti-hyperlipidemic effects of *Gynostemma pentaphyllum* in rats. *Journal of Pharmacy and Pharmaceutical Sciences*, **8**(3): 507-515.

Na, Q., and Xie, H. (2008). Effects of panax notoginsenosides on the expression of cytochrome P450 2E1 in liver tissues in rats with nonalcoholic fatty fiver. *Journal of Clinical Hepatology*, **4**(11): 233-235.

Nagao, K., Inoue, N., Inafuku, M., Shirouchi, B., Morooka, T., Nomura, S., Nagamori, N., and Yanagita, T. (2010). Mukitake mushroom (*Panellus serotinus*) alleviates nonalcoholic fatty liver disease through the suppression of monocyte chemoattractant protein 1 production in db/db mice. *The Journal of Nutritional Biochemistry*, **21**: 418-423.

Nakanishi, T., Oikawa, D., Koutoku, T., Hirakawa, H., Kido, Y., Tachibana, T., and Furuse, M. (2004). Gamma-linolenic acid prevents conjugated linoleic acid-induced fatty liver in mice. *Nutrition (Burbank, Los Angeles County, Calif.)*, **20**(4): 390-393.

Namikawa, C., Zhang, S.-P., Vyselaar, J.R., Nozaki, Y., Nemoto, Y., Ono, M., Akisawa, N., Saibara, T., Hiroi, M., Enzan, H., and Onishi, S. (2004). Polymorphisms of microsomal triglyceride transfer protein gene and manganese superoxide dismutase gene in non-alcoholic steatohepatitis. *Journal of Hepatology*, **40**(5): 781-786.

Noto, A., Zahradka, P., Yurkova, N., Xie, X., Nitschmann, E., Ogborn, M., and Taylor, C.G. (2006). Conjugated linoleic acid reduces hepatic steatosis, improves liver function, and favorably modifies lipid metabolism in obese insulin-resistant rats. *Lipids*, **41**(2): 179-188.

Oikawa, D., Tsuyama, S., Akimoto, Y., Mizobe, Y., and Furuse, M. (2008). Arachidonic acid prevents fatty liver induced by conjugated linoleic acid in mice. *British Journal of Nutrition*, **101**(10): 1558-1563.

Omagari, K., Kato, S., Tsuneyama, K., Hatta, H., Sato, M., Hamasaki, M., Sadakane, Y., Tashiro, T., Fukuhata, M., Miyata, Y., Tamaru, S., Tanaka, K., and Mune, M. (2010). Olive leaf extract prevents spontaneous occurrence of non-alcoholic steatohepatitis in SHR/NDmcr-cp rats. *Pathology*, **42**(1): 66-72.

Pan, L. (2005). The effect of different kinds of teas and green tea polyphenol on fatty liver in rats fed high-fat diet. *Pharmacology and Clinics of Chinese Materia Medica*, **21**: 24-25.

Pan, M., Song, Y.-L., Xu, J.-M., and Gan, H.-Z. (2006). Melatonin ameliorates nonalcoholic fatty liver induced by high-fat diet in rats. *Journal of Pineal Research*, **41**(1): 79-84.

Park, H.J., Dinatale, D.A., Chung, M.Y., Park, Y.K., Lee, J.Y., Koo, S.I., O'Connor, M., Manautou, J.E., and Bruno, R.S. (2010). Green tea extract attenuates hepatic steatosis by decreasing adipose lipogenesis and enhancing hepatic antioxidant defenses in ob/ob mice. *The Journal of Nutritional Biochemistry*, (DOI: 10.1016/j.jnutbio.2010.03.009).

Petta, S., Muratore, C., and Craxi, A. (2009). Non-alcoholic fatty liver disease pathogenesis: the present and the future. *Digestive and Liver Disease*, **41**(9): 615-625.

Purushotham, A., Shrode, G.E., Wendel, A.A., Liu, L.F., and Belury, M.A. (2007). Conjugated linoleic acid does not reduce body fat but decreases hepatic steatosis in adult Wistar rats. *The Journal of Nutritional Biochemistry*, **18**(10): 676-684.

Quercioli, A., Montecucco, F., and Mach, F. (2009). Update on the Treatments of Non-Alcoholic Fatty Liver Disease (NAFLD). *Cardiovascular and Haematological Disorders-Drug Targets*, **9**(4): 261-270.

Raju, J., and Bird, R. (2006). Alleviation of hepatic steatosis accompanied by modulation of plasma and liver TNF- levels by *Trigonella foenum graecum* (fenugreek) seeds in Zucker obese (fa/fa) rats. *International Journal of Obesity*, **30**(8): 1298-1307.

Rapavi, E., Kocsis, I., Fehér, E., Szentmihályi, K., Lugasi, A., Székely, E., and Blázovics, A. (2007). The effect of citrus flavonoids on the redox state of alimentary-induced fatty liver in rats. *Natural Product Research*, **21**(3): 274-281.

Reddy, J.K., and Rao, M.S. (2006). Lipid metabolism and liver inflammation. II. Fatty liver disease and fatty acid oxidation. *American Journal of Physiology - Gastrointestinal and Liver Physiology*, **290**(5): G852-G858.

Ren, Y., Xu, Z., Liang, R., Li, X., Zhang, Z., and Yuan, Y. (2008). Studies on dose-response relationship and safety of curcumin for preventing and treating duck models of fatty liver. *Liaoning Journal of Traditional Chinese Medicine*, **35**: 1753-1755.

Ren, Y., Xu, Z., Liang, R., Liu, P., Li, Y., and Su, J. (2008). Mechanism and interventional effects of curcumin on liver lipid and serum lipid in model ducks with fatty liver. *Lishizhen Medicine and Materia Medica Research*, **19**(10): 2327-2329.

Roskams, T., Yang, S.Q., Koteish, A., Durnez, A., DeVos, R., Huang, X., Achten, R., Verslype, C., and Diehl, A.M. (2003). Oxidative stress and oval cell accumulation in mice and humans with alcoholic and nonalcoholic fatty liver disease. *American Journal of Pathology*, **163**(4): 1301-1311.

Qiang, P., and Wang, X.-S. (2008). The main study status of traditional Chinese medicine in treating fatty liver. *Medical Recapitulate*, **24**: 3789-3791.

Sabuncu, T., Nazligul, Y., Karaoglanoglu, M., Ucar, E., and Kilic, F.B. (2003). The effects of sibutramine and orlistat on the ultrasonographic findings, insulin resistance and liver enzyme levels in obese patients with non-alcoholic steatohepatitis.

Saller, R., Meier, R. and Brignoli, R. (2001). The use of silymarin in the treatment of liver diseases. *Drugs*, **61**(14): 2035-2063.

Santos, V.N., Lanzoni, V.P., Szejnfeld, J., Shigueoka, D., and Parise, E.R. (2003). A randomized double-blind study of the short-time treatment of obese patients with nonalcoholic fatty liver disease with ursodeoxycholic acid. *Brazilian Journal of Medical and Biological Research*, **36**: 723-729.

Satapathy, S.K., Sakhuja, P., Malhotra, V., Sharma, B.C., and Sarin, S.K. (2007). Beneficial effects of pentoxifylline on hepatic steatosis, fibrosis and necroinflammation in patients with non-alcoholic steatohepatitis. *Journal of Gastroenterology and Hepatology*, **22**(5): 634-638.

Savel, J., and Leroi, E. (1964) Action of betaine citrae on hepatic steatosis of alimentary origin in rats. *Pathologie-Biologie*. **12**: 837-841.

Schwimmer, J.B., Middleton, M.S., Deutsch, R., and Lavine, J.E. (2005). A phase 2 clinical trial of metformin as a treatment for non-diabetic paediatric non-alcoholic steatohepatitis. *Alimentary Pharmacology and Therapeutics*, **21**(7): 871-879.

Shang, J., Chen, L.L., and Xiao, F.X. (2008a). Resveratrol improves high-fat induced nonalcoholic fatty liver in rats. *Chinese Journal of Hepatology*, **16**(8): 616-619.

Shang, J., Chen, L.L., Xiao, F.X., Sun, H., Ding, H.C., and Xiao, H. (2008b). Resveratrol improves non-alcoholic fatty liver disease by activating AMP-activated protein kinase1. *Acta Pharmacologica Sinica*, **29**(6): 698-706.

Shao, L., Han, Z., Wu, W., and He, C. (2006). Effect of garlicin on protecting nonalcoholic fat liver in SD rats induced by high fat diet. *Chinese Journal of Clinical Pharmacology and Therapeutics*, **12**: 571-574.

Shen, F., Lv, J., and Pan, J. (2008). Effect of *Artemisia capillaris* Thunb on fatty liver rats with insulin resistance. *Chinese Traditional Patent Medicine*, **30**: 28-31.

Shi, Z., Zhang, J., Zheng, Y., Chen, Z., Zhu, X., and Feng, Y. (2009). Influences of fresh fistular onion stalker extract on preventing nonalcoholic fatty liver. *Chinese Journal of Integrated Traditional and Western Medicine on Liver Diseases*, **19**(04): 229-231.

Shou, Z., and Fan, H. (2008). Effect of aconine on leptin insulin resistance in rats with nonalcoholic hepatosteatosis. *Journal of Shandong University of TCM*, **32**(002): 166-168.

Song, F., Xie, M., Zhu, L., Zhang, K., Xue, J., and Gu, Z. (2008). Regulatory mechanism of osthole on lipid metabolism in alcohol-induced fatty liver rats. *Chinese Pharmacological Bulletin*, **24**: 979-980.

Song, Y.-L., Zeng, M.-D., Lu, L.-G., Fan, Z.-P., and MAO, Y.-M. (2007). Preventive and therapeutic effects of *Lycium barbarum* polysaccharide on rat nonalcoholic fatty liver induced by high fat feeding. *Anhui Medical and Pharmaceutical Journal*, **11**(3): 202-205.

Song, Z., Deaciuc, I., Zhou, Z., Song, M., Chen, T., Hill, D., and McClain, C.J. (2007). Involvement of AMP-activated protein kinase in beneficial effects of betaine on high-sucrose diet-induced hepatic steatosis. *American Journal of Physiology-Gastrointestinal and Liver Physiology*, **293**(4): G894-G902.

Spadaro, L., Magliocco, O., Spampinato, D., Piro, S., Oliveri, C., Alagona, C., Papa, G., Rabuazzo, A.M., and Purrello, F. (2008). Effects of *n-3* polyunsaturated fatty acids in subjects with nonalcoholic fatty liver disease. *Digestive and Liver Disease*, **40**(3): 194-199.

Sun, F., Xie, M.L., Xue, J., and Wang, H.B. (2010). Osthol regulates hepatic PPAR [alpha]-mediated lipogenic gene expression in alcoholic fatty liver murine. *Phytomedicine*, **17**(8-9): 669-673.

Sun, L., and Huang, M. (2007). Protective effect of Danshen injection on lipid injury of non-alcoholic fatty liver rats. *Chinese Journal of Traditional Medical Science and Technology*, **27**: 517-519.

Sun, Y., Sun, L., Li, Y., Li, X., and Wu, J. (2006). Experimental research of *Fructus lycii* on preventing the fatty liver of rat. *Journal of Qiqihar Medical College*, **17**: 2049-2051.

Sun, Y.-Q., Gao, T.-Y., Zhou, J., Hong, B.-B., and Ding, H. (2007). Protective effect of ligustrazine on acute injury fatty liver in mice. *Chinese Journal of Clinical Pharmacology and Therapeutics*, **12**: 540-543.

Tan, D., Fu, W., Zhou, Z., Huang, G., Zhang, S., and Chen, X. (2007). Experimental study of effect of curcumin treatment on rat non-alcoholic fatty liver disease. *Chongqing Medicine*, **36**(16): 1626-1628.

Tan, H. (2006). Experimental investigation of Gynostemma on preventing Japanese white rabbits from fatty liver induced by high fatty feeding. *Chinese Journal of Traditional Medicine Science and Technology*, **13**: F0003.

Tandy, S., Chung, R.W.S., Wat, E., Kamili, A., Berge, K., Griinari, M., and Cohn, J.S. (2009). Dietary krill oil supplementation reduces hepatic steatosis, glycemia and hypercholesterolemia in high-fat fed mice. *Journal of Agricultural and Food Chemistry*, **57**(19): 9339-9345.

Tang, J., Ye, X., Liu, J., Li, P., Zhang, Q., and Hu, J. (2009). Effects of total flavonoids in Gingko Biloba on glucose and lipid metabolism and liver function in rats with insulin resistance. *Journal of Shanghai Jiaotong University(Medical Science)*, **29**(2): 150-153.

Torres-Durán, P.V., and Paredes-Carbajal, M.C. (2006). Protective effect of *Arthrospira maxima* on fatty acid composition in fatty liver. *Archives of Medical Research*, **37**(4): 479-483.

Trappoliere, M., Tuccillo, C., Federico, A., Di Leva, A., Niosi, M., D'Alessio, C., Capasso, R., Coppola, F., D'Auria, M., and Loguercio, C. (2005). The treatment of NAFLD. *European Review for Medical and Pharmacological Sciences*, **9**(5): 299-304.

Ulicná, O., and Brixová, E. (1985). The effect of silymarin on lipids in the blood and liver in steatosis. *Vnitr ní Lékar Ství*, **31**(1): 15-19.

Uzun, M.A., Koksal, N., Aktas, S., Gunerhan, Y., Kadioglu, H., Dursun, N., and Sehirli, A.O. (2009). The effect of ursodeoxycholic acid on liver regeneration after partial hepatectomy in rats with non-alcoholic fatty liver disease. *Hepatology Research*, **39**(8): 814-821.

Vivekanandan, P., Gobianand, K., Priya, S., Vijayalakshmi, P., and Karthikeyan, S. (2007). Protective effect of picroliv against hydrazine-induced hyperlipidemia and hepatic steatosis in rats. *Drug and chemical toxicology*, **30**(3): 241-252.

Wada, S., Yamazaki, T., Kawano, Y., Miura, S., and Ezaki, O. (2008). Fish oil fed prior to ethanol administration prevents acute ethanol-induced fatty liver in mice. *Journal of Hepatology*, **49**(3): 441-450.

Wang, J., Liu, R., Yan, X.,. He, J.C., Wang, J.Y., Ma, Z.Y., and Liu, S-X. (2007). Effects of berberine hydrochloride on nonalcoholic fatty liver disease in rats. *Journal of Lanzhou University (Medical Sciences)*, **33**(4): 8-11.

Wang, J.Q., Li, J., Zou, Y.H., Cheng, W.M., Lu, C., Zhang, L., Ge, J.F., Huang, C., Jin, Y., Lv, X.W., Hu, C.M., and Liu, L.P. (2009). Preventive effects of total flavonoids of *Litsea coreana* leve on hepatic steatosis in rats fed with high fat diet. *Journal of Ethnopharmacology*, **121**(1): 54-60.

Wang, Q., Zeng, T., YU, L., and Xie, K. (2007). Preventive effect of garlic oil on fatty liver in experimental rats. *Journal of Toxicology = Dulixue Zazhi*, **21**(6): 450-453.

Wang, T., and Wang, Y.G. (2008). To explore the effect of *Cordyceps sinesis* on alcoholic fatty liver in rats. *Guide of China Medicine*, **6**(19): 31-32.

Wang, X., Xie, G., Shi, X., Shao, Y., Wang, R., and Huang, Z. (2006). The Effect of Different Kinds of Chinese Herb Medicine Such as Padix Polygoni Multiflori on Blood Biochemical Indexes in Rats of Fatty Liver. *Journal of Anhui Traditional Chinese Medical College,* **25**: 39-40.

Wang, Z., Yao, T., Pini, M., Zhou, Z., Fantuzzi, G., and Song, Z. (2010). Betaine improved adipose tissue function in mice fed a high-fat diet: a mechanism for hepatoprotective effect of betaine in nonalcoholic fatty liver disease. *American Journal of Physiology- Gastrointestinal and Liver Physiology,* **298**(5): G634-G642.

Wei, H.F., Liu, T., Xing, L.J., Zheng, P.Y., and Ji, G. (2009). Distribution pattern of traditional Chinese medicine syndromes in 793 patients with fatty liver disease. *Zhong Xi Yi Jie He Xue Bao= Journal of Chinese Integrative Medicine,* **7**(5): 411-417.

Wei, J., Wu. J., Wang, S., and Wang, Z. (2004). Clinical study on improvement of type diabetes mellitus complicated with fatty liver treated by berberine. *Chinese Journal Of Integrated Traditional and Western Medicine on Liver Diseases,* **14**: 334-336.

Wei, L., and Zhao, C. (2010). Effects of lycopene on nonalcoholic fatty liver in rats. *China Pharmaceuticals,* **19**(3): 3-5.

Wu, Y., Tong, Q., and Luo, D. (2006). Study on the effect of chondroitin sulfate on fatty liver induced by alcohol in mice. *Chinese Journal of Gastrornterology and Hepatology,* **15**(4): 387-389.

Xiao, F., Chen, L., Sun, H., and Shang. J. (2008). Effect of resveratrol on serum level of tumor necrosis factor-α in fatty liver rats induced by high fat diet. *Chinese Journal of Rehabilitation,* **23**: 377-379.

Xiao, H., Zhang, J., and Zheng, J. (2008). Resveratrol down-regulates hepatic cyclooxygenase-2 expression in mice with nonalcoholic steatohepatitis. *World Chinese Journal of Digestology,* **16**(19): 2092-2096.

Xing, M., Liu, L., Qian, D., Fang, J., Qi, J., Song, P., and Tian, D. (2008). Clinical research of *Fructus lycii* glucopeptide on patients with nonalcoholic fatty liver disease. *Chinese Journal of Integrated Traditonal and Western Medicine on Liver Diseases,* **18**: 83-85.

Xu, K.Z.-Y., Zhu, C., Kim, M.S., Yamahara J., and Li, Y. (2009). Pomegranate flower ameliorates fatty liver in an animal model of type 2 diabetes and obesity. *Journal of Ethno-pharmacology,* **123**(2): 280-287.

Xu, Z., Lu, Z., Chen, J., Deng, X., Mao, Y., and Ho, X. (2007). The effect of rhubarb ethanol extract on hyperlipidemia and liver fatty in rabbits. Chinese Journal of Applied Physiology, **23**: 375-380.

Xu, Z., Tan, J., Chen, J., Ho, X., Deng, X., Zhang, D., and Jian, X. (2009). Investigation of Perilla leaf extract on fatty liver of rabbits. *Heilongjiang Animal Science and Veterinary Medicine,* **5**: 100-101.

Xu, Z.-N., Xie, M.-L., Lu, L.-G., Tian, X., Zhu, L.-J., Xue, J., Zhang, K.-P., Chen, W.-H., Liu, M., Mao, Y.-M., and Zeng, M.-D. (2006). Effect of betaine on alcoholic fatty liver in alcohol-fed rat. *Chinese Hepatology,* **11**(3): 163-166.

Yamada, K., Hosokawa, M., Yamada, C., Watanabe, R., Fujimoto, S., Fujiwara, H., Kunitomo, M., Miura, T., Kaneko, T., Tsuda, K., Seino, Y., and Inagaki, N. (2008). Dietary corosolic acid ameliorates obesity and hepatic steatosis in KK-Ay mice. *Biological and Pharmaceutical Bulletin*, **31**(4): 651-655.

Yan, M.-X., Chen, Z.-Y., and He, B.-H. (2009). Effect of total flavonoids of Chinese hawthorn leaf on expression of NF-κB and its inhibitor in rat liver with non-alcoholic steato-hepatitis. *China Journal of Traditional Chinese Medicine and Pharmacy*, (2): 139-143.

Yanagita, T., Wang, Y.-M., Nagao, K., Ujino, Y., and Inoue, N. (2005). Conjugated linoleic acid-induced fatty liver can be attenuated by combination with docosahexaenoic acid in C57BL/6N mice. *Journal of Agricultural and Food Chemistry*, **53**(24): 9629-9633.

Yang, J., Zou, J., and Bai, L. (2007). Clinical observation of taurine treatment on non-alcoholic fatty liver. *Shaangxi Medicine*, **36**: 354-355.

Yang, S.F., Tseng, J.K., Chang, Y.Y., and Chen, Y.C. (2009). Flaxseed oil attenuates non-alcoholic fatty liver of hyperlipidemic hamsters. *Journal of Agricultural and Food Chemistry*, **57**(11): 5078-5083.

Yang, Z., Wei, Z. Yin, J., and Yan, W. (2007). Effect of Ash bark extract on the treatment of experimental fatty liver and its mechanism. *Chinese Journal of Gerontology*, **14**: 168-170.

Yarnell, E., and Abascal, K. Herbal medicine and nonalcoholic fatty liver disease. (2010). *Alternative and Complimentary Therapies*, **16**(1): 15-21.

Ye, B., Wang, Z., Zhong, W., Lu, B., and Chen, M. (2008). Protective and therapeutic effects of andrographolide on nonalcoholic steatohepatitis. *Anhui Medical and Pharmaceutical Journal*, **12**: 582-584.

Ye, W.S. (2004). The recognition and treatment of patients with fatty liver by traditional Chinese medicine. *China Tropical Medicine*, **6**: 1023-1024.

Ye, X.-Y., Xu, M.-H., Li, X.-F., and Wang, Y.-F. (2009). Effects of hawthorn leaf flavonoids on reducing blood lipids and preventing fatty liver in the quails. *Fudan University Journal of Medical Sciences*, **36**(**2**): 142-148.

Yeh, E., Wood, R.D., Leeson, S., and Squires, E.J. (2009). Effect of dietary omega-3 and omega-6 fatty acids on clotting activities of Factor V, VII and X in Fatty Liver Haemorrhagic Syndrome-susceptible laying hens. *British Poultry Science*, **50**(3): 382-392.

Yi, X., and Wang Y. (2008). Berberine decreases plasma lipids and liver weight in hypercholesterolemic rats. *The FASEB Journal*, **22**(2_Meeting Abstracts): 754.

Yin, H.Q., Je, Y.T., Kim, Y.C., Shin, Y.K., Sung, S., Lee, K., Jeong, G.S., Kim, Y.C., and Lee, B.H. (2009). *Magnolia officinalis* reverses alcoholic fatty liver by inhibiting the maturation of sterol regulatory element–binding protein-1c. *Journal of Pharmacological Sciences*, **109**: 486-495.

Yin, H.Q., Kim, Y.C., Chung, Y.S., Kim, Y.C., Shin, Y.K., and Lee, B.H. (2009). Honokiol reverses alcoholic fatty liver by inhibiting the maturation of sterol regulatory element binding protein-1c and the expression of its downstream lipogenesis genes. *Toxicology and Applied Pharmacology*, **236**(1): 124-130.

Ying, W., Zhu, C., and Li, R. (2007). Effects of rhein on nonalcoholic steatohepatitis in rats. *Chinese Journal of Hepatology = Zhonghua Gan Zang Bing Za Zhi*, **15**(11): 869-870.

Yokohama, S., Yoneda, M., Haneda, M., Okamoto, S., Okada, M., Aso, K., Hasegawa, T., Tokusashi, Y., Miyokawa, N., and Nakamura, K. (2004). Therapeutic efficacy of an angiotensin II receptor antagonist in patients with nonalcoholic steatohepatitis. *Hepatology*, **40**(5): 1222-1225.

Yu, X.-H., Zhu, J.-S., Gu, G.-M., and Shi, J.-P. (2007). Clinical effect of oxymatrine combined with metformin on insulin resistance and serum TNF-a in patients with non-alcoholic fatty liver. *Chinese Journal of Clinical Hepatology*, **3**: 195-196.

Yu, Z., and Zhao, J. (2007). Some recognition and thinking on the development of integrative traditional Chinese and western medicine. *Chinese Journal of Integrated Traditional and Western Medicine*, **27**(8): 749-752.

Yuan, R., and Lin, Y. (2000). Traditional Chinese medicine: an approach to scientific proof and clinical validation. *Pharmacology and Therapeutics*, **86**(2): 191-198.

Zelber-Sagi, S., Kessler, A., Brazowsky, E., Webb, M., Lurie, Y., Santo, M., Leshno, M., Blendis, L., Halpern, Z., and Oren, R. (2006). A double-blind randomized placebo-controlled trial of orlistat for the treatment of nonalcoholic fatty liver disease. *Clinical Gastroenterology and Hepatology*, **4**(5): 639-644.

Zhang, J., Tan, S., Jiang, L., Zhu, W., and Cheng, J. (2007). Effects of quercetin on the expression of nuclear factor kappaB in alcoholic fatty liver of rats. *WorldChinese Journal of Digestology*, **15**(22): 2399-2402.

Zhang, S. (1992). Progress of study on Chinese herbal drugs in treating fatty liver. *Chinese Journal of Integrated Traditional and Western Medicine = Zhongguo Zhong Xi Yi Jie He Za Zhi*, **12**(12): 758-759.

Zhang, X., Pei, X., and Da, H. (2009). Current situations of TCM new drug application against fatty liver and discussion on the existed questions. *Traditional Chinese Drug Research and Clinical Pharmacology*, **20**: 180-182.

Zhang, Y., Huang, X., Xu, J., and Wen, C. (2008). Experimental study of effects of curcumin solid dispersion preparation on fatty liver in rat. *China Pharmaceutical*, **17**: 7-9.

Zhan, B. (2006). Erigeron injection in the treatment of chronic hepatitis B patients with fatty liver rats. *Guangdong Medical Journal*, **27**: 278-279.

Zhang, D.Y., Jia, Z.H., Fu, M.Z., and Liu, L. (2008). New methods on active componets and pharmacological effects of traditional Chinese medicine. *Progress in Veterinary Medicine*, **29**(12): 89-93.

Zhang, G.L., Shi, X.F., Liu, Q., and Luo, Q. (2004). The effect of lipid extract of mildew fungus Mortierella against experimental NAFLD Wistar rats. *Pharmacology and Clinics of Chinese Materia Medica*, **20**(6): 22.

Zhang, J., Hao, J., Shi, Z., Chang, Q., and Bing, F. (2007). Effects of a preparation of Chinese *Allium fistulosum* L on the morphology and metabolism of lipids in fatty liver rats. *World Chinese Journal of Digestology*, **15**(22): 2447-2452.

Zhang, M., Chen, S., Zheng, W., and Chen, F. (2006). The dosage-effect relationship of seaweed decoction [*Sargassum fusforme* (Harv.) Seteh] on rat fatty livers induced by high fatty feeding. *Zhejiang Journal Of Clinical Medicine*. **8**(5): 452-452.

Zhang, W., Zhang, C., Wang, D., and Ying, X. (2008). Study on the antifatty liver of the extract of the leaves of *Crataegus pinnatifida* Bge. *var.* major. *Chinese Archives of Traditional Chinese Medicine*, **26**: 559-561.

Zhang, Y., Zhang, Y., Li, L., Yang, W., Ran, X., Yang, Y., and Mao, X. (2006). Therapeutic effects of *Trigonella foenum-greacum* saponin on rats with alcoholic fatty livers. *Chinese Journal of Hepatology*, **14**: 854-856.

Zhao, W., Duan, R., and Miao, M. (2005). Study of Radix on the insulin resistance and leptin in fatty liver model rats. *Journal of Sichuan Traditional Chinese Medicine*, **23**: 33-34.

Zhao, X. (2004). Advances in diagnosis and treatment of hepatic steatosis. *Journal of Traditional Chinese Medicine*, **24**(1): 64-69.

Zeng, T., Guo, F.F., Zhang, C.L., Zhao, S., Dou, D.D., Gao, X.C., and Xie, K.Q. (2008). The anti-fatty liver effects of garlic oil on acute ethanol-exposed mice. *Chemico-Biological Interactions*, **176**(2-3): 234-242.

Zheng, B., Zheng, F., and Pu, W. (2005).The influence of tablets preparation of *Phyllanthus urinaria* L, a Dai minority medicine, on the blood lipids of the patients with fatty liver. *Chinese Medicine and Western Medicine Intergrating*, **2**: 29-30.

Zheng, H., Chang, Y., Cao, B., and Qi, Y. (2008). Study on therapeutic effect of chicory polysaccharides on fatty liver function of rat. *Food Science*, **29**: 575-579.

Zheng, P., Ji, G., Ma, Z., Liu, T., Xin, L., Wu, H., Liang, X., and Liu, J. (2009). Therapeutic effect of puerarin on non-alcoholic rat fatty liver by improving leptin signal transduction through JAK2/STAT3 pathways. *American Journal of Chinese Medicine*, **37**(1): 69-83.

Zheng, P., Ma, Z., Liu, T., Xing, L., and Ji, G. (2008). Effect of puerarin on hepatic lipid of nonalcoholic fatty liver disease rats. *Shanghai Journal of Traditional Chinese Medicine*, **42**: 61-63.

Bioactive Phytochemicals: Perspectives for Modern Medicine Vol. 1 (2012) *Pages* **177–214**
Editor: **V.K. Gupta**
Published by: **DAYA PUBLISHING HOUSE, NEW DELHI**

5

Phytochemicals Against Liver Disease II: Recent Progress in the Treatment of Liver Fibrosis by Natural Drug Products and their Active Chemical Entities, in China and Other Countries

Pengfei Gao[1], Lu Xu[1], Mengxi Xu[1], Xiumei Wu[1], Hui Li[1], Yan Xu[2], Guangming Liu[1,*] Guoping Yang[1], Xiaoman Lv[1], Ping Gan[1], Li Lu[1], Shawn Spencer[3], Yu Zhao[1,2*] and Xiaojiang Hao[4]

ABSTRACT

This chapter presents a current review of bioactive natural products with potential utility in the treatment of Liver Fibrosis. This Review covers 79 bioactive natural preparations or active chemical species often utilized in Traditional Chinese Medicine (TCM), however includes phytochemicals used in other countries. The medicinal agents discussed are categorized

1 Key Laboratory of Yunnan Insect Drug R&D, Pharmacy School of Dali College, Wanhua Road, Dali 671000, China.

2 Department of TCM and Natural Drug Research, College of Pharmaceutical Sciences, Zhejiang University, Yu Hang Tang Road 388, Hangzhou 310058, China.

3 College of Pharmacy and Pharmaceutical Sciences, Florida A&M University, FL 32307, USA.

4 The Key Laborotory of Chemistry and Natural Products of Guizhou Province and Chinese Academy of Sciences, Sha Chong Nan Road 202, Guiyang 550002, China

* *Corresponding author*: E-mail: lgm888999@yahoo.com.cn (Liu, G) or dryuzhao@126.com (Zhao, Y.)

according to their basic structure, in an attempt to be used as a basis for developing quantitative structure-activity relationships (QSAR). Some progress using QSAR in liver disease is also reviewed, followed by the outlook for future research in the field.

Keywords: Active hits, Anti-hepatofibrotic drugs, Effective extracts, Liver fibrosis, Natural drugs, New drug R&D, QSAR.

Introduction

Liver fibrosis is a wound-healing response to various chronic liver injuries, including alcoholism, persistent viral and helminthic infections, and hereditary metal overload (Friedman, 2008; Kisseleva and Brenner, 2008). Hepatitis B viral (HBV) infection is the major cause of liver fibrosis in China, whereas the main causes of liver fibrosis in industrialized countries are chronic Hepatitis C viral infection (HCV), alcohol abuse, and nonalcoholic steatohepatitis (NASH). Prolonged unresolved hepatic fibrosis can lead to severe complications such as cirrhosis and hepatocellular carcinoma (HCC). Control or resolution of hepatic fibrosis is an important issue to block the development of end-stage liver diseases (Ginès *et al.*, 2004; Cheung *et al.*, 2009). The pathogenesis of liver fibrosis involves the activation of hepatic stellate cells (HSCs), the over-expression and over-secretion of collagens, and consequently an excessive accumulation of extracellular matrix (ECM) proteins (Wells, 2005). Research has been focused on the management of liver fibrosis including the elimination of primary diseases, immunomodulation, suppression of hepatocyte inflammation, prevention of death and damage of hepatocytes, inhibition of over-secretion and accumulation of ECM proteins, promotion of ECM degradation, improvement of microcirculation and metabolism of liver and remission of complications (Friedman, 2003). Some researches suggest advanced liver fibrosis is reversible (Friedman, 2007). However, effective therapies against liver fibrosis are still limited up to present.

There is no clinical diagnosis as liver fibrosis in ancient Chinese medicinal literature. According to its clinical manifestations, such as distending pain on flank, jaundice mass in the area of flank and so on, it is considered to be flank pain, jaundice, and amass by modern traditional Chinese medicine (TCM) clinicians (Qi, 2009). However, they have different views on the cause and mechanism of it. In some modern TCM clinicians' view, liver fibrosis is thought to be caused by poor blood circulation, toxin stagnation and a deficiency of healthy energy (Feng *et al.*, 2009), some of them consider that the treatment of liver fibrosis should be based on syndrome differentiation. It is important to understand that the concepts of liver, spleen, and kidney in TCM are different from those in western medicine, which are more related to an accumulation of some physiological function than the meaning of anatomy.

Treatments of liver fibrosis with single natural drug and active natural products have been under intensive research worldwide, however, there are little reviews on this topic. This review provides an overview about its recent research on the type of compounds or extracts.

Single Natural Drug and Active Natural Products Used to Treat Liver Fibrosis

Seven Kinds of Alkaloids from Natural Medicine Used to Treat Liver Fibrosis

Berberine (Ranunculaceae/Coptis Salisb.)

Zhang *et al.* (2008) investigated the therapeutic effect of berberine on hepatic fibrosis in rats induced by multiple hepatotoxic factors, including carbon tetrachloride (CCl_4), ethanol and high cholesterol. Berberine (50, 100 or 200 mg/kg b.w., i.g., daily for 4 weeks) was administered to the treated rats. The results showed that, compared with the fibrotic control group, serum levels of alanine aminotransferase (ALT), aspartate aminotransferase (AST), hepatic content of malondialdehyde (MDA) and hydroxyproline (Hyp) were significantly decreased, but the activity of hepatic superoxide dismutase (SOD) was markedly increased in berberine-treated groups in a dose-dependent manner. In addition, histopathological changes, such as steatosis, necrosis and myofibroblast proliferation, were reduced and the expression of alpha-smooth muscle actin (SMA), transforming growth factor (TGF)-beta1 were apparently downregulated in the berberine-treated groups ($P < 0.01$). It suggests that berberine could be used to prevent experimental liver fibrosis. Sun *et al.* (2009) incubated activated rat hepatic stellate cells (CFSCs) with various concentrations (0-20 μg/mL) of berberine. The results showed that berberine significantly inhibited CFSC proliferation and induced cell cycle arrest in G1 phase after 48 h incubation. In addition, Real-time PCR and Western blotting revealed that both p21 and p27 expression were markedly reduced by berberine. Berberine also decreased Akt phosphorylation and FoxO1 phosphorylation, which led to FoxO1 nuclear translocation. It suggests berberine is able to prevent liver fibrosis by inhibiting hepatic stellate cell proliferation.

Pentoxifylline (Sterculiaceae/Theobroma)

Yang *et al.* (2008) studied the effect of pentoxifylline (PTX) in the prevention of experimental hepatic fibrosis in rats induced by bile duct occlusion, the rats in the treatment groups were administered 16 mg/kg b.w. PTX, intragastrically, daily for 6 weeks. In comparison with the model group, PTX treatment could reduce the histological scoring in liver fibrosis and downregulate the expression of collagen I mRNA. This suggests PTX could attenuate hepatic fibrosis in rats induced by bile duct occlusion.

Oxymatrine, Matrine (Leguminosae/Sophora L.)

Zeng *et al.* (2005) evaluated the effect of oxymatrine in the prevention of experimental hepatic fibrosis in rats induced by CCl_4, the rats in the treatment group received celiac injection of oxymatrine at a dose of 10 mg/kg b.w. twice per week for 8 weeks. The results showed that, compared with the model group, the semi-quantitative histological scores, average area of collagenous fibre, the positive rates of Mothers Against DPP Homolog (Smad) 4 mRNA and Smad 4 protein were decreased; meanwhile, the positive rate of Smad 7 mRNA and Smad 7 protein were increased considerably in oxymatrine-treated group (all $P < 0.05$). It demonstrates that oxymatrin has potential effect in preventing experimental liver fibrosis. Wu *et al.* (2008) explored the anti-fibrotic effect of oxymatrine on CCl_4-induced liver fibrosis in rats. The treated rats received oxymatrine via celiac injection at a dosage of 10 mg/kg twice a week for 8 weeks. Compared with the model group, oxymatrine reduced significantly the collagen deposition and rearrangement of the parenchyma in the liver tissue in oxymatrine-treated group. Moreover, the semi-quantitative histological scores, average area of collagen and the expression of Smad 3 mRNA, cAMP response element-binding (CREB)-binding protein (CBP) mRNA were markedly decreased in oxymatrine-treated group, whereas the expression of Smad 7 mRNA was increased considerably. It suggests oxymatrine is effective against CCl_4-induced liver fibrosis in rats. Ma *et al.* (2007) studied the effect of matrine on the expression of inducible nitric oxide synthase (iNOS) in $CC1_4$-induced liver injury in mice, the mice in the treatment group received administration of matrine (100 mg/kg b.w., i.g., daily for 8 weeks). The mice were sacrificed at fourth and eighth weeks, the results showed the liver tissue was obviously improved in matrine-treated group at all time points, the score of iNOS-IR hepatocytes in $CC1_4$ group was significantly higher than that in matrine-treated group ($P < 0.01$). It suggests matrine inhibits expression of iNOS in injured hepatocytes and attenuates hepatic fibrosis in mice induced by CCl_4.

Chelerythrine (Papaveraceae/Macleaya R. Br.)

Li *et al.* (2009) observed the anti-fibrotic effects of chelerythrine in rats with CCl_4-induced hepatic fibrosis, the rats in the treatment groups were administered with chelerythrine (0.2, 0.6 or 2.0 mg/kg b.w., i.g., daily for 8 weeks). The results showed that the expression of TGF-beta1 and alpha-SMA in the liver tissue in chelerythrine-treated groups were ameliorated significantly compared with the model group (both $P < 0.01$), whereas the expression of them in the liver tissue were not obviously different between chelerythrine-treated groups and γ-INF-treated group (both $P > 0.05$). It indicates chelerythrine can attenuate the hepatic injuries in rats with CCl_4-induced hepatic fibrosis.

Corydalis saxicola Bunting Alkaloids (Papaveraceae/Corydalis)

Liang *et al.* (2008) studied the effect of *Corydalis saxicola* Bunting alkaloids (CSA) in the prevention of experimental hepatic fibrosis in rats induced by CCl_4, the rats in the treatment groups were administered 50, 75 or 100 mg/kg b.w. CSA, intragastrically, daily for 12 weeks. The results showed that the parameters reflecting liver function were improved in CSA-treated groups, whereas hepatic content of hydroxyproline was obviously declined in it. In addition, histopathological findings revealed that the development of liver fibrosis was prevented in CSA-treated groups, while hepatic levels of TGF-beta1 and Matrix metallopeptidase 9 (MMP-9) in CSA-treated groups were significantly lower than those in the model group. The results suggest that CSA is effective for the treatment of hepatic fibrosis in rats induced by CCl_4.

Tetrandrine (Menispermaceae/Cocculus DC.)

Yin *et al.* (2007) investigated the therapeutic effect of tetrandrine on liver fibrosis *in vivo* and *in vitro*. The *in vitro* study disclosed the effect of tetrandrine on the apoptosis of rat hepatic stellate cells transformed by simian virus 40 (T-HSC/Cl-6), which retains the features of activated cells. In the *in vivo* study, hepatic fibrosis was induced in the rats by thioacetamide. Tetrandrine (5, 10 or 20 mg/kg b.w., daily for 4 weeks) was given orally to rats compared with intraperitoneal injection of interferon-γ (IFN-γ). The results of *in vitro* study indicated that the activation of caspase-3 in T-HSC/Cl-6 cells dose-dependently induced by 5, 10 or 25 mg/mL of tetrandrin. The *in vivo* study also showed both tetrandrine and IFN-γ treatments reduced serum levels of AST, ALT, total bilirubin (T-Bil), decreased the levels of liver hydroxyproline, hyaluronic acid (HA), laminin (LN) in liver and improved histological findings. The effects of tetrandrine at the concentration of 20 mg/kg were better than the other concentration groups. These indicated that tetrandrine might ameliorate the development of liver fibrosis.Hsu *et al.* (2007) investigated the *in vitro* and *in vivo* effects of tetrandrine (Tet) (an alkaloid isolated from the Chinese medicinal herb *Stephania tetrandra*) on hepatic fibrosis. A cell line of rat hepatic stellate cells (HSC-T6) was stimulated with TGF-beta1 or tumor necrosis factor-alpha (TNF-alpha). The inhibitory effects of Tet on the nuclear factor kappaB (NFkappaB) signaling cascade and molecular markers including intercellular adhesion molecule-1 (ICAM-1) and alpha-SMA secretion were assessed. In the *in vivo* study, liver fibrosis was induced by dimethylnitrosamine (DMN) administration to the rats for 4 weeks. The rats in the treatment groups were intragastrically administered 1, 5 mg/kg b.w. Tet twice daily for 3 weeks starting after 1 week of DMN administration. The results showed that in the *in vivo* study, Tet (0.5-5.0 μM) concentration-dependently inhibited NFkappaB transcriptional activity induced by TNF-alpha, including IkappaBalpha phosphorylation and mRNA expressions of ICAM-1 in HSC-T6 cells. In addition, Tet also inhibited TGF-beta1-induced alpha-SMA secretion and collagen deposition in HSC-T6 cells. In the *in vivo* study, fibrosis scores of livers from DMN-treated rats with high-dose Tet were significantly reduced in comparison with DMN-treated rats receiving saline. Hepatic collagen content of DMN-treated rats was significantly reduced by either Tet or silymarin treatment. Double-staining results showed that alpha-SMA and NFkappaB-positive cells were decreased in the fibrotic livers by Tet or silymarin treatments. In addition, mRNA expression of ICAM-1, alpha-SMA and TGF-beta1 were attenuated by Tet treatment. Moreover, levels of plasma AST and ALT were reduced by Tet or silymarin treatment. All these data suggest tetrandrine exerts a direct effect on preventing liver fibrosis.

Betaine (Chenopodiaceae/Beta Linn)

Erman *et al.* (2004) studied the effect of betaine or taurine on liver fibrogenesis and lipid peroxidation in rats. Fibrosis was induced by treatment of the rats with drinking water containing 5 per cent ethanol and CCl_4. The results indicated that ethanol plus CCl_4 treatment caused increased lipid peroxidation and disturbed antioxidant system in the liver. Histopathological findings suggested that the development of liver fibrosis was prevented in the rats treated with betaine or taurine (1 per cent v/v in drinking water) together with ethanol plus CCl_4 for 4 weeks. Betaine or taurine was also found to decrease serum transaminase activities and hepatic lipid peroxidation without any change in hepatic antioxidant system in the rats with hepatic fibrosis. The results showed that administration of betaine or taurine exerted anti-fibrotic effect in rats with CCl_4-induced liver fibrosis.

Nine Kinds of Total Flavonoids and Total Phenolic Acids from Natural Medicine Used to Treat Liver Fibrosis

Total Flavonoids of Litsea coreana Leve. (Lauraceae/Litsea)

Zhu *et al.* (2009) investigated the anti-liver fibrotic effect of total flavonoids of (TFLC) in rats induced by CCl_4, the rats in the treatment groups were administered 100, 200 or 400 mg/kg b.w. TFLC, intragastrically, daily for 6 weeks. The results indicated TFLC (200, 400 mg/kg b.w.) not only reduced the levels of ALT, AST, HA, LN, collagen IV (CIV) and procollagen III N-terminal peptide (PIIINP) in serum and the degree of liver fibrosis significantly, but also decreased the mRNA expression of TGF-beta1 and connective tissue growth factor (CTGF) in liver tissue obviously. The authors suggested that TFLC prevented the development of liver fibrosis in rats induced by CCl_4.

Total Flavones of Bidens bipinnata L. (Asteraceae/Bidens)

Yan *et al.* (2008) explored the therapeutic effect of total flavones of *Bidens bipinnata* L. (TFB) on liver fibrosis in rats induced by CCl_4. The rats in the treatment groups were administered 40, 80 or 160 mg/kg b.w. TFB, intragastrically, daily for 10 weeks. The results showed TFB significantly reduced serum levels of HA, CIV, procollagen III (PCIII) and hepatic hydroxyproline content, ameliorated the liver pathologic injury, increased collagen hyperplasia, inhibited the activation and proliferation of HSC and promoted the apoptosis of HSC in liver in the treatment groups compared with the model group. In addition, TFB significantly inhibited the proliferation of HSC and increased the apoptosis of isolated and cultured HSC in the *in vitro* study. This suggests TFB has a significantly therapeutic effect on the liver fibrosis rats.

Total Flavones of Cudrania cochin chinensis (Moraceae/Cudrania)

Yang and Teng (2009) investigated the anti-liver fibrotic effect of total flavones of *Cudrania cochin chinensis* (TFC) in rats induced by CCl_4 or sterile pig serum, the rats in the treatment groups were administered 10, 20 or 30 mg/kg b.w. TFC, intragastrically, daily for 8 weeks, the results showed that TFC decreased the serum levels of ALT, AST and hepatic content of MDA, increased the hepatic activity of SOD in TFC-treated groups compared with the model group. The results implied that TFC could prevent the progress of liver fibrosis in rats induced by CCl_4.

Total Flavonoids of Ampelopsis megalophylla Diels et Gilg (Vitaceae/ Ampelopsis Michx.)

Kuang *et al.* (2009) studied the therapeutic effects of tengcha (*Ampelopsis megalophylla* Diels *et* Gilg) flavonoids (TCF) on liver fibrosis in rats induced by CCl_4, the rats in the treatment group were administered 500 mg/kg b.w. TCF, intragastrically, daily for 12 weeks, the results showed TCF treatment significantly reversed CCl_4-induced liver fibrosis and reduced the expression of collagen I, III in liver tissue compared with the model group ($P < 0.05$). It was thus suggested that TCF can ameliorate the development of hepatic fibrosis in rats induced by CCl_4.

Tanshinone IIA (Labitae/Salvia L.)

Qin *et al.* (2010) investigated the therapeutic effect of Tanshinone IIA (TSN) on liver fibrosis in rats induced by CCl_4, the rats in the treatment groups were administered 7.1, 14.2, 21.3 mg/kg b.w. TSN, intragastrically, daily for 8 weeks. The results demonstrated TSN increased the levels of albumin (ALB), total protein (TP) in serum, decreased hydroxyproline level and reduced the expression of collagen fibers in liver tissue in TSN-treated group compared with the model group. The results suggest TSN could block the liver fibrosis in rats induced by CCl_4.

Scutellaria baicalensis Stem-Leaf Total Flavonoids (Lamiaceae/Scutellaria L.)

Yang *et al.* (2006) studied the therapeutic effects of *Scutellaria baicalensis* stem-leaf total flavonoids (SSTF) on liver fibrosis in rats induced by CCl_4, the rats in the treatment group were administered 35 mg/kg b.w. SSTF, intragastrically, daily for 8 weeks. The results indicated SSTF remarkably reduced the expression of alpha-SMA, significantly ameliorated the pathological changes of liver tissue, while SSTF reduced the production of fibers apparently, and decreased the serum levels of ALT, AST and hepatic content of hydroxyproline obviously when compared with those of the model group. It was suggested that SSTF could resist CCl_4-induced hepatofibrosis in rats.

Morin (Variety of Plant Sources)

Lee *et al.* (2009) investigated the protective effect of morin on hepatic fibrosis induced by DMN in rats. The results indicated oral administration of morin remarkably prevented weight losses of the body and liver, and inhibited the elevation of serum ALT, AST and total bilirubin levels in comparison with the model group. Furthermore, morin significantly reduced the expression of collagen I, TGF-beta1 and alpha-SMA on hepatic fibrosis induced by DMN. It suggests that morin could ameliorate the development of liver fibrosis in rats induced by DMN.

Soybean Isoflavones (Leguminosae/Glycine Willd)

Zhao *et al.* (2010) studied the effect of soybean isoflavones (SI) against hepatic fibrosis in rats induced by CCl_4. A 1.8 per cent water solution of SI (90 mg/kg b.w., i.g.) was administered daily to rats for 8 weeks. The results showed that SI remarkably decreased the levels of ALT, AST, and increased the levels of ALB and TP in serum. In addition, SI eased the inflammatory pathological injury of liver parenchyma. These results implied that SI could attenuate the liver fibrosis in rats induced by CCl_4.

Total Phenolic Acids of Oenanthe javanica (Umbelliferae/Oenanthe L.)

Nian *et al.* (2010) investigated the protective effect of total phenolic acids of *Oenanthe javanica* (TPAOJ) on hepatic fibrosis in rats induced by CCl_4, the rats in the treatment groups were administered 0.75, 1.5, 3.0 mg/kg b.w. TPAOJ, intragastrically, daily for 7 weeks. The levels of hepatic function indices (ALT, AST, ALB, ALP, TP, ChE, LDH) and hepatic fibrosis indices (HA, LN, PCIII, CIV) in serum and MDA content, SOD activity in hepatic tissue were detected, liver histopathological changes and α-SMA, TGF-beta1, TMP-1 expression quantity in hepatic tissue were also observed. The results showed that the rats in the model group suffered obvious hepatic damage and chronic fibrosis, while hepatic function and hepatic fibrosis indices were improved in TPAOJ-treated groups, the degree of hepatic fibrosis was also relieved apparently. This suggested that TPAOJ was useful in preventing the development of hepatic fibrosis in rats induced by CCl_4.

Ten Kinds of Single Phenolic Acids from Natural Medicine Used to Treat Liver Fibrosis

Epigallocatechin-3-gallate (Theaceae/Camellia Linn)

Zhen *et al.* (2008) examined the protective effects of epigallocatechin-3-gallate (EGCG) on CCl_4-induced liver fibrosis in rats, the rats in the treatment group were administered EGCG (25 mg/kg b.w., i.p.) daily for 7 weeks. Compared with the model group, histopathological and hepatic hydroxyproline examination revealed that EGCG significantly arrested progression of hepatic fibrosis. In addition, EGCG caused obvious amelioration of liver injury and reduced activities of serum ALT and AST (both $P < 0.05$). Additionally, redox state was improved in CCl_4-induced hepatic fibrosis through treatment with EGCG by suppressing the thiobarbituric acid reactive substances (TBARS) formation and increasing the level of glutathione (GSH). Moreover, EGCG markedly reduced mRNA and protein expression of TGF-beta1 and CTGF in the liver tissue (both $P < 0.05$). These results indicated that EGCG can significantly arrest progression of hepatic fibrosis in rats induced by CCl_4. Yasuda *et al.* (2009) studied the effects of (-)-epigallocatechin gallate (EGCG) on liver fibrosis in rats induced by CCl_4. The results indicated that drinking water with 0.1 per cent EGCG significantly inhibited the elevated serum levels of both AST and ALT, attenuated hepatic fibrosis and decreased the amount of hydroxyproline in the experimental liver. In addition, the expressions of platelet-derived growth factor (PDGF) receptor (PDGFR) beta and insulin-like growth factor (IGF)-1 receptor (IGF-1R) mRNAs in the liver were significantly lowered by the treatment with EGCG. Furthermore, EGCG decreased the expression of PDGFRbeta and alpha-SMA proteins, thus indicating the inhibition of HSC activation. These findings suggest that EGCG is useful in preventing the development of hepatic fibrosis in rats induced by CCl_4.

Curcumin (Zingiberaceae/Curcuma)

Pinlaor *et al.* (2010) investigated the preventing effect of curcumin on hepatobiliary fibrosis using *Opisthorchis viverrini*-infected hamsters supplemented with dietary 1 per cent curcumin (w/w) as an animal model. Histopathological studies revealed that curcumin had no effect on fibrosis at the short-term infection (21 days and 1 month); however, after the long-term curcumin treatment for 3 months, curcumin significantly reduced the hepatic hydroxyproline level and mRNA expression of collagen I and III compared with the untreated group. Furthermore, the expression of TIMP-1, TIMP-2, and TNF-alpha genes was also decreased after curcumin treatment. In contrast, curcumin increased mRNA expression of MMP-13, MMP-7 (at 6 months), interleukin (IL)-1beta, and TGF-beta1. These results implied that curcumin could exert an anti-fibrotic effect on the periductal fibrosis after long-term treatment. Wu, S.J. *et al.* (2010) studied the anti-inflammatory and anti- fibrotic actions of curcumin and saikosaponin A on CCl_4-induced liver damage. Curcumin and saikosaponin A were supplemented alone or in combination with diet 1 week before CCl_4 injection for 8 weeks. The results indicated curcumin and/or saikosaponin A significantly reduced hepatic collagen deposition, obviously inhibited activated nuclear factor-kappa B expression induced by CCl_4 in the liver, considerably inhibited hepatic proinflammatory cytokines TNF-alpha, IL-1beta, and IL-6, increased markedly anti-inflammatory cytokine IL-10 in comparison with the model group. Additionally, curcumin and/or saikosaponin A apparently reduced the elevation of levels of hepatic TGF-beta1 and hydroxyproline after CCl_4 treatment. Therefore, supplementation with curcumin and/or saikosaponin A suppressed inflammation and fibrogenesis in rats with CCl_4-induced liver injury. However, the combination of them has no additive effects on anti-inflammation and anti-fibrosis. Ji *et al.* (2009) examined the effects of curcumin against hepatic fibrosis in rats induced by CCl_4, the rats in the treatment groups were administered 100, 200 or 400 mg/kg b.w. curcumin, intragastrically, three times per week for 10 weeks. The results showed that, compared with the model group, curcumin increased the dropped liver index and decreased the elevation of serum levels of AST and ALT in curcumin-treated group (both$P < 0.05$). Additionally, HE and Masson stain revealed that the lesion of liver in curcumin-treated group was more mitigated than that of the model group, and the degree of live fibrosis was also lesser ($P < 0.05$). The authors suggested that the curcumin can reduce the liver fibrosis in rats induced by CCl_4.

Rhein (Polygonaceae/Rheum)

Wan *et al.* (2009) investigated the effect of rhein (RH) in the prevention of experimental hepatic fibrosis in rats induced by porcine serum, the rats in the treatment groups were administered 100 mg/kg b.w. curcumin, intragastrically, daily for 16 weeks. The results showed that the model group exhibited typical hepatic fibrosis, the expression of CTGF and TGF-beta1 increased obviously; while the collagen area and the expression of CTGF, TGF-beta1was obviously reduced in rhein-treated group. This investigation implied that rhein could resist hepatic fibrosis in rats induced by porcine serum.

Resveratrol (Polygonaceae/Polygonum)

Lv *et al.* (2005) assessed the therapeutic effects of resveratrol on chronic liver fibrosis in rats induced by CCl_4. Resveratrol (25, 50 or 100 mg/kg b.w., i.g.) was administered to rats daily for 6 weeks. Compared with the model group, treated groups (50 and 100 mg/kg b.w.) had significant reductions in the level of serum ALT, hepatic content of hydroxyproline, MDA and liver fibrogensis. It suggests resveratrol may have a protective effects against liver fibrosis in rats induced by CCl_4. Hong *et al.* (2010) studied the protective effects of resveratrol on DMN-induced liver fibrosis in rats. The rats in the treatment group were treated with resveratrol daily by oral gavage for seven days after a single intraperitoneal injection of DMN (40 mg/kg b.w.). The results showed that resveratrol remarkably recovered the weight losses of body and liver, alleviated the infiltration of inflammatory cells and fibrosis of liver tissue, decreased the level of MDA, and increased the levels of glutathione peroxidase and SOD. Also, resveratrol significantly inhibited the mRNA expression of inflammatory mediators, including inducible nitric oxide, TNF-alpha and IL-1beta. In addition, resveratrol not only reduced mRNA expression of fibrosis-related genes such as TGF beta1, collagen I, and alpha-SMA, but also markedly decreased hepatic hydroxyproline content in rats with DMN-induced liver fibrosis. These results indicate that resveratrol could exert an anti-fibrotic effect in rats induced by CCl_4.

Silymarin (Compositae/Silybum)

Cao *et al.* (2009) observed the anti-fibrotic effect of silymarin in mice induced by alcohol and CCl_4, the mice in the treatment groups were administered 50, 100 or 200 mg/kg b.w. silymarin, intragastrically, daily for 8 weeks. The results indicated silymarin decreased the levels of serum ALT, AST and the expression of TGF-beta1, alpha-SMA and collagen I mRNA in the silymarin-treated group compared with the model group. The medium dose of silymarin had the most significant effect. It suggests silymarin is useful in preventing the development of hepatic fibrosis in mice induced by alcohol and CCl_4.

Salvianolic Acid B (Labiatae/Salvia)

Lu *et al.* (2007) investigated the anti-fibrotic effect of salvianolic acid (Sal) B in rats induced by DMN, the rats in the treatment group were administered 12.5 mg/kg b.w. salvianolic acid B, intragastrically, 3 times per week for 4 weeks. The results showed that the levels of serum ALT, AST, HA, LN and expression levels of TGF-beta1, TIMP-2 in the salvianolic acid B-treated group were significantly lower than those in the model group. It suggests salvianolic acid B could resist DMN-induced hepatic fibrosis in rats. Tsai *et al.* (2010) studied the protective effects of Sal A and B on oxidative stress and liver fibrosis in rats. A cell line of rat hepatic stellate cells (HSCs) was stimulated with PDGF factor (10 ng/mL). Liver fibrosis was induced by intraperitoneal injections of thioacetamide (TAA, 200 mg/kg b.w.) twice per week for 6 weeks. Sal A (10 mg/kg b.w.), Sal B (50 mg/kg b.w.) or S-adenosylmethionine (SAMe, 10 mg/kg b.w.), was given intragastrically twice per day consecutively for 4 weeks starting 2 weeks after TAA injection. *In vitro*, PDGF increased the accumulation of hydrogen peroxide in HSCs, which was attenuated by Sal A (10 muM) and Sal B (200 muM). Sal A and B reduced the PDGF-stimulated expression of alpha-SMA and nicotinamide adenine dinucleotide phosphate (NADPH) oxidase subunits gp91 (phox) and p47 (phox) in membrane fractions. *In vivo* studies showed that the administrations of Sal A or Sal B attenuated the increased hepatic levels of collagen, MDA, TNF-alpha, IL-6, and IL-1beta, fibrosis scores and protein expression of alpha-SMA, heme-oxygenase-1, inducible nitric oxide synthase (iNOS), gp91 (phox), and serum levels of ALT, AST, IL-6, and IL-1beta compared with TAA-intoxicated rats. These results indicate that Sal A and B treatments are effective against hepatic fibrosis in TAA-intoxicated rats.

Glycyrrhizin (Leguminosae/Glycyrrhiza)

Zhou *et al.* (2006) investigated the anti-fibrotic effects of glycyrrhizin in rats induced by CCl_4, the rats in the treatment group received intraperitoneal injections of 3 μL glycyrrhizin (0.2 per cent) twice per week. The differences of Smad7 in different stages (1, 2, 4, 8 weeks after injection of CCl_4) were assessed by immunohistochemistry. The result showed that, compared with the model group, glycyrrhizin ameliorated the histopathological changes of rat liver at any stage, especially in later stage of liver fibrosis in the treatment group, and it also increased the expression level of smad7 in late stage of liver fibrosis in the treatment group. The authors indicated that glycyrrhizin can reduce hepatic fibrosis in rats induced by CCl_4.

Quercetin (Variety of Plant Sources)

Mao *et al.* (2004) studied the effect of quercetin on the expression of CTGF and FN in HSCs stimulated with TGF-beta1, the activated HSCs were incubated with quercetin (10^{-9}-10^{-5} M) for 24, 48 and 72 h. The results showed that quercetin (10^{-8}-10^{-5} M) inhibited the expression of TGF-beta1 in HSCs; TGF-beta1 expression decreased after the HSCs being incubated with quercetin (10^{-7} M) for 48 h; TGF-beta1 increased the expression of CTGF mRNA in HSCs, but this effect was abrogated by quercetin (10^{-7} M) within 72 h; quercetin (10^{-7} M) significantly inhibited the expression of FN in HSCs also. It suggests that quercetin may have an inhibitory effect on the signal pathways of TGF-beta, including the expression of TGF-beta1, FN and CTGF. Thus, quercetin may be useful in preventing liver fibrosis.

Rosmarinic Acid (Variety of Plant Sources)

Li, G.S. *et al.* (2010) studied the therapeutic effect of rosmarinic acid (RA) on experimental liver fibrosis *in vitro* and *in vivo*. RA (2.5, 5, 10 mg/kg b.w., i.g., daily for 4 weeks) was administered to the rats. The results indicated that RA inhibits HSCs proliferation, TGF-beta1, CTGF and alpha-SMA expression in cultured HSCs. Moreover, it had marked evidence in reducing fibrosis grade, ameliorating biochemical indicator and histopathological morphology, reducing liver TGF-beta1 and CTGF expression in CCl_4-induced liver fibrosis. It indicates that RA is useful in preventing the development of hepatic fibrosis.

Chlorogenic Acid (Variety of Plant Sources)

Shi *et al.* (2009) assessed the therapeutic effects of chlorogenic acid (CGA) on liver fibrosis in rats induced by CCl_4. CGA (60 and 30 mg/kg b.w., i.g.) was administered daily for 8 weeks to the rats. Histopathological examination indicated that CGA significantly reduced liver damage and symptoms of liver fibrosis compared with CCl_4 group. CGA suppressed the increased expression of collagen I and collagen III mRNA, reduced the protein expression of alpha-SMA and glucose-regulated proteins 78 and 94 (GRP78 and GRP94). In addition, as compared with the CGA-treated group, the expression of Bcl-2, vascular endothelial growth factor (VEGF), and TGF-beta1mRNA increased in CCl_4 group, whereas Bax mRNA expression decreased. The data indicated that CGA could effectively inhibit CCl_4-induced liver fibrosis in rats.

Two Kinds of Lignanoids from Natural Medicine Used to Treat Liver Fibrosis

γ-Schisandrin (Magnoliaceae/Schisandra Michx.)

Zhao *et al.* (2008) investigated the effect of γ-schisandrin in the proliferation, collagen synthesis and procollagen gene expression in HSCs from rats, the results showed in activated HSC being cultured, γ-schisandrin significantly decreased ^{3}H-proline incorporation into HSCs at the concentration of 40 μM and reduced procollagen gene I expression at the concentration of 80 μM ($P < 0.05$). It suggests γ-schisandrin could decrease collagen synthesis of HSC *in vitro.*

Schizandrin (Magnoliaceae/Schisandra Michx.)

Wang *et al.* (2008) observed the effect of schizandrin (SCH) on cytokines released by kupffer cells in rats with hepatic fibrosis. The results showed SCH significantly inhibited kupffer cells from delivering TNF-alpha, IL-6, and IL-8 (all $P < 0.05$). It suggests schizandrin can be used to attenuate liver fibrosis.

Seven Kinds of Glycosides Natural Medicine Used to Treat Liver Fibrosis

Total Saponins of Panax notoginseng (Araliaceae/Panax L.)

Zhang *et al.* (2007) investigated the effect of total saponins of *Panax notoginseng* (PNS) in the prevention of experimental hepatic fibrosis in rats induced by multiple hepatotoxic factors, including bovine serum albumin (BSA) and high fat diet. PNS (30 or 60 mg/kg b.w.) was administered intracutaneously daily for 6 weeks. The results showed the BSA injection significantly increased the serum levels of ALT and AST, whereas PNS treatment markedly down-regulated them; the positive staining of the collagen I, III and TGF-beta1 were stronger in hepatic fibrosis model group than that in PNS treatment group; the hepatic content of collagen was identical to the immunohistochemical results. It suggests PNS has the protective effect against liver fibrosis

Salidroside (Crassulaceae/Rhodiola L.)

Wu *et al.* (2009) observed the therapeutic effects of salidroside on CCl_4-induced liver fibrosis in rats. Salidroside (0.5 mg/kg b.w., i.p.) was administered to the rats twice per week for 8 weeks. The results showed that, compared with the model group, the expression of ROCK I, ROCK II and ROCK I mRNA, ROCK II mRNA decreased significantly in salidroside-treated group. It suggests salidroside could interfere with the signal transduction of Rho-ROCK pathway and inhibit CCl_4-induced liver fibrosis in rats.

Saikosaponin-d (Umbelliferae/Bupleurum L.)

Guo *et al.* (2009) investigated the anti-fibrotic effects of saikosaponin-d (SSd) with the relationship between MDA, SOD in liver tissue and zine, calcium content in the serum of rats with DMN-induced liver fibrosis. SSd (1.8 mg/kg b.w., i.p., daily for 4 weeks) was administered to the rats. Compared with the model group, SSd significantly reduced the expression of TGF-beta1 and alpha-SMA, improved the degree of fibrosis, decreased the hepatic content of MDA, increased the activity of SOD gradually and adjusted the serum contents of Zn and Ca in the SSd-treated group. It suggests SSd can evidently ameliorate the progression of hepatic fibrosis in rats induced by DMN.

Cucurbitacin B (Variety of Plant Resources)

Xu and Tong (2009) studied the inhibitory effect of cucurbitacin B on the liver fibrosis in mice due to *Schistosoma japonicum* infection, the mice in the treatment group were administered cucurbitacin B 0.2 mg/kg b.w., intragastrically, daily for 8 weeks. The results showed cucurbitacin B relieved the degree of hepatic fibrosis, reduced the contents of hepatic MDA, VEGFmRNA, VEGF, collagen I and III obviously and markedly elevated the activity of SOD in comparison with those in the model group; but those did not get back to normal level. It suggests cucurbitacin B may be useful in inhibiting the progress of liver fibrosis in mice due to *S. japonicum* infection.

Astrogalosides (Leguminosae/Astragalus L.)

Ding *et al.* (2008) investigated the therapeutic effect of astrogalosides on liver fibrosis in mice induced by *Schistosomiasis japonica*, the mice in the treatment groups were administered 10, 20 mg/kg b.w. astrogalosides, intragastrically, daily from 6th week of the experiment. The results showed that at the end of either 10th or 14th week of the experiment, in groups receiving high or low dose of astrogalosides, the mean area of Schistosome eggs nodules was decreased significantly, the degree of liver fibrosis and the expression of collagen I and III were also reduced in comparison with those in the model group; meanwhile, there was a significantly difference in the protein expression of collagen III between the high and low dose astrogaloside groups at the end of 10th week of the experiment ($P < 0.01$). It suggests astrogaloside exerts therapic effects on hepatic fibrosis in mice induced by *S. japonica.*

Total Glucosides of Paeony (Ranunculaceae/Paeonia L.)

Li, R.L. *et al.* (2007) studied the effect of total glucosides from paeony root (TGP) in the prevention of experimental hepatic fibrosis in rats induced by CCl_4, the rats of treatment groups were administered with TGP (40, 80, 160 mg/kg b.w., i.g.) daily for 8 weeks. Compared with the model group, TGP significantly decreased the serum levels of ALT, AST, ALP, HA and PCIII, increased albumin level and ratio of albumin over globulin (A/G) in TGP-treated groups. TGP (60, 120, 240 mg/L) markedly decreased the levels of HA and PCIII, escalated the HSC apoptosis and ameliorated the hepatic lesions. It suggests TGP could ameliorate the progress of hepatic fibrosis in rats induced by CCl_4.

Baicalin, Baicalein (Labiatae/Scutellaria L.)

Cheng and Yang (2010) investigated the protective effect of baicalin against CCl_4-induced hepatic fibrosis in mice. Baicalin (1, 2 g/kg b.w., s.c., once a week for 4 weeks) was administered to the KM mice. The results showed baicalin significantly reduced serum levels of ALT/GPT, AST/GOT, AKP, hepatic content of hydroxyproline and liver index in baicalin-treated groups compared with the model group. It suggests baicalin has a protective effect on hepatic fibrosis induced by CCl_4 in mice. Sun *et al.* (2010) studied the therapeutic effect of baicalein on liver fibrosis induced by CCl_4 in rats. CCl_4 treatment increased levels of AST, ALT, HA, LN and PCIII in serum, as well as hydroxyproline and MMPs in liver of rats. Baicalein treatment (20, 40, or 80 mg/kg b.w., daily for 10 weeks) dose-dependently decreased levels of these markers. Additionally, baicalein reduced inflammation, destruction of liver architecture and collagen accumulation and significantly inhibited protein synthesis of PDGF-beta receptor. The results suggest that baicalein is useful in inhibiting the progress of liver fibrosis induced by CCl_4 in rats.

Four Kinds of Amino Acids and Heterocyclic Natural Medicine Used to Treat Liver Fibrosis

Taurine (Single Amino Acid) (Bovidae/Genus Bos)

Deng *et al.* (2007) explored the protective effect of natural taurine on mitochondria of hepatic fibrosis in rats induced by CCl_4, the rats in the treated group were administered 600 mg/kg b.w. natural taurine, intragastrically, daily for 12 weeks. The results showed that membrane potential, cyt-c and SOD activity were obviously increased and the contents of MDA, TGF-beta1 and Ca^{2+} were markedly decreased in the natural taurine-treated group compared with those in the model group. In addition, hepatic pathologic tissue was ameliorated also. It suggests natural taurine is effective in resisting hepatic fibrosis in rats induced by CCl_4. Miyazaki *et al.* (2005) investigated the effects of taurine on hepatic fibrogenesis and in isolated HSC. The rats of the hepatic damage (HD) group were administered CCl_4 for 5 weeks and a subgroup received, in addition, a 2 per cent taurine containing diet for 6 weeks. The results indicated that taurine treatment reduced the loss of hepatic taurine concentration, the hepatic histological damage and fibrosis (particularly in the pericentral region) compared with the model group. Furthermore, the hepatic alpha-SMA, lipid hydroperoxide and 8-OHdG levels in serum and liver, as well as hepatic TGF-beta1 mRNA and hydroxyproline levels were significantly increased in the HD group, and most of these parameters were significantly reduced following taurine treatment. In addition, the lipid hydroperoxide and hydroxyproline concentrations, as well as TGF-beta1 mRNA level were significantly reduced by taurine in activated HSC. It demonstrates that oral taurine administration enhances hepatic taurine accumulation, reduces oxidative stress and prevents progress of CCl_4-induced hepatofibrosis in HD rats, as well as inhibits transformation of the HSC. Lakshmi and Anuradha (2010) examined the influence of taurine on mitochondrial damage, oxidative stress and apoptosis in experimental liver fibrosis. The results demonstrated that hepatocytes isolated from ethanol plus iron-treated rats showed decreased cell viability and redox ratio, increased reactive oxygen species formation, lipid peroxidation, DNA fragmentation, and formation of apoptotic bodies. Additionally, liver mitochondria showed increased susceptibility to swell, diminished activities of mitochondrial respiratory chain complexes and antioxidants. Moreover, taurine administration to fibrotic rats restored mitochondrial function, reduced reactive oxygen species formation, and prevented DNA damage and apoptosis. It suggests that taurine might ameliorate the process of liver fibrosis.

Hirudin (Leech from Hirudinidae)

Jia *et al.* (2009) observed the effect of hirudin on CTGF mRNA expression in CCl_4-induced fibrotic liver of rats. The rats in the treated group were administered with himdin (60 mg/kg b.w., i.g.) daily for 12 weeks. The results showed the CTGF mRNA expression in himdin group was down-regulated compared with the model group ($P < 0.05$). It suggests himdin has a protective effect on hepatic fibrosis induced by CCl_4 in rats.

Tetramethylpyrazine (Umbelliferae/Ligusticum L.)

Hua *et al.* (2007) investigated the effects of tetramethylpyrazine (TMP) for chronicity liver fibrosis in rats induced by porcine serum, the rats in the treated group were injected intraperitoneally 10, 20, 40 mg/kg b.w. TMP, daily for 8 weeks. The result showed that compared with the model group, the degree of liver fibrosis indexes were improved significantly; the serum ALT, AST and ALP levels were depressed, the level of A/G were enhanced; the expression of TGF-beta1, TIMP-1 were reduced whilst the serum HA, LN, C-IV and PIIINP levels were decreased in TMP-treated group. It suggests TMP could ameliorate liver fibrosis in rats induced by porcine serum.

Melatonin (From High Class of Animals)

Zhao *et al.* (2009) studied the mechanism of melatonin against liver fibrosis in rats induced by CCl_4. The rats in the treatment group were administered melatonin (10mg/kg b.w., i.p.) daily for 3 months. The results showed that compared with the model group, melatonin decreased the score of rat liver fibrosis and the number of activated HSCs in the treatment group. It suggests melatonin could reduce rat liver fibrosis induced by CCl_4. Ye *et al.* (2007) explored the influence of melatonin (MT) on the apoptosis and function of hepatic stellate cells (HSC). The model of rat hepatic fibrosis was induced by CCl_4. *In vivo*, the rats in the treatment groups were administered MT (0.125, 0.5, 2.0 mg/kg b.w., i.g.) daily for 8 weeks. *In vitro*, HSC isolated from the model group rats was exposed to MT (10^{-9}, 10^{-7} or 10^{-5} moL/L). The results showed that in the *in vivo* experiment, liver pathological changes induced by CCl_4 were relieved when compared with the model group, and the levels of serum HA and PCIII were reduced in each dose of MT-treated groups; *in vitro*, the apoptosis of HSC was significantly induced by MT of 10 μmoL/L, and the levels of HA and PCIII were reduced by MT of all concentrations. It suggests melatonin could relieve rat hepatic fibrosis.

Three Kinds of Terpenoids and Steroids of Natural Medicine Used to Treat Liver Fibrosis

Ursolic Acid (Variety of Plant Sources)

Ouyang *et al.* (2009) investigated the effect of ursolic acid (UA) on the expression of TGF-beta1 mRNA, protein and alpha-SMA protein in liver fibrosis of rats induced by DMN. UA (10, 20 or 40 mg/kg b.w., i.p.) was administered daily to rats for 4 weeks in the treatment groups. The results indicated that the degree of hepatic cell necrosis and fibrous tissue hyperplasia were decreased markedly in the U2 (medium dose UA) and U3 (high dose UA) groups. The expression levels of TGF-beta1 protein in the U1 (low-dose UA) group and colchine group were lower than those in the model control group, while the expression levels of TGF-beta1 protein in the U2 (medium-dose UA) and U3 (high-dose UA) groups were not only significantly lower than that in the model control group (both $P < 0.01$), but also lower than that in the colchine group ($P < 0.05$ or 0.01). Furthermore, the expression levels of TGF-beta1 mRNA in the U2 and U3 groups wee lower than those in the model control group (both$P < 0.01$) and colchine group ($P < 0.05$ or 0.01). The expression levels of alpha-SMA protein in the U1, U2 and U3 groups were significantly lower than those in the model control group (all $P < 0.01$) and colchine group (all $P < 0.01$). It suggests UA could significantly ameliorate DMN-induced liver fibrosis in rats.

Ganoderma Triterpene (Polyporaceae/Ganoderma Karst.)

Chen *et al.* (2008) studied the protective effect of *Ganoderma* triterpene on hepatic fibrosis in rats induced by CCl_4. The rats in the treated groups were administered with 45, 90, 180 mg/kg b.w. of *Ganoderma* triterpene, intragastrically, daily for 7 weeks. Compared with model group, *Ganoderma* triterpene significantly decreased serum levels of AST, ALT, GGT, and the expression of TGF-beta1 mRNA, MMP-2 in liver tissue in *Ganoderma* triterpene-treated group; in addition, liver pathological changes induced by DMN were obviously attenuated. It suggests*Ganoderma* triterpene has a protective effect on hepatic fibrosis in rats induced by DMN.

Beta1-elemene (Zingiberaceae/Curcuma L.)

Hu *et al.* (2007) investigated the effect of Zedoary rhizome extract (beta1-elemene) on the expression of TGFbeta1, alpha-SMA and collagen I in rats with hepatic fibrosis induced by CCl_4. The rats in the treatment group were intraperitonealy administered 1 mL/kg b.w. beta1-elemene (percent by volume: 95 per cent) daily for 8 weeks. The results showed that the area percentages were significantly lower in the treatment group than those in the model and control group (both$P < 0.01$), and the histological remission and collagen fiber diminishment were also better in the treatment group, the expression of collagen I was significantly lower in the treatment group than that in the model and control group ($P < 0.01$) too, the levels of alpha-SMA and TGF-beta1 expression were significantly different between the treatment group and the model group (both $P < 0.01$). It suggests that beta1-elemene can reverse the pathologic progression of CCl_4-induced liver fibrosis in rats.

A Kind of Polysaccharide from Natural Medicine Used to Treat Liver Fibrosis

Corydyceps Polysaccharide (Clavicipitaceae/Cordyceps)

Li *et al.* (2006) studied the effect of corydyceps polysaccharide (CP) against liver fibrosis in rats induced by DMN. The rats in the treated group were adminstered CP (60 mg/kg b.w., i.p.) daily for 4 weeks. Compared with the model group, CP improved the hepatic function indices (ALT, AST, ALB and TBIL), decreased the hepatic content of MDA and increased the activity of SOD in CP-treated group. Moreover, compared with normal control group, hydroxyproline and collagen IV contents, TIMMP-2 level were increased and MM-2 level was decreased in liver tissue of the model group, while CP depressed these histopathological changes at different degrees. It suggests CP could exert good effect against liver fibrosis in rats induced by DMN.

Coumarin of Natural Medicine Used to Treat Liver Fibrosis

Lycopene (Solanaceae/Lycopersicon Mill.)

Zhang *et al.* (2008) studied the therapeutic effect of lycopene on hepatic fibrosis in KM mice induced by concanavalin A. The mice in the treatment group were intragastriclly administered 15 mg/kg b.w. lycopene twice a week and were killed in batch in 1, 2, 3, 4, 5 weeks later. Histopathological examination showed that the mice in control group did not catch hepatic fibrosis whereas the mice in placebo group did, and the mice in treatment group were cured after 5 weeks. It suggests lycopene has a therapeutic effect on hepatitis fibrosis induced by concanavalin A.

Thirty Two Kinds of Single Herbal Drugs Used to Treat Liver Fibrosis

Root

Yam (Dioscoreaceae/Dioscorea L.)

Chan *et al.* (2010) investigated the hepatic protection of yam in the CCl_4-induced hepatic fibrosis of rats. Yam (0.5, 1 or 2 g/kg b.w., i.g., daily for 8 weeks) was administered to the treated rats. The results showed that treatment with yam significantly decreased the ratio of liver/body weight, levels of gamma-glutaminotranspeptidase (GGT), low-density lipoprotein, and triglyceride in serum compared with those administered CCl_4 alone, while treatment with yams significantly elevated antioxidant activities of glutathione peroxidase (GSH-Px) and SOD in livers. Microscopically, yam-treated groups presented with low histoscores of CCl_4-induced liver injury and fibrosis. Additionally, yam treatment reduced the area of GGT-positive foci and the index of proliferating cell nuclear antigen (PCNA) in liver. It suggests daily administration of yam can ameliorate the CCl_4-induced hepatic fibrosis in rats in a dose-dependent manner.

Salvia miltiorrhiza (Labiatae/Salvia L.)

Lee *et al.* (2003) studied the effects of long-term *Salvia miltiorrhiza* administration in CCl_4-induced hepatic injury in rats. *S. miltiorrhiza* (10, 25 or 50 mg/kg b.w., twice a day) was given for 9 weeks, beginning at the same time as the injections of CCl_4. The results showed that *S. miltiorrhiza* administration increased the hepatic glutathione level and decreased the peroxidation products in a dose-dependent manner. Additionally, it reduced the mRNA expression of markers (TGF-beta1, TIMP-1 and procollagen I) for hepatic fibrogenesis. In conclusion, long-term administration of *S. miltiorrhiza* in rats ameliorates the CCl_4-induced hepatic injury that probably related to a reduced oxidant stress and degree of hepatic fibrosis.

Rhei rhizome (Polygonaceae/Rheum L.)

Jin *et al.* (2005) investigated the therapeutic effect of herbal medicine Rhei rhizome, extract powder from herbs, on the development of liver fibrosis. In an *in vivo* study, the effects of Rhei rhizome were examined using the choline-deficient L-amino acid-defined (CDAA) diet-induced liver fibrosis model. In an *in vitro* study, the effects of Rhei rhizome on procollagen I mRNA expression, alpha-SMA, MMPs and TIMPs of isolated HSCs were examined. The *in vivo* results exhibited that Rhei rhizome prevented fibrosis in a dose-dependent manner up to 1.0 per cent (w/w) with a reduced number of activated stellate cells. Moreover, the *in vitro* experiment demonstrated that Rhei rhizome prevented stellate cell activation resulting in reduced procollagen in mRNA, alpha-SMA and TIMP-1, 2 expressions. These results indicated that Rhei rhizome can significantly reduces liver fibrosis.

Radix ampelopsis Sincae (Ampelidaceae/Ampelopsis Michx.)

Cheng *et al.* (2008) investigated the effect of *Radix ampelopsis* Sincae extract-containing rat semen on the apoptosis and expression of Bax/Bcl-2 gene in cultured HSC/T_6 cells. The results showed the apoptotic rates were 8.50 per cent, 14.30 per cent, 22.60 per cent after treatment with 5 per cent, 10 per cent, 20 per cent *R. ampelopsis* extract-containing rat semen, which were more than those treated with control semen. Moreover, the gene expression of Bax was up-regulated and that of Bcl-2 was down-regulated after treatment with the extract-containing rat semen. It suggests *R. ampelopsis* extract-containing rat semen has the potential anti-fibrotic effect.

Aqueous Garlic Extract (Liliaceae/Allium L.)

Gedik *et al.* (2005) evaluated the antioxidant and anti-fibrotic effects of chronic administration of aqueous garlic extract on liver fibrosis induced by biliary obstruction in rats. Liver fibrosis was induced in male Wistar albino rats by bile duct ligation and scission (BDL). Aqueous garlic extract (AGE, 1 mL/kg b.w., i.p., corresponding to 250 mg/kg b.w.) or saline was administered daily for 28 days. The results showed that AGE treatment significantly reduced the elevated levels of serum AST, ALT, LDH, and TNF-alpha, elevated the depressed hepatic GSH level, and reduced the increases in tissue free radical, MDA level, MPO activity and hepatic collagen content back to control levels as compared to control group. Since AGE administration alleviated the BDL-induced oxidative injury of the liver and improved the structure and function of liver, it suggests that AGE may have potential therapeutic value in protecting the liver from fibrosis and oxidative injury due to biliary obstruction. Shinkawa *et al.* (2009) investigated the anti-fibrotic effects of S-allylcysteine (SAC), an ingredient of aged garlic extract, on liver fibrosis in male Wistar rats induced by porcine serum (PS). SAC (0.15 per cent of basal diet) or N-acetylcysteine (NAC, 0.45 per cent of basal diet) was orally administered to the rats for 12 weeks. The results revealed that both SAC and NAC markedly attenuated the development of hepatic fibrosis and significantly suppressed the PS-induced increase in alpha-SMA expression. It suggests oral administration of SAC reduces PS-induced hepatic fibrosis in rats via inhibition of HSC activation. D'Argenio *et al.* (2010) investigated the anti-fibrotic effect of garlic extract and cystamine as specific tissue transglutaminase inhibitors, which are considered to contribute to liver damage in the development of hepatic fibrosis. Rat liver fibrosis was induced by intraperitoneal injection of CCl_4 for 7 weeks. Cystamine or garlic extract was administrated by daily intraperitoneal injection, starting from the day after the first administration of CCl_4. The results indicated that cystamine and garlic extract decreased the elevation of transglutaminase activity ($P < 0.05$), reduced the the liver fibrosis and collagen deposition, particularly in the garlic extract group ($P < 0.01$). Additionally, the liver damage improved and serum ALT was decreased ($P < 0.05$). Moreover, tissue transglutaminase immunolocalised with collagen fibres and was mainly found in the ECM of damaged liver; Alpha-SMA, IL-1beta, tissue transglutaminase mRNA and tissue transglutaminase protein were down-regulated in the cystamine and garlic extract groups compared to controls. These findings may identify garlic cystamine-like molecules as a potential therapeutic strategy in the treatment of hepatic fibrosis.

Alchornea trewioides (Benth.) Muell. Arg. (Euphorbiaceae/Alchornea)

Lü *et al.* (2007) observed the therapeutic effect of Hongbeiyegen [the root of *Alchornea trewioides* (Benth.) Muell.-Arg.] on alcohol-induced liver fibrosis in rats. Aqueous Hongbeiyegen extract (9, 18 or 36 mg/kg b.w., i.g.) was administered daily for 90 days to the treated rats. Compared with the control group, Hongbeiyegen could significantly reduce the levels of TGF-beta1, TIMP-1, HA, LN, PCIII, CIV, ALT and AST in rats treated with it. It suggests Hongbeiyegen can ameliorate liver fibrosis possibly by inhibiting the expression of TGF-betal and TIMP-1.

Stephania tetrandra (Menispermaceae/Cocculus DC.)

Chor *et al.* (2009) investigated the preventive effects of *Stephania tetrandra* (ST) on hepatic fibrosis in rats induced by CCl_4. As compared with the CCl_4-only rats, ST significantly decreased serum ALT activity ($P < 0.01$), and prevented or reversed the hepatic fibrosis ($P < 0.01$) induced by CCl_4. Moreover, ST reduced protein expression of alpha-SMA in prevention ($P < 0.05$) and regression ($P < 0.01$) experiments. Additionally, the double-color staining of alpha-SMA and TUNEL indicated that ST increased HSC apoptosis. It suggests *S. tetrandra* may effectively prevent and reverse hepatic fibrosis through activating HSC apoptosis in rats.

Leaf

Piper Betel Leaves (Piperaceae/Piper L.)

Young *et al.* (2007) evaluated the antihepatotoxic effect of piper betel leaves (PBL) extract on the CCl_4-induced liver injury in a rat model. The results indicated that PBL extract significantly inhibited the elevated AST and ALT activities, attenuated total glutathione S-transferase (GST) activity and GST alpha isoform activity, whereas enhanced SOD and catalase (CAT) activities. In addition, the histological examination showed the PBL extract protected liver from the damage induced by CCl_4 by decreasing alpha-SMA expression, inducing active MMP2 expression through Ras/Erk pathway, and inhibiting TIMP2 level that consequently attenuated the fibrosis of liver. The data of this study support a chemopreventive potential of PBL against liver fibrosis.

Gingko biloba (Ginkgoaceae/Ginkgo L.)

Shi *et al.* (2006) investigated the effects of *Gingko biloba* extract (GBE) on CCl_4 induced liver fibrosis in rats. The rats in the treatment group were intragastrically administered with GBE (0.4 g/kg b.w.) daily for 8 weeks. The results showed that compared with the model group, GBE treatment decreased the grade of liver fibrosis ($P < 0.05$), significantly improved the serum levels of ALT, AST and ALB (all $P < 0.05$), markedly reduced mRNA and protein levels of activin A (both $P < 0.01$), decreased the apoptosis index ($P < 0.01$) in the treatment group. It suggests GBE can markedly attenuate the degrees of hepatic fibrosis. Zhou *et al.* (2008) studied the therapeutic effect of *Gingko* leaves on hepatic fibrosis in rats induced by multiple hepatotoxic factors, including CCl_4, high-fat, low-protein diet and alcohol. The rats in the treated groups were administered with the extract of *Gingko* leaves (50, 100 mg/kg b.w., i.g.) daily for 8 weeks. Compared with normal control group, the serum level of HA and hepatic hydroxyproline content increased in spontaneous recovery group ($P < 0.05$), while decreased in the two treated groups compared with the spontaneous recovery group ($P < 0.05$); the expressions of TGF-beta1 and alpha-SMA in spontaneous recovery group were higher than those in normal control group ($P < 0.05$); compared with spontaneous recovery group, the expressions of TGF-beta1 and alpha-SMA decreased remarkably and showed a direct correlation in the two treated groups ($r = 0.735$ and $P < 0.05$ in high dose treated group; $r = 0.936$ and $P < 0.01$ in low dose treated group). It suggests the extracts of *Gingko* leaves may palliate the hepatic fibrosis by regulating the activity of HSCs through TGF-beta1 pathway.

Green Tea (Theaceae/Camellia)

Kim *et al.* (2009) studied the protective effect of green tea extract (GT) on hepatic fibrosis *in vitro* and *in vivo* in DMN-induced rats. HSC-T6, a rat hepatic stellate cell line, was used as an *in vitro* assay system. GT (100 mg/kg) was administered in drinking water which was calculated according to the amount of water consumed in the previous day for 4 weeks, which prevented the development of hepatic fibrosis in the rat model of DMN-induced liver fibrosis. These results were confirmed by both ameliorated liver histology and quantitative measurement of hepatic hydroxyproline content, a marker of liver collagen deposition. Accordingly, inhibition of proliferation, reduced collagen deposition, and collagen I expression were observed in activated HSC-T6 cells following GT treatment. These results implied that green tea administration can effectively attenuate liver fibrosis in rats caused by DMN.

Fruit

Actinidia rubricaulis (Actinidiaceae/Actinidia Lindl.)

Liao *et al.* (2007) assessed the antioxidant activity and hepatoprotective effect of ethanol extracts of *Actinidia rubricaulis* (AR) on chronic liver injury induced by CCl_4 in rats. AR was administered to rats for 8 weeks. The results showed AR reduced the elevated levels of serum glutamate-oxalate-transaminase (sGOT) and glutamate-pyruvate-transaminase (sGPT) caused by CCl_4 at weeks 1, 3, 6, and 8. The biochemical data were also consistent with those of the histological observations. Moreover, the AR extract recovered the CCl_4-induced liver injury and showed antioxidant effect in assays of antioxidant enzyme activity, such as SOD, GSH-Px and GSH-Rd. Based on these results, it was suggested that the AR has the hepatoprotective effect and could attenuate liver fibrosis caused by CCl_4.

Phaseolus trilobus (Leguminosae/Vicia L.)

Fursule *et al.* (2010) studied the effect of *Phaseolus trilobus* as hepatoprotective and antioxidant agents. The hepatoprotective activity of methanol and aqueous extract of *P. trilobus* was evaluated by bile duct ligation induced liver fibrosis. The results indicated that methanol and aqueous extracts of *P. trilobus* reduced elevated level of ALT, AST, ALP, LDH, bilirubin and hydroxyproline significantly ($P < 0.01$) in bile duct ligated Wistar rats, proving it's hepatoprotective activity comparable with silymarin. Moreover, both the extracts decreased the elevation of serum TBARS level and elevate superoxide scavenging radical activity, proving antioxidant activity comparable with ascorbic acid. Additionally, it was found to elevate the reduced level of glutathione in liver proving antioxidant activity comparable with silymarin. The data suggest *P. trilobus* possesses anti-hepatic fibrosis property.

Coffee (Rubiaceae/Coffea L.)

Shi *et al.* (2010) evaluated the effects of a coffee preparation on liver fibrosis induced by CCl_4. Coffee preparation (300 and 150 mg/kg) was intragastrically administered to the two coffee preparation groups daily for 8 weeks. The results indicated that coffee preparation treatment significantly reduced liver damage and symptoms of liver fibrosis upon histopathological examination. In addition, the mRNA expressions of collagen I, collagen III, Bcl-2, VEGF and TGF-beta1 were markedly increased by CCl_4 treatment, but they were suppressed by coffee preparation treatment. Whereas compared with the CCl_4 group, the mRNA expression of Bax increased in the coffee preparation group. Moreover, administration of a coffee preparation reduced the protein expression of alpha-SMA and the glucose-regulated proteins (GRP) 78 and 94 in rats increased by CCl_4. It suggests coffee exerts a protective effect against liver fibrosis. Shin *et al.* (2010) examined the protective effect of coffee against liver fibrosis in rats induced by DMN. Compared to the rats treated with DMN and water, coffee administration significantly prevented the deterioration of body weight, organ weight, and serum biochemistry in coffee-treated rats. Histopathological examination also revealed that necrosis/inflammation and fibrotic septa decreased significantly. Furthermore, coffee treatment remarkably inhibited the accumulation of hydroxyproline ($P < 0.001$), the production of MDA ($P < 0.05$) and stellate cell activation, protected the depletion of glutathione, SOD, and catalase in liver tissue caused by DMN injection. In addition, coffee administration inhibited the gene expression of iNOS, TGF-beta, TNF-alpha, IL-1 and PDGF-beta in liver tissue, and lowered the concentration of TGF-beta and PDGF-beta in liver. It indicates that coffee can efficiently inhibit CCl_4-induced liver fibrosis in rats. Modi *et al.* (2010) investigated the preventive effects of caffeine intake on hepatic fibrosis. Caffeine intake was compared between patients with mild and advanced liver fibrosis (bridging fibrosis/cirrhosis). One hundred seventy-seven patients (99 male, 104 white, 121 with chronic HCV infection) undergoing liver biopsy completed the caffeine questionnaire on up to three occasions. The results showed that daily caffeine consumption above the 75th percentile for the cohort (308 mg = approximately 2.25 cups of coffee equivalents) was associated with reduced liver fibrosis (odds ratio [OR], 0.33; 95 per cent confidence interval [CI], 0.14-0.80; $P = 0.015$) and the protective association persisted after controlling for age, sex, race, liver disease, body mass index, and alcohol intake in all patients (OR: 0.25; 95 per cent CI: 0.09-0.67; $P = 0.006$), as well as the subset with HCV infection (OR: 0.19; 95 per cent CI: 0.05-0.66; $P = 0.009$). However, consumption of caffeine from sources other than coffee or of decaffeinated coffee was not associated with reduced liver fibrosis. It suggested that caffeine consumption above a threshold of approximately 2 coffee-cup equivalents per day, particularly from regular coffee, was useful in preventing the progress of liver fibrosis.

Black Bean (Leguminosae/Glycine Willd)

López-Reyes *et al.* (2008) examined the effects of methanolic black bean extract on CCl_4-induced liver fibrosis in rats. Black bean extract (70 mg/kg b.w., i.g.; daily for

8 weeks) was administered to the treated rats. Qualitative and quantitative histological analysis showed that administration of black bean extract reduced hepatic fibrosis index by 18 per cent compared to positive controls ($P = 0.006$), as a result of a decrease in collagen I (44.3 per cent less, $P = 0.03$) and IV gene expression (68.9 per cent less, $P = 0.049$) compared to CCl_4-injured and quercetin treated rats. These data suggest that this methanolic black bean extract ameliorates liver fibrosis in the animal model used.

Semen hoveniae (Rhamnaceae/Hovenia Thunb)

Geng *et al.* (2008) investigated the anti-liver fibrotic effect of *Semen hoveniae* extracts (SHE) in rats induced by CCl_4, the rats in the treatment groups received daily SHE (40, 80 or 160 mg/kg b.w., i.g.) for 6 weeks. The results showed the levels of serum PCIII, HA, LN decreased and liver function got improved; the histological examination also demonstrated its anti-fibrotic effect. It suggests SHE has anti-hepatic fibrosis property.

Zizyphus spinachristi (L.) (Rhamnaceae/Zizyphus Mill)

Amin and Mahmoud-Ghoneim (2009) examined the effects of the water extract of *Zizyphus spina-christi* (L.) (ZSC) on CCl_4-induced hepatic fibrosis in rats. ZSC extract (0.125, 0.250 or 0.350 g/kg b.w., oral) was daily administered to the rats for 8 weeks. The results revealed that ZSC reduced activities of serum ALT and AST, restored normal levels of MDA and retained control activities of endogenous antioxidants, such as SOD, CAT and GSH. Furthermore, it reduced the expression of alpha-SMA, the deposition of collagen I, III and improved the quality of collagen I distribution and its quantity. The data demonstrate that administration of ZSC can be used to inhibit the progression of hepatic fibrosis in rats induced by CCl_4.

Blueberry (Ericaceae/Vaccinium spp.)

Wang *et al.* (2010) evaluated the effects of blueberry on hepatic fibrosis in rats induced by CCl_4. Forty-five male Sprague-Dawley rats were randomly divided into control group (A); CCl_4-induced hepatic fibrosis group (B); blueberry prevention group (C); Dan-shao-hua-xian capsule (DSHX) prevention group (D); and blueberry + DSHX prevention group (E). Blueberry juice (15 g/kg b.w., p.o., daily for 8 weeks) was administered to treated rats. Compared with group B, liver indices, levels of serum HA and ALT of groups C, D and E reduced (all $P < 0.05$), and SOD level was significantly higher, but MDA level was lower in liver homogenates (all $P < 0.05$). Meanwhile, the stage of hepatic fibrosis was significantly weakened ($P < 0.05$). Compared with group A, the activity of GST in liver homogenates, expression levels of *Nrf2* and Nqo1 in group B elevated ($P < 0.05$). The expression level of *Nrf2* and Nqo1 in groups C, D, and E increased as compared with group B, but the difference was not significant. It suggests blueberry has therapeutic effects against CCl_4-induced hepatic fibrosis in rats.

Bark

Fraxinus rhynchophylla (Oleaceae/Fraxinus L.)

Peng *et al.* (2010) examined the effect of *Fraxinus rhynchophylla* ethanol extract (FR(EtOH)) on liver fibrosis induced by CCl_4 in rats. The rats in the treatment groups were administered daily with FR(EtOH) (0.1, 0.5 or 1.0 g/kg b.w., p.o.) for 8 weeks. The results showed that FR(EtOH) (0.1, 0.5 or 1.0 g/kg b.w.) significantly reduced the elevated activities of sGOT and sGPT, obviously increased the activities of GSH-Px, reduced the incidence of liver lesions, including hepatic cells cloudy swelling, lymphocytes infiltration, cytoplasm vacuolization hepatic necrosis and fibrous connective tissue proliferated induced by CCl_4 in rats. Moreover, FR(EtOH) (0.1 and 0.5 g/kg b.w.) inhibited the increased protein levels of uPA, MMP-2, MMP-9 and TIMP-1. Finally, the amount of esculetin in the FR(EtOH) was 33.54 mg/g extract. It suggests oral administration of FR(EtOH) has preventive effects on CCl_4-induced hepatic fibrosis in rats.

Peel

Pomegranate Peel (Punicaceae/Punica L.)

Toklu *et al.* (2007) evaluated the effect of chronic administration of pomegranate peel extract (PPE) on liver fibrosis induced by bile duct ligation (BDL) in rats. PPE (50 mg/kg b.w.) or saline was administered orally for 28 days. Compared with the control group, PPE treatment significantly decreased the elevation of serum AST, ALT, LDH and cytokines; meanwhile, it increased plasma AOC and hepatic GSH levels back to control levels; in addition, increases in tissue MDA levels, MPO activity and hepatic collagen content due to BDL were reduced back to control levels. It demonstrates PPE could alleviate the BDL-induced oxidative injury of the liver and improve the hepatic tissue structure and liver function.

Flower

Hibiscus sabdariffa L. (Malvaceae/Hibiscus)

Liu *et al.* (2006) investigated extracts of dried flower of *Hibiscus sabdariffa* L. (HSE), a local soft drink material and medicinal herb, for its protective effects against liver fibrosis induced by CCl_4 in rats. The rats in the treatment groups received various HSE doses (1-5 per cent) for 9 weeks. Compared with the control group, HSE significantly reduced the liver damage including steatosis and fibrosis in a dose-dependent manner and decreased the elevation in plasma AST, ALT. Moreover, it restored the decrease in glutathione content and inhibited the formation of lipid peroxidative products during CCl_4 treatment. In addition, HSE obviously inhibited the activation of the hepatic stellate cells in the primary culture. These results suggest that HSE may have protective effects against CCl_4-induced liver fibrosis in rats.

Grass

Saururus chinensis (Saururaceae/Saururus)

Wang *et al.* (2009) evaluated the hepatoprotective and anti-fibrotic effects of *Saururus chinensis* extract (SC-E) in CCl_4 induced liver fibrosis rats. SC-E (70 mg/kg b.w., i.g., daily for 8 weeks) was administered to the rats starting from the onset of CCl_4 treatment. The results showed SC-E effectively reduced the elevated levels of liver index, serum ALT, AST, HA, and hepatic MDA content, enhanced the reduced hepatic SOD activity in CCl_4-treated rats. Moreover, the histopathological analysis suggested that SC-E obviously alleviated the degree of liver fibrosis induced by CCl_4. These results suggest SC-E is useful in preventing the progress of liver fibrosis.

Lygodium flexuosum (Lygodiaceae/Lygodium)

Wills and Asha (2007) evaluated the protective effect of *Lygodium flexuosum* n-hexane extract against CCl_4-induced fibrosis in rats. *L. flexuosum* n-hexane extract (200 mg/kg b.w., p.o.) was administered daily for 10 weeks in preventive treatment and given daily for 2 weeks after the establishment of fibrosis for 10 weeks in curative treatment. Compared with the model group, administration of *L. flexuosum* n-hexane extract reduced the mRNA levels of proinflammatory cytokines, growth factors and other signaling molecules, which are involved in hepatic fibrosis. In addition, the elevation of expression levels of TNF-alpha, IL-1beta, TGF-beta1, procollagen-I, procollagen-III and TIMP-1 were found to be reduced to normal by the treatment of *L. flexuosum* n-hexane extract. Moreover, the increased levels of MMPs-13 in*L. flexuosum* n-hexane extract treated rats were indicative of the protective action of it. The data suggest *L. flexuosum* n-hexane extract effectively reverses CCl_4-induced hepatic fibrosis in curative treatment and reduces the effect of ongoing toxic liver injury in preventive treatment by promoting extracellular matrix degradation in the fibrotic liver.

Anoectochilus formosanus (Orchidaceae/Anoectochilus Bl.)

Shih *et al.* (2005) investigated the effects of aqueous extract of *Anoectochilus formosanus* (AFE) on liver fibrogenesis in CCl_4-induced cirrhosis. AFE (0.5 and 2.0 g/kg b.w., p.o., daily for 8 weeks) was administered to rats simultaneously. The results showed that compared with the model group, AFE increased the albumin concentration, the liver weight, the protein content and liver glutathione concentrations, whereas reduced the elevated levels of GOT and GPT, decreased the spleen weight and collagen content in rats liver in AFE-treated groups. All these results clearly demonstrated that AFE can reduce the liver fibrogensis in rats induced by CCl_4. Wu *et al.* (2010) studied the effects of a standardized aqueous extract of *A. formosanus* (SAEAF) on thioacetamide (TAA)-induced liver fibrosis in mice. An *in vitro* study showed that the inhibitory effect of kinsenoside, a major component of SAEAF, on TNF-alpha secretion from Kupffer cells might be derived at least partly from downregulation of LPS-receptor Toll-like receptor 4 (TLR4) signaling. SAEAF (1.0, 0.2 g/kg b.w., i.g., daily for 12 weeks) was administered to the treated mice. The results showed that SAEAF significantly reduced plasma ALT activity, relative liver weight and hepatic hydroxyproline content in SAEAF-treated groups in comparison with the model group. In addition, the histological examination confirmed that SAEAF reduced the degree of fibrosis caused by TAA treatment. Furthermore, RT-PCR analysis showed that SAEAF reduced mRNA expressions of collagen I, lipopolysaccharide-binding protein, CD14, TLR4, and TNF receptor 1. An immunohistochemical examination also indicated that SAEAF reduced the number of CD68-positive cells (macrophages). It suggests administration of SAEAF markedly reduces TAA-induced hepatic fibrosis in mice, probably through inhibition of hepatic Kupffer cell activation.

Aquilegia vulgaris (Ranunculaceae/Aquilegia L.)

Jodynis-Liebert *et al.* (2009) investigated the effect of ethanol extract of *Aquilegia vulgaris* (extract) on liver fibrosis induced by CCl_4 in rats. The rats in the treatment group were simultaneously administered 100 mg/kg b.w. extract daily for 6 weeks. The results showed that administration of the extract increased the activity of antioxidant enzymes, decreased the level of hydroxyproline, reduced the elevated activity of serum hepatic enzymes, and caused a fall in bilirubin and cholesterol level when compared with animals treated with CCl_4 alone. Additionally, histopathological examination revealed less-severe fibrosis in rats administered with the extract. All these results suggest ethanol extract of *A. vulgaris* can reduce the liver fibrogensis in rats induced by CCl_4.

Hsian-tsao (Labiatae/Mesona Bl.)

Shyu *et al.* (2008) evaluated the protective effect of extract of Hsian-tsao (*Mesona Procumbens* Heml.) (EHT) against liver fibrogenesis in CCl_4-injured rats, and the inhibitory effect of oleanolic acid (OA) and ursolic acid (UA), which are the active compounds in EHT, on the activation of hepatic stellate cells (HSC). The results showed that oral administration of EHT at the dose of 1.2g/kg b.w. significantly reduced the liver injury, the level of alpha-SMA and the activity of MMPs compared with the model group. Furthermore, it decreased the serum levels of AST, ALT and the deposition of collagen in the liver. In addition, experiments with the rat hepatic stellate cell line HSC-T6 showed EHT induced the expression of MMP-2 and alpha-SMA with phorbol-12-myristate-13-acetate (PMA). Treating these cells with OA (20 μM) or UA (10 μM) caused a decrease in the levels of both proteins. Taken together, the data indicated that EHT can efficiently inhibit CCl_4-induced liver fibrosis in rats.

Breviscapine (Compositae/Erigeron L.)

Du *et al.* (2009) observed protective effects of breviscapine against hepatic fibrosis *in vivo* and *in vitro*. In the *in vitro* test, breviscapine had no cytotoxicity directly on HSCs; however, it suppressed cell proliferation, activation and secretion of HA, LN and collagen I induced by TGF-beta1 in HSCs. Furthermore, in the *in vivo* experiment, administration of breviscapine (0.5 mg/kg b.w., i.g., daily for 28 days) inhibited the elevation of serum ALT, AST and the depression of SOD activity, peroxidase (POD) and catalase (CAT). In addition, breviscapine reduced hepatic hydroxyproline, collagen, MDA and TGF-beta1 content in liver tissue of rats. All these data suggested that breviscapine has certain protective effect against hepatic fibrosis.

Potentilla chinensis (Rosaceae/Potentilla)

Li, Z. *et al.* (2007) observed the curative effect of the ethanolic extract of *Potentilla chinensis* (PS) on hepatic fibrosis in rats induced by CCl_4. PS treatment group was intragastrically administered 5g/kg b.w. PS daily for 8 weeks. Compared with model control group, the serum levels of ALP, HA, and the hepatic content of MDA lowered obviously whereas the serum level of ALB and activity of SOD elevated significantly, and the hepatic fibrosis degree was relieved in PS treatment group. It suggests PS has the function of protecting liver and delaying hepatic fibrosis in rats induced by CCl_4.

Ganoderma (Polyporaceae/Ganoderma Karst.)

Lin and Lin (2006) investigated the effects of Reishi mushroom, *Ganoderma lucidum* extract (GLE) on liver fibrosis induced by CCl_4 in rats. The rats in GLE groups were treated with GLE (600 or 1,600 mg/kg b.w., i.g., daily for 8 weeks). Compared with CCl_4 group, GLE treatment significantly increased plasma albumin level and A/G ratio ($P < 0.05$) and reduced the hepatic hydroxyproline content ($P < 0.01$). Moreover, GLE (1,600 mg/kg b.w.) treatment markedly decreased the activities of transaminases ($P < 0.05$), spleen weight ($P < 0.05$) and hepatic MDA content ($P < 0.05$), while increased hepatic protein level ($P < 0.05$) and improved liver histology ($P < 0.01$). In addition, RT-PCR analysis showed that GLE treatment decreased the expression of TGF-beta1 ($P < 0.05$-0.001), changed the expression of MAT1A ($P < 0.05$-0.01) and MAT2A ($P < 0.05$-0.001). These data suggest oral administration of GLE significantly reduces CCl_4-induced hepatic fibrosis in rats.

Viola diffusa Ging (Violaceae/Viola L.)

Li, X.H. *et al.* (2010) studied the effect of *Vioal diffusa* Ging (VDG) on hepatic fibrosis induced by CCl_4 in rats, VDG group rats were administered daily with the aqueous extract of VDG (7.5g£¯kg b.w., i.g.) for 6 weeks. Compared with the model group, the serum levels of ALT, AST and ALP of VDG group were remarkably decreased ($P < 0.01$). In VDG treated group, the hepatic lobe structure was normal and the slender textile fiber gap was minor with little inflammatory cell infiltration. There were significant differences in the average grey degrees of collagen I, collagen III, alpha-SMA and TGF-beta1 between model control group and VDG group ($P < 0.01$). It suggests the aqueous extract of VDG has protective effect against liver fibrosis in rats induced by CCl_4.

Kadsura coccinea (Magnoliaceae/Schisandra Michx.)

Li, W.S. *et al.* (2010) studied the therapeutic effects of *Kadsura coccinea* on hepatic fibrosis in rats induced by multiple hepatotoxic factors, including CCl_4, rich fat and poor protein. Compared with the model group, administration of *K. coccinea* (2.5, 5 g/kg b.w., i.g., daily for 6 weeks) significantly decreased the levels of ALT, AST, HA, LN and PCIII in serum, and the hepatic contents of hydroxyproline, MDA. It also increased the level of ALB in serum and the activity of hepatic SOD in liver tissue. The degree of necrosis of liver cells, liver fats degeneration and collagen fiber hyperplasia were alleviated significantly. It suggests *K. coccinea* could attenuate liver fibrosis in rats induced by CCl_4.

Oil

Olive Oil (Burevaceae/Canarium L.)

Fang *et al.* (2008) evaluated the inhibitory effect of olive oil on liver fibrosis induced by CCl_4 in rats. The rats in the treatment groups were treated daily with olive oil (2 or 10 mL/kg b.w.) through gastrogavage for 8 weeks. RT-PCR analysis showed that olive oil decreased the hepatic mRNA expressions of lipopolysaccharide binding protein, CD14, TLR4, NADPH oxidase, nuclear factor-kappa beta, collagen I, collagen III, and TGF-beta1 in the treatment groups in comparison with the model group. Western blot analysis also supported these results. Moreover, olive oil treatment decreased the hepatic MDA and hydroxyproline levels. In addition, histological evaluations showed that olive oil could attenuate the CCl_4-induced liver fibrosis, necrosis, and expression of alpha-SMA. It is speculated that the phenolic compounds in olive oil significantly reduces CCl_4-induced hepatic fibrosis in rats.

Ginger Oil (Zingiberaceae/Zingiber Boehmer)

Geng *et al.* (2010) studied the protective effect of ginger oil against hepatic fibrosis induced by CCl_4 in rats. The rats in the ginger oil groups were treated with ginger oil (0.25, 0.5 or 1 mL/kg b.w.) daily for 4 weeks. Compared with the model group, ginger oil administration dramatically reduced the serum levels of ALT ($P < 0.05$), AST ($P < 0.01$), HA ($P < 0.01$) and LN ($P < 0.01$) and increased the levels of TP and ALB (both $P < 0.01$). In addition, ginger oil suppressed the formation of pseudo-liver-lobules and collagen deposition in hepatic fibrosis rats. It suggests ginger oil could reduce hepatic fibrosis in rats induced by CCl_4.

Three Kinds of Animal Drugs Used to Treat Liver Fibrosis

Holotrichia diomphalia (Dried Larvae Body of Scarabaeoidea)

Oh *et al.* (2003) investigated the effect of *Holotrichia diomphalia* larvae against acute liver damage and liver fibrosis in rats. The results showed that a single administration of *H. diomphalia* decreased the serum aminotransferase (ALT, AST) activities in rats with acute liver damage induced by carbon tetrachloride and beta-D-galactosamine. The hepatic cirrhosis was induced by 28 days of bile duct ligation/scission in rats. The four-week treatment with *H. diomphalia* reduced the serum ALT, AST, ALP levels, and hydroxyproline content in the liver and improved the histological appearance of the liver sections. It leads to the conclusion that *H. diomphalia* larvae can reduce the degree of hepatocellular damage.

Amydae carapax (Hydrocharitaceae/Hydrocharis L.)

Gao *et al.* (2009) investigated the preventive and therapeutic effect of *Amydae carapax* decoction on liver fibrosis in rats induced by CCl_4 or DMN. In CCl_4 experiment, the rats in the treated groups were administered *A. carapax* decoction (corresponding to 18 g/kg b.w. *A. carapax*, i.g., low dose group: once per day; high dose group: twice per day) for 4 weeks (prevention group) or 8 weeks (treatment group). In DMN experiment, the rats in the treated group were administered *A. carapax* decoction (corresponding to 18 g/kg b.w. *A. carapax*, i.g.) twice per day for 4 weeks (prevention group) or 8 weeks (treatment group). Compared with those in the model group, histopathological scores of fibrosis, collagen content in the liver tissue, liver fibrosis index and some indices in serum were significantly lower, but anti-oxidation index of liver tissue was markedly higher ($P < 0.05$-0.01) in prevention and treatment group. The effect in prevention group and high dose group were particularly good. It suggests *A. carapax* decoction possesses significant preventive and therapeutic effect on liver fibrosis.

Earthworm (Megascolecidae/Pheretima)

Lu *et al.* (2004) investigated the effect of Earthworm II (Ew) on liver fibrosis in rats induced by CCl_4. The rats in the treated groups were administered daily with Ew (25, 50 mg£¯kg b.w., i.g.) for 8 weeks. The results showed the evaluation of hepatic fibrosis in animals of Ew groups was significantly lower, while the serum markers of HA, LN and AST/ALT also reduced obviously than those in the model group. It suggests Ew can inhibit CCl_4-induced liver fibrosis in rats.

Quantitative Structure-Activity Relationship (QSAR) Studies on Anti-Hepatic Fibrosis Drugs

In QSAR studies, chemical structures or descriptors of compounds are quantitatively correlated with activities (Wold and Dunn, 1983; Hermens, 1991) Molecular descriptors, determined empirically or by computational methods, include parameters derived from various aspects of a molecule, such as hydrophobicity, topology, electronic properties and steric effects. Activities used in QSAR include various chemical properties and bio-activities. An interesting application of QSAR in drug design is modeling and predicting pharmacological activities, such as ADMET (absorption, distribution, metabolism, excretion, toxicity) properties. A properly used QSAR model can serve as an effective pre-screening of potential drugs, provide information concerning how to adjust or modify a molecule to improve its properties and cast a light on understanding of the molecular bioactivities. Recent QSAR studies on anti-hepatic fibrosis drugs are therefore reviewed.

Heightened oxidative stress is an important mechanism in the pathogenesis of liver diseases caused by exposure to environmental toxins. Based on that Ge-Gen Huang–Lian Huang-Qin (GHH) decoction may suppress hepatic lipid peroxidation (LPO), Lin (1995) developed a QSAR model on some selected flavonoids (flavones, flavonols, flavanones and flavanonols) derived from GHH and other sources:

$$Y = 0.92X1 - 0.35X2 - 0.000051X3 - 0.0046X4 - 0.21X5 - 3.26,$$
$$(r^2 = 0.95,\ r^2cv = 0.93)$$

Where Y denotes antioxidant potency; a value of 1 is assigned to X1 if a functional group is present at both positions 5 and 8 of ring A in the flavonoid structure and to X2 for at positions 3× and 4× in ring B; X3 is HOMO energy; X4 denotes electrostatic energy; X5 is bond energy; r^2 is the linear regression coefficient; r^2cv denotes cross validation coefficient. According to the above QSAR model, the protective effects of flavones were more potent than flavonols, flavanones or flavanonols in *tert*-butyl hydroperoxide-induced LPO. QSAR studies also indicated that the energy parameters are important factors in predicting the potency of flavones, flavonols, flavanones and flavanonols in suppressing LPO in liver. The same equation also applies to flavones from herbs not contained in GHH (*e.g.* morusin, cyclomuberrin, cyclomuberrochromene and others derived from *Morus alba*). Results derived from the above model would be helpful in improving current and in developing new herb formulae.

Many researchers have found that HCV is a major cause of liver fibrosis and other forms of liver dysfunction. Chen, K.X. *et al.* (2009) performed a QSAR study on anthranilic acid derivatives for their potent allosteric inhibition activities of HCV NS5B polymerase. Genetic algorithm was performed for variable selection. Highly statistically significant model with $r^2 = 0.966$ and r^2 (cross validation) $= 0.951$ was obtained with 5 descriptors. High r^2 of predicted value of 0.884 indicates the good predictive power of the best model. Important descriptors include spatial descriptors of radius of gyration, molecular volume (Vm), length of molecule in the z dimension

(Shadow-Z length), thermodynamic descriptors of the octanol/water partition coefficient (LogP) and molecular refractivity index (MR). The model gives insight on indispensable structural requirements for the activity and can be used to design more potent analogs against HCV NS5B polymerase.

As activation of the CB1 receptor triggers fibrosis progression, whereas CB2 activation promotes antifibrogenic actions in the liver, Ferreira*et al.* (2009) attempted to perform a QSAR study on the ligand selectivity of the cannabinoid CB1 and CB2 receptors in the absence of generally accepted models for their structures. Quantum-chemical descriptors based on PM3 semi-empirical calculations for a series of phenyl-substituted cannabinoids and a set of structurally similar adamantyl-substituted cannabinoids were collected. A good model for CB2 inhibition ($r^2 = 0.78$) has been developed with four explanatory variables derived from semi-empirical results. The role of the ligand dipole moment was discussed, and it was proposed that the CB2 binding pocket might possess a significant electric field. Describing the affinities with respect to the CB1 receptor was not possible with the current set of ligands and descriptors, although the attempt highlighted some important points regarding the development of QSAR models.

Conclusion and Outlook

The above overview of the 79 kinds of natural medicines could lead to the conclusion that these natural medicines have great potential in the treatment of liver fibrosis, and it is also beneficial to pharmaceutical scientists who are interested in searching for monomer composition or compound. Although most of reviewed researches focused on the liver fibrosis itself, it may serve as an important strategy to search for the natural medicines possessing therapeutic effects on both virus and liver fibrosis since viral infection hepatitis is the major cause of liver fibrosis in China (Chen and Jia, 2009; Wang and Zhou, 2003).

It is still difficult to set up specific animal models according to the TCM theory, further studies should nevertheless be carried out with the efforts on meeting both TCM and modern science's criterion. That would boost the success rate in the development of natural medicine for the treatment of liver fibrosis.

It could be noted that many compounds or extracts from Chinese medicines have been reported to have anti-liver fibrotic effects. Natural medicine in China is quite abundant, and use of Chinese medicines in the treatment for clinical manifestations of liver fibrosis has a long tradition in China. All of this merits further research and development of natural drugs for the treatment of liver fibrosis and it provides a great potential for exploitation of it.

Abbreviations

8-OHdG: 8-hydroxydeoxyguanosine; A/G: albumin over globulin; ALB: albumin; ALP: alkaline phosphatase; alpha-SMA: alpha-smooth muscle actin; ALT: alanine aminotransferase; AST: serum aspartate aminotransferase; ChE: chollnesterase; CTGF: connective tissue growth factor; cyt c: Cytochromes c; DMN: dimethylnitrosamine; GOT: glutamate-oxalate-transaminase; GPT: glutamate-pyruvate-transaminase; HA: hyaluronic acid; HSC: hepatic stellate cell; ICAM: intercellular adhesion molecule;

IL: interleukin; LDH: lactate dehydrogenase; LN: laminin; MAP: Mitogen-activated protein; MDA: malondialdehyde; MMP: Matrix metallopeptidase; PCIII: Procollagen III; PDGF: platelet derived growth factor; SOD: superoxide dismutase; TBARS: hiobarbituratic acid-reactive substance; T-Bil: total bilirubin; TGF-beta1: transforming growth factor-beta1; TLR4: Toll-like receptor 4; TNF-alpha: tumor necrosis factor-alpha; TP: total protein; uPA: urokinase-type plasminogen activator; VEGF: Vascular endothelial growth factor.

Acknowledgements

The authors thank Yunnan Province Project (Lead high-level personnel training project No. 2009CI121), Key Industries Innovation Project of Yunnan Science and Technology Department (Modernization of Chinese Technology Industry Base Construction in Yunnan Province No. 2008IF012) and Program for Innovative Research Team (in Science and Technology) in University of Yunnan Province (IRTSTYN, 2010-11) and Program for Yunnan Innovative Research Team.

References

Amin, A., and Mahmoud-Ghoneim, D. (2009). *Zizyphus spina-christi* protects against carbon tetrachloride-induced liver fibrosis in rats. *Food and Chemical Toxicology*, **47**(8): 2111-2119.

Cao, L.B., Li, B., Li, Z.J., Huang, J.J., OuYang, L.Q., Huang, H., and Liu, S.K. (2009). The effect and mechanism of Silymarin on liver fibrosis in mice. *Chinese Pharmacological Bulletin*, **25**(6): 794-796.

Chan, Y.C., Chang, S.C., Liu, S.Y., Yang, H.L., Hseu, Y.C., and Liao, J.W. (2010). Beneficial effects of yam on carbon tetrachloride-induced hepatic fibrosis in rats. *Journal of the Science of Food and Agriculture*, **90**(1): 161-167.

Chen, J., and Jia, J.D. (2009). Treatment of viral hepatitis in China: better clinical research and improved practice. *Chinese Medical Journal (English)*, **122**(19): 2236-2238.

Chen, J., Shi, Y.J., Luo, L., and Xu, J.L. (2008). Protective effect and the mechanism of *Ganoderma* triterpene on chronic hepatic fibrosis in rats. *Chinese Journal of Hospital Pharmacy*, **28**(9): 694-697.

Chen, K.X., Xie, H.Y., and Li, Z.G. (2009). 2D-QSAR Studies on anthranilic acid derivatives: a novel class of allosteric inhibitors of hepatitis C NS5B polymerase. *Chinese journal of structural chemistry*, **28**(10): 1217-1225.

Cheng, H.Q., Huang, C.H., Qiu, J.W., Zhang, C.Z., and Cheng, K.L. (2008). Effects of *Radix ampelosis* sincae extract-containing rat serum on apoptosis and expression of Bax/Bcl-2 gene in hepatic stellate cells. *Chinese Journal of New drugs*, **17**(4): 300-302.

Cheng, J., and Yang, Y.X. (2010). Protective effect of baicalin on hepatic fibrosis in mice. *West China Journal of Pharmaceutical Sciences*, **25**(1): 32-33.

Cheung, K.F., Ye, D.W., Yang, Z.F., Lu, L., Liu, C.H., Wang, X.L., Poon, R.T., Tong, Y., Liu, P., Chen, Y.C., and Lau, G.K. (2009). Therapeutic efficacy of Traditional

Chinese Medicine 319 recipe on hepatic fibrosis induced by carbon tetrachloride in rats. *Journal of Ethnopharmacology*, **124**(1): 142-150.

Chor, J.S., Yu, J., Chan, K.K., Go, Y.Y., and Sung, J.J. (2009). *Stephania tetrandra* prevents and regresses liver fibrosis induced by carbon tetrachloride in rats. *Journal of Gastroenterology and Hepatology*, **24**(5): 853-859.

D'Argenio, G., Amoruso, D.C., Mazzone, G., Vitaglione, P., Romanoa, A., Ribeccoa, M.T., D'Armiento, M.R., Mezza, E., Morisco, F., Fogliano, V., and Caporaso, N. (2010). Garlic extract prevents CCl_4-induced liver fibrosis in rats: The role of tissue transglutaminase. *Digestive and Liver Disease*, **42**(8): 571-577.

Deng, X., Liang, J., Li, Y.Z., Huang, B., and Zhang, X.L. (2007). Protective effect of natural taurine on mitochondria of hepatic fibrosis in rats. *Journal of Xi'an Jiaotong University (Medical Sciences)*, **28**(6): 648-650.

Ding, X.D., Wang, H.Q., Wu, Q., Wang, X.L., Huang, Y., Zhang, Q., and Yang, F. (2008). Effect of astrogalosides on liver fibrosis in mice with *Schistosomiasis japonica*. *World Chinese Journal of Digestology*, **16**(2): 125-131.

Du, G.J., Wang, M., Lin, H.H., Zhang, S., Ji, L.Y., and Lu, L.L. (2009). Protective effects of breviscapine against hepatic fibrosis. *Journal of Henan University (Medical Science)*, **28**(3): 170-173.

Erman, F., Balkan, J., Cevikba°, U., Koçak-Toker, N., and Uysal, M. (2004). Betaine or taurine administration prevents fibrosis and lipid peroxidation induced by rat liver by ethanol plus carbon tetrachloride intoxication. *Amino Acids*, **27**(2): 199-205.

Fang, H.L., Lai, J.T., and Lin, W.C. (2008). Inhibitory effect of olive oil on fibrosis induced by carbon tetrachloride in rat liver. *Clinical Nutrition*, **27**(6): 900-907.

Feng, Y., Cheung, K.F., Wang, N., Liu, P., Nagamatsu, T., and Tong, Y. (2009). Chinese medicines as a resource for liver fibrosis treatment. *Chinese Medicine*, **4**: 16.

Ferreira, A.M., Krishnamurthy, M., Moore, B.M. 2nd, Finkelstein, D., and Bashford, D. (2009). Quantitative structure-activity relationship (QSAR) for a series of novel cannabinoid derivatives using descriptors derived from semi-empirical quantum-chemical calculations. *Bioorganic and Medicinal Chemistry*, **17**(6): 2598-2606.

Friedman, S.L. (2008). Mechanisms of hepatic fibrogenesis. *Gastroenterology*, **134**(6): 1655-1669.

Friedman, S.L. (2007). Reversibility of hepatic fibrosis and cirrhosis-is it all hype? *Nature Clinical Practise Gastroenterology and Hepatology*, **4**(5): 236-237.

Friedman, S.L. (2003). Liver fibrosis-from bench to bedside. *Journal of Hepatology*, **38**(Suppl 1): 38-53.

Fursule, R.A., and Patil, S.D. (2010). Hepatoprotective and antioxidant activity of *Phaseolus trilobus*, ait on bile duct ligation induced liver fibrosis in rats. *Journal of Ethnopharmacology*, **129**(3): 416-419.

Gao, J.R., Zhu, Y.F., Zhang, C.Z., Liu, Y.W., Shao, Z.H., Hu, Z.L., Cai, W.M., Tao, J., Chen, J.W., Wu, H.Z., Yao, H.P., Zhang, H.Q., Tang,Y.P., and Hu, C.L. (2009). Experimental study of *Amydae carapax* Decoction on prevention and treatment of liver fibrosis in rats induced by two different causes. *Chinese Aarches Traditional Chinese Medicine*, **27**(8): 1727-1733.

Gedik, N., Kabasakal, L., Sehirli, O., Ercan, F., Sirvanci, S., Keyer-Uysal, M., and Sener, G. (2005). Long-term administration of aqueous garlic extract (AGE) alleviates liver fibrosis and oxidative damage induced by biliary obstruction in rats. *Life Sciences*, **76**(22): 2593-2606.

Geng, T., Xie, M.L., and Sun, X.F. (2010). Effects of ginger oils on hepatic fibrosis in rats. *Chinese Remedies and Clinics*, **10**(3): 280-283.

Geng, W.X., Ding, H.Y., and Yi, Y.S. (2008). Prevention and treatment of experimental liver fibrosis in rats by *semen hoveniae* extracts. *Journal of Chinese Medicinal Materials*, **31**(10): 1550-1552.

Ginès, P., Cárdena, A., Arroyo, V., and Rodés, J. (2004). Management of cirrhosis and ascites. *The New England Journal of Medicine*, **350**(16): 1646-1654.

Guo, J.Z., Wang, F., Li, X., Li, P., He, Y., Hu, Z.F., Li, K.M., and Li, H. (2009). Study of the influence about the lipoperoxidation and zine, calcium content on Saikosaponin-d against liver fibrosis in rats. *Pharmacology and Clinics of Chinese Materia Medica*, **25**(3): 11-14.

Hermens, J. (1991). QSAR in environmental sciences and drug design. *Science of the Total Environment*, **109-110**: 1-7.

Hong, S.W., Jung, K.H., Zheng, H.M., Lee, H.S., Suh, J.K., Park, I.S., Lee, D.H., and Hong, S.S. (2010). The protective effect of resveratrol on dimethylnitrosamine-induced liver fibrosis in rats. *Archives of Pharmacal Research*, **33**(4): 601-609.

Hsu, Y.C., Chiu, Y.T., Cheng, C.C., Wu, C.F., Lin, Y.L., and Huang, Y.T. (2007). Antifibrotic effects of tetrandrine on hepatic stellate cells and rats with liver fibrosis. *Journal of Gastroenterology and Hepatology*, **22**(1): 99-111.

Hu, S.J., Yang, L., Zhu, Q.J., and Peng, H.G. (2007). Effect of β-elemene on the expression of transforming growth factor-β_1, α-smooth muscle actin and collagen-I in rats with hepatic fibrosis. *World Chinese Journal of Digestology*, **15**(12): 1324-1330.

Hua, H.Y., Li, Y.Y., and Ge, S.W. (2007). Study of tetramethylpyrazine in treatment on liver fibrosis and mechanism in rats. *Pharmacology and Clinics of Chinese Materia Medica*, **23**(5): 60-62.

Ji, H., Chi, B.R., Ren, L.Q., Zhang,Y.N., Li, X.J., and Shi, Y. (2009). Prophylactic effects of curcumin on rats hepatic fibrosis. *Liaoning Journal of Traditional Chinese Medicine*, **36**(8): 1423-1425.

Jia, Y., Niu, Y.C., Zhang, Y.B., Zhou, L., and Dong, M.X. (2009). Effect of Hirudin on the expression of CTGF mRNA in fibrotic liver in rats. *Lishizhen Medicine and Materia Medica Research*, **20**(1): 95-97.

Jin, H., Sakaida, I., Tsuchiya, M., and Okita, K. (2005). Herbal medicine Rhei rhizome prevents liver fibrosis in rat liver cirrhosis induced by a choline-deficient L-amino acid-defined diet. *Life Sciences*, **76**(24): 2805-2816.

Jodynis-Liebert, J., Adamska, T., Ewertowska, M., Bylka, W., and Matlawska, I. (2009). *Aquilegia vulgaris* extract attenuates carbon tetrachloride-induced liver fibrosis in rats. *Experimental and Toxicologic Pathology*, **61**(5): 443-451.

Kim, H.K., Yang, T.H., and Cho, H.Y. (2009). Antifibrotic effects of green tea on*in vitro* and *in vivo* models of liver fibrosis. *World Journal of Gastroenterology*, **15**(41): 5200-5205.

Kisseleva, T., and Brenner, D.A. (2008). Mechanisms of fibrogenesis. *Experimental Biology and Medicine*, **233**(2): 109-122.

Kuang, M.Y., Deng, P.C., and Xu, S. (2009). The effects of Tengcha flavonoids on expression of collagen I, III of hepatic fibrosis in rats. *Progress in Modern Biomedicine*, **9**(11): 2055-2057.

Lakshmi, D.S., and Anuradha, C.V. (2010). Mitochondrial damage, cytotoxicity and apoptosis in iron-potentiated alcoholic liver fibrosis: amelioration by taurine. *Amino Acids*, **38**(3): 869-879.

Lee, H.S., Jung, K.H., Park, I.S., Kwon, S.W., Lee, D.H., and Hong, S.S. (2009). Protective effect of morin on dimethylnitrosamine-induced hepatic fibrosis in rats. *Digestive Diseases and Sciences*, **54**(4): 782-788.

Lee, T.Y., Wang, G.J., Chiu, J.H., and Lin, H.C. (2003). Long-term administration of *Salvia miltiorrhiza* ameliorates carbon tetrachloride-induced hepatic fibrosis in rats. *Journal of Pharmacy and Pharmacology*, **55**(11): 1561-1568.

Li, F.H., Liu, P., Xiong, W.G., and Xu, G.F. (2006). Effects of corydyceps polysaccharide on liver fibrosis induced by DMN in rats. *China Journal of Chinese Materia Medica*, **31**(23): 1968-1970.

Li, G.S., Jiang, W.L., Tian, J.W., Qu, G.W., Zhu, H.B., and Fu, F.H. (2010). *In vitro* and *in vivo* antifibrotic effects of rosmarinic acid on experimental liver fibrosis. *Phytomedicine*, **17**(3-4): 282-288.

Li, R.L., Ma, Y., Wei, W., Ye, G.S., Chen, W.B., and Yan, J.C. (2007). Pharmacological effects of total glucosides from Paeony root on CCl_4-induced liver fibrosis and function of hepatic stellate cells. *Chinese Journal of New Drugs*, **16**(9): 685-688.

Li, W.S., Chen, J., Wen, J.P., and Guo, L.J. (2010). Research on the preventive and therapeutic effects of *Kadsura coccinea* on experimental hepatic fibrosis in rat and the related Mechanism. *Chinese Journal of Experimental Traditional Medical Formulae*, **16**(6): 199-201.

Li, X.H., and Li, C.Y. (2010). Anti-hepatic fibrosis effect of *Viola diffusa* Ging in rats. *Chinese Journal of Public Health*, **26**(5): 546-547

Li, Y.J., Wang, Y.H., Liu, Y.M., and Liu, Y.X. (2009). Effects of chelerythrine on hepatic TGF-β_1 and α-SMA expression in rats with hepatic fibrosis. *Journal of Clinical Hepatology*, **12**(3): 167-170.

Li, Z., Cheng, L.F., Zhang, T.Q., Li, S., and Jia, Y.H. (2007). Experimental study of the ethanolic estract from *Potentilla chinensis* on rat hepatic fibrosis induced by carbon tetrachloride. *Liaoning Journal of Traditional Chinese Medicine*, **34**(8): 1157-1159.

Liang Y.H., Jia, J., Spencer, P.S., Mao, Y.A., and Tan, C.J. (2008). Protective effect of *Corydalis saxicola* alkaloids (CSA) on level of TGF-β_1, MMP-9 in rats with liver fibrosis. *Lishizhen Medicine and Materia Medica Research*, **19**(11): 2620-2622.

Liao, J.C., Lin, K.H., Cheng, H.Y., Wu, J.B., Hsieh, M.T., and Peng, W.H. (2007). *Actinidia rubricaulis* attenuates hepatic fibrosis induced by carbon tetrachloride in rats. *The American Journal of Chinese Medicine*, **35**(1): 81-88.

Lin, W.C., and Lin, W.L. (2006). Ameliorative effect of *Ganoderma lucidum* on carbon tetrachloride-induced liver fibrosis in rats. *World Journal of Gastroenterology*, **12**(2): 265-270.

Lin, Y.C. (1995). Model development of new herb formulae against hepatic lipid peroxidation. *Taipei Medical University*, PhD thesis.

Liu, J.Y., Chen, C.C., Wang, W.H., Hsu, J.D., Yang, M.Y., and Wang, C.J. (2006). The protective effects of *Hibiscus sabdariffa* extract on CCl_4-induced liver fibrosis in rats. *Food and Chemical Toxicology*, **44**(3): 336-343.

López-Reyes, A.G., Arroyo-Curras, N., Cano, B.G., Lara-Díaz, V.J., Guajardo-Salinas, G.E., Islas, J.F., Morales-Oyarvide, V., Morales-Garza, L.A., Galvez-Gastelum, F.J., Grijalva, G., and Moreno-Cuevas, J.E. (2008). Black bean extract ameliorates liver fibrosis in rats with CCl_4-induced injury. *Annals of Hepatology*, **7**(2): 130-135.

Lu, M.Q., Pan, C.W., Li, J., and Chen, Y.P. (2007). Effect of salvianolic acid B on levels of TGF-β_1, MMP-2 and TIMP-2 in rats with liver fibrosis. *World Chinese Journal of Digestology*, **15**(36): 3847-3851.

Lu, Y.Q., Liu, S.Y., Chen, H., Zhang, Z.G., and Zhao, C.G. (2004). The study of Earthworm in preventing rat hepatic fibrosis induced by CCl_4. *Chinese Journal of Gastroenterology and Hepatology*, **13**(3): 225-227.

Lü, X.Y., Liu, Q., Chen, Y.Y., Song, Y.H., and Lü, Z.P. (2007). Therapeutic effect of Hongbeiyegen on alcohol-induced rat hepatic fibrosis. *Journal of Southern Medical University*, **27**(2): 153-155.

Lv, Q.J., Xie, J.Q., Wen, L.Q., Chen, Y.Y., Zhang, M., and Ye, Q.N. (2005). Effects of resveratrol on chronic liver fibrosis in rats. *Chinese Journal of New Drugs*, **14**(7): 855-858.

Ma, N.F., Huang, H.S., Zhang, C., Guo, X.Z., Li, Y.L., and Guo, X.C. (2007). Inhibitory effects of matrine on the expression of inducible nitric oxide synthase during hepatic fibrosis induced by carbon tetrachloride in mice. *World Chinese Journal of Digestology*, **15**(32): 3367-3371.

Mao, Y.Q., Liu, X.J., Jiang, Y., and Wu, H.B. (2004). Effect of quercetin on the signal pathway of TGF-β_1 in activated hepatic stellate cells. *Journal of Sichuan University (Medical Sciences Edition)*, **35**(6): 802-805.

Miyazaki, T., Karube, M., Matsuzaki, Y., Ikegami, T., Doy, M., Tanaka, N., and Bouscarel, B. (2005). Taurine inhibits oxidative damage and prevents fibrosis in carbon tetrachloride-induced hepatic fibrosis. *Journal of Hepatology*, **43**(1): 117-125.

Modi, A.A., Feld, J.J., Park, Y., Kleiner, D.E., Everhart, J.E., Liang, T.J., and Hoofnagle, J.H. (2010). Increased caffeine consumption is associated with reduced hepatic fibrosis. *Hepatology*, **51**(1): 201-209.

Nian, G.X., Huang, Z.M., Yang, X.B., Li, R.S., and Song, J.G. (2010). Effect of total phenolics acid of *Oenanthe Javanica* on hepatic fibrosis in rats. *Pharmaceutical Journal of Chinese People's Liberation Army*, **26**(1): 22-26.

Oh, W.Y., Pyo, S., Lee, K.R., Lee, B.K., Shin, D.H., Cho, S.I., and Lee, S.M. (2003). Effect of *Holotrichia diomphalia* larvae on liver fibrosis and hepatotoxicity in rats. *Journal of Ethnopharmacology*, **87**(2-3): 175-180.

Ouyang, C.H., Zhu, X., Zhang, K.H., Dai, Y., Chen, J., He, W.H., Li, B., and Li, B.M. (2009). Effects of ursolic acid on the expression of transforming growth factor-β_1 and α-smooth muscle actin in fibrotic liver in rats. *World Chinese Journal of Digestology*, **17**(22): 2237-2243.

Peng, W.H., Tien, Y.C., Huang, C.Y., Huang, T.H., Liao, J.C., Kuo, C.L., and Lin, Y.C. (2010). *Fraxinus rhynchophylla* ethanol extract attenuates carbon tetrachloride-induced liver fibrosis in rats via down-regulating the expressions of uPA, MMP-2, MMP-9 and TIMP-1. *Journal of Ethnopharmacology*, **127**(3): 606-613.

Pinlaor, S., Prakobwong, S., Hiraku, Y., Pinlaor, P., Laothong, U., and Yongvanit, P. (2010). Reduction of periductal fibrosis in liver fluke-infected hamsters after long-term curcumin treatment. *European Journal of Pharmacology*, **638**(1-3): 134-141.

Qi, H.B. (2009). Liver fibrosis research and treatment of TCM. *Chinese Journal for Clinicians*, **37**(9): 33-34.

Qin, X.Y., Yan, L., Tang, L., and Dai, J.F. (2010). Infuence of Tanshinone II_A on expression of hepatic collagen fibers in rats with liver. *Lishizhen Medicine and Materia Medica Research*, **21**(4): 782-784.

Shi, H., Dong, L., Bai, Y., Zhao, J., Zhang, Y., and Zhang, L. (2009). Chlorogenic acid against carbon tetrachloride-induced liver fibrosis in rats. *European Journal of Pharmacology*, **623**(1-3): 119-124.

Shi, H., Dong, L., Zhang, Y., Bai, Y., Zhao, J., and Zhang, L. (2010). Protective effect of a coffee preparation (Nescafe pure®) against carbon tetrachloride-induced liver fibrosis in rats. *Clinical Nutrition*, **29**(3): 399-405.

Shi, Z.H., Liu, H., Liu, S., Zhong, J.M., and Tu, J.W. (2006). Roles of activin A and hepatocellular apoptosis in the anti-liver fibrosis process induced by *Ginkgo biloba* extract in rats. *World Chinese Journal of Digestology*, **14**(21): 2060-2066.

Shih, C.C., Wu, Y.W., and Lin, W.C. (2005). Aqueous extract of *Anoectochilus formosanus* attenuate hepatic fibrosis induced by carbon tetrachloride in rats. *Phytomedicine*, **12**(6-7): 453-460.

Shin, J.W., Wang, J.H., Kang, J.K., and Son, C.G. (2010). Experimental evidence for the protective effects of coffee against liver fibrosis in SD rats. *Journal of the Science of Food and Agriculture*, **90**(3): 450-455.

Shinkawa, H., Takemura, S., Minamiyama, Y., Kodai, S., Tsukioka, T., Osada-Oka, M., Kubo, S., Okada, S., and Suehiro, S. (2009). S-allylcysteine is effective as a chemopreventive agent against porcine serum-induced hepatic fibrosis in rats. *Osaka City Medical Journal*, **55**(2): 61-69.

Shyu, M.H., Kao, T.C., and Yen, G.C. (2008). Hsian-tsao (*Mesona procumbens* Heml.) prevents against rat liver fibrosis induced by CCl_4 via inhibition of hepatic stellate cells activation. *Food and Chemical Toxicology*, **46**(12): 3707-3713.

Sun, H., Che, Q.M., Zhao, X., and Pu, X.P. (2010). Antifibrotic effects of chronic baicalein administration in a CCl_4 liver fibrosis model in rats. *European Journal of Pharmacology*, **631**(1-3): 53-60.

Sun, X., Zhang, X., Hu, H., Lu, Y., Chen, J., Yasuda, K., and Wang, H. (2009). Berberine inhibits hepatic stellate cell proliferation and prevents experimental liver fibrosis. *Biological and Pharmaceutical Bulletin*, **32**(9): 1533-1537.

Toklu, H.Z., Dumlu, M.U., Sehirli, O., Ercan, F., Gedik, N., Gökmen, V., and Sener, G. (2007). Pomegranate peel extract prevents liver fibrosis in biliary-obstructed rats. *Journal of Pharmacy and Pharmacology*, **59**(9): 1287-1295.

Tsai, M.K., Lin, Y.L., and Huang, Y.T. (2010). Effects of salvianolic acids on oxidative stress and hepatic fibrosis in rats. *Toxicology and Applied Pharmacology*, **242**(2): 155-164.

Wan, X.Q., Zheng, Z.D., Shang, J.J., and Li, X.S. (2009). Effects of rhein on immunological hepatic fibrosis induced by porcine serum in rats. *Chongqing Medicine*, **38**(10): 1204-1206.

Wang, H., and Zhou, X.Q. (2003). Study on relationshop between serum marker and human hepatic fibrosis pathology. *Acta Universitatis Medicinalis Secondae Shanghai*, **23**(1): 93-95.

Wang, L., Cheng, D., Wang, H., Di, L., Zhou, X., Xu, T., Yang, X., and Liu, Y. (2009). The hepatoprotective and antifibrotic effects of *Saururus chinensis* against carbon tetrachloride induced hepatic fibrosis in rats. *Journal of Ethnopharmacology*, **126**(3): 487-491.

Wang, Y.P., Cheng, M.L., Zhang, B.F., Mu, M., and Wu, J. (2010). Effects of blueberry on hepatic fibrosis and transcription factor *Nrf2* in rats. *World Journal of Gastroenterology*, **16**(21): 2657-2663.

Wang, Y., Qi, H.W., Hu, Y.W., and Wang, S.C. (2008). Inhibitory effect of schizandrin on KC-mediated hepatic fibrosis. *Journal of the Fourth Military Medical University*, **29**(9): 816-818.

Wells, R.G. (2005). The role of matrix stiffness in hepatic stellate cell activation and liver fibrosis. *Journal of Clinical Gastroenterology*, **39**(4 Suppl 2): S158-161.

Wills, P.J., and Asha, V.V. (2007). Protective mechanism of *Lygodium flexuosum* extract in treating and preventing carbon tetrachloride induced hepatic fibrosis in rats. *Chemico-Biological Interactions*, **165**(1): 76-85.

Wold, S., and Dunn, W.J. 3rd. (1983). Multivariate quantitative structure-activity relationships (QSAR): conditions for their applicability. *Journal of Chemical Information and Modeling*, **23**(1): 6-13.

Wu, J.B., Chuang, H.R., Yang, L.C., and Lin, W.C. (2010). A standardized aqueous extract of *Anoectochilus formosanus* ameliorated thioacetamide-induced liver fibrosis in mice: the role of Kupffer cells. *Bioscience, Biotechnology, and Biochemistry*, **74**(4): 781-787.

Wu, S.J., Tam, K.W., Tsai, Y.H., Chang, C.C., and Chao, J.C. (2010). Curcumin and saikosaponin A inhibit chemical-induced liver inflammation and fibrosis in rats. *The American Journal of Chinese Medicine*, **38**(1): 99-111.

Wu, X.L., Zeng, W.Z., Jiang, M.D., Qin, J.P., and Xu, H. (2008). Effect of Oxymatrine on the TGFbeta-Smad signaling pathway in rats with CCl_4-induced hepatic fibrosis. *World Journal of Gastroenterology*, **14**(13): 2100-2105.

Wu, X.L., Zeng, W.Z., Jiang, M.D., Qin, J.P., Xu, H., and Wang, Z. (2009). Effects of salidroside on expression of ROCK in rats with liver fibrosis. *World Chinese Journal of Digestology*, **17**(8): 765-769.

Xu, B., and Tong, Q.X. (2009). Effect of cucurbitacin B on the expression of VEGF and oxidative stress in the liver fibrosis tissue due to *Schistosoma japonicum* infection. *Pharmacology and Clinics of Chinese Materia Medica*, **25**(6): 33-35.

Yan, B., Chen, F.H., Wu, F.R., Hu,W., Yuan, L.P., and Li, J. (2008). Therapeutic effects of total flavones of *Bidens bipinnata* L (TFB) on liver fibrosis in rats and its mechanisms. *Chinese Pharmacological Bulletin*, **24**(12): 1640-1645.

Yang, H.M., Li, S.T., Mei, L.X., and Ma, C.H. (2006). Effects of *Scutellaria baicalensis* stem-leaf total flavonoid on the activation of hepatic stellate cells. *Chinese Journal of Basic Medicine in Traditional Chinese Medicine*, **12**(1): 42-44.

Yang, J.H., Hu, J.C., Jia, J.D., Wang, Y., Mao, X.M., and Mao, H. (2008). Antifibrotic effect of pentoxifylline on rat liver fbrosis induced by bile duct occlusion. *Journal of Clinical and Experimental Medicine*, **7**(5): 53-55.

Yang, Z.Y., and Teng, H.L. (2009). Effect of TFC on two kinds of liver fibrosis model in rat. *Journal of Sichuan Traditional Chinese Medicine*, **27**(7): 30-31.

Yasuda, Y., Shimizu, M., Sakai, H., Iwasa, J., Kubota, M., Adachi, S., Osawa, Y., Tsurumi, H., Hara, Y., and Moriwaki, H. (2009). (-)-Epigallocatechin gallate prevents carbon tetrachloride-induced rat hepatic fibrosis by inhibiting the expression of the PDGFRbeta and IGF-1R. *Chemico-Biological Interactions*, **182**(2-3): 159-164.

Ye, G.S., Ma, Y., Wei, W., Li, R.L., Chen, W.B., Yan, J.C., and Ding, T.L. (2007). The influence of melatonin on the apoptosis and function of hepatic stellate cells from the rat hepatic fibrosis model induced by carbon tetrarchloride. *Acta Universitatis Medicinalis Anhui*, **42**(2): 183-185.

Yin, M.F., Lian, L.H., Piao, D.M., and Nan, J.X. (2007). Tetrandrine stimulates the apoptosis of hepatic stellate cells and ameliorates development of fibrosis in a thioacetamide rat model. *World Journal of Gastroenterology*, **13**(8): 1214-1220.

Young, S.C., Wang, C.J., Lin, J.J., Peng, P.L., Hsu, J.L., and Chou, F.P. (2007). Protection effect of piper betel leaf extract against carbon tetrachloride-induced liver fibrosis in rats. *Archives of Toxicology*, **81**(1): 45-55.

Zeng, W.Z., Wu, X.L., and Jiang, M.D. (2005). Effect of oxymarine on Smad gene expression in CCl_4-induced hepatic fibrosis in rats. *World Chinese Journal of Digestology*, **13**(8): 984-987.

Zhang, B.J., Xu, D., Guo, Y., Ping, J., Chen, L.B., and Wang, H. (2008). Protection by and anti-oxidant mechanism of berberine against rat liver fibrosis induced by multiple hepatotoxic factors. *Clinical and Experimental Pharmacology and Physiology*, **35**(3): 303-309.

Zhang, G.L., Shi, X.F., Ran, C.Q., Xu, M., and Zhu, Z.J. (2007). Effects of total saponins of *Panax notoginseng* against liver fibrosis in rats. *Acta Academiae Medicinae Militaris Tertiae*, **29**(23): 2212-2214.

Zhang, W., Fan, Y., Zhu, L.Q., Yao, G.T., and Li, Y.K. (2008). Therapeutic effect of lycopene on hepatic fibrosis in KM mice. *Lishizhen Medicine and Materia Medica Research*, **19**(7): 1743-1744.

Zhao, W.X., Yang, J.L., and Chen, Z.M. (2008). Effect of γ-schisandrin on proliferation, procollagen gene expression and collagen synthesis in hepatic stellate cells in vitro. *Chinese Journal of Comparative Medicine*, **18**(4): 25-27.

Zhao, Y.F., Huang, Y.Q., Zhang, Y.S., Xu, S., and Yang, H. (2010). Experiment on the protection of soybean isoflavones against the liver damage of hepatic fibrosis rats. *Guangming Journal of Chinese Medicine*, **25**(4): 604-606.

Zhao, Z.H., Mei, Q., Wu, J., Hu, Y.M., Xu, X.H., and Xu, J.M. (2009). An initial research on the mechanism of melatonin against rat liver fibrosis. *Anhui Medical Journal*, **30**(3): 266-267.

Zhen, M.C., Wang, X.M., Yin, Z.Y., Wang, Q., Liu, P.G., Wu, G.Y., Yu, K.K., and Li, G.S. (2008). Effect of EGCG on expression of TGF-β_1 and CTGF in rats with liver fibrosis. *World Chinese Journal of Digestology*, **16**(34): 3828-3834.

Zhou, C.H., Cai, Y., Sheng, X.Z., Zhu, T.F., and Wang, J.Y. (2006). Effects of glycyrrhizin on Smad7 in CCl_4 induced rat liver fibrosis. *Clinical Medical Journal of China*, **13**(1): 67-69.

Zhou, X.Q., He, Y., and Cheng, M.L. (2008). Effects of ginkgo leaves on hepatic fibrosis induced by CCl_4 in rats. *Medical Journal of Chinese People's Liberation Army*, **33**(9): 1117-1119.

Zhu, P.L., Li, J., Zhang, L., Huang, C., Jiang, G.L., and Liu, J. (2009). Effect of total flavonoids of *Litsea coreana* level on hepatic fibrosis and expression of TGF-β_1, CTGF mRNA in liver. *Acta Universitatis Medicinalis Anhui*, **44**(2): 232-235.

Bioactive Phytochemicals: Perspectives for Modern Medicine Vol. 1 (2012) *Pages* **215–253**
Editor: **V.K. Gupta**
Published by: **DAYA PUBLISHING HOUSE, NEW DELHI**

6

Anti-Allergic Leads from Indian Medicinal Plant

Pulok K. Mukherjee[1]* and P. Venkatesh[1]

ABSTRACT

Immediate-type allergic (anaphylactic) reaction is a life threatening syndrome induced by sudden systemic release of inflammatory mediators such as histamine, leukotrienes (LTs), 5-hydroxy tryptamine, platelet activating factor. Inhibition of these mediators upon allergen exposure is considered to be the promising strategy for the treatment of allergic disorders. Several herbal remedies including constituents derived from them have been used as a source for treatment of allergic disorders from time immemorial. Flavonoids including apigenin, kaempferol, luteolin and quercetin inhibited the release of IL-4 in purified basophils. Alkaloids like (-) vasicine, a pyrrolo [2, 1-b] quinazoline (Adhatoda vasica Nees) is reported to be a respiratory stimulant. Saponin from Albizia lebbeck (L.) has been proved for inhibition of degranulation of mast cells. Extracts from A. vasica, Clerodendron serratum Spreng., Curcuma longa L., Euphorbia hirta L., Ocimum sanctum L., Picrorhiza kurroa Royle., and Withania somnifera Dunal, Chrysanthemi sibirici herba var., Coleus forskohlii (Willd.) Briq., Curcuma mangga Valeton and van Zijp, Curcuma zedoaria (Christm.) Roscoe, Kaempferia galanga L. (Proh Hom), Kaempferia parviflora Wall. Ex. Baker, Nyctanthes arbortristis L., Plumbago zeylanica Iliee, etc. are well known plants having anti-allergic activity. This communication aims to provide a comprehensive review on the Indian medicinal plants and the phytoconstituents that have been tested for anti-allergic activity in in vitro and in vivo.

Keywords: Allergic diseases, Ayurveda, Histamine, India, Leukotrienes, Phytoconstituents.

1 School of Natural Product Studies, Department of Pharmaceutical Technology, Jadavpur University, Kolkata – 700 032, India.

* Corresponding author: naturalproductm@gmail.com; Tel: +91 33 24298313; Fax: +91 33 24146046.

List of Abbreviations

anti-DNP IgE: Anti-dinitrophenyl-immunoglobulin G
AP-1: Activating protein-1
c-AMP: Cyclic adenosine monophosphate
CCL11: Chemokine (C-C motif) ligand 11
CD_4^+: Cluster of differentiation
DSCG: Disodium cromoglycate
FBS: Fetal bovine serum
FcåRI: Fc epsilon RI
H1R: H_1 receptor
HeLa cells: Henrietta Lacks cells
IL-4: Interleukins
LTs: Leukotrienes
mRNA: Messenger RNA
NFAT: Nuclear factor of activated T cells
NF-kB: Nuclear factor kappa B
NO: Nitric oxide
OVA: Ovalbumin
PCA: Passive cutaneous anaphylaxis
PG: Prostaglandin
PGE2: Prostaglandins E2
RBL-2H3 cells: Rat basophilic leukemic cells
RPMC: Rat peritoneal mast cells
ROS: Reactive oxygen species
RPMI-1640: Roswell Park Memorial Institute-1640
TNF-α: Tumor Necrosis Factor-α

Introduction

The prevalence of allergic diseases has been significantly increased around the world. Histamine plays a crucial role in allergic inflammation, which is a complex network of cellular events involving redundant mediators and signals (Dev *et al.*, 2008). Histamine is released from the granules of FceRI+ cells (*e.g.*, mast cells and basophils) after the cross-linking of surface IgE by allergen or via IgE independent mechanism (Figure 6.1). It acts mainly through the histamine H1 receptor (H1R) (Simons, 2004; Miyoshi *et al.*, 2006). Das *et al.* (2007) reported that the activation of H1R up-regulates H1R through augmentation of H1R mRNA expression in HeLa cells.

A number of plants has been described in traditional medicine including Ayurveda in India for the treatment of allergic disorders, namely psoriasis, eczema,

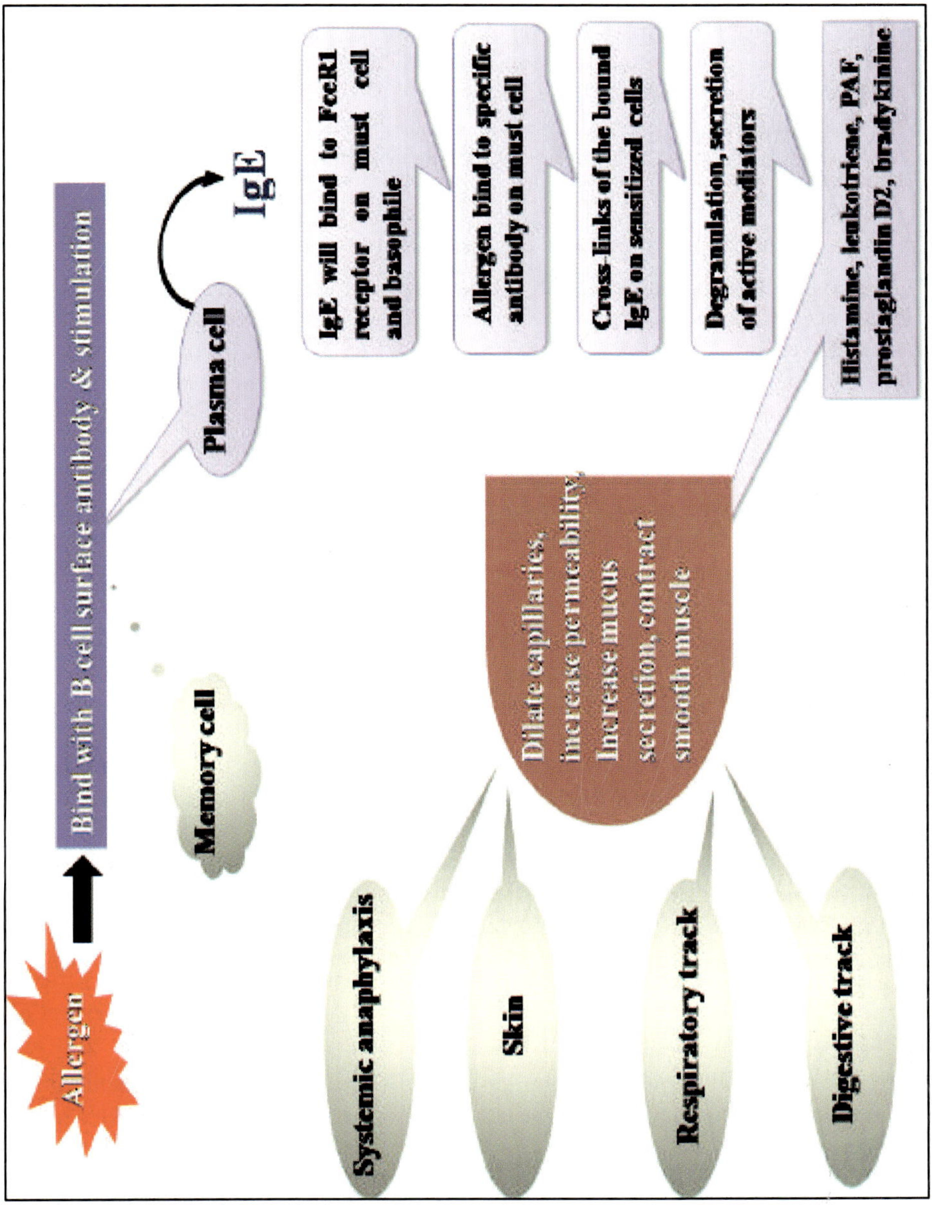

Figure 6.1 : Physiology of allergy in different body system.

bronchial asthma, etc (Mukherjee and Wahile, 2006). India being one of the 12 mega biodiversity centers with two hot-spots of biodiversity in the Western Ghats and northeastern region has several potential medicinal plants for treatment of allergy and related disorders (Mukherjee and Tamang, 2009). Anti-allergic preparations with medicinal plants of India have got enormous potentials throughout the world for a range of anti-allergic preparations. Many Indian plants have been reported for their beneficial use in different types of allergy. The search for a curative non-toxic and potent anti-allergic herbs will help to explore the biodiversity is different way for drug development from natural resources (Mukherjee, 2001). There are few inbuilt protocols available for the reliable identification of their antiallergic potential from the medicinal plants.

Plants as Source of Anti-Allergic Potential

The phytochemical and pharmacological screening of the crude drug or on the phyto moiety could help in validation of traditional claims. But continuation of the work is often ceased, which some time results in very less lead isolation of the bioactive constituents. Although the traditional claims have been followed by ancestors, the recognition for the same is unreachable to modern system of medicine until the same has been brought to and made available in pharmacy stores. There are still numerous unexplored targets had just been identified and neglected with the preliminary screening. The reason could be: (*i*) crude drugs need several trials, (*ii*) time consuming and cost factor, (*iii*) no certainty of getting the same beneficial result in subsequent trials, iv) degree of progression is aught when the screening is proceeded from *in vitro* to *in vivo* models and so on. While considering the traditional medicinal plants used for treating allergic diseases, number of clinically tested and established phytomolecules available in the hands of physician are countable. The accomplished phytomolecules like vasicine [1] (*A. vasica*), curcumin [2] (*C. longa*), forskolin [3] (*C. forskohlii*), daidzein [4] (*Pureraira lobata* (Willd.) Ohwi), quercetin [5] (*Allium cepa* L.) had undergone respective pharmacological studies and are clinically proven for their anti allergic properties. Beside search for the potential and possible target (phytomolecule) from the crude drugs, there has been considerable involvement to go forward in basic scientific research to identify the mechanism underlying in the plant extracts and their therapeutic effects (Mukherjee *et al.,* 2006). The following section narrates some of most traditionally used and potential anti-allergic plants. Several pharmacological works performed on these aspects has been explained in Table 6.1.

Adhatoda vasica Nees

A. vasica is a well known plant in Ayurveda, commonly known as Malabar nut and belong to the family Acanthaceae. It has been most frequently used for the treatment of respiratory diseases like cough, asthma and colds and herbal preparations containing *A. vasica* exists worldwide. Methanol extract of the aerial part of the plant has been shown to possess anti-allergic and anti-asthmatic activities in the guinea pig after inhalation or intragastric administration at doses of 6 mg/animal or 2.5 gm/kg, respectively (Mueller *et al.,* 1993). The frequent use of *A. vasica* has resulted in its inclusion in the WHO manual for the use of traditional medicine in primary

Table 6.1: Medicinal plants with potential anti-allergic activities.

Plant	*Activity/Dosage*	*Mechanism of Action*
Acanthopanax senticosus (Rupr.& Maxim.) Harms/Araliaceae	*Acanthopanax senticosus* (Rupr.& Maxim.) Harms root (2.0 g/kg) (methanol) inhibited PCA to 53.17±6.62 per cent and the treatment of root extract blocked the production (TNF-α) in a concentration-dependent manner (Yi *et al.*, 2001).	Inhibition of PCA activated by anti-dinitrophenyl (DNP) IgE (Yi *et al.*, 2001).
Adhatoda vasica Nees/Acanthaceae	Anti-allergic and anti-asthmatic activity of whole plant (methanolic) extract at 6mg/animal (guinea-pig) or 2.5 gm/kg, i.g. (Mueller *et al.*, 1993).	The protective effect against bronchospasm induced by histamine mediated through H_1 receptor antagonism (Kumar and Ramu, 2002).
Amomum cardamomum Willd./Zingiberaceae	The fruit extract of *Amomum cardamomum* Willd. (hexane) inhibited release of histamine up to 66.85±6.49 per cent at 0.5 mg/ml (Ikawati *et al.*, 2001).	Inhibiting histamine release from rat basophilic leukemia cell line, a tumor analog of mast cells (Ikawati *et al.*, 2001).
Asystasia gangetica (L.) T.Anderson/Acanthaceae	The leaf extracts (ethyl acetate) of *Asystasia gangetica* (L.) T.Anderson showed inhibition of smooth muscle contraction at 2.82 mg/ml (Akah *et al.*, 2003).	The elevation of c-AMP in bronchial smooth muscles and mast cells (Kreutner *et al.*, 1985).
Bacopa monnieri L./ Scrophulariaceae	The methanolic (leaves) fraction exhibited potent mast cell stabilization activity and reduced the degranulation up to 38.0±4.2 per cent at 10 µg/ml (Samiulla *et al.*, 2001)	Ability of extract to inhibit the release of mediators from mast cells and basophils (Lee *et al.*, 2004).
Benincasa hispida Thunb./Cucurbitaceae	*Benincasa hispida* fruit pulp (methanol) increased the exposition time against histamine exposure in seconds of 702.2±5.4 at 200mg/kg (Kumar and Ramu, 2002).	The protective effect against bronchospasm induced by histamine aerosol mediated by antihistaminic activity (H_1 receptor antagonism) (Kumar and Ramu, 2002).
Capparis spinosa L./ Capparidaceae	Inhibition of histamine induced bronchospasm by flowering buds (methanol) of *Capparis spinosa* L.up to 65.5 per cent at 14.28 mg/kg, p.o. (Trombetta *et al.*, 2005).	The protective effect against bronchospasm induced by histamine aerosol mediated by antihistaminic activity (H_1 receptor antagonism) (Kumar and Ramu, 2002).
Cassia alata L./ Leguminosae	*C. alata* leaf extract (alcohol) at the dose of 1000 µg/ml significantly reduced the percentage of degranulation of mast cells induced by carbachol up to 35.8±0.4 per cent (Palanichamy *et al.*, 1991).	Ability of extract to inhibit the release of mediators from mast cells and basophils (Lee *et al.*, 2004).

Contd...

Table 6.1–*Contd...*

Plant	*Activity/Dosage*	*Mechanism of Action*
Chrysanthemi sibirici herba var. latilobum Komar/Compositae	Inhibition of mast cell degranulation from the ethanolic extracts of *C. herba* (aerial part) at IC_{50} 76 µg/ml (Lee *et al.*, 2004).	Ability of extract to inhibit the release of mediators from mast cells and basophils (Lee *et al.*, 2004).
Cimicifuga racemosa (Nutt.) L./Ranunculaceae	The berries of *Cimicifuga racemosa* (Nutt.) L. (methanol) inhibited PCA reaction in mice at 0.1 and1 g/kg (Kim *et al.*, 2004).	Inhibition of the release of chemical mediators from mast cells induced by the antigen-IgE antibody reaction (Ito *et al.*, 1998).
Cinnamomum burmannii (Nees) Blume/Lauraceae	Hexane extract of cortex of *Cinnamomum burmannii* (Nees) Blume inhibited the histamine release up to 62.97±0.82 per cent at 0.5 mg/ml (Ikawati *et al.*, 2001).	Inhibiting histamine release from rat basophilic leukemia cell line, a tumor analog of mast cells (Ikawati *et al.*, 2001).
Cissampelos pareira L./ Menispermaceae	Roots of *Cissampelos pareira* L. (50 per cent ethanol) extract inhibited the release of histamine to 15.38 per cent and 30.77 per cent *in vivo* at 200, 400 mg/kg respectively (Amresh *et al.*, 2007).	Ability of extract to inhibit the release of mediators from mast cells and basophils (Lee *et al.*, 2004).
Coleus aromaticus Benth/ Lamiaceae	Aqueous and hydroalcoholic extracts of leaves (100µg/ml) of *Coleus aromaticus* Benth inhibited mast cell degranulation to 67.8 and 63.8 per cent respectively (Kumar *et al.*, 2007).	Ability of extract to inhibit the release of mediators from mast cells and basophils (Lee *et al.*, 2004).
Coleus forskohlii (Willd.) Briq./Lamiaceae	Percentage inhibition of PCA reaction by *C. forskohlii* (root) aqueous extract (50mg/kg) to 75 per cent was reported by Gupta *et al.* (1993).	Potentiation of c-AMP in turn inhibits basophil and mast cells degranulation and histamine release (Marone *et al.*, 1986).
Curculigo orchioides Gaertn/Amaryllidaceae	75.73 per cent protection resulted from the ethanol extract of *C. orchioides* (rhizome) on histamine-induced bronchoconstriction at 300mg/kg, p.o. (Pandit *et al.*, 2008)	Inhibition of bronchoconstriction and airway inflammation which leads to bronchial hyper responsiveness to various stimuli, in which many cell types play a role, more important being mast cells, eosinophils and T-lymphocytes (Pandit *et al.*, 2008).
Curcuma mangga Valeton and van Zijp,/Zingiberaceae	Inhibition of β-hexosaminidase release (RBL-2H3 cells) by rhizome of *C. mangga* (aqueous and ethanol extracts) at IC_{50} 36.1 and 36.7 µg/ml, respectively (Tewtrakul and Subhadhirasakul, 2007).	Inhibition of the release of enzyme stored in the secretory granules of mast cells and basophils (RBL-2H3 cells) upon their activation (Teshima *et al.*, 1986).

Contd...

Table 6.1–*Contd...*

Plant	*Activity/Dosage*	*Mechanism of Action*
Curcuma zedoaria (Christm.) Roscoe/Zingiberaceae	*C. zedoaria* (rhizome, 80 per cent aqueous acetone) inhibited the PCA reaction in mice at 100mg/kg up to a percentage of 27.6 (Matsuda *et al.,* 2004b).	Inhibition of the release of chemical mediators from mast cells, induced by the antigen-IgE antibody reaction (Ito *et al.,* 1998).
Curcuma zedoaria (Christm.) Roscoe/Zingiberaceae	Rhizome of *C. zedoaria* (80 per cent aqueous acetone and ethyl acetate soluble fraction) inhibited β-hexosaminidase release in RBL-2H3 cells at IC_{50} 48 and 35 μg/ml, respectively (Matsuda *et al.,* 2004b).	Inhibition of the release of chemical mediators from mast cells, induced by the antigen-IgE antibody reaction (Ito *et al.,* 1998).
Dioscorea membranacea Pierre/Disocoreaceae	*Dioscorea membranacea* Pierre (rhizome, ethanol) extract inhibited β-hexosaminidase release in RBL-2H3 cells at 37.5 mg/ml (Tewtrakul and Itharat, 2006).	Inhibition of the release of enzyme stored in the secretory granules of mast cells and basophils (RBL-2H3 cells) upon their activation (Teshima *et al.,* 1986).
Eucalyptus globules Labill./ Myrtaceae	Leaves (hexane and ethanol) extract of *Eucalyptus globules* Labill. inhibited histamine release to 84.85±6.18 and 85.39± 1.70 per cent at 0.5 mg/ml, respectively (Ikawati *et al.,* 2001).	Inhibiting histamine release from rat basophilic leukemia cell line, a tumor analog of mast cells (Ikawati *et al.,* 2001).
Eucalyptus globules Labill./ Myrtaceae	Fruit (ethanol) extract of *Eucalyptus globules* Labill. inhibited histamine release to 93.21±1.42 per cent at 0.5 mg/ml (Ikawati *et al.,* 2001).	Inhibiting histamine release from rat basophilic leukemia cell line, a tumor analog of mast cells (Ikawati *et al.,* 2001).
Euphorbia hirta L./ Euphorbiaceae	Inhibition of TNF-α and IL-6 by *E. hirta* (leaves, ethanol) extract at the doses ranging 100 to 1000 mg/kg (Youssouf *et al.,* 2007).	Inhibition of the activation of basophils and eosinophils upon the release of interleukins (ILs) (Bousquet *et al.,* 2001).
Glycyrrhiza glabra L./ Leguminosae	Mast cell stabilizing activity of ethanol extract (200 and 400 mg/kg b.w) of *Glycyrrhiza glabra* L. was found to inhibit degranulation of mast cells to an extent of 59.25±2.96 and 67.34±3.50 per cent, respectively (Choudhary *et al.,* 2007).	Ability of extract to inhibit the release of mediators from mast cells and basophils (Lee *et al.,* 2004).
Glycyrrhiza uralensis Fisch./ Leguminosae	80 per cent ethanolic extract of *Glycyrrhiza uralensis* Fisch. inhibited the release of β-hexosaminidase in RBL-2H3 cells up to 86.8 per cent at 100μg/ml (Lee *et al.,* 2007).	Inhibition of the release of enzyme stored in the secretory granules of mast cells and basophils (RBL-2H3 cells) upon their activation (Teshima *et al.,* 1986).

Contd...

Table 6.1–*Contd...*

Plant	*Activity/Dosage*	*Mechanism of Action*
Gymnema sylvestre (Retz.) R.Br/Asclepiadaceae	The ethanolic extract of *Gymnema sylvestre* (Retz.) R.Br root (150 and 200mg/kg) inhibited histamine induced rat paw oedema and the percentage inhibition is found to be 37.33 per cent and 41.08% respectively (Ravi Shankar and Ganga Rao, 2008).	Inhibition of serotonin induced edema in the tissues (Mukherjee *et al.,* 1997).
Justicia gendarusa L./ Acanthaceae	Inhibition of histamine release by *Justicia gendarusa* L. (leaves, ethanol) extract up to 41.78±0.01 per cent at 0.5 mg/ml (Ikawati *et al.,* 2001).	Inhibiting histamine release from rat basophilic leukemia cell line, a tumor analog of mast cells (Ikawati *et al.,* 2001).
Kaempferia parviflora Wall. Ex. Baker/ Zingiberaceae	*K. parviflora* rhizome (aqueous and ethanol) inhibited β-hexosaminidase release in RBL-2H3 cells at IC_{50} 48.4 and 10.9 µg/ml, respectively (Tewtrakul and Subhadhirasakul, 2007).	Inhibition of the release of enzyme stored in the secretory granules of mast cells and basophils (RBL-2H3 cells) upon their activation (Teshima *et al.,* 1986).
Kaempferia galanga L. (Proh Hom)/Zingiberaceae	*K. galanga* rhizome (aqueous) inhibited β-hexosaminidase release in RBL-2H3 cells at IC_{50} 49.5 µg/ml (Tewtrakul and Subhadhirasakul, 2007).	Inhibition of the release of enzyme stored in the secretory granules of mast cells and basophils (RBL-2H3 cells) upon their activation (Teshima *et al.,* 1986).
Lycopersicon esculentum Mill./Solanaceae	Ethanol extract of *Lycopersicon esculentum* Mill. (skin) inhibited the release of histamine at IC_{50} 500 µg/ml (Yamamoto *et al.,* 2004).	To suppress an allergic reaction through the inhibition of histamine release. However, the mechanism for this histamine-release inhibition by naringenin [23] is not clear (Yamamoto *et al.,* 2004).
Lycopus lucidus Turcz./ Labiatae	The whole plant of *Lycopus lucidus* Turcz. extract (aqueous) inhibited TNF-α and IL-6 secretion at doses 0.01, 0.1 and 1 mg/ml dose dependently (Shin *et al.,* 2005).	Inhibition of the activation of basophils and eosinophils upon the release of ILs (Bousquet *et al.,* 2001).
Melia azedarach L. var. Japonica/Meliaceae	80 per cent ethanolic extract of *Melia azedarach* L. var. Japonica inhibited the release of β-hexosaminidase in RBL-2H3 cells up to 85.1 per cent at 100µg/ml.The extract exhibited the most potent activity in mast cells at IC_{50} 29±1.5 µg/ml for antigen stimulation and 57±3.4 µg/ml for thapsigargin stimulation. It inhibited compound-48/80-induced systemic anaphylaxis by 52.9 per cent at a dose of 300 mg/kg in mice; it also inhibited the expression of the proinflammatory mediator TNF-α (Lee *et al.,* 2007).	Inhibition of the release of enzyme stored in the secretory granules of mast cells and basophils (RBL-2H3 cells) upon their activation (Teshima *et al.,* 1986).

Contd...

Table 6.1–*Contd...*

Plant	*Activity/Dosage*	*Mechanism of Action*
Mentha arvensis L./ Labiatae	The whole plant of *Mentha arvensis* L. extract (aqueous) inhibited PCA reaction at doses 0.001 to 1 g/kg (Shin, 2003).	Inhibition of the release of chemical mediators from mast cells, induced by the antigen-IgE antibody reaction (Ito *et al.*, 1998).
Momordica dioica Roxb. ex Willd/Cucurbitaceae	65 per cent (50mg/kg) of inhibition of PCA reaction exhibited by root extracts (hydroalcohol) of *Momordica dioica* Roxb. ex Willd (Gupta *et al.*, 1993).	Inhibition of the release of chemical mediators from mast cells, induced by the antigen-IgE antibody reaction (Ito *et al.*, 1998).
Nelumbo nucifera Gaertn./ Nymphaceae	Methanol extract of *Nelumbo nucifera* Gaertn. (rhizome) at doses of 200 and 400 mg/kg, p.o. reduced serotonin induced rat paw edema *in vivo* (Mukherjee *et al.*, 1997).	Inhibition of serotonin induced edema in the tissues (Mukherjee *et al.*, 1997).
Nyctanthes arbortristis L./ Oleaceae	The hydroalcoholic extract of *N. arbortristis* (flower) inhibited the PCA reaction to 76 per cent at 50mg/kg and leaf extract inhibited to 64 per cent at 50mg/kg (Gupta *et al.*, 1993).	Inhibition of the release of chemical mediators from mast cells, induced by the antigen-IgE antibody reaction (Ito *et al.*, 1998).
Ocimum sanctum L./ Lamiaceae	The seed oil (3 ml/kg, i.p.) produced a significant increase in anti-sheep red blood cells (SRBC) antibody titre and a decrease in percentage histamine release from peritoneal mast cells of sensitized rats (humoral immune responses) (Mediratta *et al.*, 2002).	The extract modulates both humoral and cell-mediated immune responsiveness and these immunomodulatory effects may be mediated by GABAergic pathways (Mediratta *et al.*, 2002).
Perilla frutescens (L.) Britton/Labiatea	61 per cent of inhibition of PCA reaction exhibited by leaves extract (500mg/kg) (ethanol) of *Perilla frutescens* (L.) Britton (Makino *et al.*, 2003).	Inhibition of the release of chemical mediators from mast cells, induced by the antigen-IgE antibody reaction (Ito *et al.*, 1998).
Phyllanthus emblica Gaertn./Euphorbiaceae	The cough suppressive activity of *P. emblica* (fruit) is dose-dependent *i.e.* 50 and 200 mg/kg (Nosál'ová *et al.*, 2003).	It is supposed that the antitussive activity of the dry extract of *P. emblica* is due to its effect on mucus secretion in the airways (Nosál'ová *et al.*, 2003).
Picrorhiza kurroa Royle. ex Benth.,/Scrophulariaceae	Glycoside fraction obtained from root and rhizome of *P. kurroa* (Picroliv) extract inhibited PCA reaction to 82 per cent at 25mg/kg (Baruah *et al.*, 1998).	Inhibition of the release of chemical mediators from mast cells, induced by the antigen-IgE antibody reaction (Ito *et al.*, 1998).
Plantago major L./ Plantaginaceae	Extract of *Plantago major* L. obtained from leaves (ethanol) inhibited histamine release to 87.61±0.57 per cent at 0.5 mg/ml (Ikawati *et al.*, 2001).	Inhibiting histamine release from rat basophilic leukemia cell line, a tumor analog of mast cells (Ikawati *et al.*, 2001).

Contd...

Table 6.1–*Contd...*

Plant	*Activity/Dosage*	*Mechanism of Action*
Plumbago zeylanica lliee./ Plumbaginaceae	Dose dependent inhibition of *P. zeylanica* (stem, ethanol) against PCA reaction in mice at the doses 5, 20, 50 mg/ml was reported by Dai *et al.*, 2004.	Inhibition of the release of chemical mediators from mast cells, induced by the antigen-IgE antibody reaction (Ito *et al.*, 1998).
Prunella vulgaris L./ Labiateae	The aqueous extract of *Prunella vulgaris* L. (leaves) inhibited the PCA reaction in doses ranging from 0.001 to 1 g/kg (Shin *et al.*, 2001).	Inhibition of the release of chemical mediators from mast cells, induced by the antigen-IgE antibody reaction (Ito *et al.*, 1998).
Pterocarpus santalinus L.f/Fabaceae	65 per cent of inhibition of PCA reaction exhibited by stem bark (50mg/kg) (hydroalcohol) extract of *Pterocarpus santalinus* L.f (Gupta *et al.*, 1993).	Inhibition of the release of chemical mediators from mast cells, induced by the antigen-IgE antibody reaction (Ito *et al.*, 1998).
Rheum palmatum L./ Polygonaceae	80 per cent ethanolic extract of *Rheum palmatum* L. inhibited the release of β-hexosaminidase in RBL-2H3 cells up to 82.4 per cent at 100μg/ml (Lee *et al.*, 2007)	Inhibition of the release of enzyme stored in the secretory granules of mast cells and basophils (RBL-2H3 cells) upon their activation (Teshima *et al.*, 1986).
Rheum undulatum L./ Polygonaceae	Dried rhizome of *Rheum undulatum* L. (Methanol) extract exhibited inhibition of histamine release to 47.4 per cent at 200 μg/ml (Matsuda, 2001).	Inhibition of chemical mediators such as histamine and LTs released from mast cells and basophils by an IgE related mechanism (Matsuda, 2001).
Rubia cordifolia L./ Rubiaceae	65 per cent of inhibition of PCA reaction exhibited by root (hydroalcohol) extract of *Rubia cordifolia* L. at 50mg/kg (Gupta *et al.*, 1993).	Inhibition of the release of chemical mediators from mast cells, induced by the antigen-IgE antibody reaction (Ito *et al.*, 1998).
Solanum Xanthocarpum Schrader et Wendl.,/ Solanaceae	The protection of mast cells were observed at a dose of 50 and 100 mg/kg, i.p. by 74.39 per cent and 78.26 per cent respectively by flowers (ethanolic) extract as compared to DSCG shown protection by 83.81% (Vadnere *et al.*, 2008).	Ability of extract to inhibit the release of mediators from mast cells and basophils (Lee *et al.*, 2004).
Syzygium cumini (L.) Skeels/Myrtaceae	100 mg/kg of the aqueous leaf extract significantly inhibited eosinophil accumulation in allergic pleurisy from 7.662±1.524 to 1.89±0.336 x 10^6/cavity (Brito *et al.*, 2007).	The inhibition of eosinophil accumulation in the allergic pleurisy model is probably due to an impairment of CCL11/eotaxin and IL-5 production (Brito *et al.*, 2007).
Thymus vulgaris L./ Lamiaceae	*Thymus vulgaris* L. (leaves, hexane) extract inhibited the release of histamine up to 46.22±0.08 per cent at 0.5 mg/ml (Ikawati *et al.*, 2001).	Inhibiting histamine release from rat basophilic leukemia cell line, a tumor analog of mast cells (Ikawati *et al.*, 2001).

Contd...

Table 6.1–*Contd...*

Plant	*Activity/Dosage*	*Mechanism of Action*
Vitex trifolia L./Lamiaceae	Inhibition of histamine release exhibited by leaves of *Vitex trifolia* L. (hexane and ethanol) to 80.13±3.95 and 81.58±0 .24 per cent at 0.5 mg/ml, respectively (Ikawati *et al.,* 2001).	Inhibiting histamine release from rat basophilic leukemia cell line, a tumor analog of mast cells (Ikawati *et al.,* 2001).
Withania somnifera Dunal/Solanaceae	Root extract of *W. somnifera* (aqueous) inhibited PCA reaction at 0.05 mg (Amara *et al.,* 1999).	Inhibition of the release of chemical mediators from mast cells, induced by the antigen-IgE antibody reaction (Ito *et al.,* 1998).
Zingiber cassumunar Roxb./Zingiberaceae	*Z. cassumunar* rhizome (aqueous and ethanol) inhibited the release of β-hexosaminidase in RBL-2H3 cells at IC_{50} 44.4 and 12.9 μg/ml, respectively (Tewtrakul and Subhadhirasakul, 2007).	Inhibition of the release of enzyme stored in the secretory granules of mast cells and basophils (RBL-2H3 cells) upon their activation (Teshima *et al.,* 1986).
Zingiber officinale Roscoe/Zingiberaceae	Ethanol extract of *Z. officinale* (rhizome) inhibited release of β-hexosaminidase in RBL-2H3 cells at IC_{50} 40.3 μg/ml (Tewtrakul and Subhadhirasakul, 2007).	Inhibition of the release of enzyme stored in the secretory granules of mast cells and basophils (RBL-2H3 cells) upon their activation (Teshima *et al.,* 1986).

health care, which is intended for health workers in South-East Asia to keep them informed of the therapeutic utility of their surrounding flora (WHO, 1990). Some herbal preparations containing *A.vasica* used world wide for the treatment of asthma and allergy are 'Kada' (asthma) (India); Femiforte (leucorrhoea) (India); Salus Tuss (dry cough, bronchitis) (Germany); Kan Jang (alleviation of symptoms of colds, antitussive) (Sweden) (Iyengar *et al.,* 1994; Shete, 1993; Rote, 1977; Farnlof, 1998). Apart from vasicine [1], other isolated alkaloids include vasicinone, anisotine, adhatodine, vasicolinone, vasicoline, and vasicinol and leaves contain betaine, steroids and alkanes (Huq, 1967).

Albizia lebbeck (L.) Benth.

A. lebbeck commonly known as Siris in India is a tree well known in the Indian subcontinent for its several range of uses belongs to the family Fabaceae. Clinical studies showed that *A. lebbeck* acts as an antidote to animal poison, which were most histaminic in nature and produced allergic dermatitis, urticaria and anaphylactic shock, suggesting its use in bronchial asthma (Sharma *et al.,* 2000) further saponins isolated from *A. lebbeck* found to accord protection to sensitized guinea pigs against histamine as well as antigen micro-aerosols. The decoction of bark of *A. lebbeck* was found to be potent vasoconstrictor. The decoction of the bark and the flowers have antiasthmatic and anti anaphylactic activities (Gupta, 2003). A novel botanical formulation, Aller-7/NR-A2, was developed for the treatment of allergic rhinitis; it is a combination of medicinal plant extracts from *A. lebbeck, Phyllanthus emblica* Gaertn., *Terminalia chebula* Retz., *Terminalia bellerica* Roxb., *Piper nigrum* L., *Zingiber officinale* Roscoe and *Piper longum* L., which has demonstrated potent antihistaminic, anti-inflammatory, antispasmodic, antioxidant, and mast-cell-stabilization activities (Pratibha *et al.,* 2004).

Clerodendron serratum Spreng.

C. serratum belongs to the family Verbenaceae, commonly called as 'Bharangi mool' in India is widely used for the treatment of asthma and cough by traditional practitioners. The isolation of phytoconstituents from this plant afforded saponin, mannitol, serratagenic acid and γ-sitosterol are reported. Gupta (1968) observed the antihistamine and anti-allergic activity of the extract. The effect of saponin on the mast cells of rat mesentery was reported by Gupta*et al.* (1971). Further saponins from *C. serratum* and *A. lebbeck* have been shown to protect sensitized mast cells from degranulation on antigen shock (Tripathi *et al.,* 1978).

Curculigo orchioides Gaertn

C. orchioides is a tiny herbal plant widely distributed in India. The scope of selecting this plant for further exploration is the Type 4 hypersensitivity of the same has been established by Bafna and Mishra (2006). Further, the effect of ethanol extract (rhizome) on histamine-induced broncho constriction is reported and inhibition of compound 48/80 induced anaphylaxis at IC_{50} 0.385 g (Venkatesh *et al.,* 2008), this effect may be the presence of curculigoside A [10], curculigoside B, curculigoside C (Fu *et al.,* 2004), orcinol glycoside (Li *et al.,* 2003).

Curcuma longa L.

The rhizomes of *C. longa* (Fam: Zingiberaceae) is a perennial herb, commonly known as haldi is extensively cultivated in all parts of India. This is most commonly used as a spice in curries and other South Asian and Middle Eastern cuisine, for dyeing, and to impart color to mustard condiments and is reported to contain curcumin [2], a diferuloylmethane. The extracts of *C. longa, Z. officinale, P. longum, P. emblica* Gaertn., *T. bellerica, O. sanctum, A. vasica* and *Cyperus rotundus* L. are the main constituents of HK-07, a polyherbal formulation, which is known for their mast cell stabilizing potential against Ag-Ab reaction and/or due to the suppression of IgE antibody production (Gopumadhavan *et al.*, 2005).

Euphorbia hirta L.

E. hirta (Fam: Euphorbiaceae) popularly known as asthma weed is a herbaceous wild plant which grows in the hotter parts of India. In traditional Ayurvedic medicines the whole aerial parts is used in bronchial and respiratory diseases (asthma, bronchitis, hay fever), gastrointestinal disorders (diarrhoea, dysentery, intestinal parasitosis) (Mhaskar *et al.*, 2000). Youssouf *et al.* (2007) proved the inhibitory activity of *E. hirta*, against TNF-α and IL-6 secretion showed the dose dependent activity from 100 to 1000 mg/kg. It is reported to contain flavonoid, quercitrin [6] (Galvez *et al.*, 1993).

Ocimum sanctum L.

In Ayurveda, *O. sanctum* (Fam: Lamiaceae) commonly known as 'Tulsi' has been well documented for its therapeutic potentials and described as 'Dashemani Shwasaharni' (antiasthmatic). Eugenol [7] is an essential oils extracted from different parts of this plant (Sen, 1993). *O. sanctum* has been reported to protect against histamine, pollen-induced bronchospasm in guinea pigs and inhibition of antigen-induced histamine release from sensitized mast cells (Palit *et al.*, 1983). Other plants of genus *Ocimum* are known for their therapeutic potentials *viz., Ocimum gratissimum* L. (Ram Tulsi), *Ocimum canum* L. (Dulal Tulsi), *Ocimum basilicum* L. (Ban Tulsi) etc. It is reported to contain several other constituensts as carvacrol, caryophyllene, nerol and camphene, eugenol [7], eugenol methyl ether, methyl chavicol, cineole and linalool (Anonymous, 2001; Prajapati *et al.*, 2004).

Picrorhiza kurroa Royle. ex Benth.

P. kurroa (Fam: Scrophulariaceae) is commonly known as kutki. Its standardized fraction, Picroliv, from the root and rhizome consisting of picroside I and kutkoside in a ratio of 1:1.5 is well known plant exerting anti-allergic activity (Baruah *et al.*, 1998). Inhibition of membrane-protease release by *P. kurroa* was suggested through the study of gastric secretion and exhibition of saturable synergism with di-isopropyl fluoro phosphate on inhibition of anaphylactic degranulation; further the pH-independence of mast cell stabilizing effect negates any *P. kurroa* influence on phospholipid transmethylation (Pandey *et al.*, 1989). The medicinal properties have been attributed to kutkin [8], an active glucosidic bitter principle.

Withania somnifera Dunal

W. somnifera (Fam: Solanaceae), a well known in India as Ashwagandha and also as Indian ginseng. It is very well known in Ayurveda for their immunomodualtory, antiallergic activities (Kirtikar and Basu, 1999). Amara *et al.* (1999) has reported the dose dependent inhibition of TNF-α and IL-6 secretion by 'Aswagandha' root at concentration of 0.01, 0.1 and 1 mg/ml. The root extract (aqueous) was examined for its effect on down regulation of antigen-specific IgE antibody response in mice and also studied for identification of immunomodulatory effects using turkey egg ovalbumin (OVA) as an allergen. The extract was found to downregulate the anti-OVA IgE antibody response in a murine model (Amara *et al.*, 1999). It contains mainly withaferinA [9] (steroidal lactone), withanine (alkaloid), withananine (alkaloid) and withanolides A-Y (steroidal lactones) (Pramanick *et al.*, 2008).

Plants Under Euphorbiaceae Family

The ethnobotanical survey by Muthu *et al.* (2006) on traditional healers on the use of medicinal plants in Kancheepuram district of Tamil Nadu state, India have reported that the traditional healers of this region used 85 varieties of plants belonging to 76 genera belonging to 41 families to treat various diseases. In this study the most dominant family was Euphorbiaceae *viz., Euphorbia antiquorum* L. (Triangular spruge), *E. hirta* (Asthma weed), *Euphorbia tirucalli* L. (Indian Tree Spurge/pencil tree), *Phyllanthus amarus* Schum. and Thnn., *P. emblica* (Amla) and *Ricinus communis* L. (Castor oil) were most frequently used for the treatment of allergic diseases. *Acalypha indica* L. (Indian acalypha) common annual shrub in Indian gardens, has been used as paste (leaf) applied topically to treat skin diseases. It is reported to contain alkaloids-acalypus and acalyphine. *Baliospermum montanum* Muell Arg. of this family is commonly known as Danti, is found in tropical and subtropical Himalaya. Root of this is reported to contain axillarenic acid, baliospermin and montanin [11] which possess a wide range of activities such as anthelmintic, diuretic, purgative, bronchitis (Kirtikar and Basu, 1999).

Plants Under Zingiberaceae Family

Z. officinale (Ginger) has been found to exert anti-inflammatory activity and is reported to be a potent inhibitor of inflammatory mediators such as prostaglandins and LTs (Kiuchi *et al.*, 1992). Tewtrakul and Subhadhirasakul (2007) reported the inhibition of β-hexosaminidase release of some species from Zingiberaceae family and their activity has been derived in terms of IC_{50} value. The result supported that *Kaempferia parviflora* Wall. Ex. Baker. (Krachaidum), *Zingiber cassumunar* Roxb. (Cassumunar ginger), *C. mangga* (Temu Pauh), have shown potent enzyme inhibitory activity and ranging from 10.9 to 36.7 μg/ml. Three compounds were isolated from the n-hexane-soluble fraction of *Z. cassumunar* and the chemical structures of these compounds were identified as (E)-1-(3, 4-dimethoxyphenyl) but-1-ene, (E)-1-(3, 4-dimethoxyphenyl) butadiene and zerumbone. The anti-inflammatory activity of the crude drug was assumed to be the presence of (E)-1-(3, 4-dimethoxyphenyl) but-1-ene (Ozaki *et al.*, 1991). The rhizome extracts of plants from Zingiberaceae family *viz., C. longa, C. mangga, C. zedoaria* (zedoary), *K. parviflora, K. galanga* (Resurrection lily), *Z. cassumunar, Z. officinale* are used in traditional system for the treatment of allergic disorders. Most of these plants have been tested for inhibition of release of key enzymes like histamine and β-hexosaminidase and significant inhibition of the enzymes shown by extracts from *C. longa*, *C. zedoaria* and *K. parviflora*.

Ethnomedicinal survey on different parts of Madhya Pradesh and Chhattisgarh, India revealed that several medicinal plant species of these regions possesses anti-allergic properties *viz.*, *Boerhavia diffusa* L., *Evolvulus alsinodes* L., *Solanum indicum* L., *Solanum nigrum* L. and *Tephrosia purpurea* L. (Jain *et al.*, 2006). Anti-allergic potentials of several medicinal plants along with the reported mechanisms of action and other profiles of some specific plants have been summarized in Table 6.1.

Several precise, sensitive and specific methods for estimation of histamine has been reported while considering the experimental design for the possible targets, of which the spectrofluorimetric method reported by Shore *et al.* (1959) is widely employed. This method involves extraction of histamine into n-butanol from alkalinized perchloric acid tissue extracts, histamine returns to an aqueous solution and condensation with o-phthalaldehyde to yield a product with strong and stable fluorescence which is measured in a spectroflourimeter. The fluorescent intensity is measured at 438 nm (excitation at 353 nm); whereas for *in vitro* experiments, the rat basophilic leukemia (RBL-2H3) cell line has been widely used to estimate various local mediators. Conjugates of these derivatives with macromolecules were examined by Hemmerich and Pecht (1988) for their binding to cells of RBL-2H3, which is widely employed as a model for immunologically induced mast cell degranulation. When these cells are seeded in diversified medium often produce controversial or unreliable results therefore appropriate medium *viz.*, minimum essential medium with 10 per cent FBS or RPMI-1640 medium with 10 per cent FBS (Eccleston *et al.*, 1973) are commonly used.

Phytoconstituents with Anti-Allergic Potential

Work on new bioactive compounds from medicinal plants has led to the isolation and structure elucidation of a number of exciting new pharmacophores (Mukherjee *et al.*, 2007b). Middleton and Anne (1995) have reported that the structure activity relationship of phytoconstituents determines the fundamental structure for inhibitory activity of cytokine synthesis and may help in developing new anti-allergy drugs by side chain modification. The major groups of phytonutrients found in our diets include, flavonoids, terpenes, amines, phenols, polysaccharides organic acids organosulfurs etc. are observed to have higher degree of anti-allergic activity. The anti-allergic effects of any phytoconstituents may be through [or either] the inhibition of degranulation of mast cells, basophils and neutrophils, tyrosine kinase and nitric oxide synthase while modulating NF-kβ, the inflammatory mediator, the release of histamine and other mediators of allergic reaction, possibly by stabilizing cell membranes so that they are less reactive to allergens (Middleton and Anne, 1995) (Figure 6.2). Activation stimuli (inflammatory cytokines *e.g.* TNF-α, IL-1, IL-6) at the cell surface begin the process of NF-kB activation and initiate a cellular cascade that results in the release of active NF-kB subunits (Bremner and Heinrich, 2005).

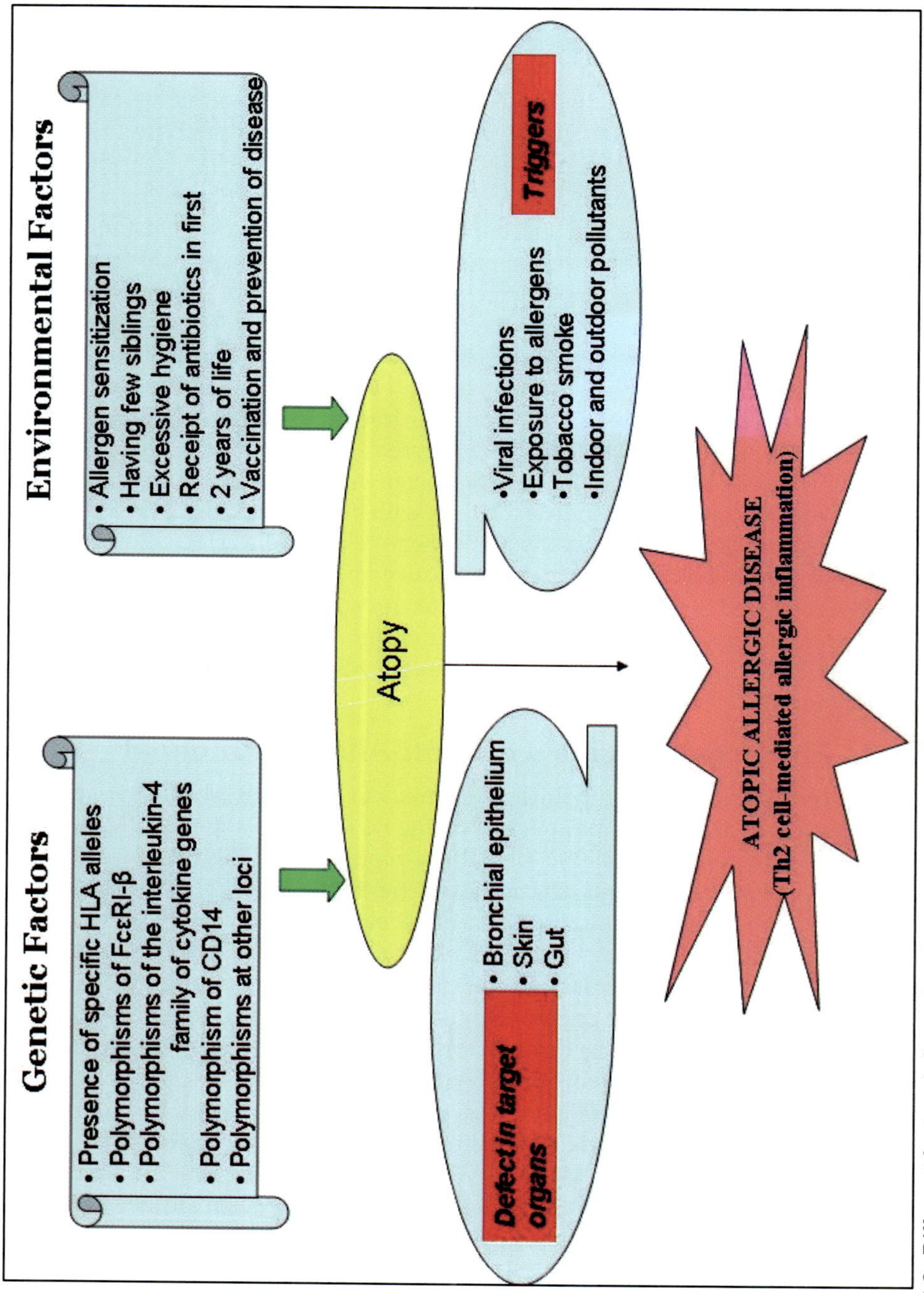

Figure 6.2: Different factors influencing the occurrence of allergic reactions.

Alkaloids

Vasicine [1], a bitter quinazoline alkaloid, from the well known Indian plant *A. vasica* has been found to be biologically active (Atal, 1980) and the pharmacologically most studied chemical component present in the leaves, roots and flowers. The yield of vasicine [1] ranges from 0.0541 to 1.105 per cent w/w. Tylophora alkaloids obtained from *Tylophora indica* (Burm.f.) Merill are reported to inhibit cellular immune responses like contact sensitivity to dinitro-flurobenzene and delayed hypersensitivity to sheep red blood cells, *in vivo*. The alkaloid mixture suppressed IL-2 production in Concanavalin A stimulated splenocytes at the inhibitory or higher concentrations and enhanced production at the lower concentrations (Ganguly *et al.*, 2001).

Terpenes

Diterpenes

The PCA inhibitory activity of andrographolide [12], and neo andrographolide proved to have anti-allergic activity (Gupta *et al.*, 1998). Coleonol or forskolin [3] has been found to have significant anti-allergic activity as shown by anti-PCA and mast cell stabilizing activity. Earlier it has been shown that coleonol has the ability to relax air way smooth muscle and inhibit the release of LTs and histamine *in vitro* and elicit bronchodilation *in vivo* (Kreutner *et al.*, 1985). Both these effects are due to the elevation of c-AMP by coleonol in bronchial smooth muscles and mast cells. Forskolin [3] activates the c-AMP which inhibits human basophil and mast cell degranulation resulting in subsequent bronchodilation (Lichey *et al.*, 1984).

Suregada multiflora (A. Juss.) Baill (Syn. Gelonium multiflorum), distributed in the tropical and subtropical areas of Asia and Africa. Bark of this plant is one potent traditional medicine used to treat inflammation and skin diseases (Wutthithamavet, 1997). The diterpenes (Ent-16-aurene-3β,15β,18-triol; Ent-3-oxo-16-kaurene-15β,18-diol; Ent-16-kaurene-3β,15β-diol; Helioscopinolide A and I; 10-gingerol [13]; 6-gingerol [14]) isolated from *S. multiflora* were tested for inhibition of β-hexosaminidase release in RBL-2H3 cells and their results supported their potential anti-allergic effect.

Sesquiterpenes

Curcumin [2], bisdemethoxy curcumin obtained from *C. zedoaria* have shown potent inhibitory potential of TNF-α and IL-4 or IL-5 synthesis at IC_{50} 38mM and 34mM; IC_{50} 20mM and 18mM (Matsuda *et al.*, 2004b) respectively. Curcumin [2] is also found to be a potent blocker of nuclear transcription factor, NF-kB, which is linked to a variety of diseases including allergy and asthma (Bharti *et al.*, 2003). The anti-allergic and antioxidative activities of curcumin-related compounds (glycosides, reductants and bis demethoxy analogs) were investigated to elucidate the underlying active mechanisms and structural features of Curcumin [2] in exerting these activities (Suzuki *et al.*, 2005).

Flavonoids

Flavonoids (apigenin [15], kaempferol [16], luteolin [17] and quercetin [5]) have been proved to have potent inhibitory potential of IL-4 synthesis in purified basophils at IC_{50} 3.1mM, 15.7mM, 2.7mM, 18.8mM, respectively (Kawai *et al.*, 2007). The promising anti-PCA activity has been shown by an isoflavone, daidzein [4] at 73 per cent (50mg/kg). The rhizome of *Pueraria lobata* (Willd.) Ohwi (Fam: Leguminosae) is useful against allergy in tarditional practice in India. Some isoflavones, puerarin, and daidzin, have been reported from this plant as the major bioactive component (Shibata *et al.*, 1959).

Glycosides

The percentage protection of mast cell degranulation (92 per cent at 10mg/kg) was achieved from the glycoside (Arbortristoside A [18], Arbortristoside C) obtained from *N. arbortristis* (Gupta *et al.*, 1995). Diosgenin [19], a cardiac glycoside, Dioscorealide A [20] and B [21], a naphthofuranoxepins, Dioscoreanone [22] a phenanthraquinone, obtained from *Dioscorea membranacea* Pierre proved to have inhibitory potential against β-hexosaminidase release at IC_{50} 29.9 μM, 27.9 μM, 5.7 μM and 7.7 μM, respectively.

Polyphenols

Polyphenols obtained from various sources are reported to have potential antiallergic activitiy. Eugenol [7], Naringenin [23], Rosmarinic acid, 6-dehydrogingerdione [24] are the main constituents of different traditionally used plant, which has been proved to have effect against various forms of allergy. Tannins and their related polyphenols are well known to have anti-oxidative properties and also inhibited histamine release induced by superoxide in rat mast cells and the most effective inhibition was exhibited by agrimoniin and euphorbin C (IC_{50} 0.68 and 0.80 μM), which have dehydrodigalloyl and euphorbinoyl groups, respectively (Kanoh *et al.*, 2000).

Saponins

Albizia saponins from *A. lebbeck* have potential protective effect from degranulation of mast cell from the toxicant and have been proved to have 27.40±11.40 per cent of protection at 10 mg/kg, p.o. (Gupta, 1994). Clerodendron saponins from *C. serratum* protected mast cell from degranulation up to 26.59 per cent at 10 mg/kg, p.o. (Gupta, 1994). This effect is due to the ability of saponin to inhibit the release of mediators from mast cells and basophils (Lee *et al.*, 2004).

Stilbenes

Stilbenes are known for their antiallergic activity which was proved by Matsuda *et al.* (2004a). Six stilbenes have been reported from tubers of *Gymnadenia conopsea* (L.) R.Br., which exert inhibition of the antigen-induced degranulation in RBL-2H3 cells. Matsuda *et al.* (2001) proved the activity of several other stilbenes including rhapontigenin [25], piceatannol, piceatannol 3′-β-D-glycoside isolated from *Rheum undulatum* L., have been reported to inhibit the release of histamine.

A list of phytoconstituents with significant anti-allergic activity has been provided in Table 6.2 and structures of some lead compounds have been shown in Figure 6.3.

Table 6.2: Phytoconstituents with reported anti-allergic activity.

Constituent	*Source*	*Work Done*	*Mechanism of Action*
Arbortristoside Glycoside	*Nyctanthes A/ arbortristis* L./ Oleaceae	At 10mg/kg, Arbortristoside A [18] obtained from alcoholic extract of seeds of the *N. arbortristis* showed 92 per cent of protection of mast cell degranulation (Gupta *et al.*, 1995).	Ability of extract to inhibit the release of mediators from mast cells and basophils (Lee *et al.*, 2004).
Arbortristoside C/ Glycoside	*Nyctanthes arbortristis* L./ Oleaceae	92 per cent of protection of mast cell degranulation showed at 10mg/kg by Arbortristoside C obtained from seeds of the *N. arbortristis* (alcoholic extract) (Gupta *et al.*, 1995).	Ability of extract to inhibit the release of mediators from mast cells and basophils (Lee *et al.*, 2004).
Albizia saponins/ Saponins	*A. lebbeck*/ Fabaceae	Albizia saponins from *A. lebbeck* stem bark showed 27.40± 11.40 per cent protection from degranulation of mast cell at 10 mg/kg, p.o. (Gupta, 1994).	Ability of extract to inhibit the release of mediators from mast cells and basophils (Lee *et al.*, 2004).
Andrographolide/ Diterpenes	*Andrographis paniculata* (Burm. F) Wall./Acanthaceae	Andrographolide [12] from *Andrographis paniculata* (Burm. F) Wall. showed the 60 per cent inhibition of PCA reaction at 50mg/kg (Gupta *et al.*, 1998).	Inhibition of the release of chemical mediators from mast cells, induced by the antigen-IgE antibody reaction (Ito *et al.*, 1998).
Apigenin/ Flavonoid	*Apium graveolens* L./Apiaceae	Inhibition of IL-4 synthesis showed by a flavonoid apigenin [15] from *Apium graveolens* L. at IC_{50} 3.1mM was reported (Kawai *et al.*, 2007).	The inhibitory activity of flavonoids on IL- 4, IL-13 and CD_{40} ligand expression may be mediated through their inhibition of transcriptional factors such as AP-1 (activating protein-1) and NFAT (nuclear factor of activated T cells) (Kawai *et al.*, 2007).
Bisdemethoxy curcumin/ Sesquiterpene	*Curcuma zedoaria* (Christm.) Roscoe/ Zingiberaceae	Bisdemethoxycurcumin inhibited the synthesis of TNF-α and IL-4 at IC_{50} 38mM and 34mM (Matsuda *et al.*, 2004b).	Inhibition of the activation of basophils and eosinophils upon the release of ILs (Bousquet *et al.*, 2001).
Clerodendron Saponins/Saponins	*C. serratum/* Verbenaceae	Clerodendron saponins protected from degranulation of mast cell up to 26.59 per cent at 10 mg/kg, p.o. (Gupta, 1994).	Ability of extract to inhibit the release of mediators from mast cells and basophils (Lee *et al.*, 2004).
Coleonol (Forskolin)/ Diterpene	*C. forskohlii*/ Lamiaceae	Inhibition of PCA reaction i.p. was observed from coleonol [3] to 54 per cent at 0.1 mg/kg, p.o. (Gupta *et al.*, 1994).	Inhibition of the release of chemical mediators from mast cells, induced by the antigen-IgE antibody reaction (Ito *et al.*, 1998).
Coleonol hemisuccinate/ Diterpene	*C. forskohlii*/ Lamiaceae	Inhibition of PCA reaction was observed from Coleonol hemisuccinate to 48.75 per cent at 0.1mg/kg, p.o. (Gupta *et al.*, 1994).	Inhibition of the release of chemical mediators from mast cells, induced by the antigen-IgE antibody reaction (Ito *et al.*, 1998).

Contd...

Table 7.2–*Contd...*

Constituent	*Source*	*Work Done*	*Mechanism of Action*
Curcumin/ Sesquiterpene	*Curcuma zedoaria* (Christm.) Roscoe./ Zingiberaceae	Curcumin [2] inhibited the synthesis of TNF-α and IL-4 at two doses *i.e.* IC_{50} 20 mM and 18 mM (Matsuda *et al.,* 2004b).	Inhibition of the activation of basophils and eosinophils upon the release of ILs (Bousquet *et al.,* 2001).
Daidzein/ Isoflavone	*Pureraira lobata* (Willd.) Ohwi/ Leguminosae	Daidzein [4], inhibited the PCA reaction to73 per cent at 50mg/kg (Choo *et al.,* 2002).	Inhibition of the release of chemical mediators from mast cells, induced by the antigen-IgE antibody reaction (Ito *et al.,* 1998).
Dioscorealide A/ Naphthofura-noxepins	*Dioscorea membranacea* Pierre/ Disocoreaceae	Dioscorealide A [20] and B [21] inhibited the release of β-hexosaminidase in RBL-2H3 cells at IC_{50} 27.9 µM and 5.7 µM, respectively (Tewtrakul and Itharat, 2006).	Inhibition of the release of enzyme stored in the secretory granules of mast cells and basophils (RBL-2H3 cells) upon their activation (Teshima *et al.,* 1986).
Dioscoreanone/ Phenanthraquinone	*Dioscorea membranacea* Pierre/ Disocoreaceae	Dioscoreanone [22] inhibited the release of β-hexosa-minidase in RBL-2H3 cells at IC_{50} 7.7 µM (Tewtrakul and Itharat, 2006).	Inhibition of the release of enzyme stored in the secretory granules of mast cells and basophils (RBL-2H3 cells) upon their activation (Teshima *et al.,* 1986).
Diosgenin/ Cardiac glycoside	*Dioscorea membranacea* Pierre/ Disocoreaceae	Inhibition of the release of β-hexosaminidase in RBL-2H3 cells was observed from Diosgenin [19] at IC_{50} 29.9 µM (Tewtrakul and Itharat, 2006).	Inhibition of the release of enzyme stored in the secretory granules of mast cells and basophils (RBL-2H3 cells) upon their activation (Teshima *et al.,* 1986).
Eugenol/ Phenol	*Syzygium aromaticum* (L.) Merrill and Perry/Myrtaceae	Eugenol [7] inhibited compound 48/80-induced systemic anaphylaxis 100 per cent at 10 µg/g b.w in rats; inhibited PCA activated by anti-DNP IgE. Eugenol [7] dose dependently inhibited histamine release from RPMC activated by compound 48/80 or had a significant inhibitory effect on anti-DNP IgE-induced TNF-α production at 10 µg/ml (Kim *et al.,* 1997).	Inhibition of the release of chemical mediators from mast cells, induced by the antigen-IgE antibody reaction (Ito *et al.,* 1998).
Luteolin/ Flavonoid	*Capsicum annum* L./Solanaceae	Inhibition of IL-4 synthesis by luteolin [17] at IC_{50} 2.7mM (Kawai *et al.,* 2007).	The inhibitory activity of flavonoids on IL- 4, IL-13 and CD_{40} ligand expression may be mediated through their inhibition of transcriptional factors such as AP-1 and NFAT (Kawai *et al.,* 2007).

Contd...

Table 7.2–*Contd...*

Constituent	*Source*	*Work Done*	*Mechanism of Action*
Naringenin/ Polyphenol	*Lycopersicon esculentum* L./ Solanaceae	Naringenin [23] inhibited the release of histamine at IC_{50} 68 mg/ml (Yamamoto *et al.*, 2004).	Inhibition of the release of chemical mediators from mast cells, induced by the antigen-IgE antibody reaction (Ito *et al.*, 1998).
Neoandro-grapholide/ Diterpenes	*Andrographis paniculata*/ Acanthaceae	Neo-andrographolide inhibited the PCA reaction to 77% at 50mg/kg (Gupta *et al.*, 1998).	Inhibition of the release of chemical mediators from mast cells, induced by the antigen-IgE antibody reaction (Ito *et al.*, 1998).
Piceatannol/ Stilbenes	*Rheum undulatum* L./Polygonaceae	Inhibition of histamine release to 86 per cent at 20 mg/ml showed by piceatannol (Matsuda *et al.*, 2001).	Inhibition of the release of chemical mediators from mast cells, induced by the antigen-IgE antibody reaction (Ito *et al.*, 1998).
Piceatannol 3'-β-D-glycoside/ Stilbenes	*Rheum undulatum* L./Polygonaceae	64.1 per cent of inhibition in the release of histamine achieved at 20 mg/ml of piceatannol 3'-β-D-glycoside (Matsuda *et al.*, 2001).	Inhibition of the release of chemical mediators from mast cells, induced by the antigen-IgE antibody reaction (Ito *et al.*, 1998).
Psoralidine/ Coumestan derivative	*Psoralea corylifolia* L./Papillionaceae	Inhibition of β-hexosaminidase release in RBL-2H3 cells were observed from psoralidine at IC_{50} 100mM (Matsuda *et al.*, 2007).	Inhibition of the release of enzyme stored in the secretory granules of mast cells and basophils (RBL-2H3 cells) upon their activation (Teshima *et al.*, 1986).
Puerarin/ Isoflavones	*Pueraria lobata* (Willd.) Ohwi/Leguminosae	Puerarin inhibited the PCA reaction to 46 per cent at 50mg/kg, i.p. (Choo *et al.*, 2002).	Inhibition of the release of chemical mediators from mast cells, induced by the antigen-IgE antibody reaction (Ito *et al.*, 1998).
Quercetin/ Flavonoid	*Allium cepa* L./ Alliaceae	Inhibition of IL-5 synthesis was achieved at IC_{50} >18.8 mM by quercetin [5] (Kawai *et al.*, 2007).	The inhibitory activity of flavonoids on IL- 4, IL-13 and CD_{40} ligand expression may be mediated through their inhibition of transcriptional factors such as AP-1 and NFAT (Kawai *et al.*, 2007).
Rabdosiin/ Tetramer of caffeic acid	*Rabdosia japonica* (Burm.f.) Hara/ Labiateae	Inhibition of β-hexosaminidase release in RBL-2H3 cells were observed from Rabdosiin [27] to > 90 per cent at 2mM (Ito *et al.*, 1998).	Inhibition of the release of enzyme stored in the secretory granules of mast cells and basophils (RBL-2H3 cells) upon their activation (Teshima *et al.*, 1986).

Contd...

Table 7.2–*Contd...*

Constituent	*Source*	*Work Done*	*Mechanism of Action*
Rhapontigenin/ Stilbenes	*Rheum undulatum* L./Polygonaceae	Inhibition of histamine release to 89 per cent at 20 mg/ml showed by rhapontigenin [25] (Matsuda *et al.*, 2001).	Inhibition of the release of chemical mediators from mast cells, induced by the antigen-IgE antibody reaction (Ito *et al.*, 1998).
Rosmarinic acid/ Polyphenol	*Perilla frutescens* (L.) Britton/Labiateae	Rosmarinic acid inhibited the PCA reaction to 50 per cent at 19mg/kg, i.p. (Makino *et al.*, 2003).	Inhibition of the release of chemical mediators from mast cells, induced by the antigen-IgE antibody reaction (Ito *et al.*, 1998).
Tylophora alkaloids/ Alkaloids	*Tylophora indica* (Burm.f.) Merill/ Asclepiadaceae	*Tylophora alkaloids* inhibited the mast cell degranulation to 32.90 per cent at 1mg/ml (Geetha *et al.*, 1981).	Ability of extract to inhibit the release of mediators from mast cells and basophils (Lee *et al.*, 2004).
Ent-16-aurene-3β, 15β,18-triol/ Diterpenes	*Suregada multiflora* (A. Juss.) Baill/ Euphorbiaceae	Ent-16-kaurene-3β, 15β, 18-triol inhibited the release of β-hexosaminidase in RBL-2H3 cells at IC_{50} 22.5 μM (Cheenpracha *et al.*, 2006).	Inhibition of the release of enzyme stored in the secretory granules of mast cells and basophils (RBL-2H3 cells) upon their activation (Teshima *et al.*, 1986).
Ent-3-oxo-16-kaurene-15β,18-diol/Diterpenes	*Suregada multiflora* (A. Juss.) Baill/ Euphorbiaceae	Ent-3-oxo-16-kaurene-15β, 18- diol inhibited the release of β-hexosaminidase in RBL-2H3 cells at IC_{50} 22.9 μM (Cheenpracha *et al.*, 2006).	Inhibition of the release of enzyme stored in the secretory granules of mast cells and basophils (RBL-2H3 cells) upon their activation (Teshima *et al.*, 1986).
Ent-16-kaurene-3β, 15β-diol/ Diterpenes	*Suregada multiflora* (A. Juss.) Baill/ Euphorbiaceae	Ent-16-kaurene-3β, 15β-diol inhibited the release of β-hexosaminidase in RBL-2H3 cells at IC_{50} 28.7 μM (Cheenpracha *et al.*, 2006).	Inhibition of the release of enzyme stored in the secretory granules of mast cells and basophils (RBL-2H3 cells) upon their activation (Teshima *et al.*, 1986).
Helioscopinolide A/Diterpenes	*Suregada multiflora* (A. Juss.) Baill/ Euphorbiaceae	Helioscopinolide A inhibited the release of β-hexosaminidase in RBL-2H3 cells at IC_{50} 26.5 μM (Cheenpracha *et al.*, 2006).	Inhibition of the release of enzyme stored in the secretory granules of mast cells and basophils (RBL-2H3 cells) upon their activation (Teshima *et al.*, 1986).
Helioscopinolide I/Diterpenes	*Suregada multiflora* (A. Juss.) Baill/ Euphorbiaceae	Helioscopinolide I inhibited the release of β-hexosaminidase in RBL-2H3 cells at IC_{50} 29.3 μM (Cheenpracha *et al.*, 2006).	Inhibition of the release of enzyme stored in the secretory granules of mast cells and basophils (RBL-2H3 cells) upon their activation (Teshima *et al.*, 1986).

Contd...

Table 7.2–*Contd...*

Constituent	*Source*	*Work Done*	*Mechanism of Action*
Kaempferol/ Flavonoid	*Nelumbo nucifera* Gaertn./ Nymphaeceae	Inhibitory effect of kaempferol [16] on the cell surface expression of FcåRI (KU812F cells) was reduced from 32.5 per cent to 30.6 per cent, 27.8 per cent, 21.0 per cent, and 13.4 per cent when treated with 0, 3.5, 8.8, 17.5, and 35.0 µM, respectively (Shim *et al.,* 2009).	Suppressive effects of kaempferol [16] on intracellular Ca^{2+} concentration and histamine release from anti-FcåRI α-chain antibody-stimulated cells in a concentration-dependent manner (Shim *et al.,* 2009).
Betulinic acid/ Triterpenoid	*Nelumbo nucifera* Gaertn./ Nymphaeceae	Betulinic acid reduced serotonin induced rat paw edema *in vivo* at doses of 50 mg/kg and 100 mg/kg, p.o. (Mukherjee *et al.,* 1997).	Inhibition of serotonin induced edema in the tissues (Mukherjee *et al.,* 1997).
Glucan A and Phosphatidyl-lycorine/Poly-saccharide and alkaloid	*Crinum latifolium* L./Amaryllidaceae	The rate of degranulation of mast cells was inhibited by the different combinations of glucan A and phosphatidyllycorine (5-20 and 5-10 µg/mL, respectively) The combination (10-20 mg/kg), *in vivo,* also provided protection against compound 48/80-induced degranulation of mast cells (Ghosal *et al.,* 1988).	Inhibition of the release of chemical mediators from mast cells, induced by the antigen-IgE antibody reaction (Ito *et al.,* 1998).
Hexahydro-curcumin/ Diarylheptanoid	*Z. officinale*/ Zingiberaceae	The degree of antigen-induced degranulation in RBL-2H3 cells was determined by inhibition of β-hexosaminidase release, *i.e.* dose and time dependent manner (~100 per cent inhibition at 200 µm) (Chen *et al.,* 2009).	Inhibition of the release of enzyme stored in the secretory granules of mast cells and basophils (RBL-2H3 cells) upon their activation (Teshima *et al.,* 1986).
6-dehydrogin-gerdione/Phenol	*Z. officinale*/ Zingiberaceae	The degree of antigen-induced degranulation in RBL-2H3 cells was determined by inhibition of β-hexosaminidase release, *i.e.* 60-70 per cent at 1 µm of 6-dehydrogingerdione [24] (Chen *et al.,* 2009).	Inhibition of the release of enzyme stored in the secretory granules of mast cells and basophils (RBL-2H3 cells) upon their activation (Teshima *et al.,* 1986).
10-gingerol/ Diterpenoid	*Z. officinale*/ Zingiberaceae	The degree of antigen-induced degranulation in RBL-2H3 cells was determined by inhibition of β-hexosaminidase release, *i.e.* 60-70 per cent at 1 µm (Chen *et al.,* 2009).	Inhibition of the release of enzyme stored in the secretory granules of mast cells and basophils (RBL-2H3 cells) upon their activation (Teshima *et al.,* 1986).

Contd...

Table 7.2–*Contd...*

Constituent	*Source*	*Work Done*	*Mechanism of Action*
6-shogaol/ Alkanone	*Z. officinale*/ Zingiberaceae	The degree of antigen-induced degranulation in RBL-2H3 cells was determined by inhibition of β-hexosaminidase release, *i.e.* 60-70 per cent at 1 μm of 6-shogaol [28] (Chen *et al.*, 2009).	Inhibition of the release of enzyme stored in the secretory granules of mast cells and basophils (RBL-2H3 cells) upon their activation (Teshima *et al.*, 1986).
6-gingerol/ Diterpenoid	*Z. officinale*/ *Zingiberaceae*	The degree of antigen-induced degranulation in RBL-2H3 cells was determined by inhibition of β-hexosaminidase release, *i.e.* 60-70 per cent at 1 μm (Chen *et al.*, 2009).	Inhibition of the release of enzyme stored in the secretory granules of mast cells and basophils (RBL-2H3 cells) upon their activation (Teshima *et al.*, 1986).

Figure 6.3: Some anti-allergic phytoconstituents found in plants.

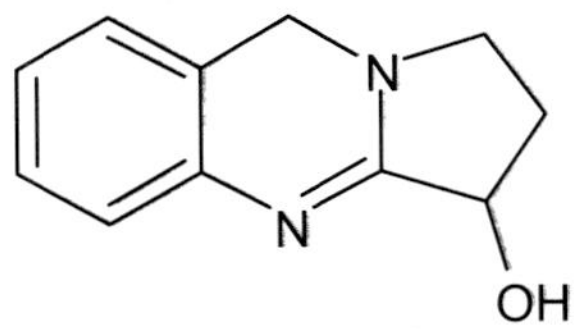

Vasicine [1]

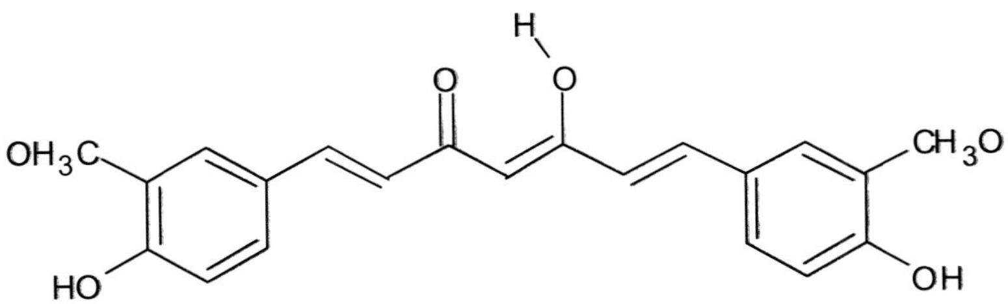

Curcumin [2]

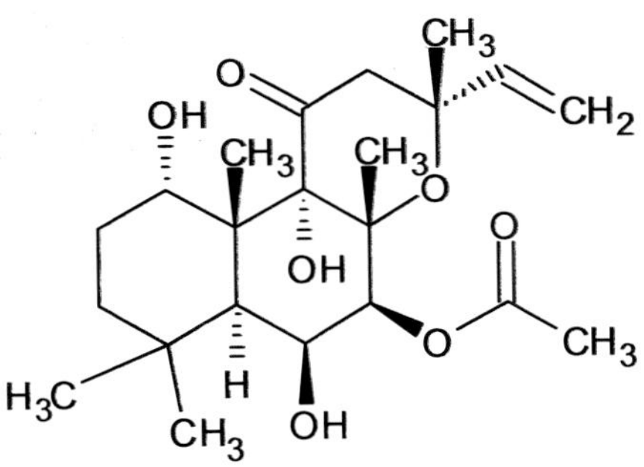

Forskolin [3]

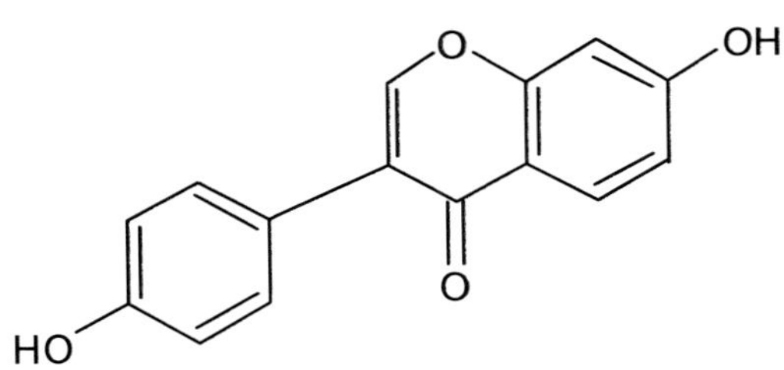

Daidzein [4]

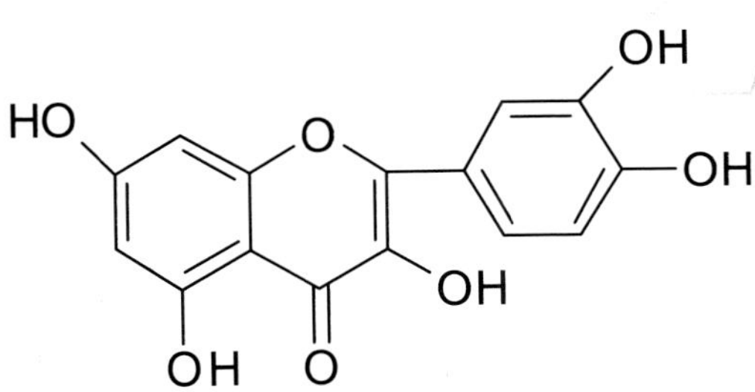

Quercetin [5]

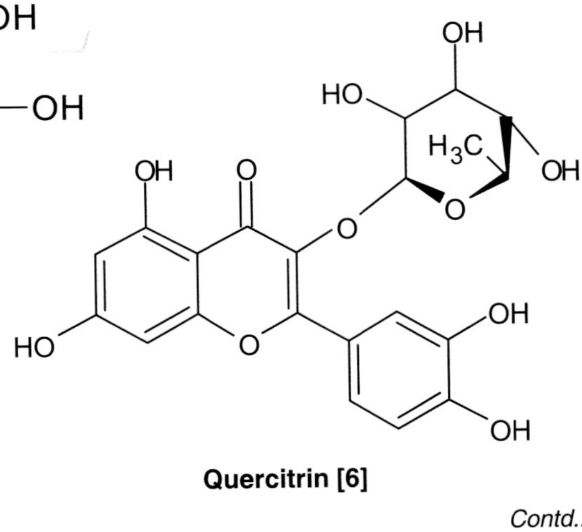

Quercitrin [6]

Contd...

Figure 6.3–*Contd...*

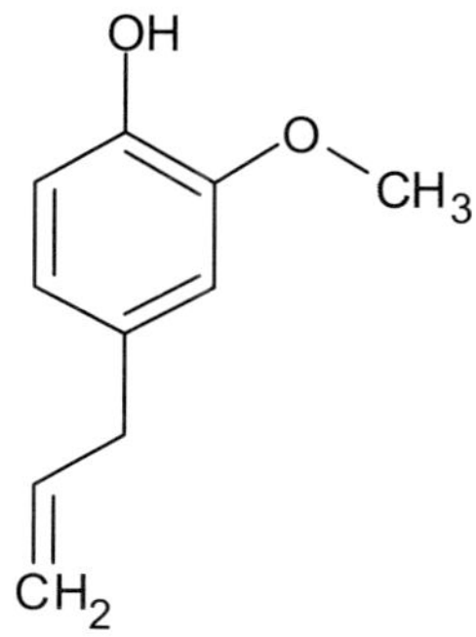

Eugenol [7]

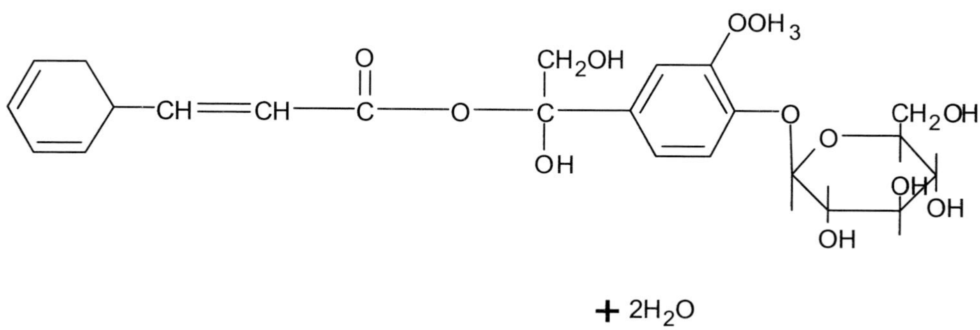

Kutkin [8]

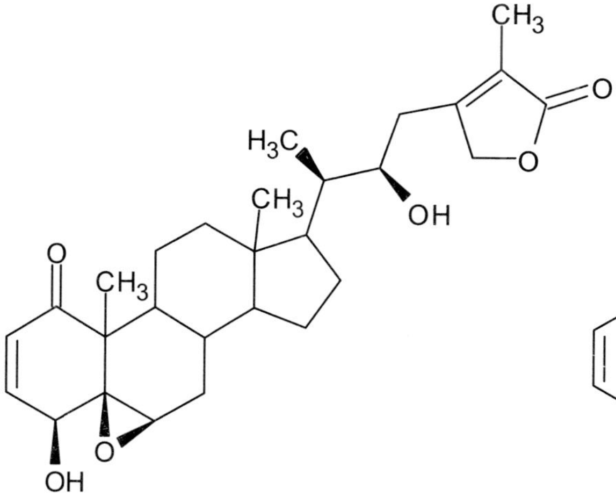

Withaferin A [9]

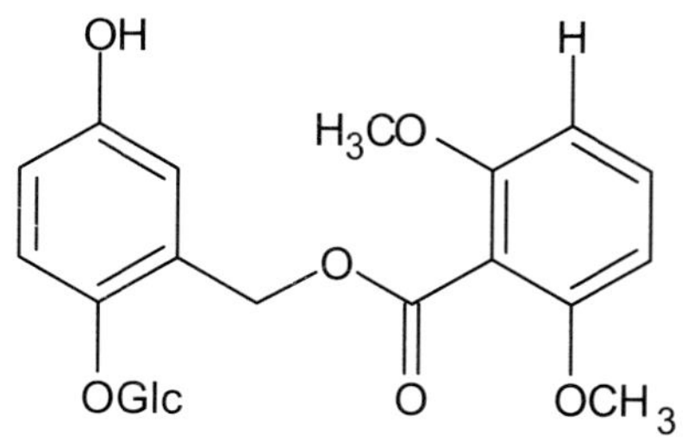

Curculigoside A [10]

Contd...

Figure 6.3–*Contd...*

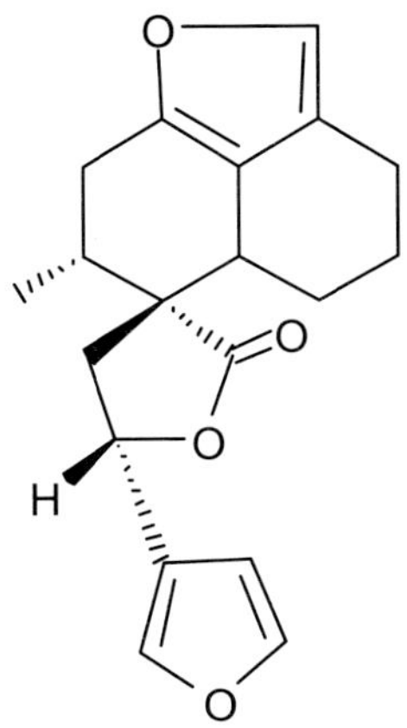

Montanin [11]

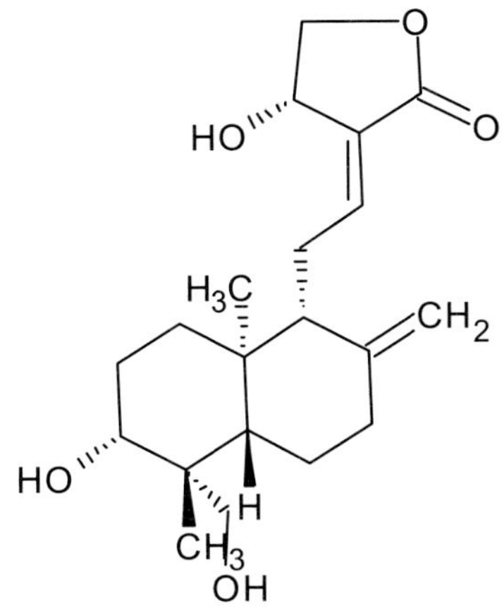

Andrographolide [12]

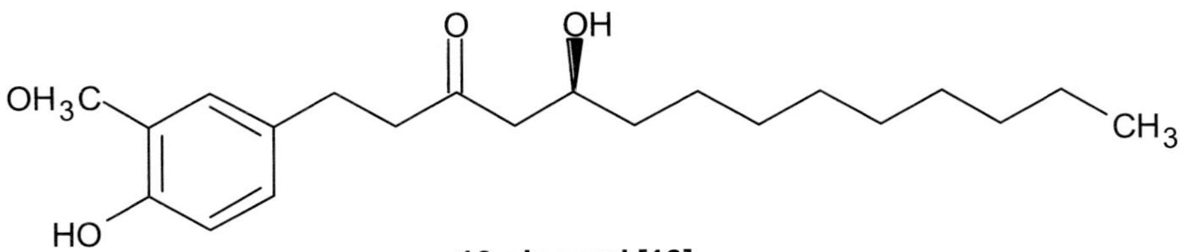

10-gingerol [13]

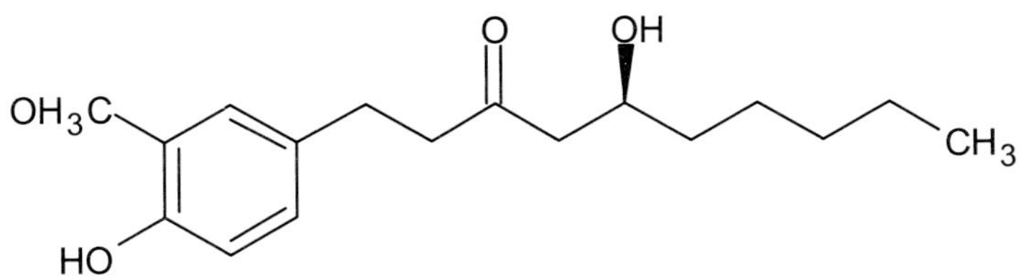

6-gingerol [14]

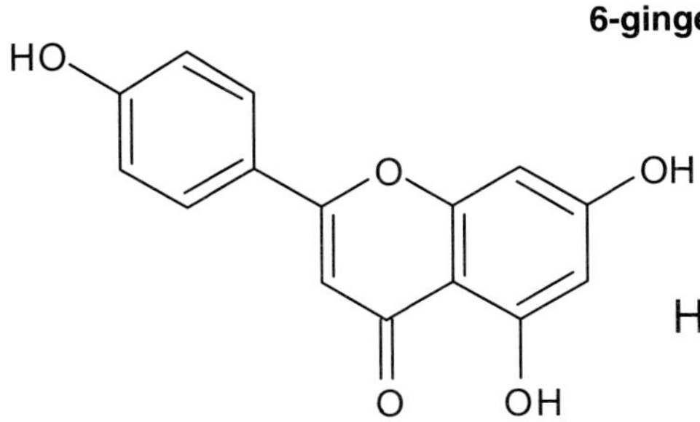

Apigenin [15]

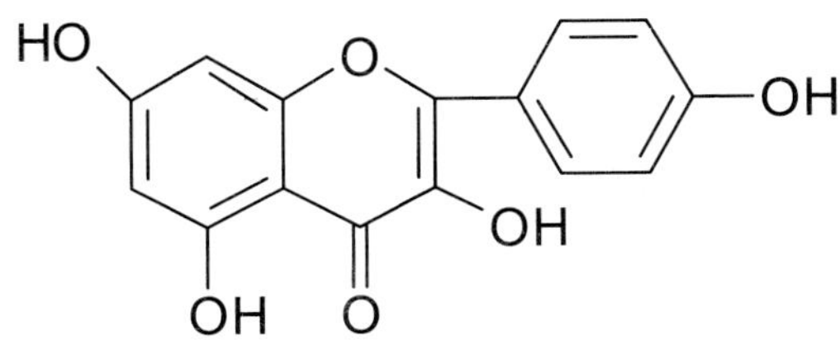

Kaempferol [16]

Contd...

Figure 6.3–*Contd...*

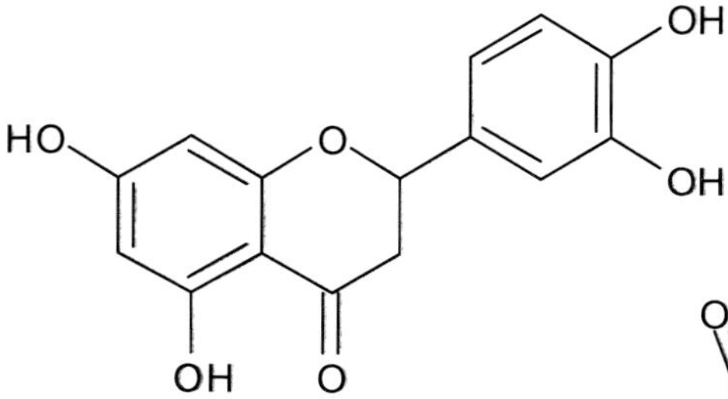

Luteolin [17]

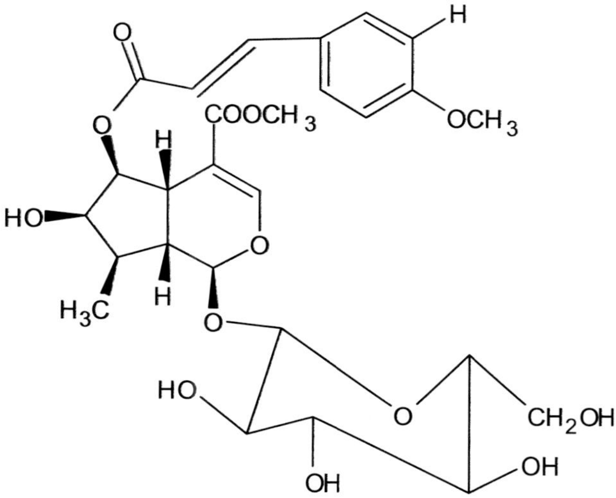

Arbortristoside-A [18]

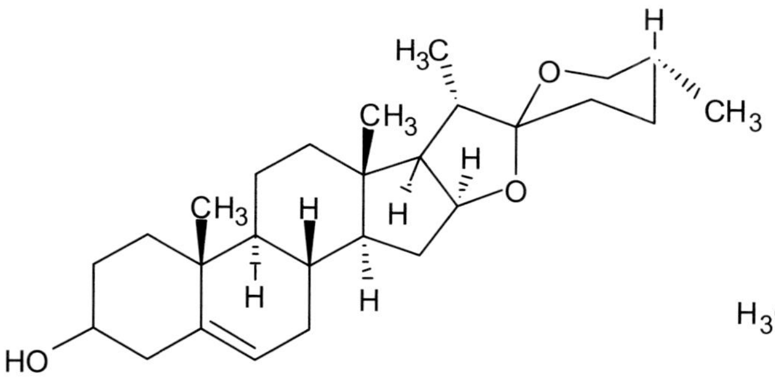

Diosgenin [19]

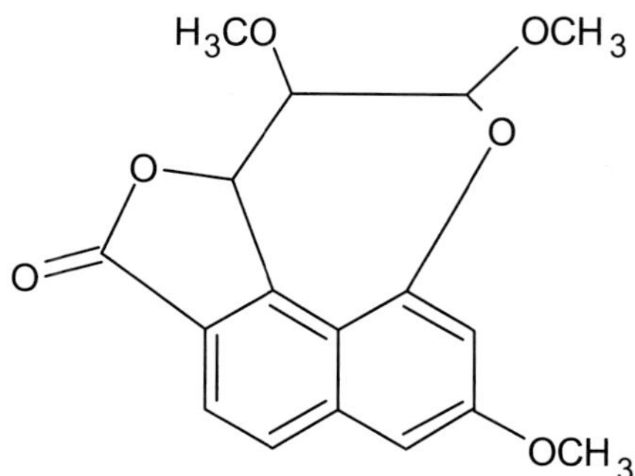

Dioscorealide A [20]

Contd...

Figure 6.3–*Contd...*

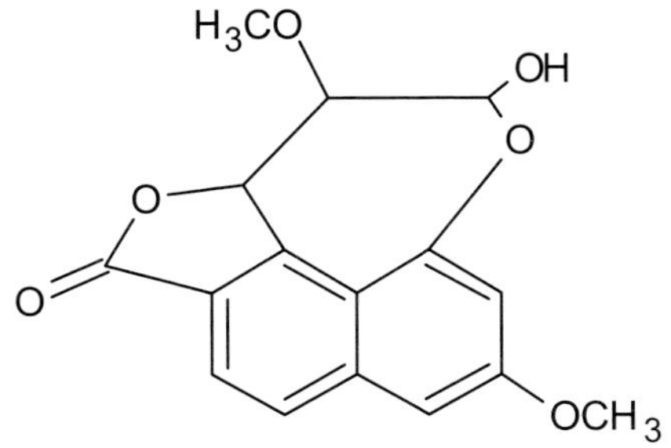

Dioscorealide B [21]

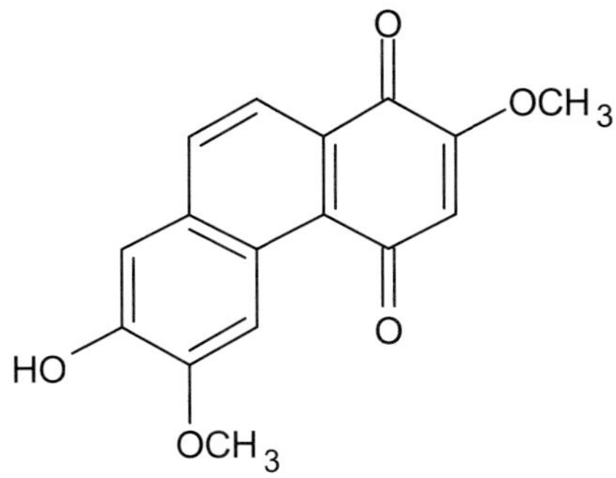

Dioscoreanone [22]

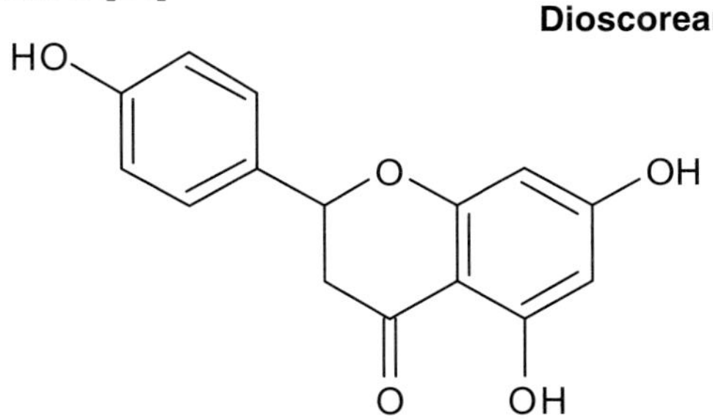

Naringenin [23]

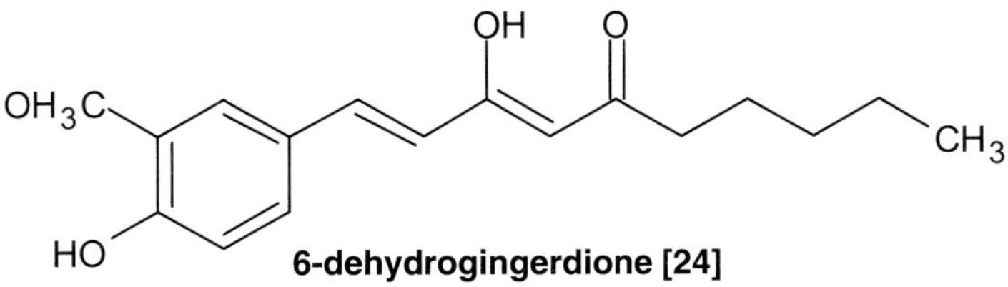

6-dehydrogingerdione [24]

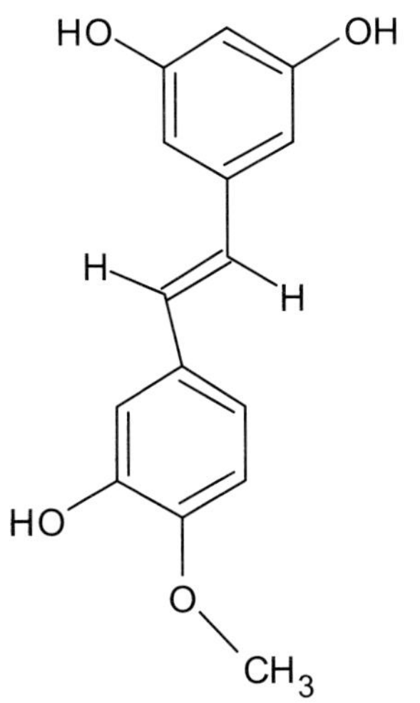

Rhapontigenin [25]

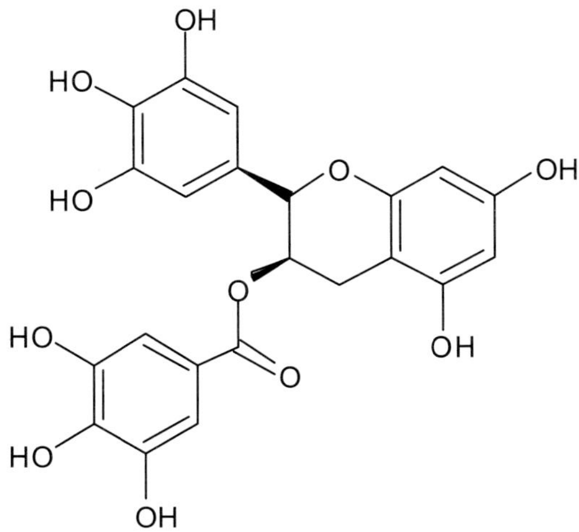

Epigallocatechin-3-O-gallate [26]

Contd...

Figure 6.3–*Contd...*

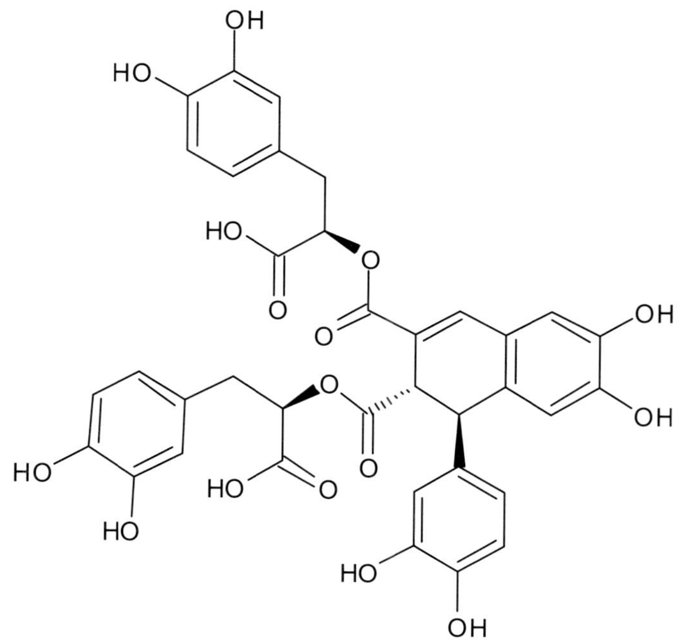

Rabdosiin [27]

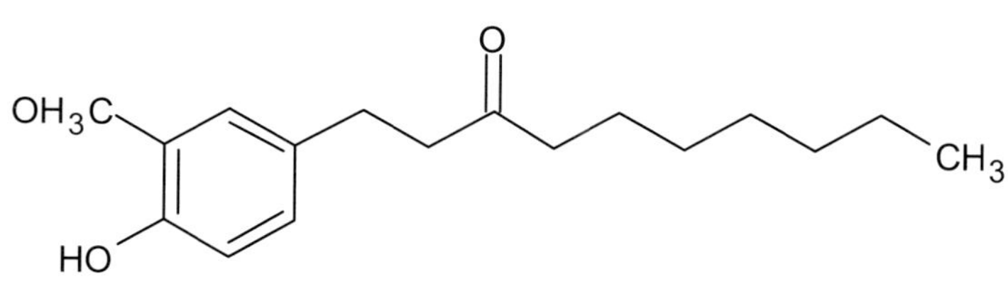

6-shogaol [28]

Concluding Remarks

Several plant species including *A. vasica*, *A. lebbeck*, *C. serratum*, *C. longa*, *E. hirta*, *O. sanctum*, *P. kurroa* and *W. somnifera* have been proven and scientifically well established as lead target for different allergic diseases. *C. herba*, *C. aromaticus*, *C. forskohlii*, *C. mangga*, *C. zedoaria*, *K. galanga*, *K. parviflora* *N. arbortristis*, *P. zeylanica*, *Tylophora indica* (Burm.f.) Merill., *Z. cassumunar*, *Z. officinale* and many other plants (Table 6.1) have been proven for their antiallergic activities. Several phytoconstituents like flavonoids (quercetin [5], luteolin [17], kaempferol [16], apigenin [15]), glycosides (arbortristoside A [18], arbortristoside C, diosgenin [19]), diterpenes (andrographolide [12], neo-andrographolide, coleonol, derivatives of ent-16-kaurene, helioscopinolide, gingerol) saponins (albizia saponin, clerodendron saponin), Sesquiterpenes (bisdemethoxy curcumin, Curcumin[2]) and alkaloids (vasicine [1], Tylophora alkaloids, phosphatidyllycorine) and other phytoconstituents (Table 6.2) have been proved for their potent anti-allergic action. Nair *et al.* (2006) showed that a possible mechanism of quercetin [5] mediated suppression of TNF-α gene and protein expression is mediated by down-regulating gene expression for NF-kβ1 and their findings suggest that the cytokine TNF-α can be inhibited by quercetin [5], which may be of clinical significance in host defense mechanisms against various infections. A decrease in endogenous TNF-α production by quercetin [5] indicates that flavonoids have immunomodulatory response, anti-inflammatory activity and the suppressive effect of epigallocatechin-3-O-gallate [26] against transcriptional up-regulation of the histamine H1 receptor and IL-4 genes were determined (Matsushita *et al.*, 2008).

Although it is a known fact that *in vitro* experiments of a hierarchy of the inhibitory action of flavonoids, it does not simply imply that an increase in the intake of flavonoids with higher activity can be recommended, since glycosylation of flavonoids commonly increases the absorption from the small intestine but lessens their inhibitory activity on IL-4 synthesis (Manach *et al.*, 2004). Therefore, progress in research regarding the bioavailability of flavonoids will be essential for establishment of dietary management for allergic or other diseases (Williamson *et al.*, 2005). Integrated multi-disciplinary research on indigenous medicinal plants from different countries has been made by public and private sponsorships under several schemes. However, in spite of all these efforts, very few drugs of plant origin could reach Stage 1 of clinical trial or could gain confidence for clinical use by the practitioners of modern medicine (Mukherjee *et al.*, 2007a). There are several constrains in the use of herbal medicinal products for their quality and consistency, which includes: (*i*) herbs of different origin are often known by the same popular name, (*ii*) plants growing in different climatic soil and seasonal conditions do not have identical chemical constituents or therapeutic effect, (*iii*) process of collection (fresh, shade or sun dried), extraction, processing and storage of herbal medicines cause variation in potency and safety, (*iv*) no specific standards for herbal medicines have been prescribed and (*v*) non-availability of these herbal medicines in suitable dosage form and others create difficulty in administration. These shortcomings have delayed the integration of some of the well recognized traditional recipes in the modern system of medicine (Mukherjee *et al.*, 2009; Gupta, 1994). So for development of herbal drugs these aspects need to be considered for production of uniform amount of the bioactive secondary metabolites.

The well-documented evidence published to date on a beneficial effect involving the inhibitory action of natural compounds on mast cells has focused on the naturally occurring phytoconstituents. The potential candidates from plant origin that have undergone *in vitro* and *in vivo* studies have revealed the discovery of target. This need to be explored further through various phases of clinical trial, which will lead to the invention of potent anti-allergic molecule from natural resources for effective treatment of various forms of allergy.

Acknowledgments

The authors wish to express their gratitude to the All India Council for Technical Education, New Delhi Govt. of India for financial support through AICTE –MODROBS project grant (F. No – 8024/RID/BOR/MOD-74./2008-09).

References

Akah, P.A., Ezike, A.C., Nwafor, S.V., Okoli, C.O., Enwerem, N.M. (2003). Evaluation of the anti-asthmatic property of *Asystasia gangetica* leaf extracts. *Journal of Ethnopharmacology*, **89**: 25-36.

Amara, S., Kumar, S.P., Athota, R.R. (1999). Suppressive effect of *Withania somnifera* root extract on the induction of anti-ovalbumin IgE antibody response in mice. *Pharmaceutical Biology*, **37**: 253-259.

Amresh, G., Reddy, G.D., Rao, Ch. V., Singh, P.N. (2007). Evaluation of anti-inflammatory activity of *Cissampelos pareira* root in rats. *Journal of Ethnopharmacology*, **110**: 526-531.

Anonymous. (2001). The Ayurvedic Pharmacopoeia of India, Part I, Vol I, First edition, Ministry of Health and Family Welfare, India, p 45.

Atal, C.K. (1980). Chemistry and pharmacology of Vasicine- A new oxytocic and abortifacient. Regional Research Laboratory, Jammu-Tawi, p 58.

Bafna, A.R., Mishra, S.H. (2006). Immunostimulatory effect of methanol extract of *Curculigo orchioides* on immunosuppressed mice. *Journal of Ethnopharmacology*, **104**: 1-4.

Baruah, C.C., Gupta, P.P., Amarnath Late, G.K., Patnaik, Dhawan, B.N. (1998). Anti-allergic and anti-anaphylactic activity of picroliv-a standardized iridoid glycoside fraction of *Picrorhiza kurroa*. *Pharmacological Research*, **38**: 487-492.

Bharti, A.C., Donato, N., Singh, S., Aggarwal, B.B. (2003). Curcumin (diferuloylmethane) down-regulates the constitutive activation of nuclear factor-kB and IkBa kinase in human multiple myeloma cells, leading to suppression of proliferation and induction of apoptosis. *Blood*, **101**: 1053-1062.

Bousquet, J., Van Cauwenberge, P., Khaltaev, N. (2001). Allergic rhinitis and its impact on asthma. *Journal of Allergy and Clinical Immunology*, **108**: S147-334.

Bremner, P., Heinrich, M. (2005). Natural products and their role as inhibitors of the pro-inflammatory transcription factor NF-κB. *Phytochemistry Reviews*, **4**: 27-37.

Brito, F.A., Lima, L.A., Ramos, M.F., Nakamura, M.J., Cavalher-Machado, S.C., Siani, A.C., Henriques, M.G., Sampaio, A.L. (2007). Pharmacological study of anti-allergic activity of *Syzygium cumini* (L.) skeels. Braz*ilian Journal of Medical and Biological Research*, **40**: 105-115.

Cheenpracha, S., Yodsaoue, O., Karalai, C., Ponglimanont, C., Subhadhirasakul, S., Tewtrakul, S., Kanjana-opas, A. (2006). Potential anti-allergic ent-kaurene diterpenes from the bark of *Suregada multiflora*. *Phytochemistry*, **67**: 2630-2634.

Chen, B.H., Wu, P.Y., Chen, K.M., Fu, T.F., Wang, H.M., Chen, C.Y. (2009). Antiallergic potential on RBL-2H3 cells of some phenolic constituents of *Zingiber officinale* (Ginger). *Journal of Natural Products*, **72**: 950–953.

Choo, M.K., Park, E.K., Yoon, H.K., Kim, D.H. (2002). Antithrombotic and antiallergic activities of Daidzein, a metabolite of Puerarin and Daidzin produced by human intestinal microflora. *Biological and Pharmaceutical Bulletin*, **25**: 1328-1332.

Choudhary, G.P., Chaturvedi, S.C., Bharti, S. (2007). Mast cell stabilizing activity of *Glycyrrhiza glabra* Linn. *The Science Journal of the American Association for Respiratory Care.* Past open forum abstracts.

Dai, Y., Hou, L.F., Chan, Y.P., Cheng, L., But, P.P. (2004). Inhibition of immediate allergic reactions by ethanol extract from *Plumbago zeylanica* stems. *Biological and Pharmaceutical Bulletin,* **27**: 429-432.

Das, A.K., Yoshimura, S., Mishima, R., Fujimoto, K., Mizuguchi, H., Dev, S., Wakayama, Y., Kitamura, Y., Horio, S., Takeda, N., Fukui, H. (2007). Stimulation of histamine H1 receptor up-regulates histamine H1 receptor itself through activation of receptor gene transcription. *Journal of Pharmacological Science,* **103**: 374-382.

Dev, S., Mizuguchi, H., Das, A.K., Matsushita, C., Maeyama, K., Umehara, H., Ohtoshi, T., Kojima, J., Nishida, K., Takahashi, K., Fukui, H. (2008). Suppression of histamine signaling by probiotic Lac-B: a possible mechanism of its anti-allergic effect. *Journal of Pharmacological Science,* **107**: 159-166.

Eccleston, E., Leonard, B.J., Lowe, J.S., Welford, H.J. (1973). Basophilic leukaemia in the *albino rat* and demonstration of the basopoietin. *Nature New Biology,* **244**: 73-76.

Farnlof, A., 1998. *Naturlakemedel och Naturmedel. Halsokos tradets Forlag, Stockholm;* **109**: p. 132.

Fu, D.X., Lei, G.Q., Chen, X.W., Chen, J.K., Zhou. (2004). Curculigoside C, a new phenolic glucoside from rhizomes of *Curculigo orchioides. Acta Botanica Sinica* **46**: 621-624.

Galvez, J., Zarzuelo, A., Crespo, M. E., Lorente, M. D., Ocete, M. A., Jiménez, J. (1993). Antidiarrhoeic activity of *Euphorbia hirta* extract and isolation of an active flavonoid constituent. *Planta Medica* **59**: 333-336.

Ganguly, T., Badheka, L.P., Sainis, K.B. (2001). Immunomodulatory effect of *Tylophora indica* on Con A induced lymphoproliferation. *Phytomedicine* **8**: 431-437.

Geetha, V.S., Viswanathan, S., Kameswaran, L. (1981). Comparison of total alkaloids of *Tylophora indica* and disodium chromoglycate on mast cell stabilization. *Indian Journal of Pharmacology* **13**: 199-201.

Ghosal, S., Shanthy, A., Das, P.K., Mukhopadhyay, M., Sarkar, M.K. (1988). Mast cell stabilizing effect of glucan A and phosphatidyllycorine isolated from *Crinum latifolium. Phytotherapy Research* **2**: 76-79.

Gopumadhavan, S., Rafiq, M., Venkataranganna, M.V., Mitra, S.K. (2005). Antihistaminic and antianaphylactic activity of HK-07, a herbal formulation. *Indian Journal of Pharmacology* **37**: 300-303.

Gupta, A.K. (2003). Quality Standards of Indian Medicinal Plants. In: Neeraj Tandon, Madhu Sharma. Indian Council of Medical Research, New Delhi, Vol 1, p 1.

Gupta, P.P., Srimal, R.C., Neeraj Verma, Tandon, J.S. (1994). Passive cutaneous anaphylactic inhibitory and mast cell stabilizing activity of coleonol and its derivative. *Indian Journal of Pharmacology,* **26**: 150-152.

Gupta, P.P., Srimal, R.C., Srivastava, M., Singh, K.L., Tandon, J.S. (1995). Antiallergic activity of Arbortristosides from *Nyctanthes arbortristis*. *Pharmaceutical Biology*, **33**: 70-72.

Gupta, P.P., Srimal, R.C., Tandon, J.S. (1993). Antiallergic activity of some traditional Indian medicinal plants. *International Journal of Pharmacognosy*, **31**: 15-18.

Gupta, P.P., Tandon, J.S., Patnaik, G.K. (1998). Antiallergic activity of andrographolides isolated from *Andrographis paniculata* (Burm. F) Wall. *Pharmaceutical Biology*, **36**: 72-74.

Gupta, S.S. (1968). Development of antihistamine and anti-allergic activity after prolonged administration of a plant saponin from *Clerodendron serratum*. *Journal of Pharmacy and Pharmacology*, **20**: 801-802.

Gupta, S.S. (1994). Prospects and perspectives of natural plants products in medicine. *Indian Journal of Pharmacology*, **26**: 1-12.

Gupta, S.S., Bhagwat, A.W., Modh, P.R. (1971). Effect of *Clerodendron serratum* saponin on the mast cells of rat mesentery. *Indian Journal of Medical Sciences*, **25**: 29-31.

Hemmerich, S., Pecht, I. (1988). Isolation and purification of an Fåe receptor activated ion channel from the rat mast cell line RBL-2H3. *Biochemistry*, **27**: 7488-7498.

Huq, M.E., Ikram, M., Warsi, S.A. (1967). Chemical composition of *Adhatoda vasica* Linn. II. *Pakistan Journal of Scientific and Industrial Research*, **10**: 224-225.

Ikawati, Z., Wahyuono, S., Maeyama, K. (2001). Screening of several Indonesian medicinal plants for their inhibitory effect on histamine release from RBL-2H3 cells. *Journal of Ethnopharmacology*, **75**: 249-256.

Ito, H., Miyazaki, T., Ono, M., Sakurai, H. (1998). Antiallergic activities of Rabdosiin and its related compounds: Chemical and Biochemical evaluations. *Bioorganic and Medicinal Chemistry*, **6**: 1051-1056.

Iyengar, M.A., Jambaiah, K.M., Kamath, M.S., Rao, G.O. **1994**. Studies on an antiasthma Kada: a proprietary herbal combination, Part I. Clinical study. *Indian Drugs*, **31**: 183-186.

Jain J.B., Kumane, S.C., Bhattacharya. (2006). Medicinal flora of Madhya Pradesh and Chhattisgarh – a Review. *Indian Journal of Traditional Knowledge*, **5**: 237-242.

Kanoh, R., Hatano, T., Ito, H., Yoshida, T., Akagi, M. (2000). Effects of tannins and related polyphenols on superoxide-induced histamine release from rat peritoneal mast cells. *Phytomedicine*, **7**: 297-302.

Kawai, M., Hirano, T., Higa, S., Arimitsu, J., Maruta, M., Kuwahara, Y., Ohkawara, T., Hagihara, K., Yamadori, T., Shima, Y., Ogata, A., Kawase, I., Tanaka, T. (2007). Flavonoids and related compounds as anti-allergic substances. *Allergology International*, **56**: 113-123.

Kim, C.D., Lee, W.K., Lee, M.H., Cho, H.S., Lee, Y.K., Roh, S.S. (2004). Inhibition of mast cell-dependent allergy reaction by extract of black cohosh (*Cimicifuga racemosa*). *Immunopharmacology and Immunotoxicology*, **26**: 299-308.

Kim, H.M., Lee, E.H., Kim, C.Y., Chung, J.G., Kim, S.H., Lim, J.P., Shin, T.Y. (1997). Antianaphylactic properties of Eugenol. *Pharmacological Research*, **36**: 475-480.

Kirtikar K.R., Basu B.D. (1999). Indian Medicinal Plants. 2nd ed. Vol.III Dehradun. International Book Distributors.

Kiuchi, F., Iwakami, S., Shibuya, M., Hanaoka, F., Sankawa, U. (1992). Inhibition of prostaglandin and leukotriene biosynthesis by gingerols and diarylheptanoids. *Chemical and Pharmaceutical Bulletin*, **40**: 387-391.

Kreutner, W., Chapman, R.W., Gulbenkian, A., Tozzi, S. (1985). Bronchodilator and antiallergic activity of forskolin. *European Journal of Pharmacology*, **111**: 1-8.

Kumar, A., Elango, K., Markanday, S., Undhad, C.V., Kotadiya, A.V., Savaliya, B.M., Vyas, D.N., Datta, D. (2007). Mast cell stabilization property of *Coleus aromaticus* leaf extract in rat peritoneal mast cells. *Indian Journal of Pharmacology*, **39**: 119-120.

Kumar, D.A., Ramu, P. (2002). Effect of methanolic extract of *Benincasa hispida* against histamine and acetylcholine induced bronchospasm in guinea pigs. *Indian Journal of Pharmacology*, **34**: 365-366.

Lee, J.H., Ko, N.Y., Kim, N.W., Mun, S.H., Kim, J.W., Her, E., Kim, B.K., Seo, D.W., Chang, H.W., Moon, T.C., Han, J.W., Kim, Y.M., Choi, W.S. (2007). *Meliae cortex* extract exhibits anti-allergic activity through the inhibition of Syk kinase in mast cells. *Toxicology and Applied Pharmacology*, **220**: 227-234.

Lee, J.H., Seo, J.Y., Ko, N.Y., Chang, S.H., Her, E., Park, T., Lee, H.Y., Han, J.W., Kim, Y.M., Choi, W.S. (2004). Inhibitory activity of *Chrysanthemi sibirici herba* extract on RBL-2H3 mast cells and compound 48/80-induced anaphylaxis. *Journal of Ethnopharmacology*, **95**: 425-430.

Li, N., Zhao, Y.X., Jia, A.Q., Liu, Y.Q., Zhou. (2003). Study on the chemical constituents of *Curculigo orchioides*. *Natural Product Research and Development*, **15**: 208-211.

Lichey, I., Friedrich, T., Priesnitz, M., Biamino, G., Usinger, P., Huckauf, H. (1984). Effect of forskolin on methacholine-induced bronchoconstriction in extrinsic asthmatics. *Lancet*, **2**: 167.

Makino, T., Furuta, Y., Wakushima, H., Fujii, H., Saito, K., Kano, Y. (2003). Anti-allergic effect of *Perilla frutescens* and its active constituents. *Phytotherapy research*, **17**: 240-243.

Manach, C., Scalbert, A., Morand, C., Remesy, C., Jimenez, L. (2004). Polyphenols: food sources and bioavailability. *Americal Journal of Clinical Nutrition*, **79**: 727-747.

Marone G, Columbo M, Triggiani M, Vigorita S, Formisano S. (1986). Forskolin inhibits the release of histamine from human basophils and mast cells. Agents Actions, **18**: 96-99.

Matsuda, H., Morikawa, T., Xie, H., Yoshikawa, M. (2004a). Antiallergic phenanthrenes and stilbenes from the tubers of *Gymnadenia conopsea*. *Planta Medica*, **70**: 847-855.

Matsuda, H., Sugimoto, S., Morikawa, T., Matsuhira, K., Mizuguchi, E., Nakamura, S., Yoshikawa, M. (2007). Bioactive constituents from Chinese natural medicines XX. Inhibitors of antigen-induced degranulation in RBL-2H3 cells from the seeds of *Psoralea corylifolia*. *Chemical and Pharmaceutical Bulletin,* **55**: 106-110.

Matsuda, H., Tewtrakul, S., Morikawa, T., Nakamura, A., Yoshikawa, M. (2004b). Anti-allergic principles from Thai zedoary: structural requirements of curcuminoids for inhibition of degranulation and effect on the release of TNF-a and IL-4 in RBL-2H3 cells. *Bioorganic and Medicinal Chemistry,* **12**: 5891-5898.

Matsuda, H., Tomohiro, N., Hiraba, K., Harima, S., Ko, S., Matsuo, K., Yoshikawa, M., Kubo, M. (2001). Study on anti-oketsu activity of Rhubarb II. Anti-allergic effects of stilbene components from Rhei undulati Rhizoma (dried rhizome of *Rheum undulatum* cultivated in Korea). *Biological and Pharmaceutical Bulletin,* **24**: 264-267.

Matsushita, C., Mizuguchi, H., Nino, H., Sagesaka, Y., Fukui, H. (2008). Identification of epigallocatechin-3-O-gallate as an active constituent in tea extract that suppresses transcriptional up-regulation of the histamine H1 receptor and interleukin-4 genes. *Journal of Traditional Medicine,* **25**: 133-142.

Mediratta, P.K., Sharma, K.K., Surender Singh. (2002). Evaluation of immunomodulatory potential of *Ocimum sanctum* seed oil and its possible mechanism of action. *Journal of Ethnopharmacology,* **80**: 15-20.

Mhaskar, K.S., Blatter, E., Caius, J.F. (2000). In: Kiritikar, Basu, editors. Illustrated Indian medicinal plants, Vol 9. New Delhi: Satguru Publications, p 3031.

Middleton E Jr, Anne, S. (1995). Quercetin inhibits lipopolysaccharide-induced expression of endothelial cell intracellular adhesion molecule-1. *International Archives of Allergy and Immunology,* **107**: 435-436.

Miyoshi, K., Das, A.K., Fujimoto, K., Horio, S., Fukui, H. (2006). Recent Advances in molecular pharmacology of the histamine systems: Regulation of histamine H1 receptor signaling by changing its expression level. *Journal of Pharmacological Science,* **101**: 3-6.

Mueller, A., Antus, S., Bittinger, M., Kaas, A., Kreher, B., Neszmelyi, A., Stuppner, H., Wagner, H. (1993). Chemistry and pharmacology of antiasthmatic *Galphimia glauca*, *Adhatoda vasica*, and *Picrorhiza kurrooa*. *Planta Medica,* **59**: 586-587.

Mukherjee, P.K., Sahoo A.K., Narayanan, N., Kumar, N.S., Ponnusankar, S. (2009). Lead finding from medicinal plants with hepatoprotective potentials. *Expert Opinion on Drug Discovery,* **4**: 545-576.

Mukherjee, P.K. (2001). Evaluation of Indian traditional medicine. *Drug Information Journal,* **35**: 623-632.

Mukherjee, P.K., Kumar, V., Mal, M., Houghton, P.J. (2007a). Acetylcholinesterase inhibitors from plants. *Phytomedicine,* **14**: 289-300.

Mukherjee, P.K., Maiti, K., Mukherjee, K., Houghton, P.J. (2006). Leads from Indian medicinal plants with hypoglycemic potentials. *Journal of Ethnopharmacology,* **106**: 1-28.

Mukherjee, P.K., Rai, S., Kumar, V., Mukherjee, K., Hylands, P.J., Hider, R.C. (2007b). Plants of Indian origin in drug discovery. *Expert Opinion on Drug Discovery*, **2**: 633-657.

Mukherjee, P.K., Saha, K., Das, J., Pal, M., Saha, B.P. (1997). Studies on the anti-inflammatory activity of rhizomes of *Nelumbo nucifera*. *Planta Medica*, **63**: 367-369.

Mukherjee, P.K., Tamang, J.P. (2009). Indigenous knowledge of the ethnic people of North East India in bio-resources management. *Indian Journal of Traditional Knowledge*, **8**: 5-7.

Mukherjee, P.K., Wahile, A. (2006). Integrated approaches towards drug development from ayurveda and other Indian system of medicines. *Journal of Ethanopharmacology*, **103**: 25–35.

Muthu, C., Ayyanar, M., Raja, N., Ignacimuthu, S. (2006). Medicinal plants used by traditional healers in Kancheepuram district of Tamil Nadu, India. *Journal of Ethnobiology and Ethnomedicine*, **2**: 43-52.

Nair, M.P., Mahajan, S., Reynolds, J.L., Aalinkeel, R., Nair, H., Schwartz, S.A., Kandaswami, C. (2006). The flavonoid quercetin inhibits proinflammatory cytokine (Tumor Necrosis Factor Alpha) gene expression in normal peripheral blood mononuclear cells via modulation of the NF-kb system. *Clinical and Vaccine Immunology*, **13**: 319-328.

Nosál'ová, G., Mokrý, J., Hassan, K.M. (2003). Antitussive activity of the fruit extract of *Emblica officinalis* Gaertn. (Euphorbiaceae). *Phytomedicine*, **10**: 583-589.

Ozaki,Y., Kawahara, N., Harada, M. (1991). Anti-inflammatory effect of *Zingiber cassumunar* Roxb. and its active principles. *Chemical and Pharmaceutical Bulletin*, **39**: 2353-2356.

Palanichamy, S., Amala bhaskar, E., Nagarajan, S. (1991). Effect of *Cassia alata* leaf extract on mast cell stabilization. *Indian Journal of Pharmacology*, **23**: 189-191.

Palit, G., Singh, S.P., Singh, N., Kohli, R.P., Bhargava, K.P. (1983). An experimental evaluation of anti-asthmatic plant drugs from ancient Ayurvedic medicine. *Aspects of Allergy and Applied Immunology*, **16**: 36-41.

Pandey, B.L., Das, P.K., Gambhir, S.S. (1989). Immunopharmacological studies on *Picrorhiza kurroa* Royle ex Benth. Part VI: Effect on anaphylactic activation events in rat peritoneal mast cells. *Indian Journal of Physiology and Pharmacology*, **33**: 47-52.

Pandit, P., Singh, A., Bafna, A., Kadam, P., Patil, M. (2008). Evaluation of antiasthmatic activity of *Curculigo orchioides* Gaertn. Rhizomes. *Indian Journal of Pharmaceutical Sciences*, **70**: 440-444.

Prajapati. (2004). A Hand Book of Medicinal Plants, A Complete Source Book. In: Purohit, Sharma, Kumar. Agrobios, India, Section II, p 367.

Pramanick S, Roy A, Ghosh S, Majumder HK, Mukhopadhyay S. (2008). Withanolide Z, a new chlorinated withanolide from *Withania somnifera*. *Planta Medica*, **74**: 1745-1748.

Pratibha, N., Saxena, V.S., Amit, A., D'Souza, P., Bagchi, M., Bagchi, D. (2004). Anti-inflammatory activities of Aller-7, a novel polyherbal formulation for allergic rhinitis. *International Journal on Tissue Reaction,* **26**: 43-51.

Ravi Shankar, K., Ganga Rao, B. (2008). Anti-arthritic activity of *Gymnema sylvestre* root extract. *Biosciences Biotechnology Research Asia,* **5**: 469-471.

Rote Liste. (1977). Bundesverband der Pharmazeutischen Industrie e.V., Frankfurt a.M.

Sen, P., 1993. Therapeutic potentials of Tulsi: from experience to facts. *Drugs News and Views* **1**: 15-21.

Samiulla, D.S., Prashanth, D., Amit, A. (2001). Mast cell stabilising activity of *Bacopa monnieri. Fitoterapia,* **72**: 284-285.

Sharma, P.C. (2000). Database on medicinal plants used in Ayurveda. In: Yelne M.B., Dennis D.J. Central Council for Research in Ayurveda and Siddha, Vol1, p 445.

Shete, A.B. (1993). Femiforte, indigenous herbomineral formulation in the management of non-specific leucorrhoea. *Doctor's News* **2**: 13-14.

Shibata S., Murakami T., Nishikawa Y. (1959). *Yakugaku Zasshi,* **79**: 757-761.

Shim, Sun-Yup, Jae-Sue Choi, Dae-Seok Byun. (2009). Kaempferol isolated from *Nelumbo nucifera* stamens negatively regulates FcåRI expression in human basophilic KU812F cells. *Journal of Microbiology and Biotechnology,* **19**: 155-160.

Shin, T.Y. (2003). Inhibition of immunologic and nonimmunologic stimulation-mediated anaphylactic reactions by the aqueous extract of *Mentha arvensis. Immunopharmacology and Immunotoxicology,* **25,** 273-283.

Shin, T.Y., Kim, S.H., Suk, K., Ha, J.H., Kim, I., Lee, M.G., Jun, C.D., Kim, S.Y., Lim, J.P., Eun, J.S., Shin, H.Y., Kim, H.M. (2005). Anti-allergic effects of *Lycopus lucidus* on mast cell-mediated allergy model. *Toxicology and Applied Pharmacology,* **209**: 255-262.

Shin, T.Y., Kim, Y.K., Kim, H.M. (2001). Inhibition of immediate-type allergic reactions by *Prunella vulgaris* in a murine model. *Immunopharmacology and Immunotoxicology,* **23**: 423-435.

Shore, P.A., Burkhalter, A., Cohn, V.H Jr. (1959). A method for the fluorometric assay of histamine in tissues. *Journal of Pharmacology and Experimental Therapeutics,* **127**: 182-186.

Simons, F.E. (2004). Advances in H1-antihistamines. *The New England Journal of Medicine,* **351**: 2203-2217.

Suzuki, M., Nakamura, T., Iyoki, S., Fujiwara, A., Watanabe, Y., Mohri, K., Isobe, K., Ono, K., Yano, S. (2005). Elucidation of anti-allergic activities of curcumin-related compounds with a special reference to their anti-oxidative activities. *Biological and Pharmaceutical Bulletin,* **28**: 1438-1443.

Tamaoki, J., Kondo, M., Sakai, N., Aoshiba, K., Tagaya, E., Nakata, J., Isono, K., Nagai, A. (2000). Effect of suplatast tosilate, a Th2 cytokine inhibitor, on steroid-dependent asthma: a double-blind randomised study. Tokyo Joshi-Idai Asthma Research Group. *Lancet,* **356**: 273-278.

Teshima, R., Suzuki, K., Ikebuchi, H., Terao, T. (1986). Possible involvement of phosphorylation of a 36,000-dalton protein of rat basophilic leukemia (RBL-2H3) cell membranes in serotonin release. *Molecular Immunology,* **23**: 279-284.

Tewtrakul, S., Itharat, A. (2006). Anti-allergic substances from the rhizomes of *Dioscorea membranacea*. Bioorganic and Medicinal Chemistry, **14**: 8707-8711.

Tewtrakul, S., Subhadhirasakul, S. (2007). Anti-allergic activity of some selected plants in the Zingiberaceae family. *Journal of Ethnopharmacology,* **109**: 535-538.

Tripathi, R.M., Sen, P.C., Das, P.K. (1978). Studies on the mechanism of action of *Albizia lebbeck* an indigenous drug used in the treatment of atopic allergy. *Journal of Ethnopharmacology,* **1**: 385-396.

Trombetta, D., Occhiuto, F., Perri, D., Puglia, C., Santagati, N.A., De Pasquale, A., Saija, A., Bonina, F. (2005). Antiallergic and antihistaminic effect of two extracts of *Capparis spinosa* L. flowering buds. *Phytotherapy Research,* **19**: 29-33.

Vadnere, G.P., Gaud, R.S., Singhai, A.K. (2008). Evaluation of anti-asthmatic property of *Solanum xanthocarpum* flower extracts. *Pharmacologyonline,* **1**: 513-522.

Venkatesh, P., Mukherjee, P.K., Bandyopadhyay, A. (2008). Effect of *Curculigo orchioides* Gaertn on Compound 48/80 induced systemic anaphylaxis in mice. 7th Joint meeting of AFERP, ASP, GA, PSE and SIF. *Planta medica,* **74**: 992.

Williamson, G., Barron, D., Shimoi, K., Terao, J. (2005). *In vitro* biological properties of flavonoid conjugates found *in vivo*. *Free Radical Research,* **39**: 457-469.

World Health Organization. (1990). The use of traditional medicine in primary health care. A manual for Health Workers in South-East Asia, SEARO Regional Health Papers, No 19, New Delhi, pp. 1-2.

Wutthithamavet, W. (1997). Thai Traditional Medicine, revised ed. Odean Store Press, Bangkok, Thailand, p. 155.

Yamamoto, T., Yoshimura, M., Yamaguchi, F., Kouchi, T., Tsuji, R., Saito, M., Obata, A., Kikuchi, M. (2004). Anti-allergic activity of *Naringenin chalcone* from a tomato skin extract. *Bioscience, Biotechnology, and Biochemistry*, **68**: 1706-1711.

Yi, J.M., Kim, M.S., Seo, S.W., Lee, K.N., Yook, C.S., Kim, H.M. (2001). *Acanthopanax senticosus* root inhibits mast cell-dependent anaphylaxis. *Clinica Chimica Acta*, **312**: 163-168.

Youssouf, M.S., Kaiser, P., Tahir, M., Singh, G.D., Singh, S., Sharma, V.K., Satti, N.K., Haque, S.E., Johri, R.K. (2007). Anti-anaphylactic effect of *Euphorbia hirta*. *Fitoterapia,* **78**: 535-539.

Bioactive Phytochemicals: Perspectives for Modern Medicine Vol. 1 (2012) *Pages* **255–275**
Editor: **V.K. Gupta**
Published by: **DAYA PUBLISHING HOUSE, NEW DELHI**

7
Essential Oils from Brazilian Amazonia

Valdir F. Veiga Junior[1*], Ana P. M. Rodrigues-Bastos[1], André L. Rüdiger[1], Iuri B. Barros[1], Joelma M. Alcântara[1], Klenicy K.L. Yamaguchi[1], Lidiam M. Leandro[1], Priscilla A. Oliveira[1] And Roosevelt H. Leal[1]

ABSTRACT

The essential oils have a prestigious position among the vegetal products of human utilization. The populations from Amazonia largely utilize these products as repellent, cosmetics and even for medicinal and religious purposes. Some of these oils are distilled for concentration of the active compounds that find their market in several industries, fragrances, insecticides, drugs and even narcotics. Phenylpropanoids, such as coumarin, safrole, dillapiol and eugenol; monoterpenes, such as linalool; and sesquiterpenes caryophyllene and humulene are some of these substances. Lauraceae, Piperaceae, Burseraceae, Annonaceae and Fabaceae families are some of the main providers of essential oils that have commercial utilization in Amazonia, as well as the oleoresins from copaiba (Copaifera sp.) and breu (Protium sp.); the oils from tonoga-bean (Dipetryx odorata) and puxuri (Licaria puchury-major) seeds; those extracted from casca-preciosa (Aniba canelilla) and rosewood (Aniba rosaeodora) barks; and oils extracted from long-pepper (Piper hispidinervum) and monkey-pepper (Piper aduncum) leaves. Some of the species that have greater economic utilization are in danger of extinction, such as rosewood and copaiba, which is already protected by the State. The rational utilization of the vegetal diversity of Amazonia necessarily includes the sustained utilization of these species. The initiatives in this direction are preliminary at this point, yet disconnected from multidisciplinary studies that would allow its use in large scale. The chemical composition of

1 Chemistry Department – Amazonas Federal University, Av. Gal. Rodrigo Octávio, 3.000, ICE, Japiim, 69077-000, Manaus – AM, Brazil.

* *Corresponding author*: E-mail: valdirveiga@ufam.edu.br

ethnobotanical indicators and pharmacological properties, already confirmed to these oils, are presented in this chapter.

Keywords: Amazonia, Essential oils, Monoterpenes, Phenylpropanoids, Sesquiterpenes.

Introduction

The history of the Amazon discovery and exploration is greatly associated with vegetable extractives, especially the essential oils. If the main reason that brought Portuguese to the new world was the necessity of a new way to get species from the East, the reason that brought the first Europeans to the equatorial region of the newly discovered continent, and gave the name of the world's largest river, was the search for cinnamon (*Cinnamomum zeylanicum*). The essential oils of these spices, extremely aromatic and with antimicrobial properties act as preservatives for food and were use by Europeans to preserve meat and to disguise the odor and taste acquired over time.

In 1541 a great expedition captained by the Spanish commander Gonzalo Pizarro left with the goal of finding the mythical "Kingdom of Cinnamon" and the "Eldorado" on the eastern side of the Andes. From Quito the expedition navigated the Napo River and experienced setbacks from the humid equatorial forest, which resulted in the death of 4,000 Indians and 140 Spanish. This caused great frustration to Pizarro's plans. Thus, Francisco de Orellana took command of the expedition when Pizarro returned to Quito through the forest and arrived at the outfall of the huge river, which crosses the continent from west to east. In the region where the city of Manaus now stands, the expedition saw a group of female warriors whom the chronicler of the expedition, the jesuit Gaspar Carvajal, gave the name Amazon women. These women were tall and strong, had long black hair, no clothes, and fought like 10 men each. The name given by Carvajal comes from the mythological Greek female warriors who had one bosom excised (a-mazo) to their bows for better manipulation. The river quickly became known as the Amazon River.

Orellana, the first European man to cross the Amazon River, became known by a name attributed to the scientific name of the plant from which the Indians from Mexico to Paraguay obtain the dye to paint themselves. This name, given by Linnaeus, was the "urucu" (red, in Tupi), called *Bixa orellana* L. The female warriors have never been seen again and the cinnamon sought by the Spanish has never been found. Such was the beginnings of the adventures and failures of the Amazon vegetable extractivism. This has subsequently been repeated by the fall of the great cycle of rubber (*Hevea brasiliensis*) and several other initiatives related to essential oils, which will be related in this chapter.

In the mid-twentieth century, various regions of the Brazilian Amazon (Coari, Manaus, and Silves) had factories producing essential oils, especially rosewood (*Aniba rosaeodora*) and "casca preciosa" (*Aniba canelilla*). These aromatic oils were supplied to Europe as a feedstock for the production of perfumes, such as "Channel No. 5". When asked what she wore to bed Marilyn Monroe related that the only thing that touched her skin was a single drop from this perfume. Since then the essential oil of rosewood has evolved into the dreams of an entire generation of men and women.

The extensive exploration of rosewood and "casca-preciosa" (precious-bark) has caused these species to approach near extinction in a little more than one generation. Thus, the factories were closed and the few trees remaining in the twenty-first century now belong to controlled management plans or distant points of virgin forests. Today other Amazon products occupy the shelves, such as "white-breu" (*Protium* sp.), tonga-bean (*Dipetryx odorata*), copaiba (*Copaifera* sp.) and priprioca oils (*Cyperus articulatus*). However, none of these have aggregation technology that would provide for the survival of Amazonian people on their land without deforestation or the desired self-sustained development.

Essential Oils

To understand what the essential oils are, it is necessary to distinguish them from other plant products. Essential oils are mixtures of lipids from plant origins that receive this name for two reasons: they are insoluble in water, and very volatile and aromatic. Thus, plants that have large amounts of essential oils are called aromatics and their aroma is noted by our sense of smell. There are other oils derived from plants, such as edible oils *e.g.* olive oil, soybeans, corn, sunflowers and many others used in human consumption. The term "essence" is sometimes confused with the term "extract", however. The name "extract" is given to products obtained from plants in a solubilization process with organic solvents (hexane, for example, is used in the extraction of soybean oil) or even in water, such as teas.

The essential oils are obtained through steam drag both in small scale and industrial processes. This simple process is the passage of water in the vapor phase over the plant part that is to be extracted, which is basically dragging the aromatic constituents. The steam is condensed and the essential oil is obtained by separating it from the water.

In plants, essential oils play several functions related primarily to defense and communication, such as antibiotics, phytophagous repelling, pollinators' attraction, plant-plant signaling, etc. These oils are produced in differentiated cells into structures such as secretory and glandular trichomes and glands, as well as in the lysogenous and schizogenous internal channels (Appezzato-da-Glória and Carmello-Guerreiro, 2006).

The production of essential oils can occur in different parts of the plant. Mint (*Mentha suaveolens*) and peppermint (*Mentha piperita*), which are used as condiments and spices, have their major aromatic constituent menthol in several parts of the plant. However, their essential oils come mainly from the leaves. This same aromatic plant part is observed in lemongrass (*Cymbopogon citratus*) and the "brazilian cidreira" (*Lippia alba*), used to prepare teas, whose flavor comes from citral present in the leaves. Aromatic oils can be obtained from some seeds, such as from tonga-bean (*Dipteryx odorata*), which are rich in coumarin and "puxuri" (*Licaria puchury-major*) mixtures of safrole and eugenol. In some species the most aromatic part is found in the stem or on their bark. "Casca preciosa" (*Aniba canelilla*) and rosewood (*Aniba

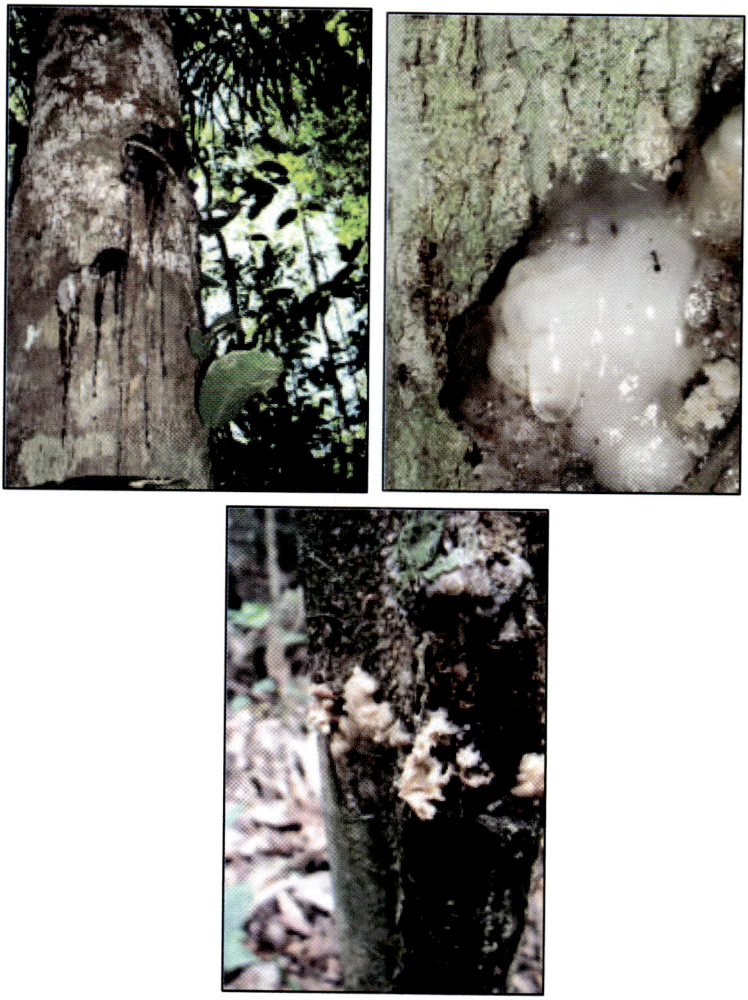

Figure 7.1: Oleoresin of the Burseraceae.

rosaeodora) are examples. In these cases, obtaining the essential oil usually leads to death of the tree. In other cases, the essential oil source is released outside of the plant, as in the oleoresin of Burseraceae species, called "breus". This oleoresin is produced when a little aggression occurs in the trunk, such as when a small fly lays its eggs inside the bark. The aromatic resins of this family are found in large clusters on the outside of the trunk and roots that can reach several kilograms. This extraction causes no damage to the plant.

Brazil is one of the world's leading producers of essential oils from oranges and lemons, which are by-products from citric juice industries. However, the Amazon's region has a very small contribution in the volume exported and consumed by the country. The major highlights are the oils of rosewood (*Aniba rosaeodora*), tonga-bean

(*Dipteryx odorata*) and copaiba (*Copaifera* spp.). Although the volume traded is extremely lower than the region's potential.

Breu, Oleoresins from Burseraceae Family

Texts about essential oils are found in many books, but one of the most famous stories appears in the Holy Bible. Following a star, three Mage Kings traveled through the desert to see God's newborn son. One of the Kings delivered gold, as a present. The other two presented him with incense and myrrh. Myrrh is a resin that has aromatic oils extracted from an Asian species of Burseraceae, *Commiphora myrrha* and the incense used at the time, or frankincense, was the aromatic resin of the genus *Boswellia*. This also belongs to the same family that was gathered in the mountains of Abyssinia or Ethiopia. The Burseraceae family (Sapindales) is one of the most important resiniferous botanic families with about 19 genus and 700 species distributed in tropical and subtropical regions (Weeks *et al.*, 2005; Thulin *et al.*, 2008).

In the Amazon, *Protium* is the most heterogeneous genus of seven belonging of this family present at region with 135 species (Ribeiro and Daly, 1999), and receives popular names related to appearance, such as "breu", "white-breu" and "black-breu". Also, the smell of resin, such as "mango-breu", "lemonn-gum", "almiscar" and "almecega" (Gentry, 1993; Silva, Lisbon, Lisbon, 1977; Pio Correa, 1984, Ribeiro and Daly, 1999). In folk medicine various uses are assigned to these oleoresins, such as healing, anti-inflammatory and analgesics, tonics, stimulants, haemostatics, anti-rheumatics, and for the treatment of pulmonary diseases (Silva *et al.*, 1977; Pio Correa, 1984; Costa, 1975) (Figure 7.1).

In Burseraceae species, the fresh oleoresin may contain 20 to 30 per cent essential oils. Sometime after exudates, the oleoresin begins to oxidize and polymerize, and the volatile portion of the essential oils begins to evaporate, reducing its content to approximately 7 to 8 per cent (Costa, 1975).

Protium heptaphyllum, one of the most commonly studied trees of this family throughout Brazil as well as in various regions of the Amazon. The essential oil extracted from the oleoresin is composed mainly of monoterpenes such as *p*-cymene (36 per cent), terpinolene (21 per cent) and still α and γ-terpinene (18 and 12 per cent respectively). The same species is found in northeastern Brazil and its essential oil is constituted differently, with high values of terpinolene (28 per cent), α-phellandrene (17 per cent), limonene (17 per cent) and α-pinene (10 per cent) (Bandeira *et al.*, 2001).

The differences observed in the chemical composition from essential oils that occur within a species are also observed among subspecies. In subspecies *P. heptaphyllum* ssp. *ullei* and *P. heptaphyllum* ssp. *heptaphyllum*, collected in Cruzeiro do Sul, Acre, Brazil, the terpinolene amount was observed to be ten times greater in *P. heptaphyllum* ssp. *ullei* than in *P. heptaphyllum* ssp. *heptaphyllum* (42.3 per cent and 4.2 per cent, respectively). Moreover, *p*-cimene was observed in greater quantities in *P. heptaphyllum* ssp. *heptaphyllum*, with 33.9 per cent, compared with *P. heptaphyllum* ssp. *ullei*, (4.7 per cent). The presence of some compounds was observed only in one or another species. Limonene and *p*-cymene-8-ol were observed only in *P. heptaphyllum* ssp. *ullei* (11.8 per cent and 13.6 per cent, respectively) and dihidro-4-carene, and ntetradecane was observed only in *P. heptaphyllum* ssp. *heptaphyllum* (11.6 per cent and 13.3 per cent, respectively) (Marques *et al.*, 2010).

In the species *P. paniculatum* var. *nova* were observed in the monoterpenes *p*-cymene (69 per cent) and α-terpinene (11 per cent) as major constituents from the essential oil of the breu. In other varieties of *P. paniculatum*, *P. paniculatum* var. *riedelianum,* the major constituents described were *p*-ment-3-ene (31 per cent), α-phellandrene (24 per cent), 1,8-cineole (11 per cent), β-phellandrene (12 per cent) and only 9 per cent of *p*-cymene (Ramos *et al.*, 2000).

The *Protium hebetatum* species produces large amounts of oleoresin and shows dark color. The essential oil composition of oil-resin is mainly *p*-cymene (75 per cent), and like several other Burseraceae essential oils, α-pinene (16 per cent), β-phellandrene (11 per cent), β-phellandrene (5 per cent) and α-terpinene (5 per cent) are minor constituents. In the *P. altsoni* species - which is taxonomically and phylogenetically similar to *P. hebetatum* - α-pinene (61 per cent), *p*-cymene (33 per cent), α-phellandrene (22 per cent) and 1,8-cineole (11 per cent) were observed (Ramos *et al.*, 2000).

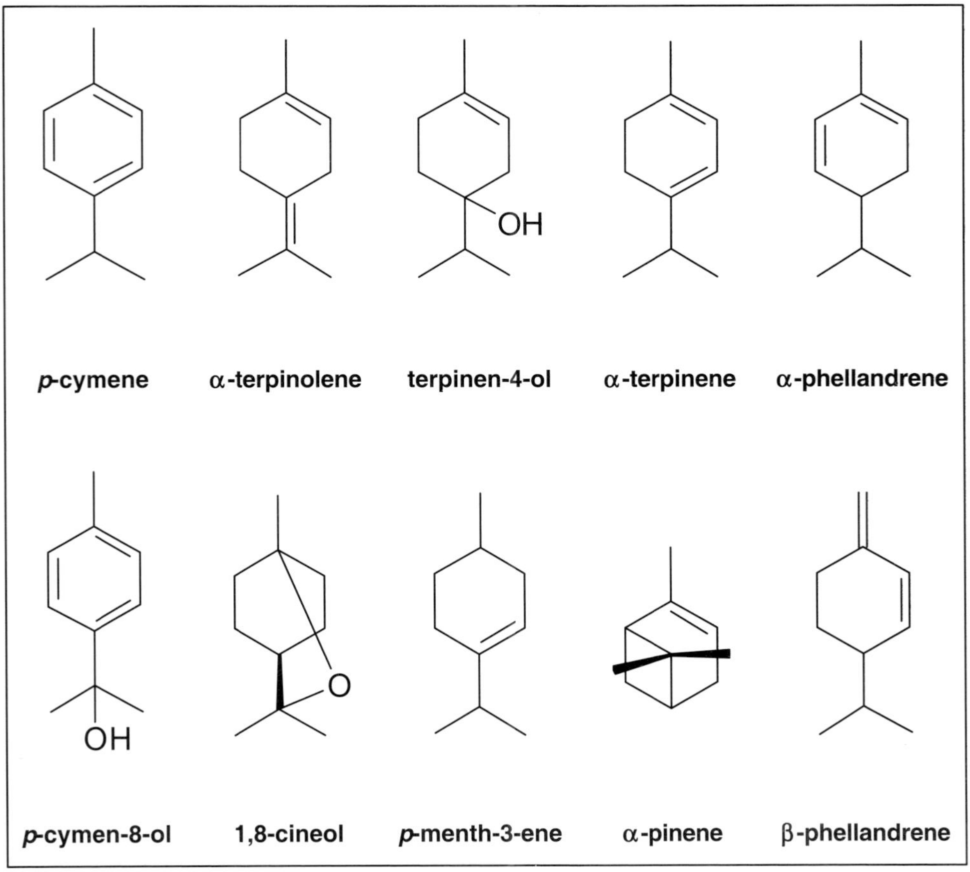

Figure 7.2: Majority monoterpenes of the "Breu" oleoresin.

It is interesting to observe that different parts of the same plant can produce essential oils with different compositions. While the essential oils obtained from the oleoresin are composed almost exclusively of monoterpenes (mainly *p*-cymene) in the leaves of the Burseraceae species, essential oils are constituted in the majority of sesquiterpenes. In *Protium hebetatum* leaves essential oils were described as the major constituents sesquiterpenes β-caryophyllene (12 per cent) and δ-cadinene (7 per cent) and in smaller quantities the monoterpenes p-cymene (2 per cent), *p*-cimenene (8 per cent) and linalool (3 per cent) (Siani *et al.*, 1999).

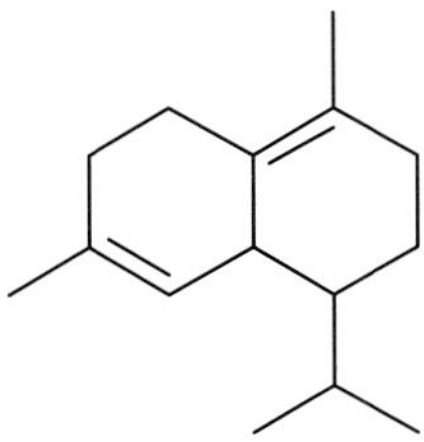

δ-cadinene

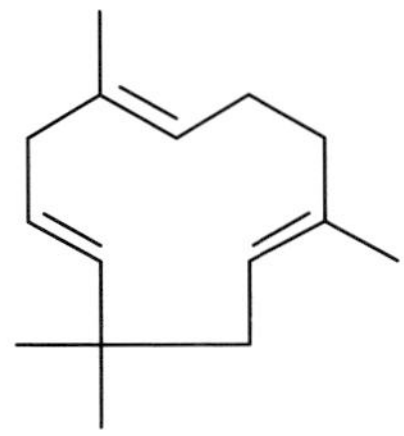

α-humulene

Figure 7.3: Majority sesquiterpenes of the Burseraceae leaf.

Currently, the breu from Amazonia are almost exclusively used in caulking in the regional boats market. A few companies use small amounts of oleoresin as incense and in making cosmetics and perfumes. The magic of those resins, already known 2,000 years ago, has not yet provided laurels for Amazonian entrepreneurs.

Winners take the Laurels

The Lauraceae family trees are known and used by mankind for thousands of years. In antiquity Greeks and Romans used to honor their warriors and victorious athletes with crowns of cinnamon and laurel (*Laurus nobilis*), considered a symbol of wisdom. In India and China they were used to flavor wine for religious purposes.

The Lauraceae family is constituted by approximately 50 genera and about 2,500 species with a pantropical distribution. In Brazil, there are about 25 genera and 400 species, often found in rain forests, sandbanks and "cerrado" areas. The Amazonian species are included primarily in the genus *Aniba*, *Cinnamomum*, *Ocotea* and *Licaria*, with essential oils of economic importance applied in perfumery industry and cosmetics, cleaning materials, food and medicine.

With around 350 species from most of the essential oil producers, *Cinnamomum* is one of major genera of this family. Its name "kayu manis" seems to have originated in Indonesia, which means "sweet wood", and evolved into "quinnamon" in Hebrew, and "Kinnamon" in Greek. In the global market the most important essential oils of sweet wood are obtained from cinnamom.

For many centuries cinnamon has been the most popular spice in Europe. During the Great Navigations, in the fifteenth and sixteenth centuries Ceylon cinnamon was strongly sought. Their lucrative trade was dominated by Portugal when they discovered the route to India and Ceylon (actual Sri Lanka) until they were expelled by the Dutch in the seventeenth century, which in turn, were expelled by the English in the late eighteenth century.

Among the various essential oils with commercial interest we can highlight those obtained from the leaves and bark of the trunk of cinnamon (*Cinnamon verum*), China cinnamon (*C. cassia*) and sassafras (*C. camphora*). The most widespread cinnamon, and of greater importance, is *C. zeylanicum*, which is known as "India cinnamon" or "Ceylon cinnamon". Originating from these two countries, the cinnamic aldehyde, is responsible for its aroma, and can exceed 80 per cent.

The chemistry variability observed in this species has caused much confusion and hindered the substitution of the Asian species by others from the New World. Several studies indicate that the oil of common cinnamon, *C. zeylanicum*, can have five different patterns that modify their chemical smells, called chemotypes: cinnamaldehyde (Variyvar and Bandyopadhyay, 1989; Senanayake, 1978, Bernard *et al.*, 1989; Möllenbeck *et al.*, 1997), eugenol (Thomas *et al.*, 1987; Senanayake, 1978), methyl benzoate (Rao *et al.*, 1988), linalool (Jirovetz *et al.*, 2001) and camphor (Senanayake, 1978).

Works performed with Amazon species showed the chemical pattern with eugenol as the major constituent (60 per cent), similarly to those obtained from the leaves of specimens collected in India and Sri Lanka, with percentages from 70.1 per cent to 94.5 per cent of eugenol (Senanayake *et al.*, 1978; Ross, 1976; Rabha *et al.*, 1979).

Oils with high content of eugenol have interest to the pharmaceutical industry, and are used in various medications, as well as in dentistry as an analgesic for toothaches and antiseptics, as well as in perfumes, soap manufacturing, and as a clarifier in histology. Eugenol is a raw material employed for the production of vanillin, used for flavoring candies, chocolates, ice cream and cigars.

Two centuries after the Orellana voyage, the German naturalist Alexander von Humboldt discovered the Amazonia cinnamon. However, it was different than expected. This was not the already known cinnamon, but another species, known as "*Orinoco cinnamon*" and "*Casca preciosa*", the *Aniba canelilla*. Soon it was observed that this American cinnamon did not have the same constituents as the cinnamic aldehyde, which is responsible for its aroma. Only in 1959, did one of the brightest Brazilian natural products chemists, Dr. Otto Gottlieb, report that the *A. canelilla* oil had eugenol and 1-nitro-2-phenylethane. This was the world's first record of a natural substance containing the nitro group. The same substance was observed as the main constituent for essential oils from other cinnamons from Brazil, as in *Ocotea pretiosa* (sassafras from Brazil southeastern).

Four centuries after the fruitless search of Orellana and Humboldt, Gottlieb found the essential oil from an ecuatorian cinnamon, *Ocotea quixos*, the cinnamic aldehyde.

The economic importance of the essential oils of the *Aniba* species began in 1875 when Samarin, in France, had the *A. duckei* essential oil obtained by distillation. Then, in 1881, Calico, also in France, separated linalool from the essential oil.

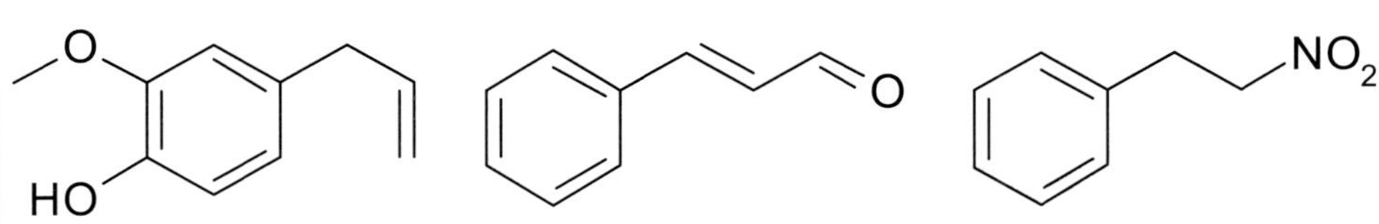

Eugenol   cinnamaldehyde   1-nitro-2-phenilethane

Figure 7.4: Phenylpropanoids of the Lauraceae.

The monoterpene linalool has an asymmetric carbon, which therefore, has two enantiomers, the licareol and the coriandrol (Figure 7.5). These molecules have a completely different fragrance. Licariol presents a scent of roses while coriandrol has an herbaceous aroma. Approximately 70 per cent of the compounds produced by the industries of cosmetics and perfumes contain mixtures of linalool isomers in their formula. Also, it is used in the composition of some drugs and has antimicrobial activity. The more pleasant aroma is that with a high content of licareol, observed in the oil of rosewood (*A. rosaeodora*).

licareol   coriandrol

Figure 7.5: Isomers of linalool found in *Aniba roseadora.*

The exploitation of linalool-producing trees has put many of them into the list of endangered species. The rosewood oil has been the third export product in the Amazon region behind only to the rubber and Brazil nuts, which currently has supply far below the demand.

Other species such as *A. fragans*, *A. canellila* and *A. parviflora* are also used in perfumery. However, *A. fragans* is the best essential oil in the perfumery and cosmetics industries. Besides the isomers of linalool, the *Aniba* essential oils are constituted with benzyl benzoate and β-caryophyllene, as major constituents. In the *A. panurensis* leaves the essential oil β-caryophyllene represents 33.5 per cent of its composition while the *A. roseadora* stem essential oil of linalool represents 86.0 per cent of its composition (Alcantara, *et al.*, 2010).

The bicyclic sesquiterpene β-caryophyllene is a fairly common Lauraceae Amazonic species and has great commercial interest due to its several biological activities, such as spasmolytic, local anesthetic, antiinflammatory and antitumor. In the leaves and stems the essential oils of the *Licaria martiniana* β-caryophyllene represents 41.7 and 21.4 per cent, respectively (Alcantara *et al.*, 2010).

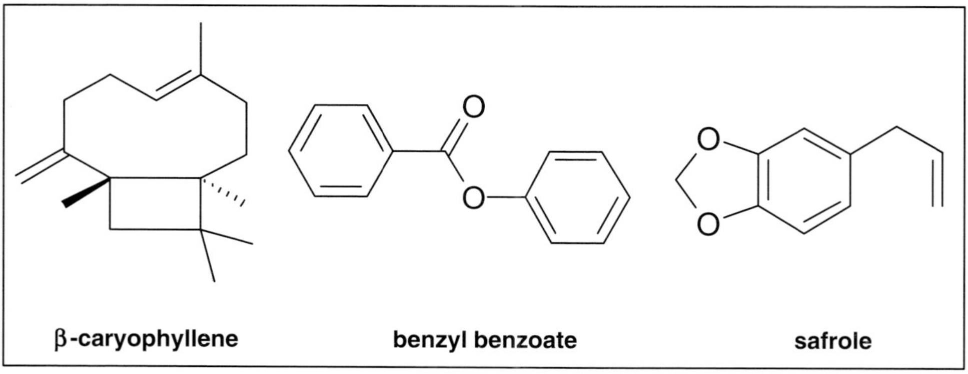

Figure 7.6: Others volatiles compounds of the Lauraceae.

Another Amazonian species of this family that deserves mention is the "puxurí" (*Licaria puchury-major*). The aromatic oil of its seeds is popularly used as a carminative in insomnia and irritability treatment. In chemical studies with the essential oil, the seeds from this specie indicated the presence of safrole, eugenol and eucalyptol. In wood it also evidences the presence of safrole and eugenol, as well as other alcohols and aldehydes. Some of the pharmacological effects of this essential oil are the reduction of motor activity and anesthesia, attributed to the presence of safrole and eugenol (Alcantara *et al.*, 2010).

Safrole is a natural allylbenzene widely distributed in the plant kingdom, present in appreciable amounts in Lauraceae species. Safrole occurs as a main component containing up to 80 per cent in the essential wood oil of "sassafras" (*Ocotea odorifera*), a Lauraceae found mainly in southern Brazil. This essential oil has figured prominently as a substitute for classic American "sassafras" oil, but due to years of exploitation the species is near extinction, which has led to the ban on its exploration in Brazil.

Some Lauraceae species occurring in the Amazon region, such as at the *Aniba* genus, also have high levels of safrole in leaves and aerial parts and could become an alternative for the production of this allylbenzene. Besides being used as a floor wax, polish, soap, detergent and perfume fragrance (Braga *et al.*, 2004), safrole is used as feedstock in the preparation of drugs of natural catechol, such as dopamine, dopa, α-methyldopa, and isoproterenol, among others. It also can be used for synthesis of hallucinogens, such as "Ecstasy" (Barreiro and Fraga, 1999). Among the products obtained from safrole is piperonal (or heliotropin), a fragrance fixative (*i.e.* serves to retard the evaporation of the essence in fine fragrances, prolonging its effect) (Leal, 1999; Mortimer, 2006).

Another product obtained from safrole is piperonyl butoxide, a stabilizing and synergistic potentiating the effects from pyrethrum (*Chrysanthemum cinerariifolium*), a natural insecticide with widespread use in industrialized countries. It is also the only formulation approved in Europe, Japan, and the United States to control pests in storage in the food processing industry and domestic use.

Safrole can be considered as one of the most abundant components in the brazillian essential oils, also found in large quantities in the Aristolochiaceae and Piperaceae families (Barreiro and Fraga, 1999; Costa, 2000). However, agronomic characteristics indicate the *Piper hispidinervium* species for the production of this compound.

Amazon Peppers

The Piperaceae family presents a pantropical distribution and is divided into 12 genera and around 1,400 species. Several species of the Piperaceae family, particularly of the genus Piper, have folk medicine application. With the large diversity of species in this genus also occurs a varied use of these plants, including the treatment of urinary tract problems, as well as epilepsy and intestinal disorders. In the essential oils of these plants is observed the presence of monoterpenes and sesquiterpenes, as well as phenylpropanoids (Navickiene *et al.*, 2006, Santos *et al.*, 1998).

Among the Piperaceae family species native to the Amazon, without a doubt one of the most notorious is *Piper hispidinervium*. Popularly known as "long pepper" (Maia *et al.*, 2000; Figueiredo *et al.*, 2004; Fazolin, Lima and Argolo, 2002), the discovery of safrole in *P. hispidinervium* leaves occurred in the 1970's by "Instituto Nacional de Pesquisas da Amazônia - INPA" researchers (Pimentel and Pinheiro, 2000). The dried leaves of *P. hispidinervium* have a content between 2.7 to 4.0 per cent of essential oil, and safrole represents 98 per cent (Braga *et al.*, 2004; Figueiredo *et al.*, 2004, Maia *et al.*, 1987; Andrade *et al.*, 2002). Not only does safrole stand out in this species, terpinolene is another constituent of the aerial parts with percentages ranging around 10 per cent. In the roots of the essential oils in this species are found the major constituents safrole (20 per cent), mirisiticine (34.9 per cent) and guaiol (10.6 per cent) (Andrade *et al.*, 2002).

Antimicrobial and insecticidal activities of the *P. hispidinervium* essential oil have been targeted for many studies on the antimicrobial activity against *Staphylococcus aureus, Proteus mirabilis, Proteus vulgaris, Klebsiella pneumoniae, Enterobacter aerogenes, Salmonella* sp. and many fungal phytopatogens as *Bipolaris sorokiniana, Fusarium oxysporum* and *Colletotrichum gloeosporiodes*. The antimicrobial activity is attributed to safrole (Lobato *et al.*, 1989; Lima *et al.*, 2009). The insecticidal activity of the *P. hispidinervum* essential oil has been evaluated against the pest *Sitophilus zeamais* that infests stored grain (Estrela*et al.*, 2006), and against *Spodoptera frugiperda*, considered the major pest of corn (Lima *et al.*, 2009).

Also known for its insecticide use, *Piper aduncum*, popularly known as the "monkeys pepper ", is very popular in folk medicine for the treatment of digestive tract disorders and in the urinary tract, as a diuretic and anti-inflammatory, among others (Duarte *et al.*, 2007; Maia *et al.*, 2000).

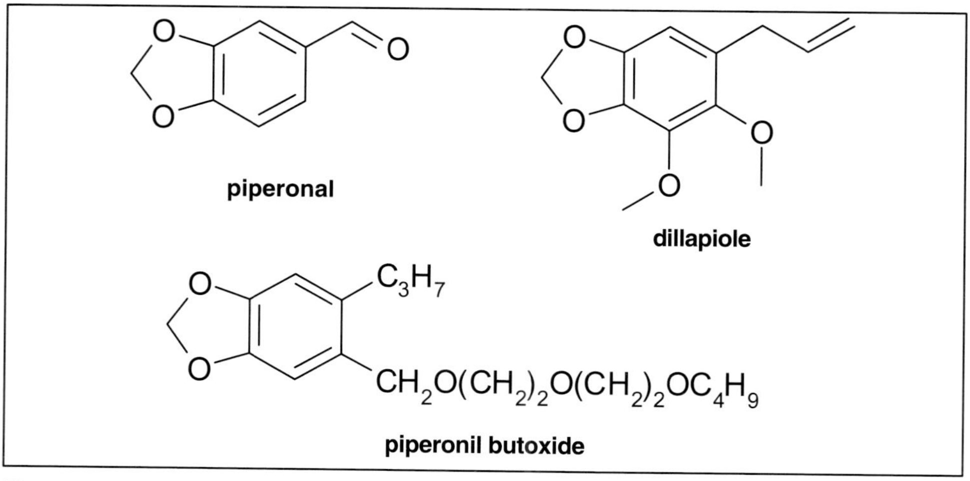

Figure 7.7: Piperaceae volatile compounds and derivatives.

The yield of the *P. aduncum* essential oil varies around 0.13 to 3.4 per cent depending on the origin of the plant material (Duarte *et al.*, 2005, Lobato *et al.*, 1989; Maia *et al.*, 2000). In specimens collected in the Amazon region, it is observed that the dillapiol (80 per cent) prevails as the major constituent of leaves essential oils (Gottlieb *et al.*, 1981). Maia and coworkers (2000), analyzing the essential oils of leaves and twigs of plants from different Amazon regions, had the amount of dillapiol reaching up to 97.3 per cent.

In terms of biological activity, the *P. aduncum* essential oil has shown activity against *Cladosporium cladosporioides*, *C. sphaerospermumas* and *Candidaalbicans* (Duarte *et al.*, 2005). Insecticide effects against *Sitophilus zeamais* are also attributed to them (Estrela *et al.*, 2006).

Throughout Brazil, street vendors offer an essential oil obtained from another Piperaceae species that is marketed for the treatment of inflammation, as well as being an astringent, digestive, antidiarrheal, hemostatic, and antiblenorrágico antileucorréico. This oil extracted from *Piper callosum* receives many popular names such as "elixir-paregórico", "eletric-oil" and "soldier herb" (Alencar *et al.*, 1971; Maia *et al.*, 2000). The yield of essential oils of leaves is about 2 per cent. Safrole is the main component (69 per cent) followed by methyleugenol (8 per cent) (Gottlieb *et al.*, 1981; Alencar *et al.*, 1971).

Piper bartlingianumm is a species with the leaves and twigs containing essential oils used as fish poison, with α-cadinol (11.2 per cent) and β-elemene (10.5 per cent) (Santos *et al.*, 1998), as the main constituents.

Another Piperaceae genus which has had its essential oils studied in the Amazon region is *Pothomorphe*. The *P. peltata* leaves essential oils, known as "caapeba", "true caapeba ", "cataié", "north caapeba " and "caapeba peuá" has low yield of only about 0.1 per cent. With many uses, such as being a tonic, an anthelmintic against internal and external inflammations, burns and tumors (Maia *et al.*, 2000) its essential oil presents β-caryophyllene (37.5 per cent), germacrene D (11.9 per cent) and heneicosane (10.2 per cent) as major constituents (Luz *et al.*, 1999).

Pothomorphe umbellata is also popularly known as "caapeba" or "pariparoba" and "malvarisco". It is used in folk medicine as a diuretic, febrifuge, anti-rheumatic, liver disease, among others (Mala *et al.*, 2000). Predominate in the leaves with twigs essential oils with germacrene D (27.4 per cent), the β-caryophyllene (14.8 per cent), the δ-cadinene (13.3 per cent) and bicyclogermacrene (11.5 per cent) (Light *et al.*, 1999).

The change of popular names is common in medicinal plants and their essential oils which is very confusing, often resulting in misuse and poisoning, and causes serious adverse effects. Although considered to be harmless, many essential oils are abortifacients, which stimulate blood flow. The widespread use of homemade teas has serious consequences for pregnant women, which makes it important to correct botanical identification.

Enviras

The Annonaceae family is distributed in South and Central America, and other tropical and sub-tropical regions of the world. The use of their species by man runs from edible fruits, fiber production from its bark, spices, applications in folk medicine, and in the perfume industry. Some of the more common species in the Amazon are *Annona, Anaxagoras, Guatteriopsis, Guatteria* and *Xylopia*. In the Amazon region, many species of this family are commonly known as envira.

Several species of this family produce essential oils with low yield and high content of caryophyllene oxide or spathulenol. In *Guatteria juruensis*, the leaves essential oil (0.2 per cent) spathulenol constitute of more than 77 per cent (Maia *et al.*, 2005a). *Guatteria poeppigiana* shows the same essential oil income, 53 per cent and 11 per cent to spathulenol and kushinol contents, respectively (Maia *et al.*, 2005a). In the *Guatteriopsis blepharophylla* the essential oil income does not change, but the main constituent is caryophyllene oxide (51.0 per cent) (Maia *et al.*, 2005a).

In *Annona foetida* leaves, known popularly as "graviola do mato", and used in northeastern Brazil against rheumatism, intermittent fevers and ulcers, the essential oil presents bicyclogermacrene as majors constituent (35.12 per cent), (E)-caryophyllene (14.19 per cent) and α-copaene (8.19 per cent). It is also used for its antimicrobial activity against various microorganisms emphasizing minimum inhibitory concentrations against *Candida albicans* and *Rhococcus equi* of 60 μgmL -1. This essential oil also has anti-Leishmania activity and low cytotoxicity against peritoneal macrophages of mice and hamsters, characterizing it as a potential source of bioactive products (Costa *et al.*, 2009).

In the *Xylopia* genus, *X. aromatica* is popularly known as the "pimenta de macaco", which is the same popular name of *Piper aduncum*. The composition of the leaves' essential oils, however, is very different with bicyclogermacrene (36.5 per cent) and spathulenol (20.5 per cent) as the main components. This species is used in folk medicine as a carminative and stimulant and is also still used as a spice (Maia *et al.*, 2005b). The high content of spathulenol is also observed in the leaves oils of

Xylopia emarginata, 73 per cent, a species known as "envira chichi" or "pinheirinho de caxiuanã" (Maia *et al.*, 2005b).

The *Anaxagoras dolichocarpa* species is one of the most abundant in the Para state, where it is known as "envira de jacu" and "marúba grande". In this species it is observed that the major components found in the leaves (yield 0.2 per cent) and branches (0.1 per cent yield) are the essential oils spathulenol (26.2, 21.2 per cent), α-pinene (16.8, 23.4 per cent) and β-pinene (12.3, 17.0 per cent) (Andrade *et al.*, 2007). Its use in the Amazon occurs not only for their essential oils, but also for its fiber, such as dental floss, fishing line, basket-making, and the use in folk medicine for its leaves and bark (Andrade *et al.*, 2007).

Other Botanic Families

Several other plant families have species that produces essential oils of commercial importance or popular usage in the Amazon. Sacaca (*Croton cajucara*, Euphorbiaceae) is a shrub extensively used for medicinal purposes. Their essential oil has large amounts of linalool and appears as a possible alternative to replace the *Aniba* species exploration that is endangered. The leaves' essential oil produces 0.8 per cent, with more than 66 per cent of it being linalool.

In the *Croton palanostigma* species, in the Brazilian Amazon, known as "marmeleiro", the essential oil from the leaves has a yield of 0.7 per cent and its mains constituents are linalool (25.4 per cent), (E)-caryophyllene (21.0 per cent) and methyleugenol (17.2 per cent). While in the fruit are found a yield of 0.5 per cent and linalool (42.7 per cent), methyleugenol (16.3 per cent) and β-elemene (6.4 per cent) are the principal components. The bark of the trunk has a better yield (2.2 per cent) and its main components are α-pinene (31.6 per cent), methyleugenol (25.6 per cent) and (E)-metilisoeugenol (23.7 per cent) (Brazil *et al.*, 2009).

Two other well-known species in the Amazon, belonging to the family Fabaceae, are "copaíba" (*Copaifera* sp.) and "cumaru" or tonga-bean (*Dypterix odorata*). While the first provides a trunk oleoresin, rich in α-copaene and β-caryophyllene (Veiga Junior and Pinto, 2003), the second provides large amounts of coumarin in its seeds, exported to perfume and cosmetic industries. Its medicinal properties were described as particularly inflammatory and wound healing. These "copaiba" properties, for example, were discovered by the Indians who watched the animals and realize that they rubbed it into their trunks when injured in fights or from snake bites.

In the Meliaceae family, four species of the *Guarea* genus: *G. convergens*, *G. humaitensis*, *G. scabra* and *G. silvatica*, had its essential oil composition and larvicidal activity against *Aedes aegypti* evaluated. The essential oils composition has been shown to have sesquiterpenes with a caryophyllene skeleton as major components. Also, larvicidal activity was observed and attributed to caryophyllene epoxide and cis-caryophyllene (Magalhães *et al.*, 2010).

The *Hyptis crenata* (Lamiaceae), popularly known as "salva de marajo", "salsa do campo" or "hortelã do campo", is used by Amazonian populations as an anti-inflammatory (Maia *et al.*, 2000; Rebelo *et al.*, 2009). In addition to its folk medicine purposes, the aroma of this species with its fragrance of green leaf, citrus and wood, shows up with potential for use in the perfume industry (Maia *et al.*, 2000). From the leaves of this species collected in several localities in Pará state were obtained essential oils that show 1,8-cineole (24 per cent), borneol (22 per cent) and β-caryophyllene (19 per cent); or α-pinene (51 per cent) 1,8-cineole (16 per cent), limonene (15 per cent) and β-pinene (10 per cent) in its composition (Zoghbi *et al.*, 2001). Another work shows α-pinene (22.0 and 19.5 per cent), 1,8-cineole (17.6 per cent and 23.2 per cent), β-pinene (17.0 per cent and 13.8 per cent) as components mainly from fresh and dried leaves, respectively. It has also been evaluated for its antioxidant activity (DPPH) and toxicity against *Artemia salina*, which showed low antioxidant activity and a minimum lethal concentration of 6.7± $0.2 mgmL^{-1}$ (Rebelo *et al.*, 2009).

Another species that has been studied is *Calyptranthes spruceana* (Myrtaceae), which occupies flooded areas on the borders of the Amazon rivers. Its aroma of orange gives it the popular name "laranjinha" (little orange), and also "cuminarana", by remembering the smell of cumin, which is attributed to the compound peryaldehyde. Its popular use is in the form of tea, which is prepared from the leaves and swallowed in case of stomach upsets (Maia *et al.*, 2000). Its leaves yield an abundant essential oil (1.8 per cent) (Correa *et al.*, 1972; Lobato *et al.*, 1989), rich in limonene (55 per cent), which provides the aroma of orange and peryaldehyde (25 per cent).

Oils rich in thymol and carvacrol are observed in "pataqueira" (*Conobea scoparioides* - Scrophulariaceae), with essential oils obtained from the leaves containing about 65 per cent thymol. Similarly profile is observed with some *Lippia* species (Verbenaceae), as in *L. grandis*, with 60 per cent of carvacrol in the leaves oil, and *L. origanoides*, "alecrin d'Angola do Pará", containing *p*-cymene (27.8 per cent), α-terpinene (22.4 per cent) and thymol (20.6 per cent) in the essential oil extracted from the set consisting of branches, leaves, flowers and fruits (Merair *et al.*, 1972).

Some species that were introduced in the Amazon are widely used by the population. An example is *Alpinia speciosa*, commonly known as "vindecá", "vindecá-grande" "colônia", "pacová" and "jardineira", has leaves and flowers used in folk medicine as a cardiovascular, hypotensive, diuretic, cleanser, carminative, for stomach disorders, and to relieve spasmodic (Maia *et al.*, 2000). The spasmogenic effects, sparmolytic and anti-inflammatory effects, as well as for CNS depression has been

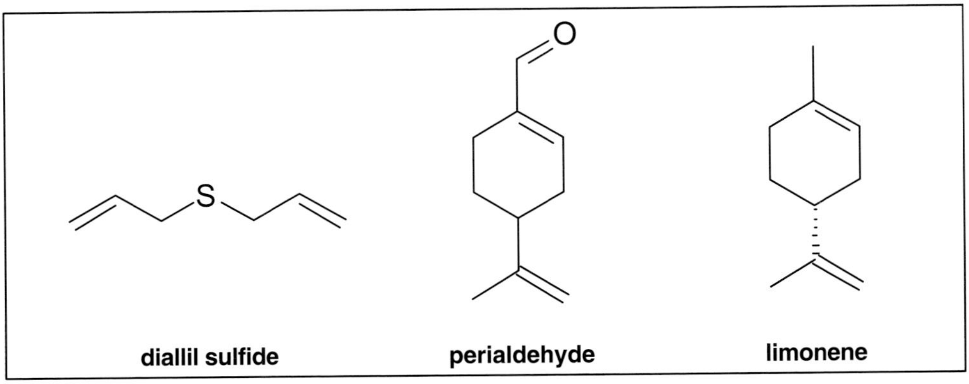

Figure 7.8: Others important volatile compounds.

reported (Brito and Souza, 1993). The whole plant is also used in cooking (Lötschert and Beese, 1983) (Maia *et al.*, 2000). There were two chemotypes of this species in the Amazon: the chemotype A with essential oil yield of 0.3 per cent with the major constituents terpinene-4-ol (20.4 per cent) and 1,8-cineole (14.9 per cent), and the chemotype B, with a yield of 0.7 per cent and limonene (25.1 per cent) and γ-terpinene (17.4 per cent) as major components. The essential oils from the leaves showed antimicrobial activity against *Staphylococcus aureus, Proteus mirabilis, P. vulgaris, Escherichia coli, Edwardsiella tarda, Klebsiella pneumoniae, Enterobacter aerogenes* and *Salmonella* sp. (Lobato *et al.*, 1989).

The "cipó-d'alho" *Adenocalymma aliaceum* Miers (Bignoniaceae) is a species known for its essential oils and aroma, which contains high levels of diallyl disulfide (31 per cent) and diallyl trisulfide (31 per cent) and has a yield of 0.1 per cent. The species is used to treat fever, flu, headache and lung problems. It is also still used in recipes as a substitute for garlic (*Allium sativum*) (Maia *et al.*, 2000).

Tanaecium nocturnum, popularly known as "cipó-vick" or "cipó-carimbo", is another Bignoniaceae. Used to combat ants and bees by Gotira Indians, as well as descongecionante airway, it had its antifungal activity tested against *Aspergillus flavus* isolated from Brazil nuts, with total inhibition at a concentration of 782ppm in contact technique and 1000ppm in the technique of fumigation. These results are attributed to the main components of this oil, benzaldehyde, benzyl alcohol and methyl benzoate (Pimentel *et al.*, 2010).

Future Prospects

More than in the Amazon, Brazil, America, and even in the history of Christianity, essential oils have been present in the history of each one. The aroma of these flowers has been associated with a first love, the maternal bouquet of spices that anticipates the satisfaction of the pleasure of hunger satiated, to be reborn in each spring, and at the dusk each summer.

In the Amazon, the aromas of the forest are part of peoples' everyday life. Using this featured plant for their survival, however, is still far from being a reality. The commercial use of the Amazon's essential oils can provide income for the population without the need for deforestation. Historically, however, the exploitation of the oil in the Amazon has led to the species' extinction.

In this chapter we have shown some of the difficulties of the commercial use of essential oils, such as low yield, biotic and abiotic variations, chemistry complexity, and their popular names. We also saw in the chemical approach, that the mixtures of monoterpenes, sesquiterpenes and phenylpropanoids produce unique flavors, although the presence of these molecules may represent the possibility for pharmacological proprieties use.

Medicinal plants have also long been used by indigenous people to treat a wide range of diseases, playing an important role in therapies that offer cultural, financial and toxicity advantages. In the Amazon the plant's essential oils have been described in different substances with economic and medicinal importance, such as safrole, eugenol, β-caryophyllene, limonene and linalool.

Finally, the analytic methods usually applied in essential oils research, such as chromatographic and spectroscopic techniques have already been well established for the most common studies. But when the very complex composition of essential oils is considered, the perception of the substances that gives the aroma oils, further studies of chiral and multidimensional chromatography, as well as olfactometry are needed.

References

Alcantara, J.M., Yamaguchi, K.K., and Veiga-Junior, V.F. (2010) Composição química de óleos essenciais de espécies de *Aniba* e *Licaria* e suas atividades antioxidantes e antiagregante plaquetária. *Química Nova*, **33**: 141-145.

Alencar, R., Lima, R.A., Corrêa, R.G.C., Gottlieb, O.R., Marx, M.C., Silva, M.L., Maia, J.G.S., Magalhães, M.T., and Assumpção, R.M.V. (1971). Óleos essenciais de plantas brasileiras. *Acta Amazonica*, **1**: 41-43.

Andrade, E.H., Guimarães, E.F., Silva, M.H.L., and Maia, J.G.S. (2002). O óleo essencial de *Piper hispidinervium* C. DC. proveniente de propagação por semente. *25a Reunião Anual da Sociedade Brasileira de Química*, Minas Gerais, Brasil.

Andrade, E.H.A., Oliveira, J. and Zoghbi, M.G.B. (2007) Volatiles of *Anaxagorea dolichocarpa* Spreng. and Sandw. and *Annona densicoma* Mart. Growing Wild in the State of Pará, Brazil. *Flavour and Fragrance Journal* **22**: 158-160.

Appezzato-da-Glória, B. and Carmello-Guerreiro (2006). Anatomia Vegetal. Editora UFV, Minas Gerais – Viçosa, 110-111pp.

Bandeira, P.N., Machado, M.I.L., Cavalcanti, F.S., and Lemos, T.L.G. (2001). Essential oil composition of leaves, fruits and resin of *Protium heptaphyllum* (Aubl.) March., *Journal of Essential Oil Research*, **13**: 33-34.

Barreiro, E.J., and Fraga, C.A.M. (1999). A utilização do safrol, principal componente químico do óleo de sassafráz, na síntese de susbstâncias bioativas na cascata do ácido araquidônico: antiinflamatórios,analgésicose anti-trombóticos. *Química Nova*, **5**: 744-759.

Braga, N.P., Cremasco, M.A. and Valle, R.C.C.R. (2004). Effects of fixed bed drying on the composition of essential oil from long pepper (*Piper hispidinervium* C. DC.) leaves. Proceedings of the 14th International Drying Symposium, vol. C: 1906-1913, São Paulo, Brazil.

Brasil, D.S.B., Müller, A.H., Guilhon, G.M.S.P., Alves, C.N., Andrade, E.H.A., Silva, J.K.R. and Maia, J.G.S. (2009). Essential oil composition of *Croton palanostigma* Klotzsch from North Brazil. *Journal of Brazilian Chemical Society*, **20**: 1188-1192.

Corrêa, R.G.C., Silva, M.L., Maia J.G.S., Gottlieb O.R., Mourão, J.C.M., Marx, M.C., Moraes, A.A., Koketsu, M., Moura, L.L. and Magalhães. M,T, (1972). Óleos essenciais de espécies do gênero *Calyptrantes*. *Acta Amazonica*, **2**: 53-54.

Costa A.F. (1975). Farmacognosia, vol.1. Fundação Calouste Gulbeukian, Lisboa.

Costa, E.V., Pinheiro, M.L., Silva, J.R.A., Lameiro, B. H., Maia, N.S., amd Duarte, M.C.T. (2009). Antimicrobial and antileishmanaial activity of essential oil from the leaves of *Annona foetida* (Annonaceae). *Química Nova*, **32**: 78-81.

Costa, P.R.R. (2000). Safrol e eugenol: estudo da reatividade química e uso em síntese de produtos naturais biologicamente ativos e seus derivados. *Química Nova*, **23**: 357-369.

Duarte, M.C.T., Figueira, G.M., Sartoratto, A., Rehder, V.L.G., and Delarmelin, C. (2005). Anti-*Candida* activity of Brazilian medicinal plants. *Journal of Ethnopharmacology*, **97**: 305-311.

Duarte, M.C.T., Leme, E.E., Delarmelina, C., Soares, A.A., Figueira, G.M. and Sartoratto, A. (2007). Activity of essential oils from Brazilian medicinal plants on*Escherichia coli*. *Journal of Ethnopharmacology*, **111**: 197-201.

Estrela, J.L.V., Fazolin, M., Catani, V., Alécio, M.R. and Lima, M.S. (2006). Toxicidade de óleos essenciais de *N12* e *Piper hispidinervum* em *Sitophilus zeamais*. *Pesquisa Agropecuária Brasileira*, **41**: 217-222.

Fazolin, M., Estrela, J.L.V., Lima, A.P. and Argolo, V.M. (2002). Boletim de Pesquisa e Desenvolvimento: Avaliação de Plantas com Potencial Inseticida no Controle da Vaquinha-do-feijoeiro (*Cerotoma tingomarianus* Bechyné). *Boletim de Pesquisa - Ministério da Agricultura Pecuária e Abastecimento* **37**: 45-45.

Figueiredo, F.J.C., Rocha-Neto, O.G. and Alves, S.M. (2004). Avaliação de Diferentes Tipos de Cortes da Biomassa Aérea de Pimenta Longa. *Boletim de Pesquisa – Embrapa*, **28**: 34-34.

Flamini, G., Cioni, P.L., Maccioni, S., Baldini, R. (2010). Essential oil composition and in vivo volatiles emission by different parts of *Coleostephus myconis capitula*. *Journal of the Brazilian Chemical Society*, **5**: 1321-4.

Gentry, A.H. (1993). Woody Plants of Northwest South America (Colombia, Ecuador, Peru). Conservation International, Washington DC.

Gobbo-Neto, L. and Lopes, N.P. (2007). Plantas Medicinais: Fatores de Influência no Conteúdo de Metobólitos Secundários. *Qu;ímica Nova*, **30**: 374-381.

Gottlieb, O.R., Koketsu, M., Magalhães, M.T., Maia, J.G.S., Mendes, P.H., Rocha, A.I., Silva. M,L, and Wilberg, V.C. (1981). Óleos essenciais da Amazônia VII. *Acta Amazonica*, **11**: 143-148.

Jirovetz, L., Buchbauer, G., Ruzicka, J., Shafi, M.P. and Rosamma, M.K. (2001). Analysis of *Cinnamomum zeylanicum* Blume leaf oil from south India. *Journal of Essential Oil Research*, **13**: 442-443.

Leal, C.M. (1999). Influência das condições de secagem no rendimento e na composição do óleo essencial de pimenta longa (*Piper hispidinervium* C.DC.). Dissertação de Mestrado, Universidade Federal do Pará, Belém. Brazil

Lima, R.K., Cardoso, M.G., Moraes, J.C., Melo, B. A., Rodrigues, V.G., and Guimarães, P.L. (2009). Atividade inseticida do óleo essencial de pimenta longa (*Piper hispidinervum* C. DC.) sobre lagarta-do-cartucho do milho *Spodoptera frugiperda* (J. E. Smith, 1797) (Lwpidoptera: Noctuidae). *Acta Amazonica*, **39**: 377 - 382.

Lobato, A.M., Ribeiro, A., Pinheiro, M.F.S. and Maia, J.G.S. (1989). Antividade Antimicrobiana de Óleos Essenciais da Amazônia. *Acta Amazonica*, **19**: 355-363.

Luz, A.I.R., Silva, J.D., Zoghbi, M.G.B., Andrade, E.H.A., Silva, M.H.L., Maia, J.G.S. (1999). The oils of *Pothomorphe umbellata* and *P. peltata*. *Journal of Essential Oil Research*, **11**: 479-481.

Magalhães, L.A., Lima, M.D., Marques, M.O.M., Facanali, R., Pinto, A.C.S., and Tadei, W.P. (2010). Chemical composition and larvicidal activity against *Aedes aegypti* larvae of essential oils from four *Guarea* species. *Molecules*, **15**: 5734-41.

Maia, J.G.S., Andrade, E.H.A., Carreira, L.M.M., Oliveira, J. and Araújo, J.S. (2005a). Essential oils of the Amazon *Guatteria* and *Guatteriopsis* species. *Flavour and Fragrance Journal*, **20**: 478-480.

Maia, J.G.S., Andrade, E.H.A., Silva, A.C.M., Oliveira, J., Carreira, L.M.M. and Araújo, J.S. (2005b). Leaf volatile oils from four Brazilian *Xylopia* species. *Flavour and Fragrance Journal*, **20**: 474-477.

Maia, J.G.S., Silva, M.L., Luz, A.I.R., Zoghbi, M.G.B. and Ramos, L.S. (1987). Espécies de *Piper* da Amazônia Ricas em Safrol. *Química Nova*, **3**: 200-204.

Maia, J.G.S., Zoghbi, M.G.B. and Andrade, E.H.A. (2000). Plantas Aromáticas na Amazônia e Seus Óleos Essenciais. Museu Paraense Emílio Goeldi (Coleção Adolpho Ducke), Belém, 186 pp.

Marques, D.D., Sartori, R.A, Lemos, T.L.G., Machado, L.L., Souza, J.S.N., Monte, F.J.Q. (2010). Chemical composition of the essential oils from two subspecies of *Protium heptaphyllum*. *Acta Amazonica*, **40**: 227-230.

Möllenbeck, S., König, T., Schreier, P., Schwab, W., Rajaonarivony, J., and Ranarivelo, L. (1997). Chemical composition and analyses of enantiomers of essential oils from Madagascar. *Flavour and Fragrance Journal*, **12**: 63-69.

Morais, A.A., Mourão, J.C., Gottlieb, O.R., Silva, M.L., Marx, M.C., Maia, J.G.S. and Magalhães, M.T. (1972). Óleos essenciais da Amazônia contendo Timol. *Acta Amazonica*, **2**: 45-46.

Mortimer, E.F. (2006). Coleção Explorando o Ensino. Ministério da Educação, Brasília, 222pp.

Navickiene, H.M.D., Morandim, A.A., Alécio, A.C., Regasini, L.O., Bergamo, D.C.B., Telascrea, M., Cavalheiro, A.J., Lopes, M.N., Bolzai, V.S., Furlan, M., Marques, M.O.M., Young, M.C.M. and Kato, M.J. (2006). Composition and antifungal activity of essential oils from *Piper aduncum, Piper arboreum and Piper tuberculatum*. *Química Nova*, **29**: 467-470.

Pimentel, F.A. and Pinheiro, P.S.N. (2000). Boletim de Pesquisa: Mapeamento e Caracterização de Habitats Naturais de Pimenta Longa (*Piper hispidinervium*) no Município de Brasiléia. *Boletim de Pesquisa – Embrapa*, **28**: 20-20.

Pimentel, F.A., Cardoso, G., Batista, L.R., Lima, L.G., Silva, D.M. (2010). Ação fungitóxica do óleo essencial de *Tanaecium nocturnum* (Barb. Rodr.) Bur. e K. Shum sobre o *Aspergillus flavus* isolado da castanha-do-Brasil (Bertholletia excelsa). *Acta Amazonica*, 40: 213 - 220.

Pio Correa, M. (1984). Dicionários de plantas úteis do Brasil e das exóticas cultivadas, vol.1. Ministério da Agricultura, Brasília.

Plowden, J.C. (2001). The ecology, management and marketing of non-timber forest products in the alto Rio Guamá Indigenous Reserve (Eastern Brasilian Amazon). PhD Thesis, The Pennsylvania State University, Pensilvania.

Ramos, M.F.S., Siani, A.C., Tappim, M.R.R., Guimarães, A.C., Ribeiro, J.E.L.S. (2000). Essential oils from oleoresin of *Protium* spp. of the Amazon region. *Flavor and Fragrance Journal*, **15**: 383-387.

Rabha, L.C., Baruah, A.K.S. and Bordoloi, D.N. (1979). Search for aroma chemicals of commercial value from plant resources of Northeast India. *Indian Perfumer*, **23**: 173-183.

Rebelo, M.M., Silva, J.K., Andrade, E.H., Maia, J.G. (2009). Antioxidant capacity and biological activity of essential oil and methanol extract of *Conobea scoparioides* (Cham. and Schltdl.) Benth. *Journal of the Brazilian Chemical Society*, **20**: 1031-1035.

Ribeiro, J.E.L. and Daly, D.C. (1999). Burseraceae. In: Flora da reserva Ducke: Guia de identificação das plantas vasculares de uma floresta de terra firme na Amazônia Central, Ed. By Ribeiro, J.E.L., Hopkins, M.J.G., Vicentini, A., Sothers, C.A., Costa, M.A.S.,

Ross, M.S.F. (1976). Analysis of cinnamon oils by high-pressure liquid chromatography. *Journal of Chromatography*, **118**: 273-275.

Santos, A.S., Andrade, E.H.A., Zoghbi, M.G.B., Luz, A.I.R., and Maia, J.G.S. (1998). Sesquiterpenos of Amazonian *Piper* Species. *Acta Amazonica*, **28**: 127-130.

Senanayake, U.M., Lee, T.H. and Wills, R.B.H. (1978). Volatile constituents of cinnamon (*Cinnamomum zeylanicum*) oils. *Journal of Agricultural and Food Chemistry*, **26**: 822-824.

Silva, M.F., Lisboa, P.L.B., and Lisboa, R.C.L. (1977). Nomes vulgares de plantas. INPA,

Thomas, J., Greetha, K. and Shylara, K.S. (1987). Studies on leaf oil and quality of *Cinnamomum zeylanicum*. *Indian Perfumer*, **31**: 249-251

Thulin, M., Beier, B.A., Razafimandimbison, S.G., Banks, H.I. (2008). Ambilobea, a new genus from Madagascar, the position of Aucoumea and comments on the ribal classification of the frankincense and myrrh family (Burseraceae). *Nordic Journal of Botany*, **26**: 218-229.

Variyar, P.S. and Bandyopadhyay, C. (1989). On some chemical aspects of *Cinnamomum zeylanicum*. *PAFAI Journal*, **10**: 35-38.

Weeks, A., Daly, D.C. and Sympson, B.B. (2005). The phylogenetic history and biogeography of the frankincense and myrrh family (Burseraceae) based on nuclear and chloroplast sequence data. *Molecular Phylogenetics Evolution*, **35**: 85-101.

Zacaroni, L.M., Cardoso, M.G., Souza, P.E., Pimentel, F.A., Guimarães, L.G.L., and Salgado, A.P.S.P. (2009). Potencial fungitóxico do óleo essencial de Piper hispidinervum (pimenta longa) sobre os fungos oxysporum e Colletotrichum gloeosporioides. *Acta Amazonica*, **39**: 193 - 198.

Zoghbi, M.G.B., Andrade, E.H.A., Silva, M.H.L., Maia, J.G.S., Luz, A.I.R. and Silva, J.D. (2001). Chemical variation in the essential oils of *Hyptis crenata* Pohl ex Benth. *Flavour and Fragrance Journal*, **17**: 5-8.

Bioactive Phytochemicals: Perspectives for Modern Medicine Vol. 1 (2012) *Pages* **277–329**
Editor: **V.K. Gupta**
Published by: **DAYA PUBLISHING HOUSE, NEW DELHI**

8

Phytochemical and Pharmacological Profile of Plants belonging to *Strychnos* Genus: A Review

P. Rajesh[1*], V. Rajesh Kannan[1], S. Latha[2] and P. Selvamani[2]

ABSTRACT

Strychnos is a medicinally important genus belonging to the family of Loganiaceae consisting of about 7 subfamily 64 genus; among one of the genus Strychnos having 394 species, which were widely distributed in tropical and subtropical India. The main goal of the present comprehensive review is to present the research carried out with species of the Strychnos genus, widely spread in the world, in order to organize the data produced as resource for reference piece. This review summarizes various reported phytoconstituents, its chemical structure and the corresponding pharmacological activities reported in various species of the Strychnos genus. There were around 185 phytoconstituents comprising alkaloids; N_b-C(21) secocuran alkaloids, zwitterionic alkaloid, quarternary alkaloid, quarternary indole alkaloid, tertiary alkaloids, trimeric indolomonoterpenic alkaloid, N_b-methylated β-carbolinium alkaloid, gluco-alkaloid, usambarine alkaloid, gluco-indole alkaloid; indole alkaloid and dimeric indole alkaloid; carbohydrates such as glucoside, iridoid glucoside, lignan glucosides and polysaccharides; glycosides namely phenolic glycosides; major flavonoids; quarternary phenolic bases, β-carboline derivatives, iridoids, pimarane diterpenoid, imidofuranyl

1 Department of Microbiology, Bharathidasan University, Tiruchirappalli – 620 024, Tamil Nadu, India.

2 Department of Pharmaceutical Technology, Anna University of Technology, Tiruchirappalli – 620 024, Tamil Nadu, India.

* *Corresponding author*: E-mail: pandiyanrajesh@rocketmail.com

carbamates, enolate methyl compounds, dimeric derivatives and trimeric derivatives. The chemical structures of reported phytoconstituents and its corresponding pharmacological activities from 37 species of the Strychnos genus were reviewed here.

Keywords: *Strychnos*, Loganiaceae, Brucine, Strychnine.

Abbreviations

TLC: Thin layer chromatography
HPLC: High performance liquid chromatography
MPLC: Medium pressure liquid chromatography
NMR: Nuclear magnetic resonance spectroscopy
IR: Infrared spectroscopy
FT-IR: Fourier transform infrared spectroscopy
UV: Ultraviolet spectroscopy
1D and 2D NMR: One dimensional and two dimensional NMR
MS: Mass spectroscopy
GLC-MS: Gas liquid chromatography and Mass spectroscopy
GC-MS: Gas chromatography and Mass spectroscopy
LC-MS: Liquid chromatography and Mass spectroscopy
ESI-MS: Electron spectroscopic imaging and Mass spectroscopy
ES-MS/MS: Electronspray mass spectroscopy
MEKC: Micellar electrokinetic chromatography
SDS: Sodium dodecyl sulphate
CCl_4: Carbon tetra-chloride
Me_2CO: Acetone
MALDI-TOFMS: Matrix assisted laser desorption ionization–mass spectroscopy

Introduction

India is richly endowed with a wide variety of plants having medicinal value. These plants are widely used by all sections of the society either directly as folk remedies or indirectly as pharmaceutical preparation of modern medicine. Its medicinal usage has been reported in the traditional systems of medicine such as Ayurveda, Siddha and Unani. *Strychnos* has been described as a rasayana herb and has been used extensively for various medicinal purposes (Gricilda Shoba *et al.*, 2001).

The genus *Strychnos,* the largest genus of the family Loganiaceae, was first described by Linnaeus on the basis of *S. nux-uomica,* the type species, and *S. colubrina* (*S. minor*). It is pantropical and comprises about 200 species, which may be subdivided into three geographically separated groups: one in Africa with 75 species; one in America with 73 species; and one in Asia (including Australia) with 44 species. The only exception is *S. potatorum* which is found both in Africa and Asia (Ohiri *et al.*, 1983).

The ethnobotanical uses of the South American species of *Strychnos* L. were reported in (Joelle Quetin Leclercq *et al.*, 1990). The study has been reported that 50 species from *Strychnos* genus among 140 samples reported to possess pyridine-indoloquinolizidinone bases (Joelle Quetin Leclercq *et al.*, 1990).

Pharmacology and Phytochemistry of the Strychnos Species

Strychnos axillaris

Five phenolic glycosides 6′-O-β-D-apiofuranosylcalleryanin **(1)**, 5′′-O-*trans*-feruloyl-6′-O-b-D-apiofuranosylcalleryanin **(2)**, 5′′-O-*trans*-feruloyl-6′-O-β-dapiofuranosylvanilloloside **(3)**, 7-O-*trans*-caffeoylvanilloloside **(4)**, 4′′-O-β-D-glucopyranosyl-caffeoylcalleryanin **(5)** and one iridoid glucoside as axillaroside **(6)** together with 22 known compounds such as tachioside **(7)**, isotachioside **(8)**, 3,4,5-trimethoxyphenol-1-O-β-D-apiofuranosyl-(1?6)-β-D-glucopyranoside **(9)**, calleryanin **(10)**, vanilloloside **(11)**, 3,5-dimethoxy-4-hydroxybenzyl alcohol 4-O-b-D-glucopyranoside **(12)**, caffeoylcalleryanin **(13)**, (7S, 8R)-balanophonin-4-O-b-D-glucopyranoside **(14)**, (+)-syringaresinol-O-β-D-glucoside **(15)**, scorzonoside **(16)**, liriodendrin **(17)**, (-)-pinoresinol-4′-O-β-D-glucopyranoside **(18)**, (+)-lariciresinol 4′-O-β-D-glucoside **(19)**, loganic acid **(20)**, loganin **(21)**, sweroside **(22)**, picconioside I **(23)**, cantleyoside **(24)**, triplostoside A **(25)**, strictosidinic acid **(26)**, 3,4-di-O-caffeoylquinic acid **(27)**, and 3,5-di-O-caffeoylquinic acid **(28)** were isolated and characterized from the dried bark and wood of methanolic extract of *Strychnos axillaris* by using reversed phase TLC (precoated Kieselgel $60F_{254}$ plates), GLC (Supelco SPB column), HPLC, MPLC (Wakogel FC-40 or Wakosil 40C18), UV and NMR analysis. The structures of the isolated compounds were characterized by spectral and chemical methods (Atsuko Itoh *et al.*, 2008).

Strychnos bicirohssa

The ethanolic extract of *Strychnos bicirohssa* reported to possess anti-inflammatory activity in carrageenan, cotton pellet and croton oil induced oedema models. The study has been reported that anti-inflammatory activity by inhibiting paw volume elevation, ear swelling and cotton pellet granuloma weight altitude (Rajesh *et al.*, 2009).

Strychnos diaboli

Strychnine **(29)**, diaboline **(30)** and deacetyldiaboline **(31)** were obtained from the bark of *Strychnos diaboli* Sandw. by using TLC and HPLC (Marini bettolo, *et al.*, 1972). The quaternary bases were also found to be flourocurarine **(32)**, alkaloids F **(33)**, G **(34)** and K **(35)** (Pellieciari *et al.*, 1966).

Strychnos diplotricha

Three new N_b, C(21)-secocuran alkaloids, *viz.*, 3-*epi*-myrtoidine **(36)**, 11-demethoxy-3-*epi*-myrtoidine **(37)** and 11-demethoxy-12-hydroxy-3-*epi*-myrtoidine **(38)** and two known compounds such as myrtoidine **(39)** and 11-demethoxymyrtoidine **(40)** were isolated and characterized from the stem bark of *Strychnos diplotricha* by using mass and NMR spectroscopy (Philippe Rasoanaivo *et al.*, 2001).

Table 8.1: Phytoconstituents classification in *Strychnos* genus.

	Nos.		*Nos.*
Alkaloids		**Flavonoids**	
Dimeric alkaloids	4	Mojor flavonoids	3
Dimeric indole alkaloid	1	**Glycosides**	
Gluco-alkaloid	2	Phenolic glycosides	5
Gluco-indole alkaloid	1	**Phenolic bases**	
Indole alkaloid	3	Dimeric derivative	11
Major/Minor alkaloids	112	Enolate methyl compounds	2
N_b C(21) secocuran alkaloids	3	Imidofuranyl carbamates	3
N_b-methylated β-carbolinium alkaloid	2	Iridoids	3
Quarternary alkaloid	2	Pimarane diterpenoid	1
Quarternary indole alkaloid	2	Quarternary base	2
Tertiary alkaloids	1	Trimeric derivative	1
Trimeric indolomonoterpenic alkaloid	2	β-carboline compounds	2
Usambarine alkaloid	5		
Zwitterionic alkaloid	1		
Carbohydrates			
Glucoside	1		
Iridoid glucoside	3		
Lignan glucosides	2		
Polysaccharides	5		

Strychnos guianensis

A zwitterionic alkaloid named guianensine **(41)** was isolated from the stem bark of the *Strychnos guianensis* and characterized by using mass spectroscopy, 1D and 2D NMR studies (Quetin Leclercq *et al.*, 1995).

A new tertiary alkaloid 9-methoxygeissoschizol **(42)** was isolated from the powdered stem bark of the *S. guianensis* by using TLC (Silica gel) on various solvent system likely ethyl acetate, isopropanol, ammonium hydroxide; MPLC (Superformance silica gel 60) on benzene, methanol solvent system and the structures were characterized through NMR studies (Helene Mavar Manga *et al.*, 1996).

Two new quaternary alkaloids, 9-methoxy-N_b-methylgeissoschizol **(43)** and guiachrysine **(44)** together with the known compounds C-alkaloid O **(45)**, fluorocurine **(46)**, C-profluorocurine **(47)**, mavacurine **(48)**, macusine B **(49)** and guiaflavine **(50)** were isolated from the stem bark of *S. guianensis* was reported. The structures of the compounds were purified by using TLC (Silica gel) on various solvents such as methanol, MeCOONa, dimethyl ester; HPLC (stationary phase: ALTIMA C8 column) on heptanesulfonic acid with acetonitrile and characterized by using NMR studies (Jacques Penelle *et al.*, 2000).

Two new quaternary indole alkaloids *viz.*, 5′,6′-dehydroguiachrysine **(51)**, 5′,6′-dehydroguiaflavine **(52)** and two known flavonoid compounds *viz.*, guiachrysine **(44)**, guiaflavine **(50)** were isolated from the stem bark of *S. guianensis* by using HPLC analysis (Jacques Penelle *et al.*, 2001).

Strychnos henningsii

Strychnos henningsii Gilg. was used in African traditional medicine for the treatment of various ailments, including rheumatism, gastrointestinal complaints and snake bites. The reported pharmacological properties might be due to the presence of minor alkaloids such as retuline **(53)**, isoretuline **(54)**, holstiine **(55)** (Monique Tits *et al.*, 1991).

Strychnos icaja

Strychnine **(29)** and 4-hydroxystrychnine **(56)** has been isolated from the branch bark of *Strychnos icaja* by using TLC analysis. Strychnine **(29)** was accompanied with other strychnine series 4-hydroxystrychnine **(56)**, colubrine **(57)** and brucine **(58)**, the pseudo series pseudostrychnine **(59)**, pseudocolubrines **(60)**, pseudobrucine **(61)** and the N-methyl-sec-pseudo series icajine **(62)**, vomicine **(63)** and novacine **(64)** were isolated (Marini Bettolo, *et al.*, 1972).

Antiplasmodial sungucine **(65)** type alkaloid such as strychnogucine B **(66)** have been isolated from the distinctively red-colored roots of *S. icaja* Baillon., which were widely used in ordeal and arrow poisons in West and Central Africa and traditionally employed to treat malaria (Frederich *et al.*, 2001).

A natural trimeric indolomonoterpenic alkaloid of trisindole alkaloid, named strychnohexamine **(67)**, was isolated from the ethyl acetate extract of *S. icaja* roots by using TLC (Silica gel) on different solvents such as ethyl acetate, 2-propanol, ammonium hydroxide; MPLC (Merck LiChroprep RP-8) on methanol, methyl cyanide, water as solvent systems and characterized by using IR, UV, 1D and 2D NMR studies. The strychnohexamine **(67)** showed significant antiplasmodial activity against *Plasmodium falciparum*, moderately active than bisnordihydrotoxiferine **(68)**. (Genevieve Philippe, 2002).

A trimeric indolomonoterpenic alkaloid, called strychnohexamine **(67)** possessing antimalarial properties, also monomeric derivative alkaloids such as strychnine **(29)**, sungucine **(45)**, strychnoguine B **(66)** and bisindole quaternary alkaloid such as guiaflavine **(50)** was isolated from *S. icaja* as used for the arrow poison or ordeals (Genevieve Philippe, 2005).

The alkaloids strychnine **(29)**, sungucine **(65)**, strychnohexamine **(67)**, protostrychnine **(69)** and strychnogucine B **(66)** were isolated from the root bark of *S. icaja*. The study also reported the interaction with the strychnine-sensitive glycine receptor evidenced by whole-cell patch-clamp recordings on glycine-gated currents in mouse spinal cord neurons in culture and by [^{3}H] strychnine **(29)** competition assays on membranes from adult rat spinal cord (Genevieve Philippe, 2006).

The methanol and dichloromethane extracts of root bark of *S. icaja* has been reported to possess significant inhibition of the growth of *Plasmodium falciparum* strains *in-vivo* (Lusakibanza *et al.*, 2010).

Figure 8.1: Chemical compounds.

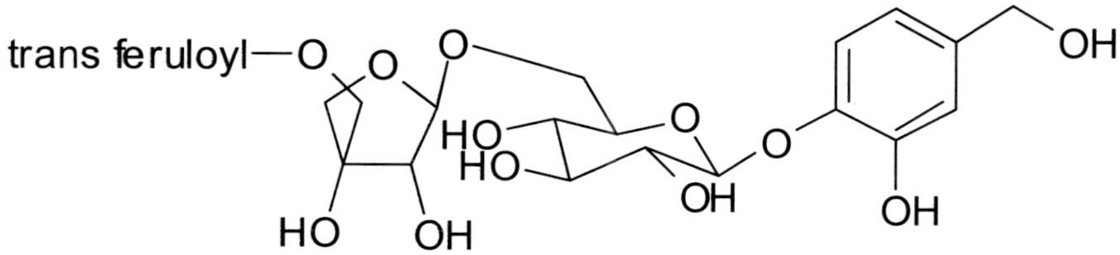

(1) 6'-O-β-D-apiofuranosylcalleryanin

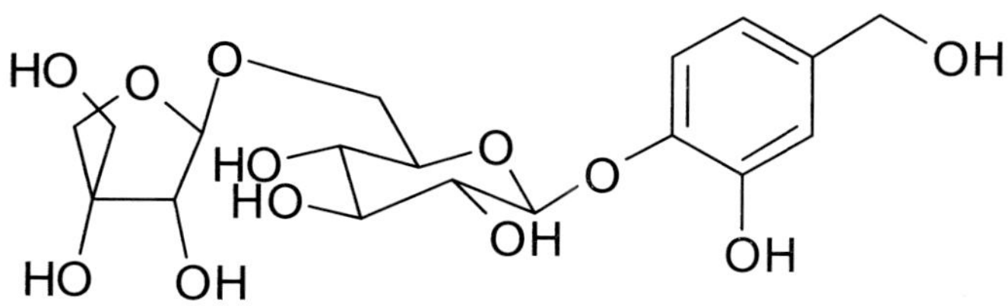

(2) 5''-O-*trans*-feruloyl-6'-O-β-D-apiofuranosylcalleryanin

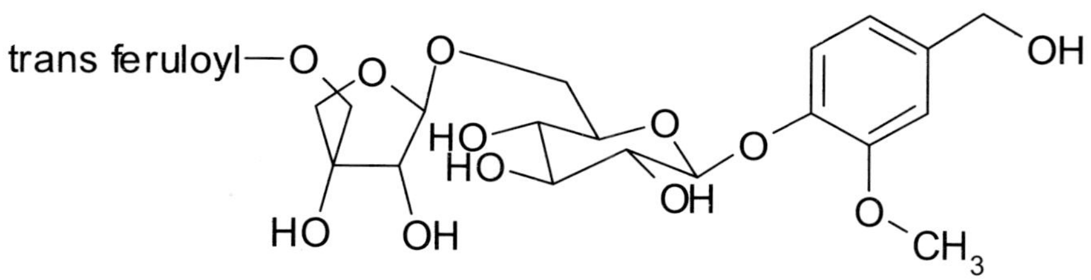

(3) 5''-O-*trans*-feruloyl-6'-O-β-dapiofuranosylvanilloloside

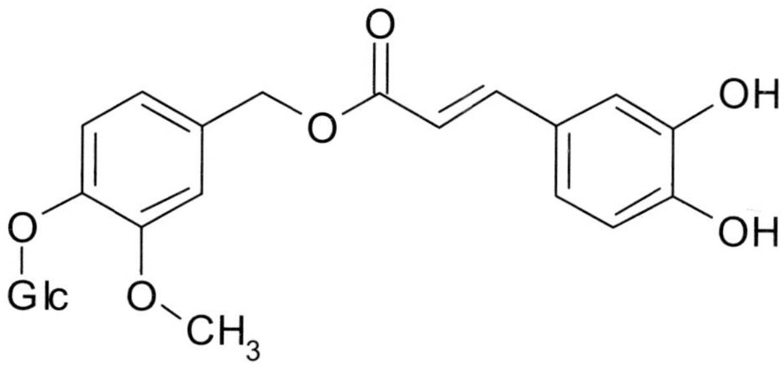

(4) 7-O-*trans*-caffeoylvanilloloside

Contd...

Figure 8.1–*Contd...*

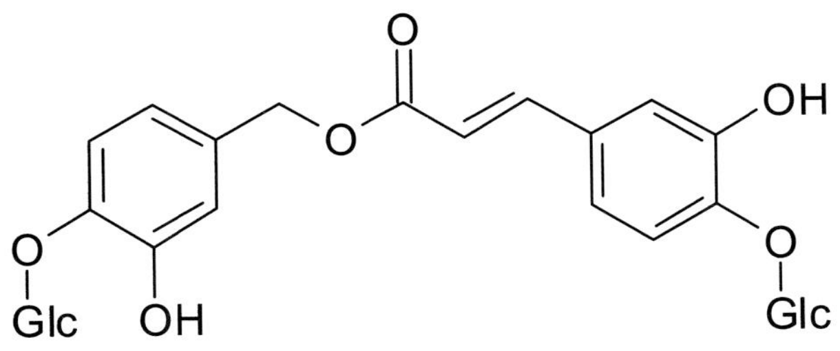

(5) 4”-O-β-D-glucopyranosyl-caffeoylcalleryanin

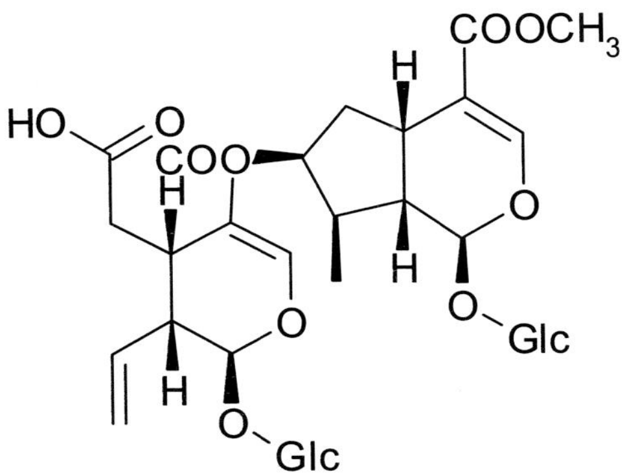

(6) Axillaroside

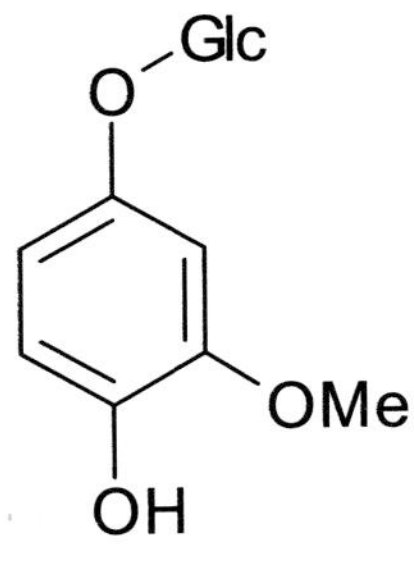

(7) Tachioside

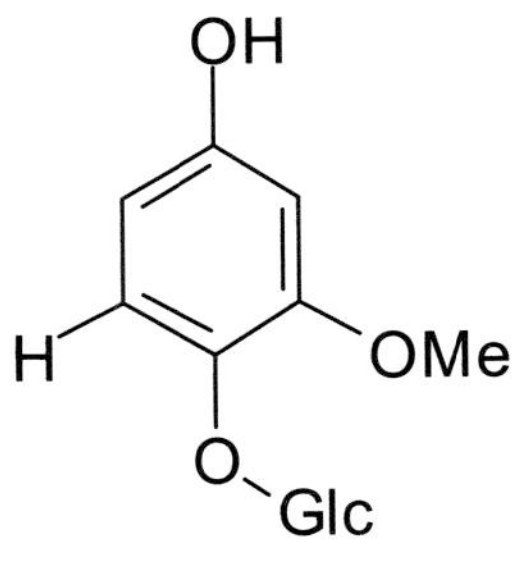

(8) Isotachioside

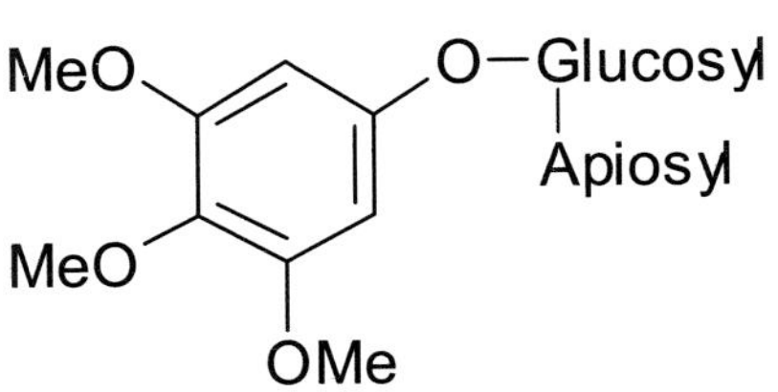

(9) 3,4,5-trimethoxyphenol-1-O-β-D-apiofuranosyl-(1-6)-b-D-glucopyranoside

Contd...

Figure 8.1–*Contd...*

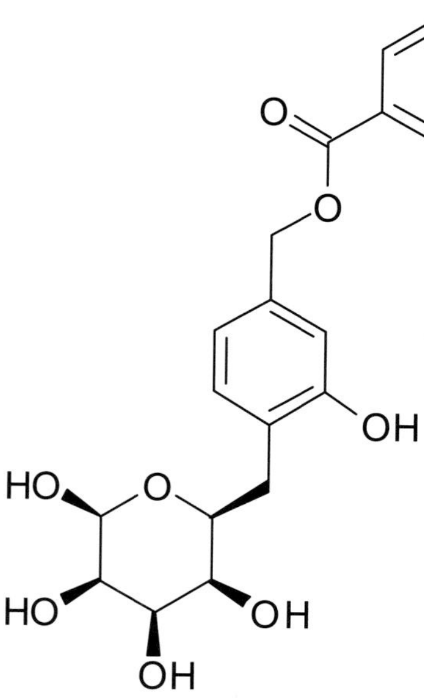

(10) Calleryanin

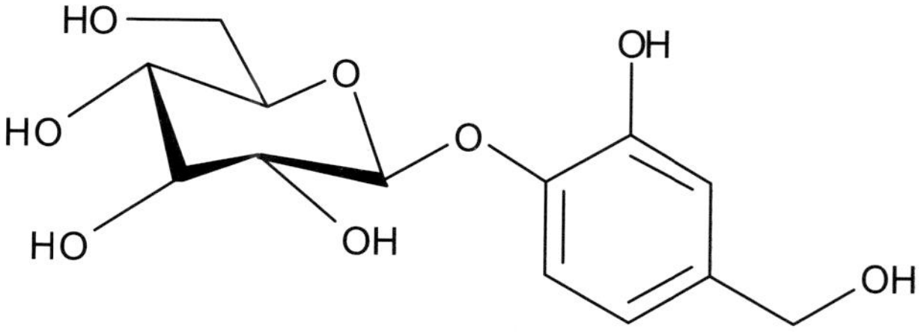

(11) Vanilloloside

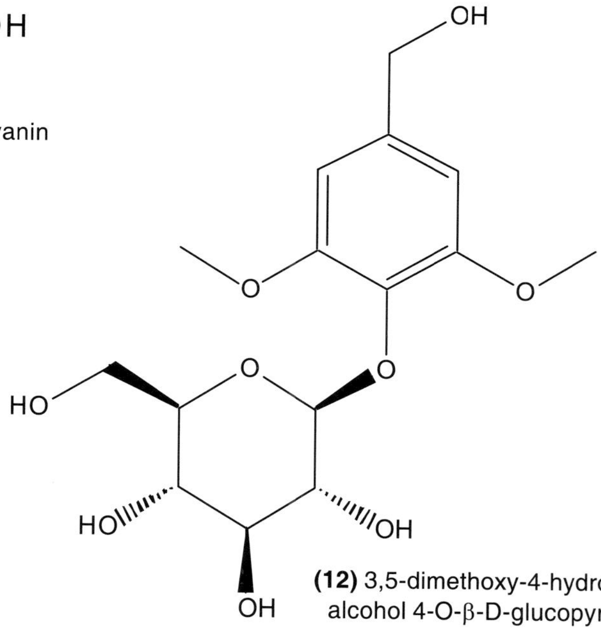

(12) 3,5-dimethoxy-4-hydroxybenzyl alcohol 4-O-β-D-glucopyranoside

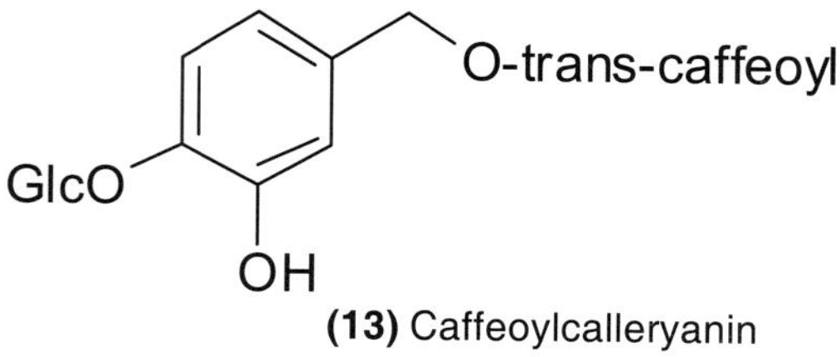

(13) Caffeoylcalleryanin

Contd...

Figure 8.1–*Contd...*

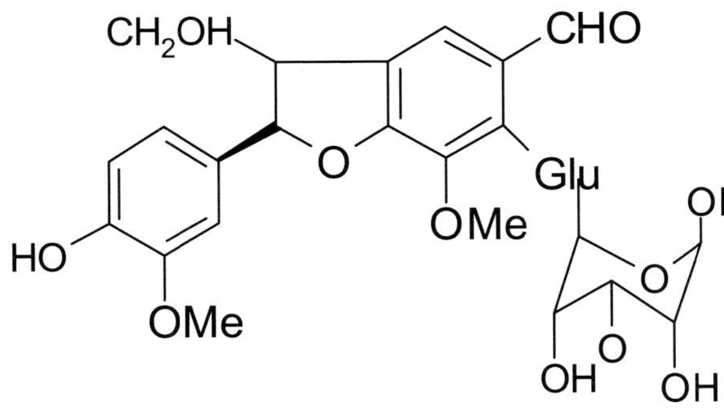

(14) (7S, 8R)-balanophonin-4-O-β-D-glucopyranoside

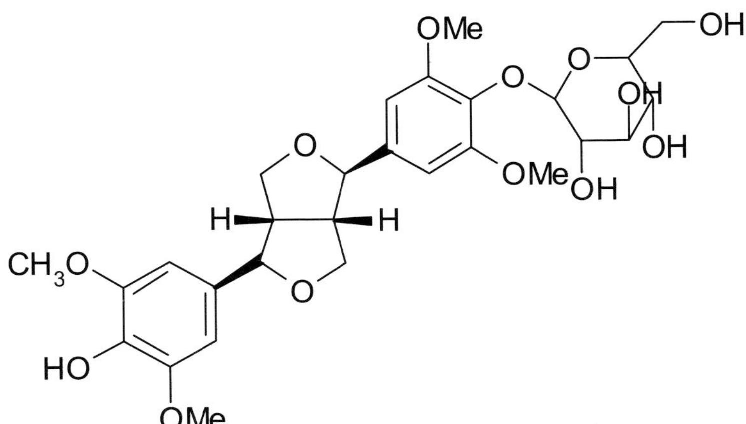

(15) (+)-syringaresinol-O-β-D-glucoside

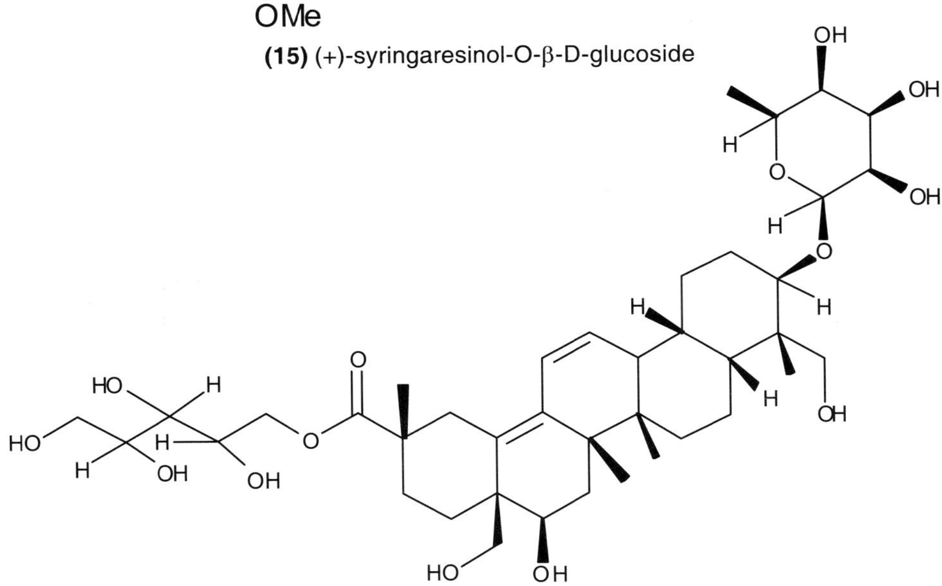

(16) Scorzonoside

Contd...

Figure 8.1–*Contd...*

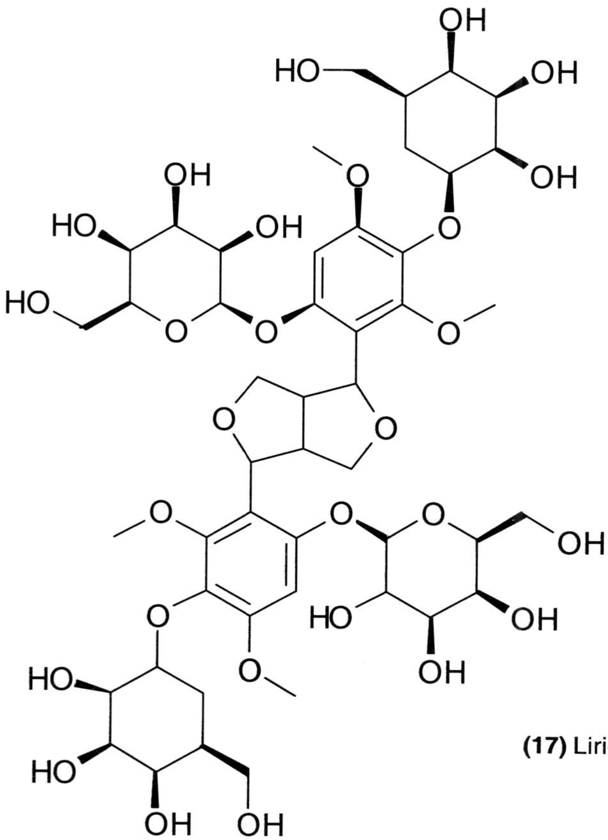

(17) Liriodendrin

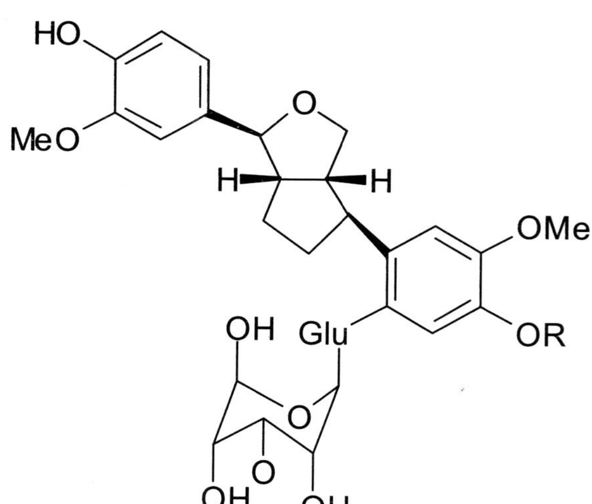

(18) (-)-pinoresinol-4'-O-β-D-glucopyranoside

Contd...

Figure 8.1–*Contd...*

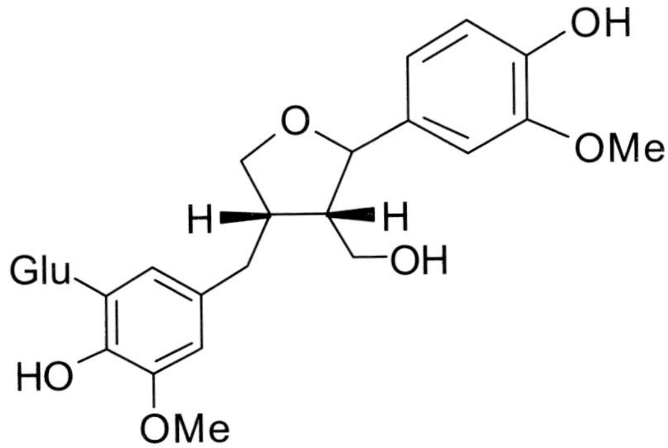

(19) (+)-lariciresinol 4'-O-β-D-glucoside

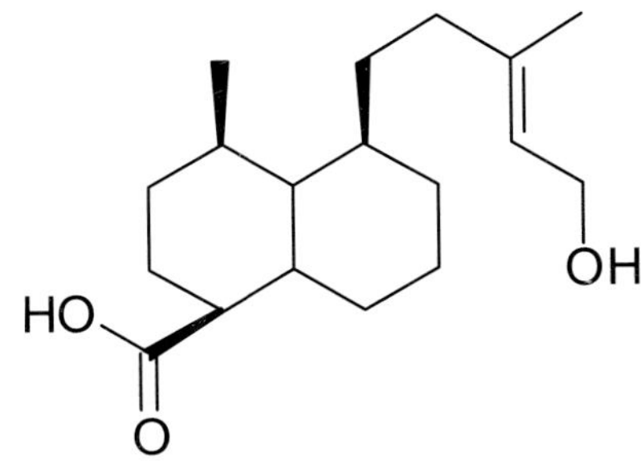

(20) Loganic acid

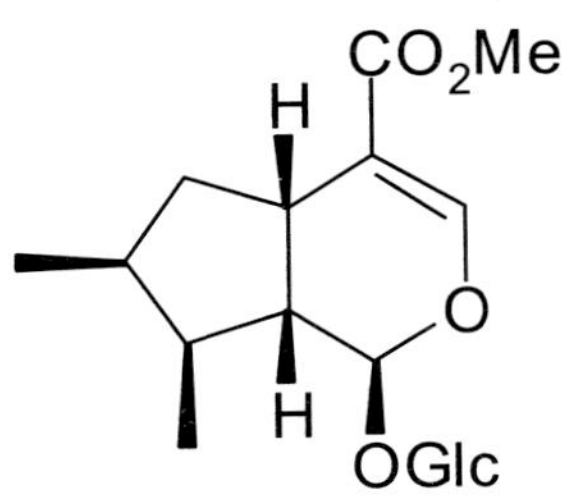

(21) Loganin

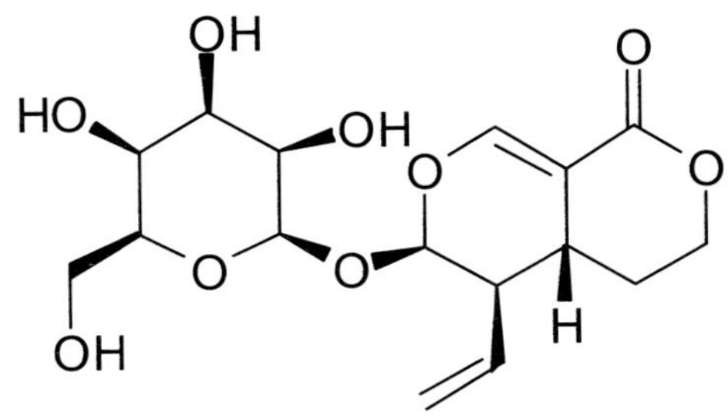

(22) Sweroside

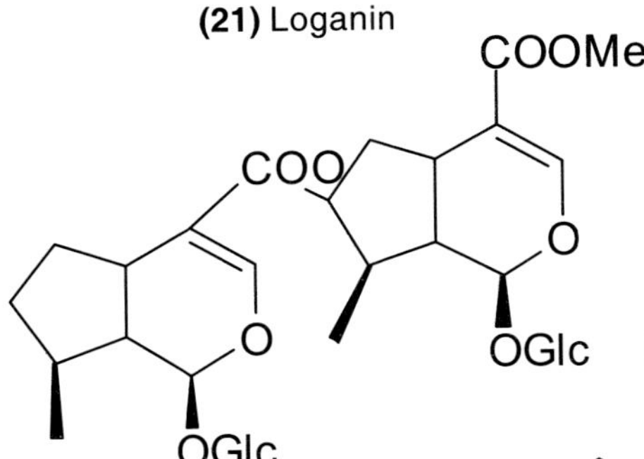

(23) Picconioside I

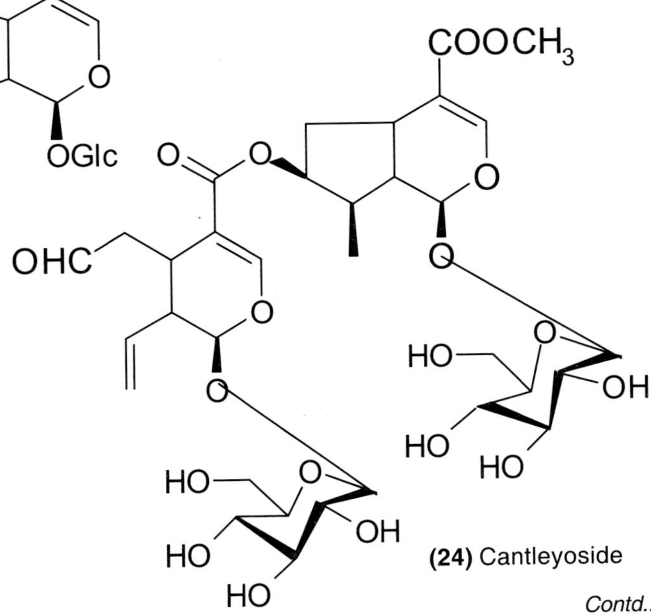

(24) Cantleyoside

Contd...

Figure 8.1–*Contd...*

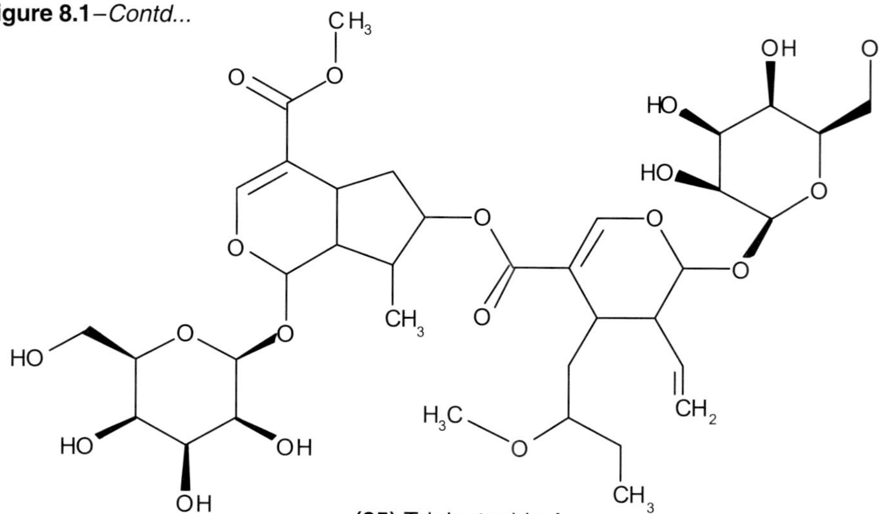

(25) Triplostoside A

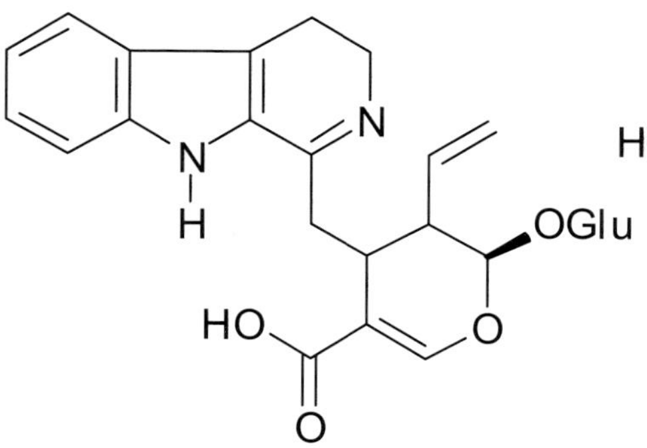

(26) Strictosidinic acid

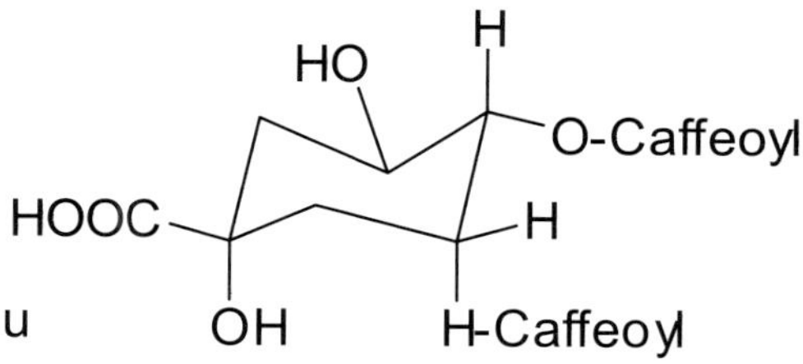

(27) 3,4-di-O-caffeoylquinic acid

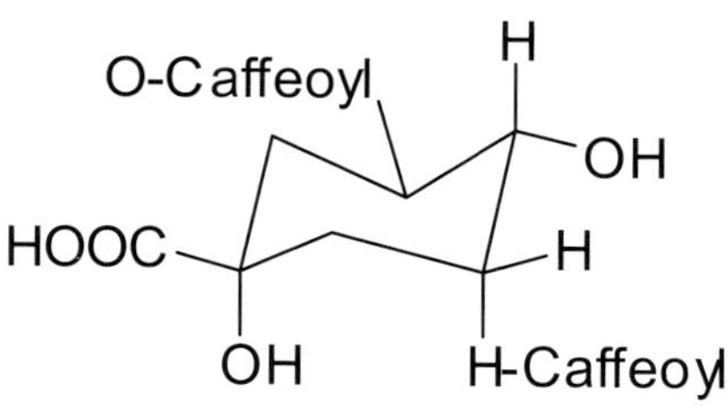

(28) 3,5-di-O-caffeoylquinic acid

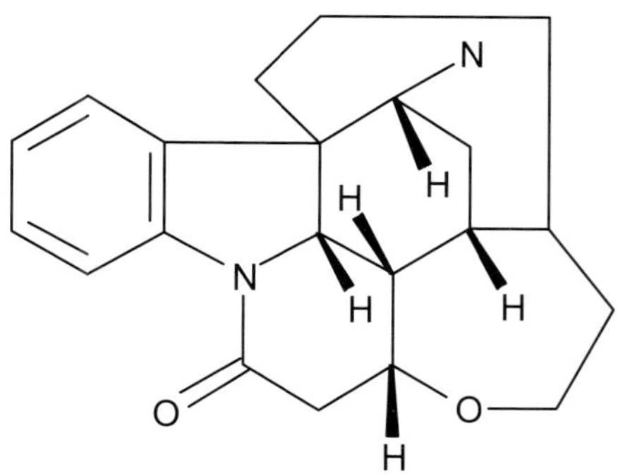

(29) Strychnine

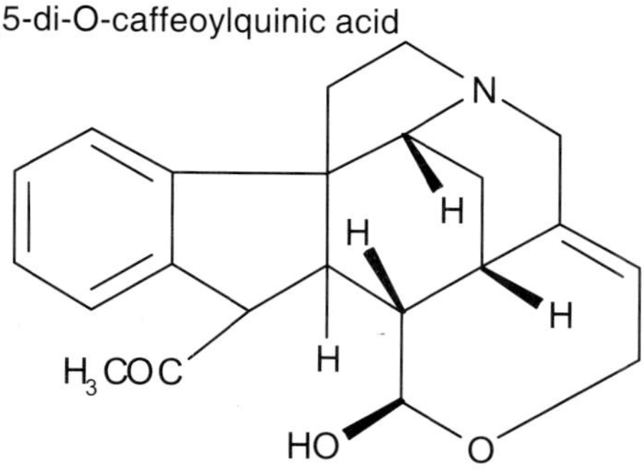

(30) Diaboline

Contd...

Figure 8.1–*Contd...*

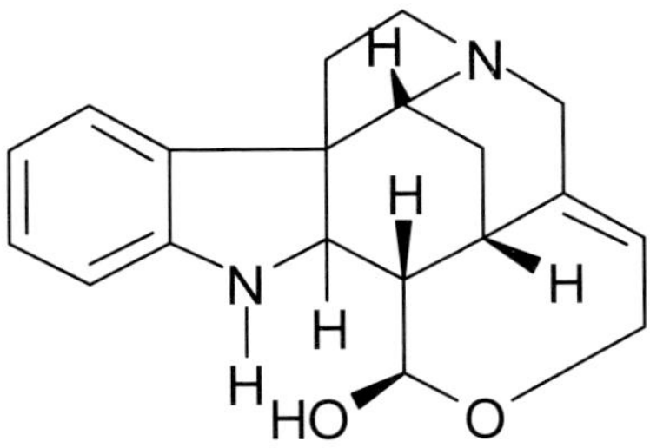

(31) Deacetyldiaboline

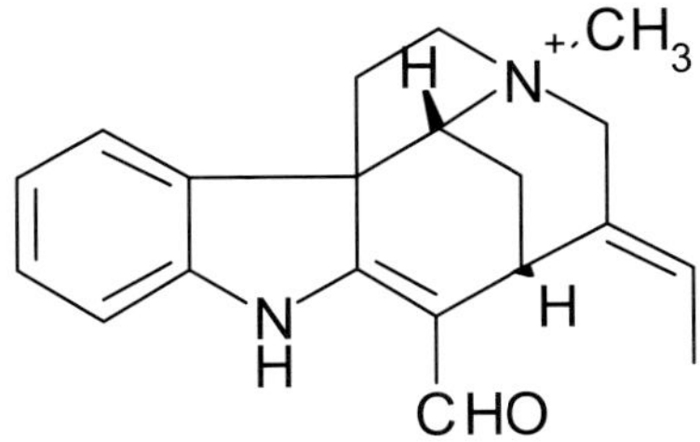

(32) Flourocurarine

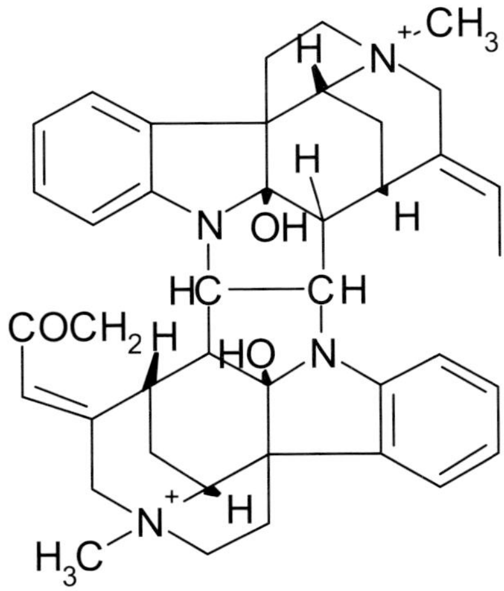

(33) Alkaloid F

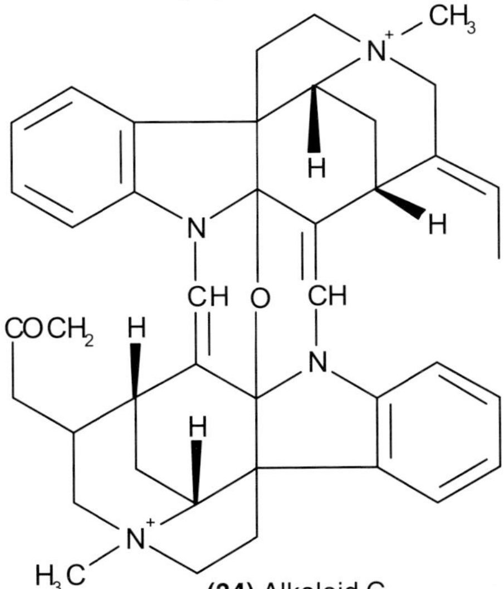

(34) Alkaloid G

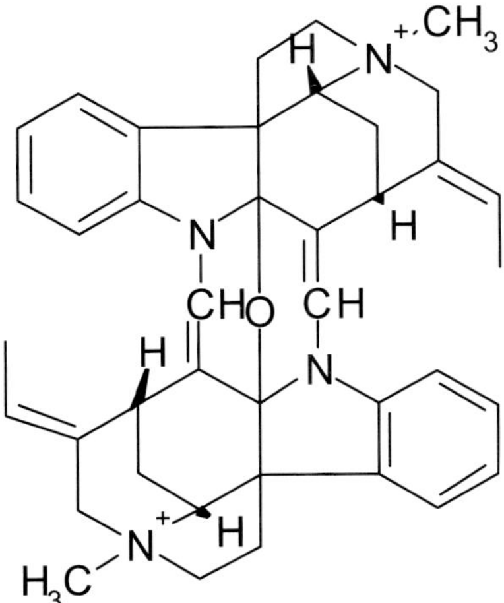

(35) Alkaloid K

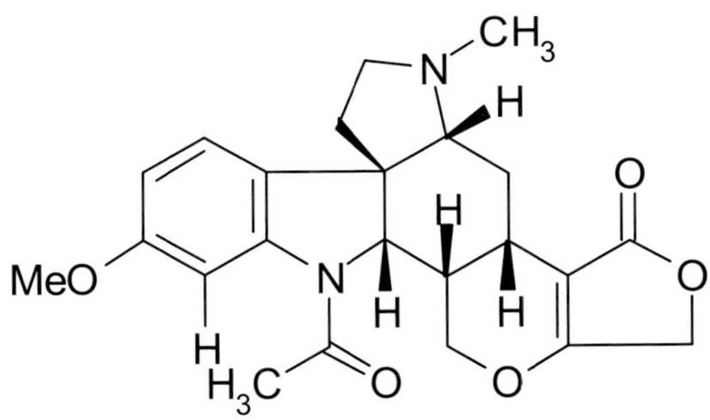

(36) 3-*epi*-myrtoidine

Contd...

Figure 8.1–*Contd...*

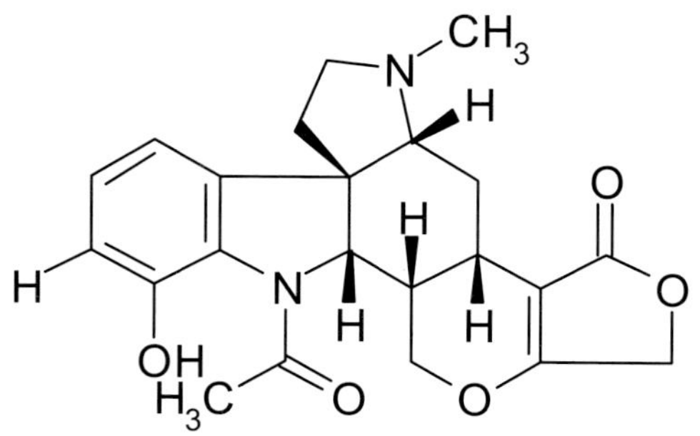

(37) 11-demethoxy-3-*epi*-myrtoidine

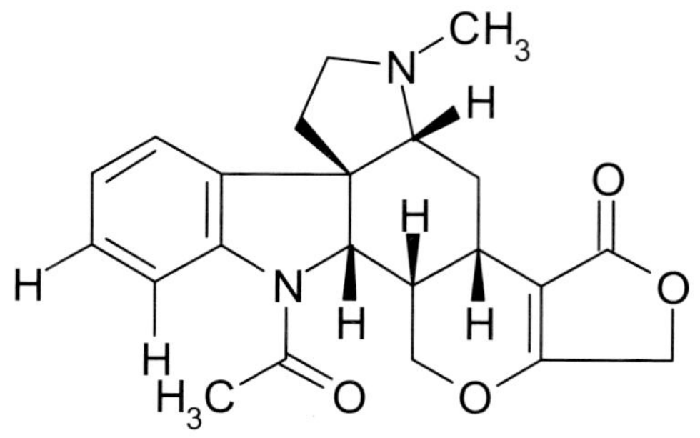

(38) 11-demethoxy-12-hydroxy-3-*epi*-myrtoidine

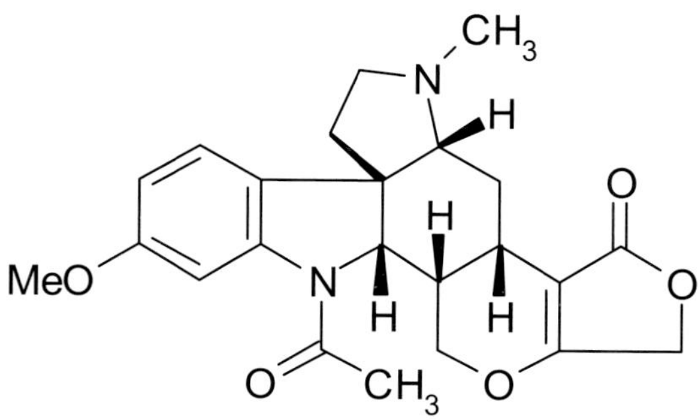

(39) Myrtoidine

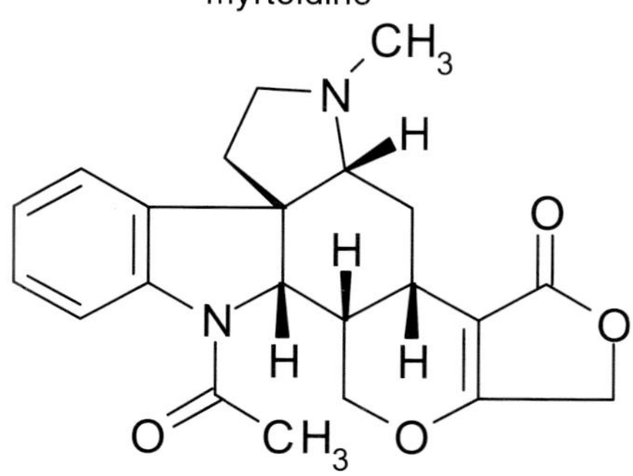

(40) 11-demethoxymyrtoidine

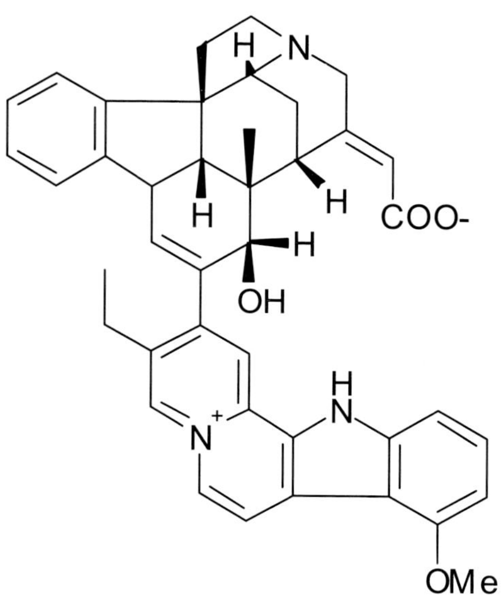

(41) Guianensine

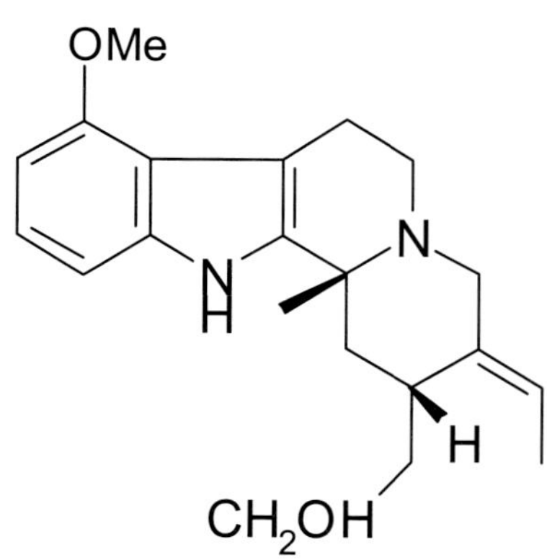

(42) 9-methoxygeissoschizol

Contd...

Figure 8.1–*Contd...*

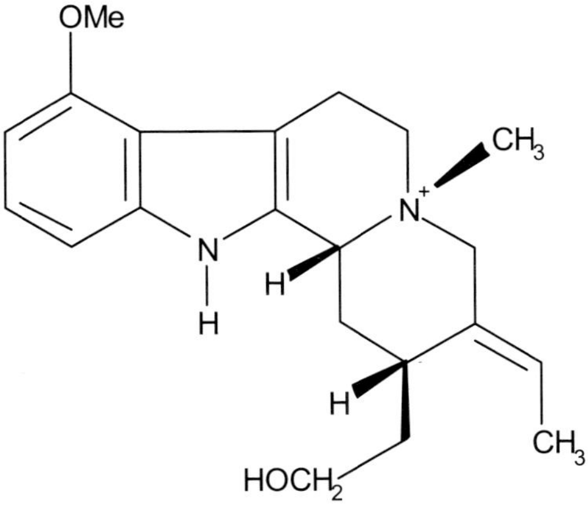

(43) 9-methoxy-N_b-methylgeissoschizol

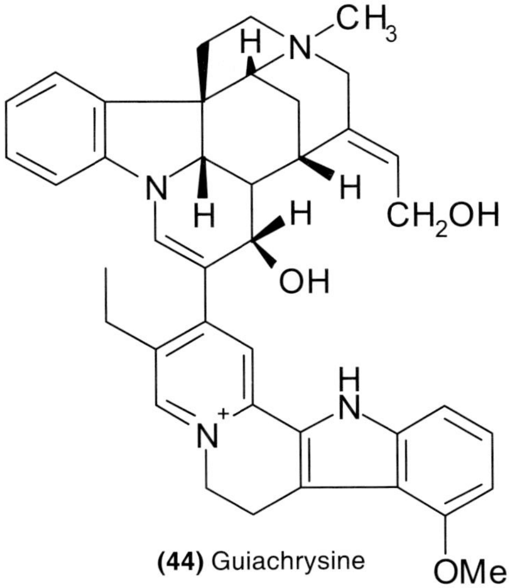

(44) Guiachrysine

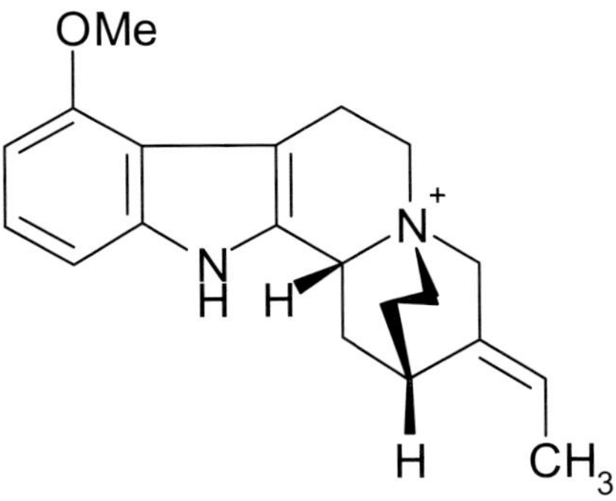

(45) C-alkaloid O

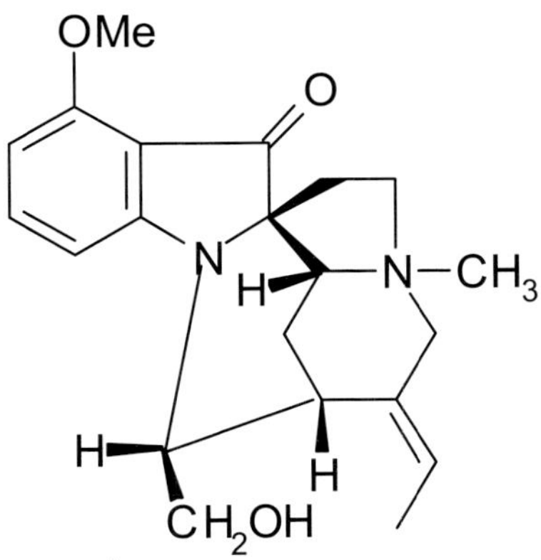

(46) Fluorocurine

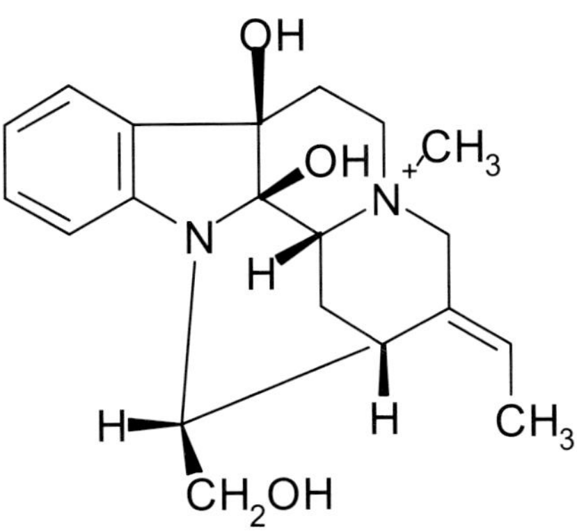

(47) C-profluorocurine

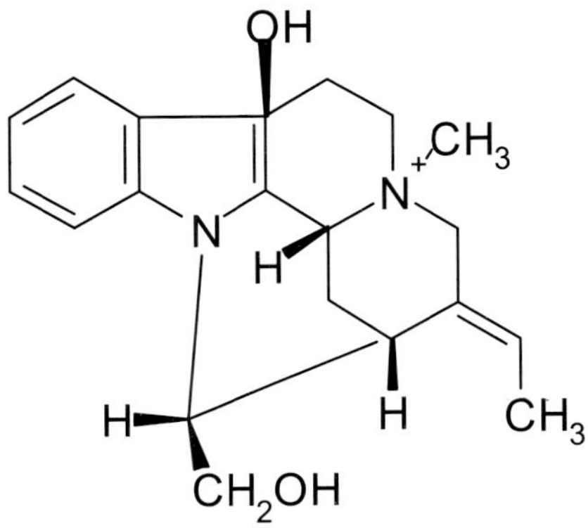

(48) Mavacurine

Contd...

Figure 8.1–*Contd...*

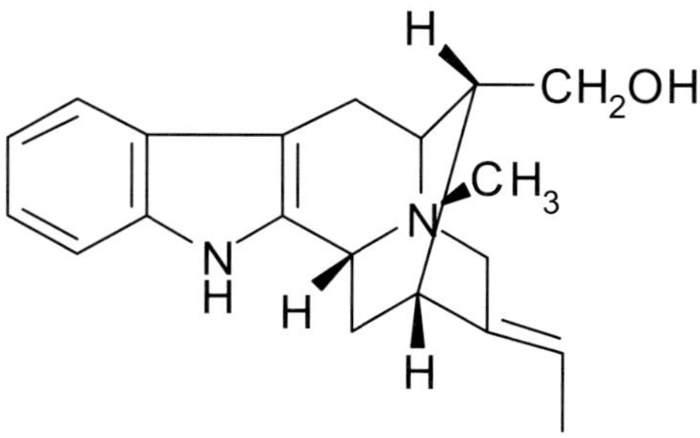

(49) Macusine B

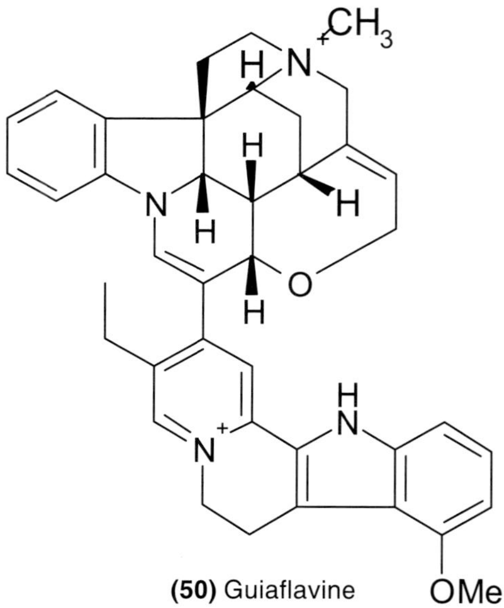

(50) Guiaflavine

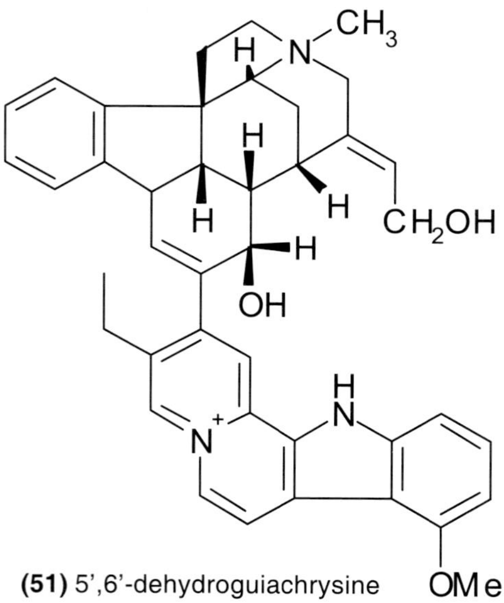

(51) 5',6'-dehydroguiachrysine

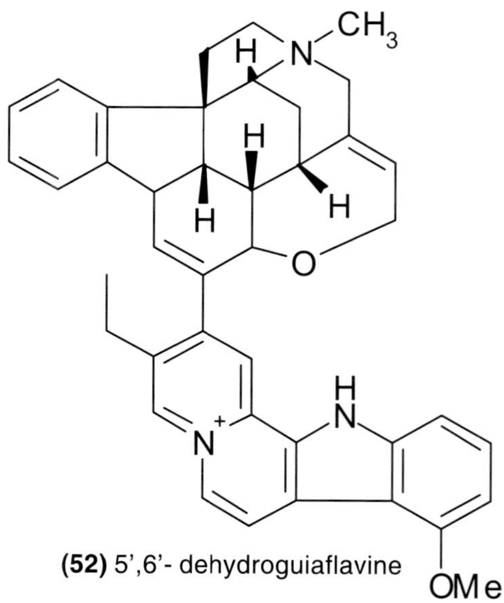

(52) 5',6'- dehydroguiaflavine

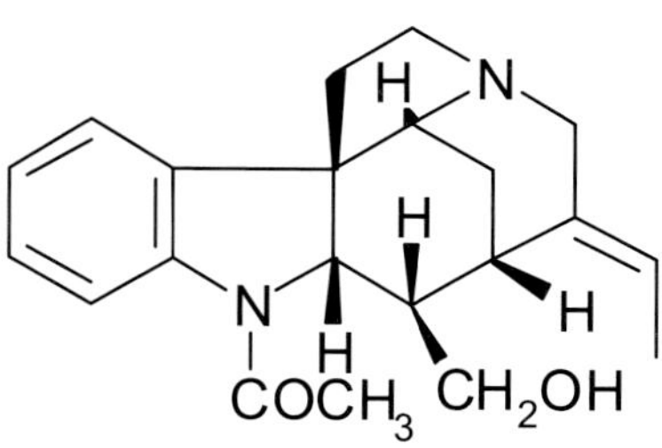

(53) Retuline

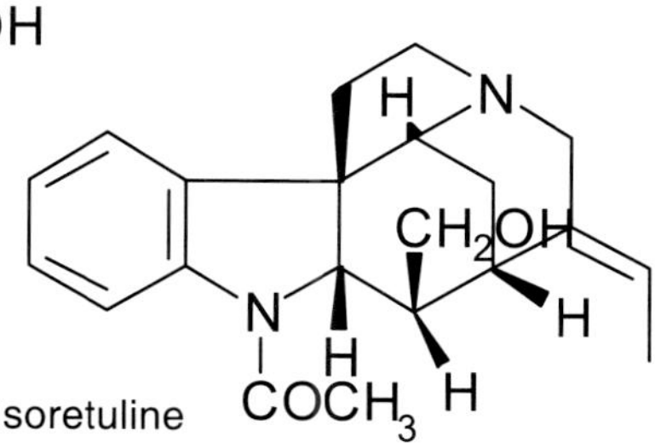

(54) Isoretuline

Contd...

Figure 8.1–*Contd...*

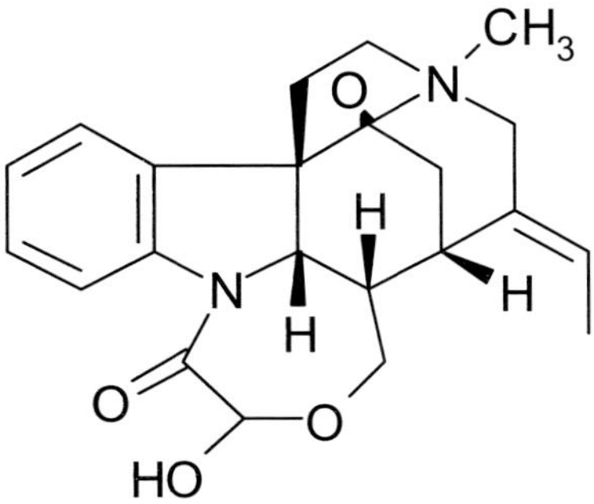

(55) Holstiine

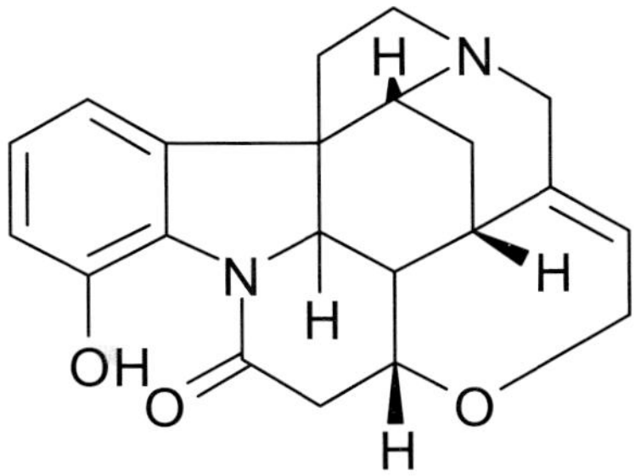

(56) 4-Hydroxystrychnine

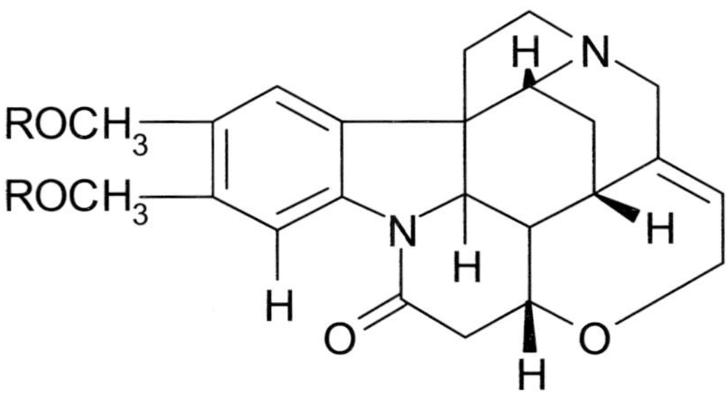

(57) Colubrine

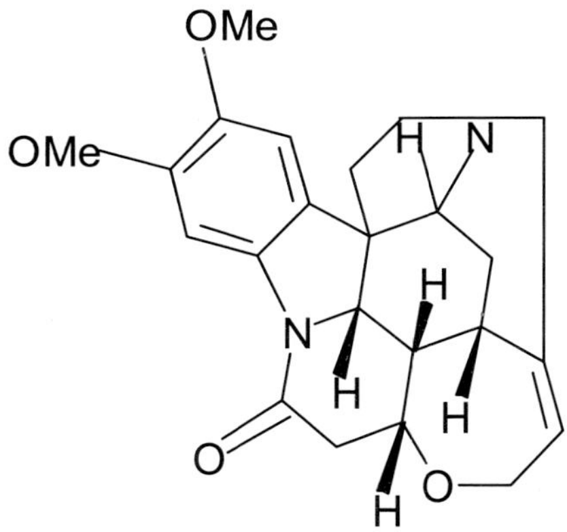

(58) Brucine

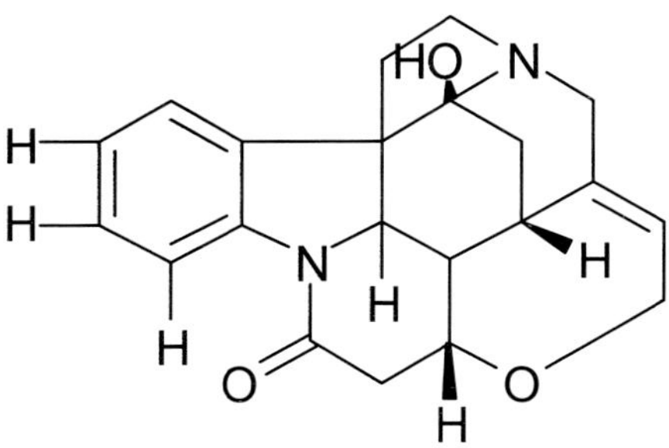

(59) Pseudostrychnine

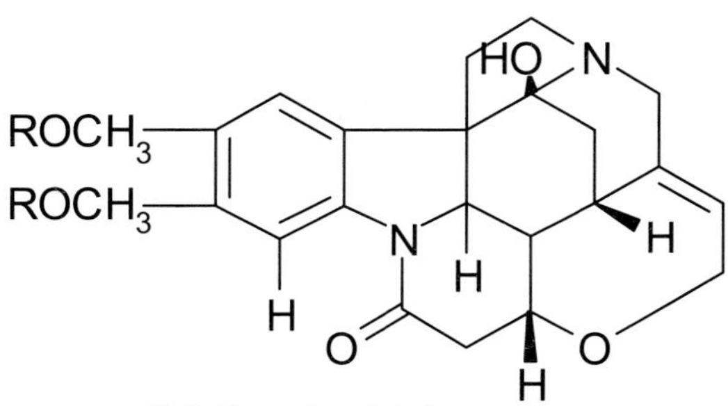

(60) Pseudocolubrine

Contd...

Figure 8.1–*Contd...*

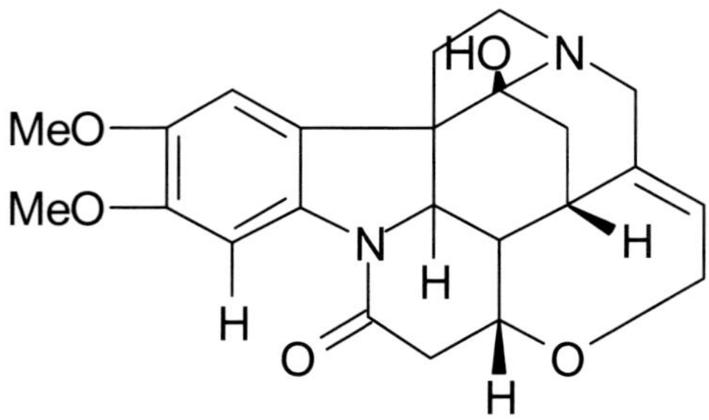

(61) Pseudobrucine

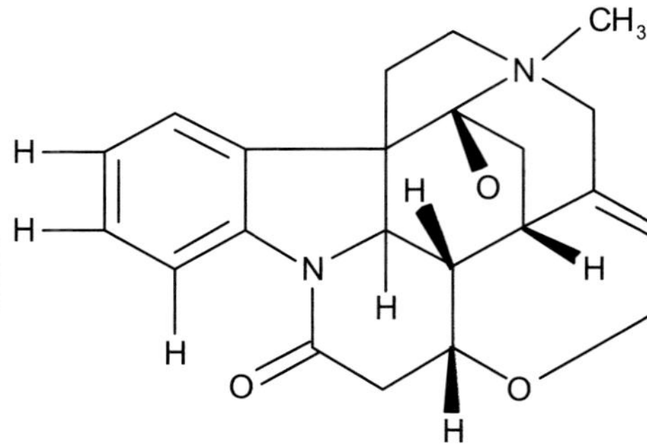

(62) Icajine

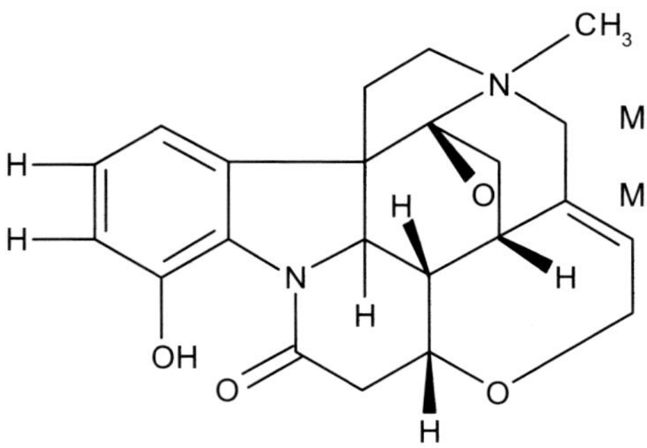

(63) Vomicine

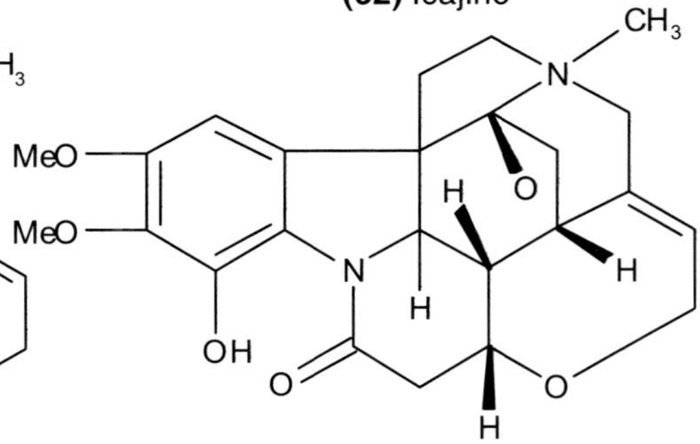

(64) Novacine

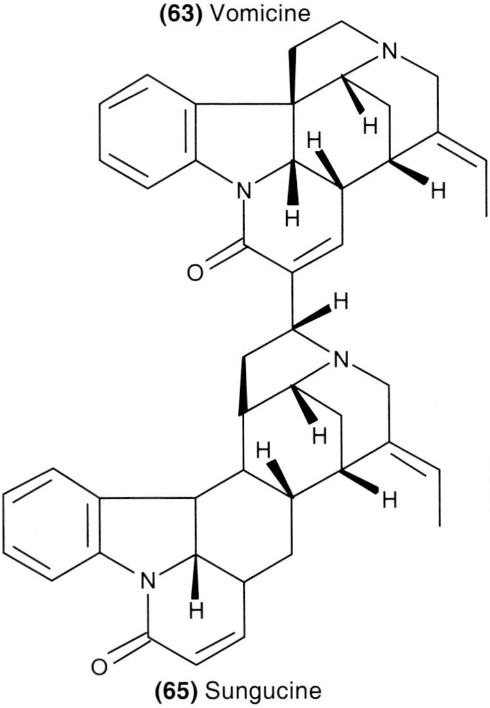

(65) Sungucine

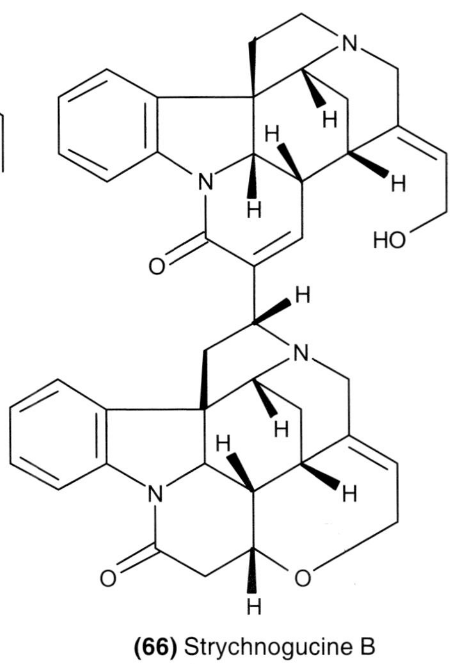

(66) Strychnogucine B

Contd...

Figure 8.1–*Contd...*

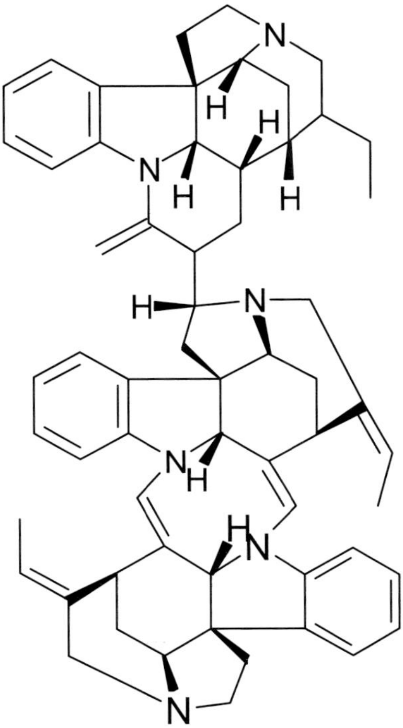

(67) Strychnohexamine

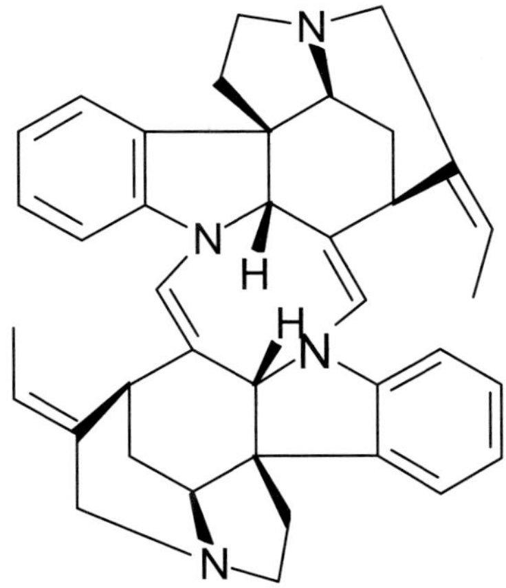

(68) Bisnordihydrotoxiferine

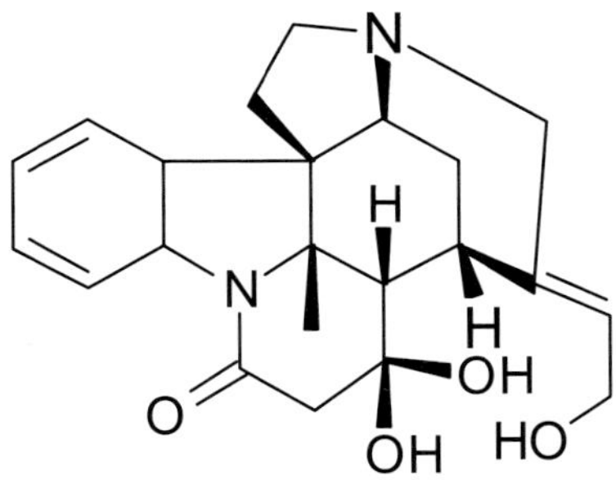

(69) Protostrychnine

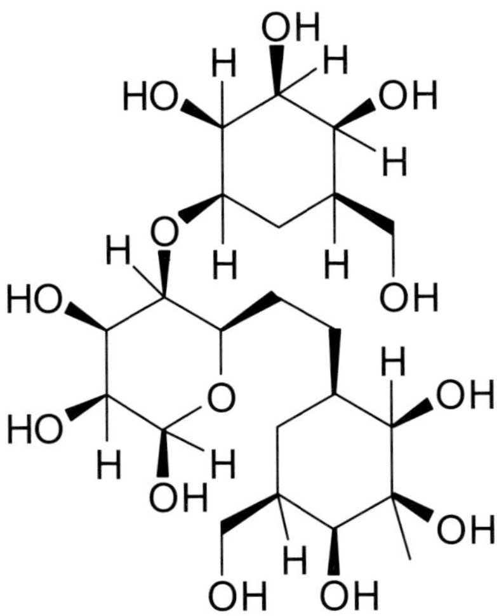

(70) Galactomannan

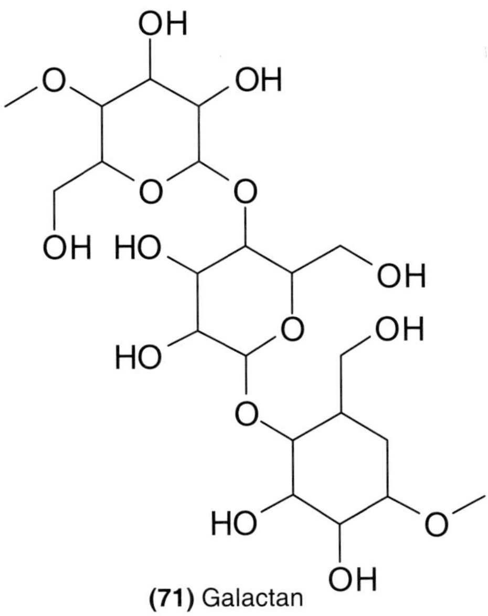

(71) Galactan

Contd...

Figure 8.1–*Contd...*

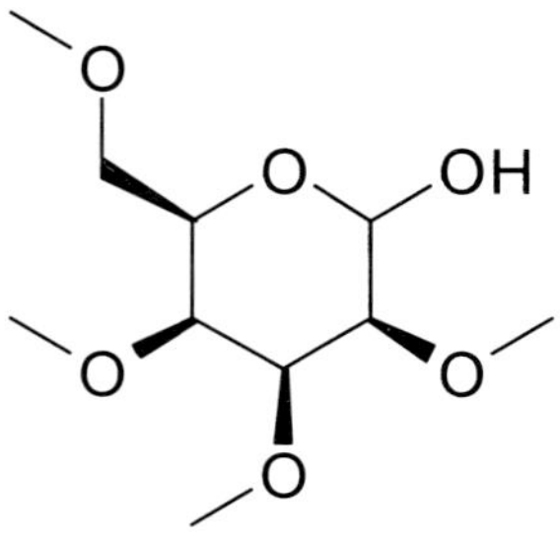

(72) 2,3,4,6-Tetra-O-methylgalactopyranose

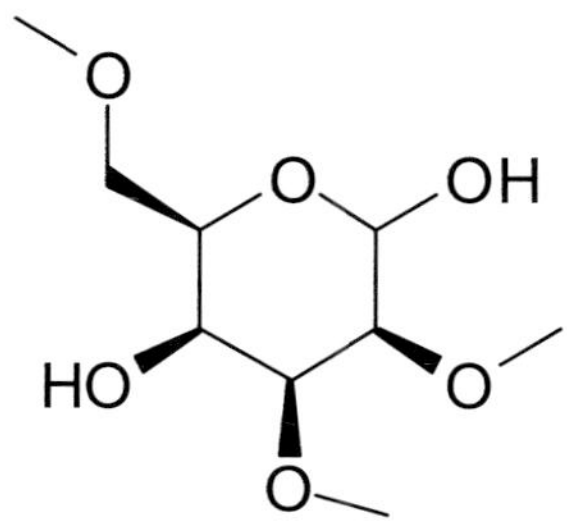

(73) 2,3,6-Tri-O-methylmannopyranose

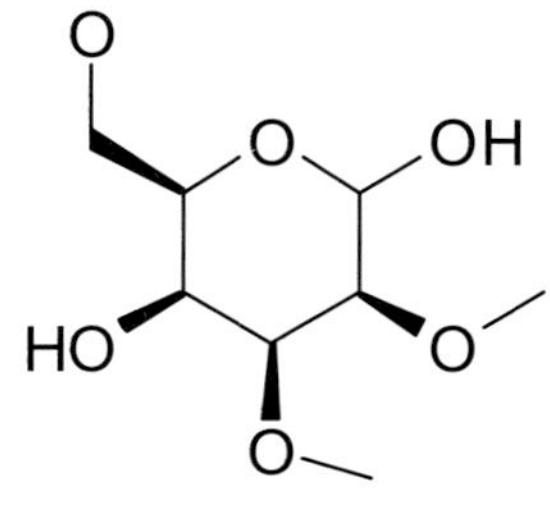

(74) 2,3-Di-O-methylmannopyranose

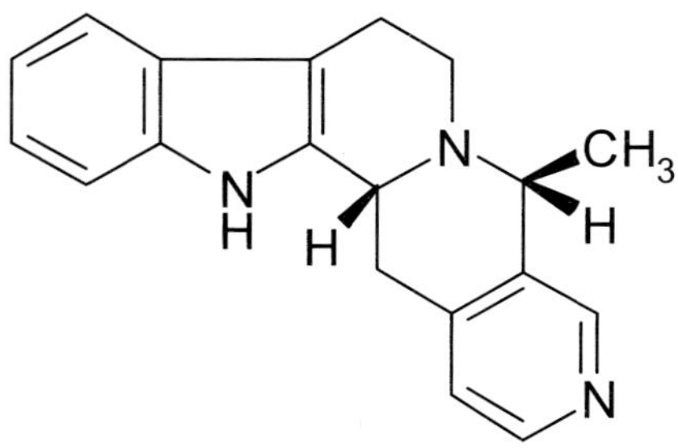

(75) Normalindine

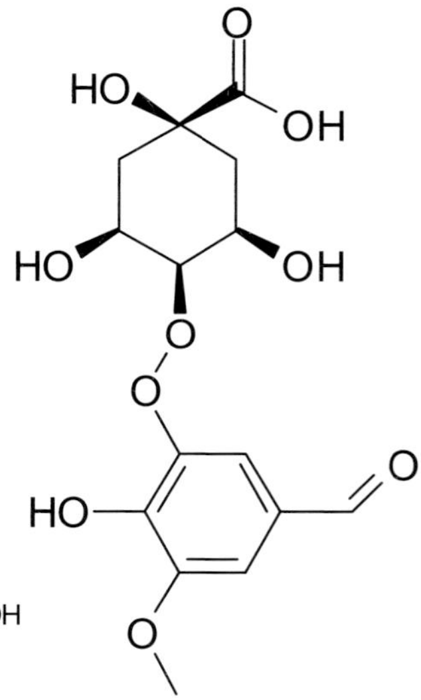

(76) 4-O-(3,5-dimethoxy-4-hydroxybenzoyl) quinic acid

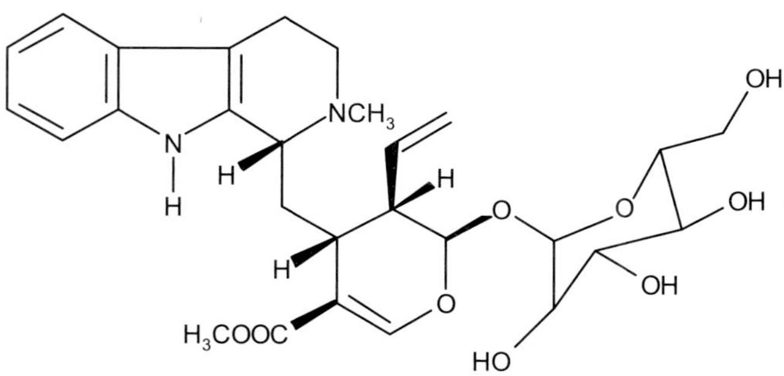

(77) 3,4,5,6-tetradehydropalicoside

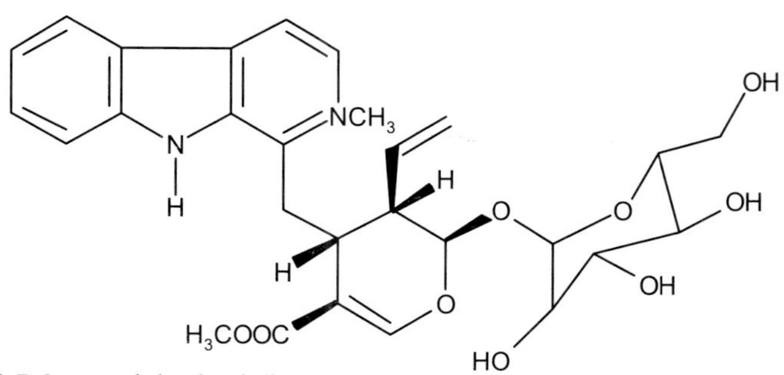

(78) 3,4,5,6-tetradehydrodolichantoside

Contd...

Figure 8.1–*Contd...*

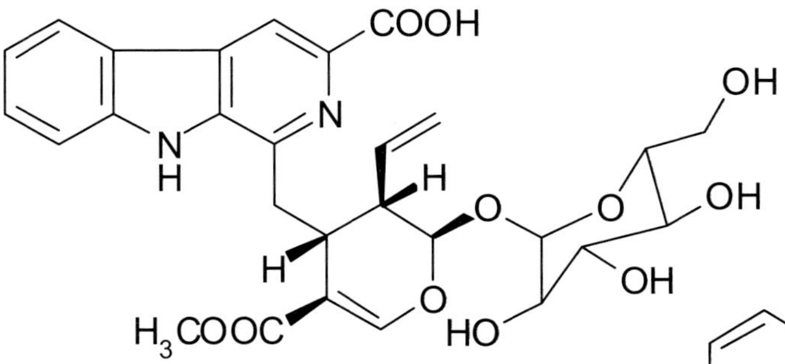

(79) Desoxycordifoline

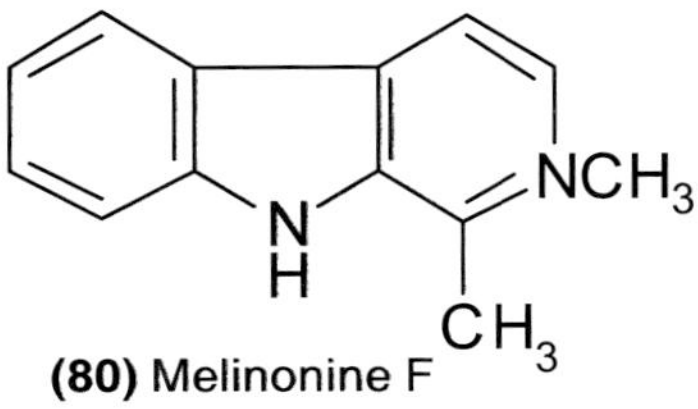

(80) Melinonine F

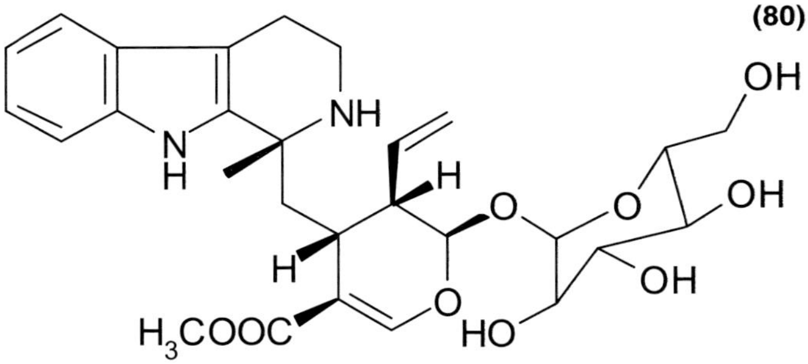

(81) Strictosidine β-glucosidase

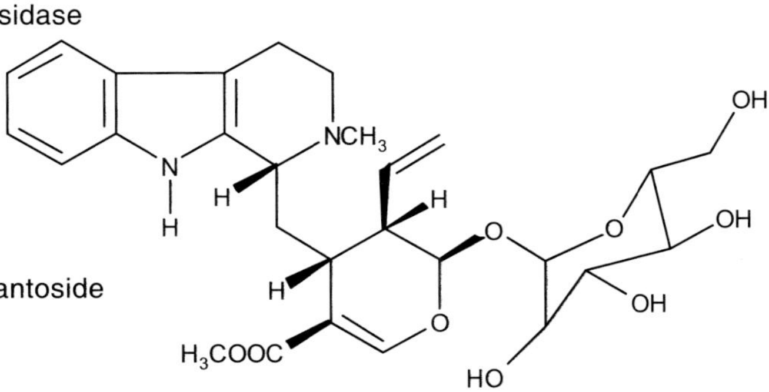

(82) Dolichantoside

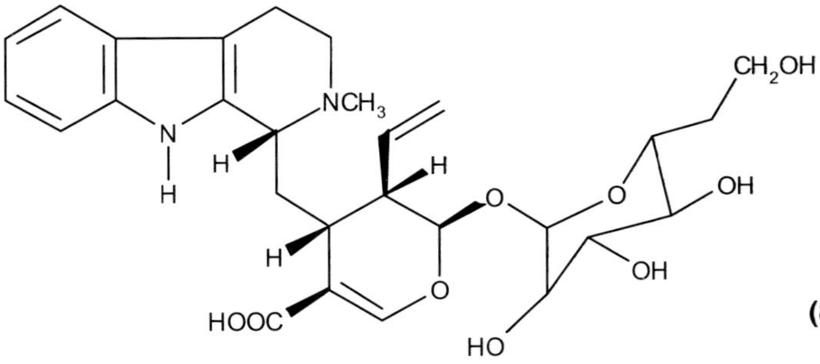

(83) Palicoside

Contd...

Figure 8.1–*Contd...*

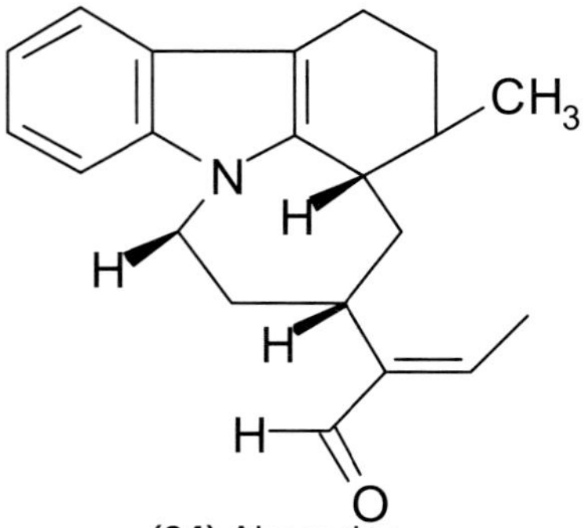

(84) Akagerine

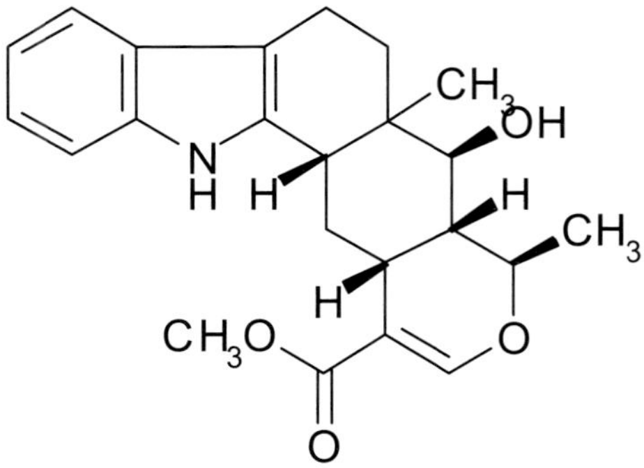

(85) N_b-methyl-21-β-hydroxy-mayumbine

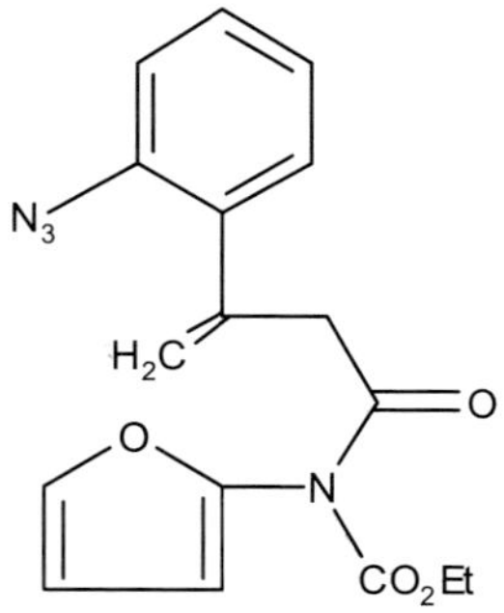

(86) Ortho-azido aryl carbamate

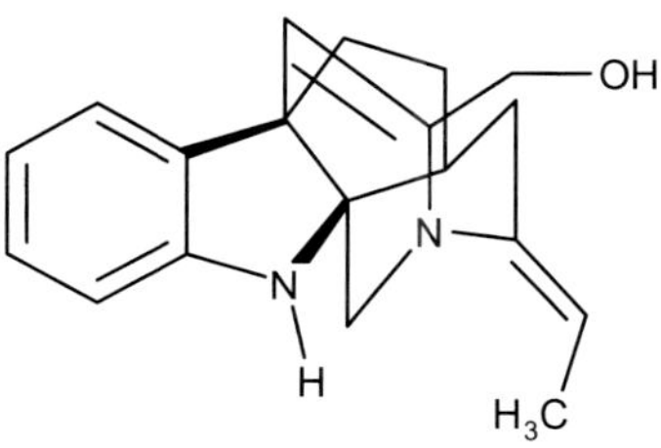

(87) Minfiensine

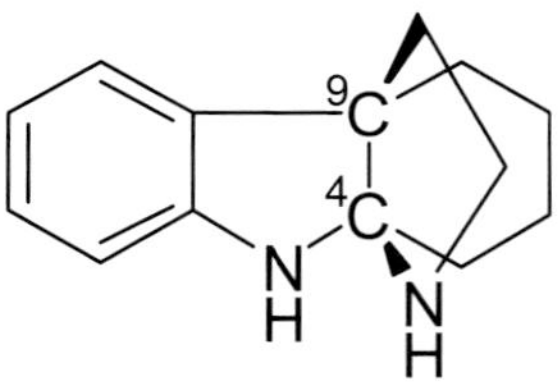

(88) 9a,4a-iminoethano-carbazole

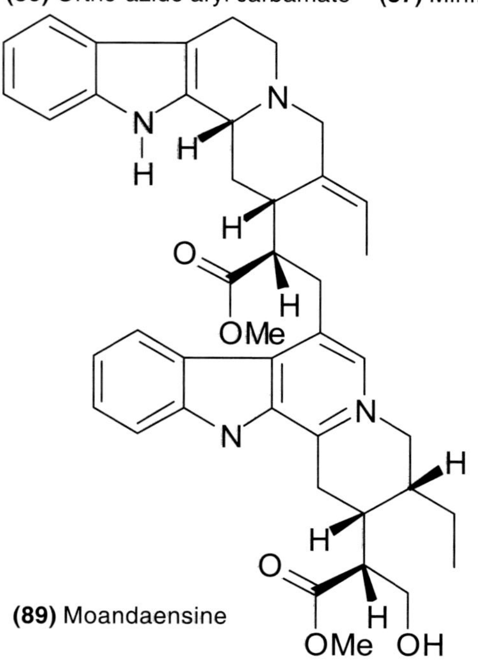

(89) Moandaensine

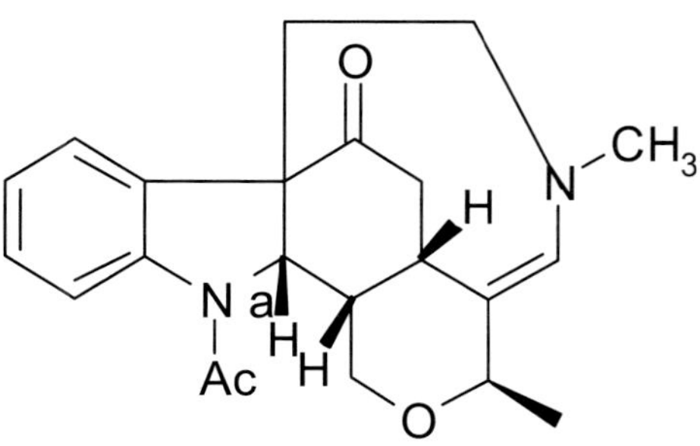

(90) Strychnobrasiline

Contd...

Figure 8.1–*Contd...*

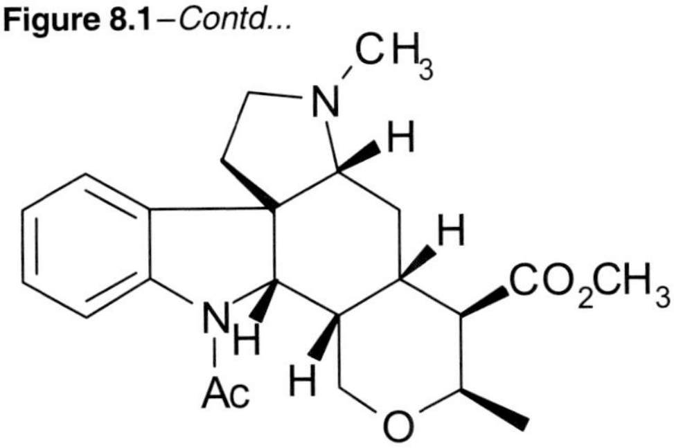

(91) Malagashanine

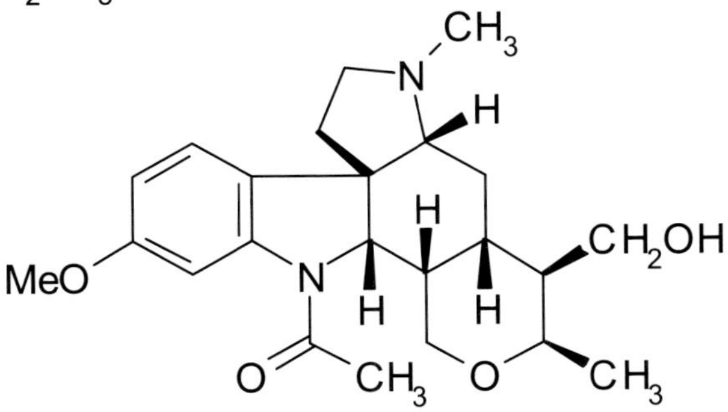

(92) Malagashanol

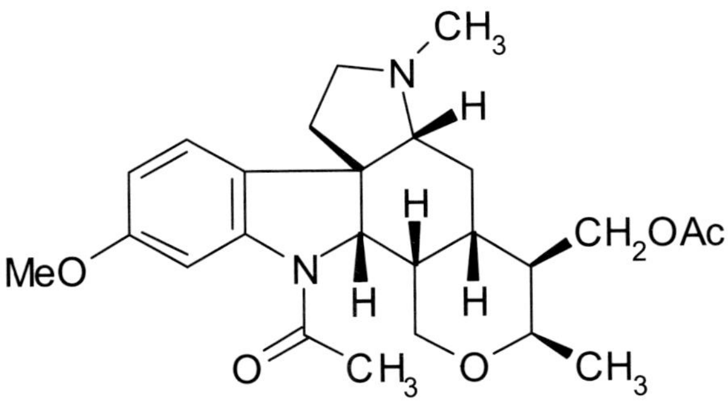

(93) Acetylmalagashanol

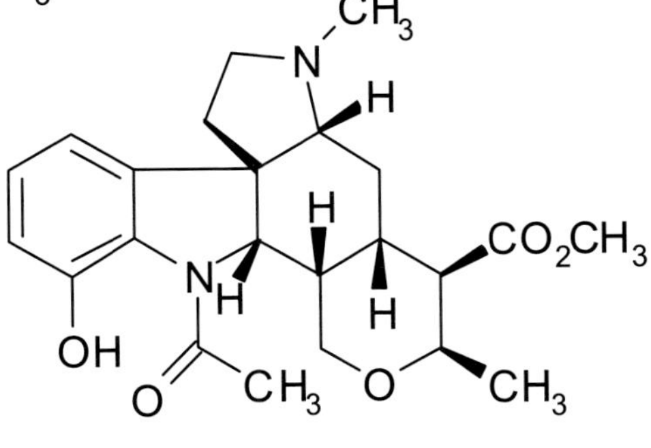

(94) 12-Hydroxymalagashanine

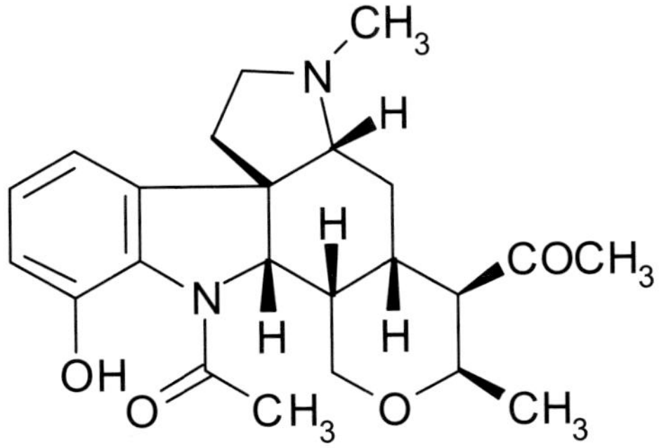

(95) 12-Hydroxy-19-*epi*-malagashanine

Contd...

Figure 8.1–*Contd...*

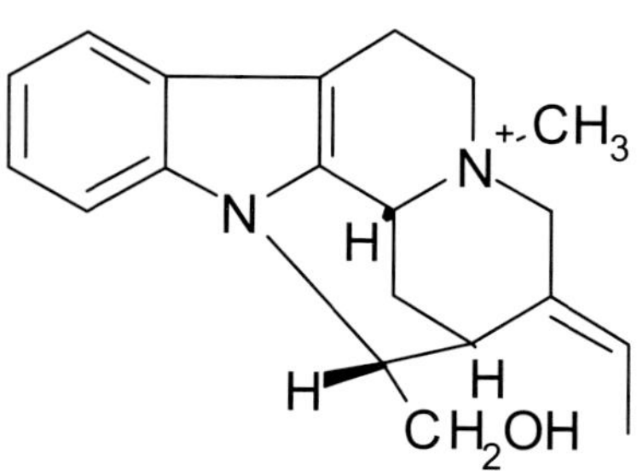

(96) C-mavacurine

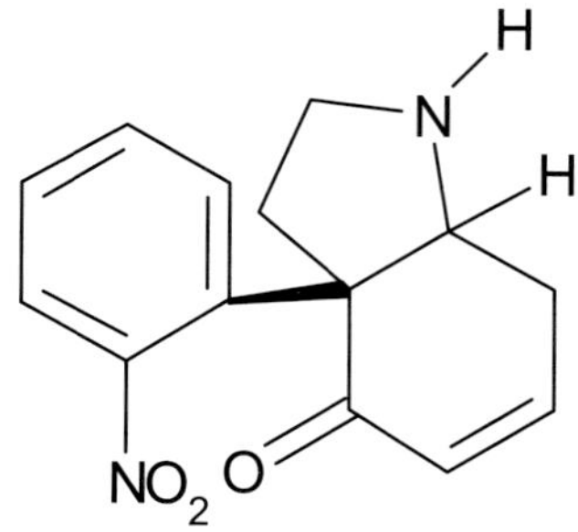

(97) *cis*-3a-(O-Nitrophenyl) hexahydroindol-4-one

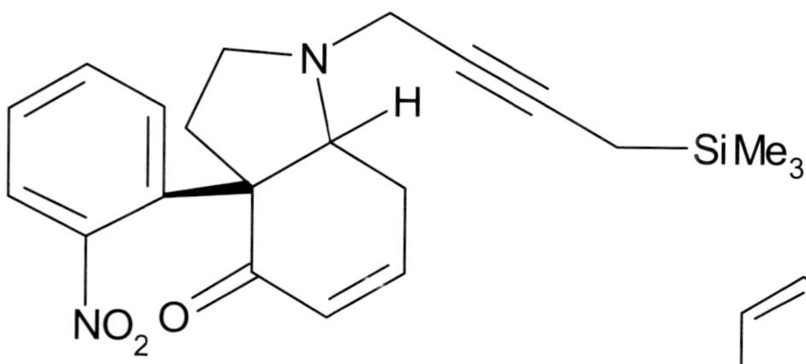

(98) Propargylic silane

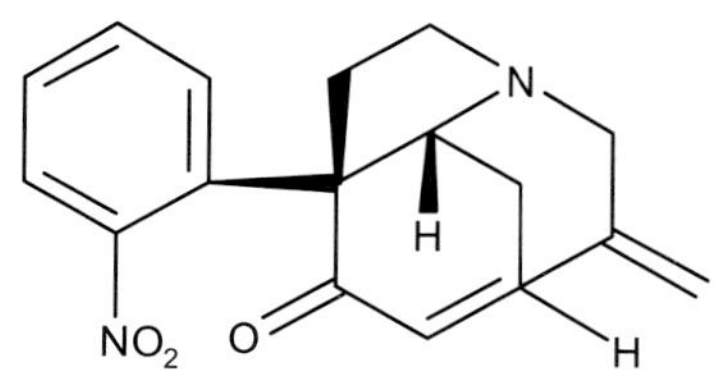

(99) Tricyclic vinylidene ketone

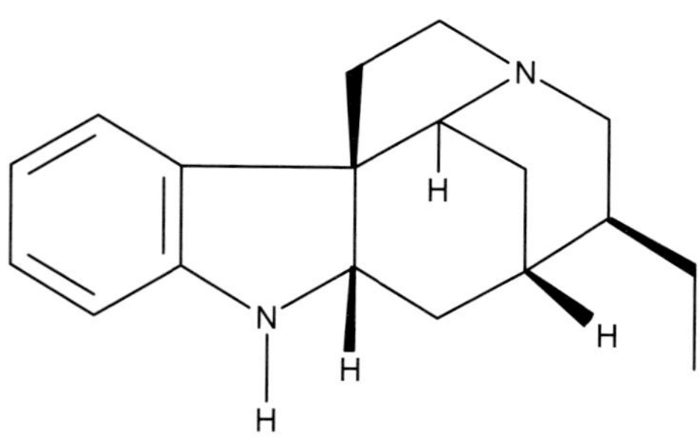

(100) Tubifolidine

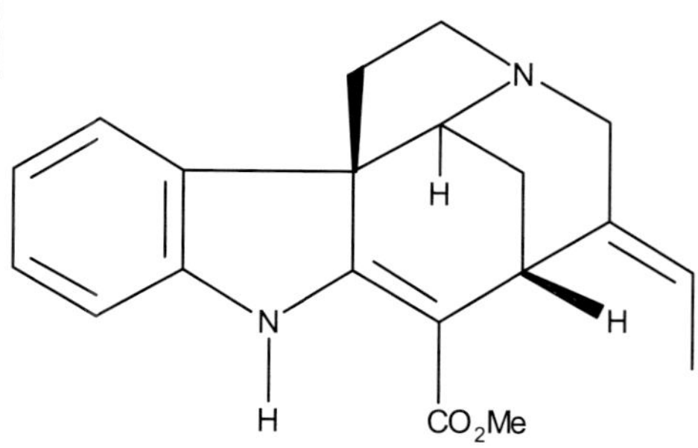

(101) Akuammicine

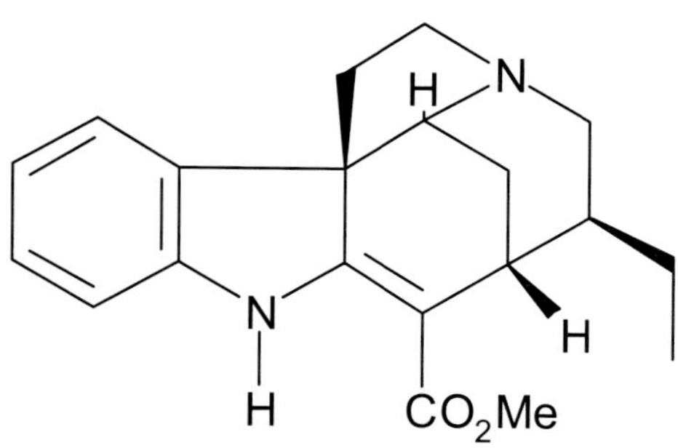

(102) 19,20-Dihydroakuammicine

Contd...

Figure 8.1–*Contd...*

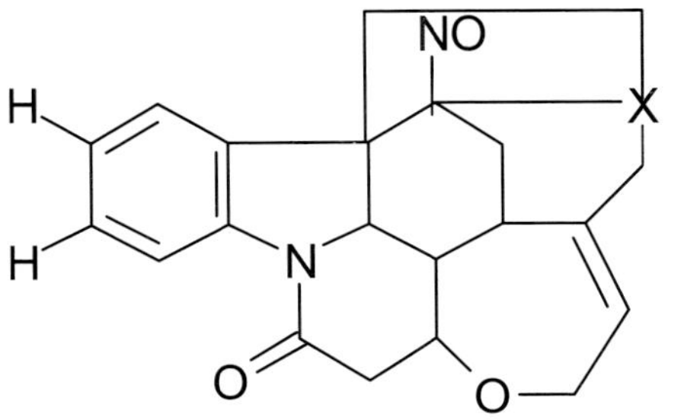

(103) Strychnine N-oxide

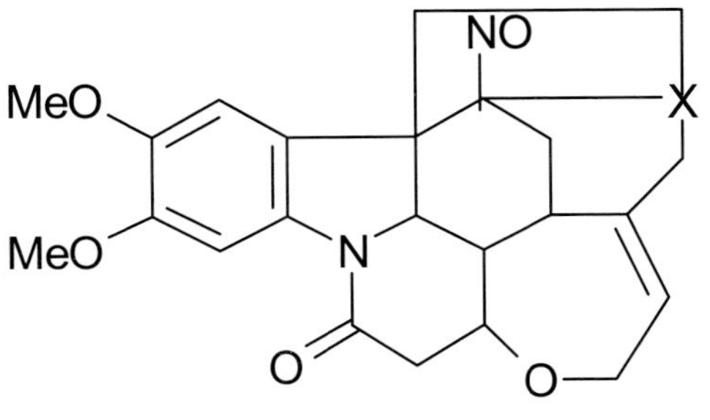

(104) Brucine N-oxide

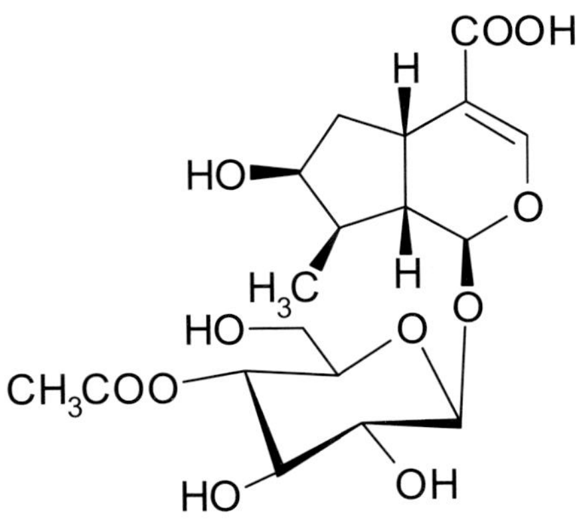

(105) 3'-O-acetylloganic acid

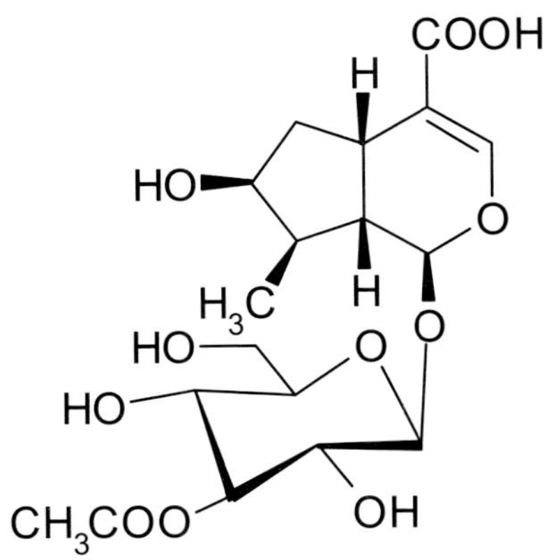

(106) 4'-O-acetylloganic acid

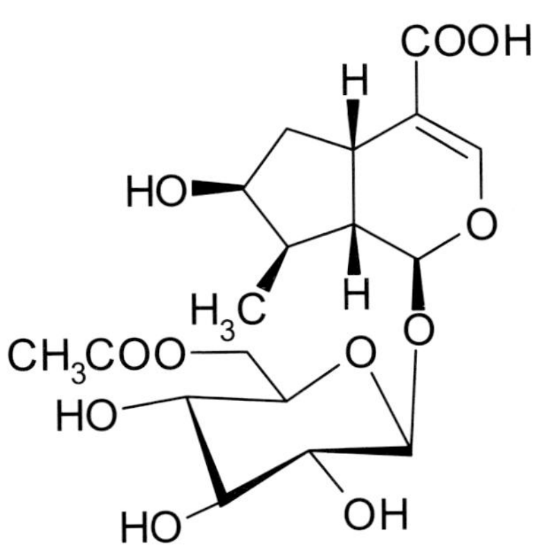

(107) 6'-O-acetylloganic acid

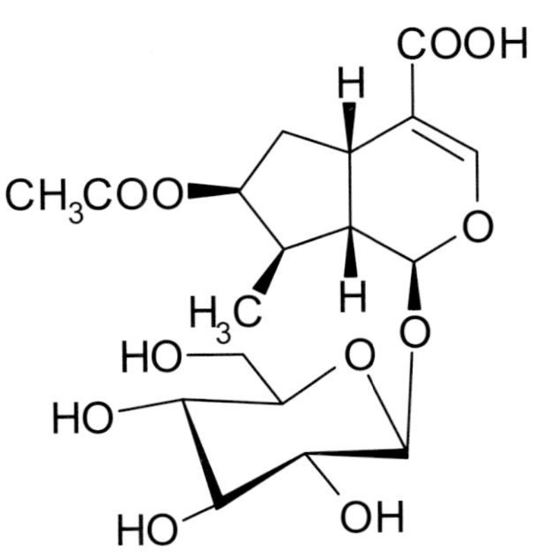

(108) 7-O-acetylloganic acid

Contd...

Figure 8.1–*Contd...*

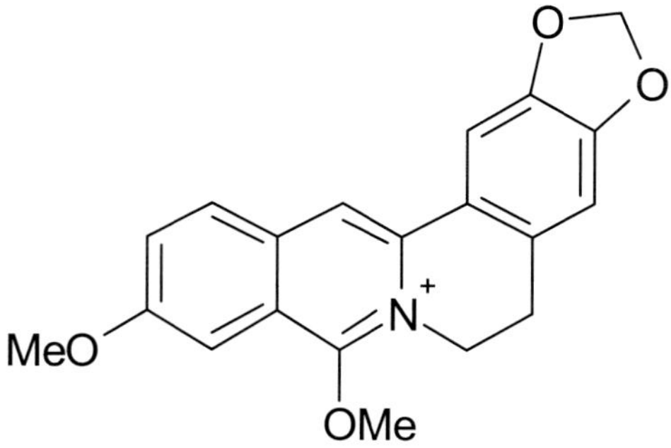

(109) Berberine

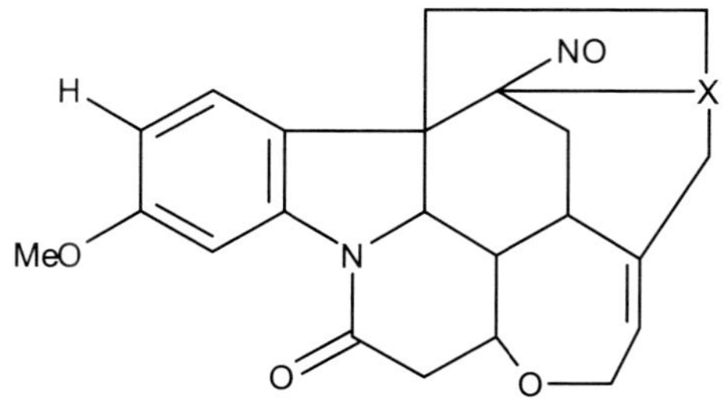

(110) 16-Hydorxy-α-colubring

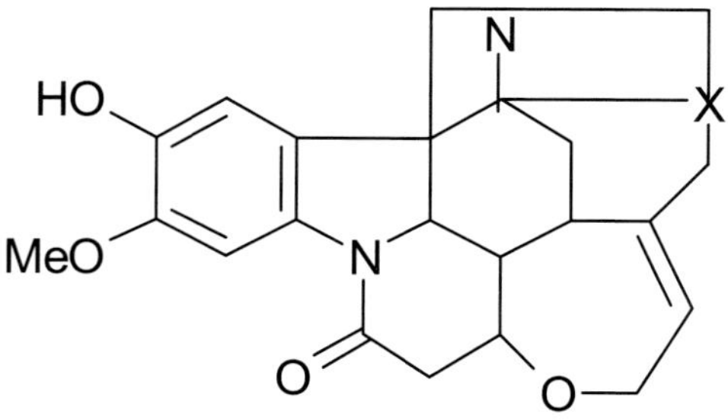

(111) 2-Hydroxy-3-methoxystrychnine

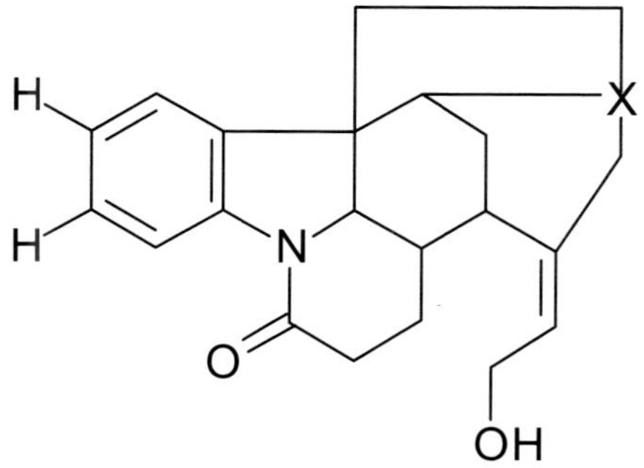

(112) Isostrychnine

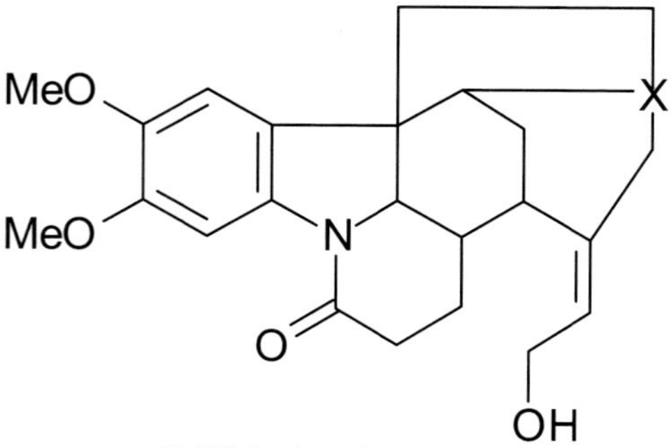

(113) Isobrucine

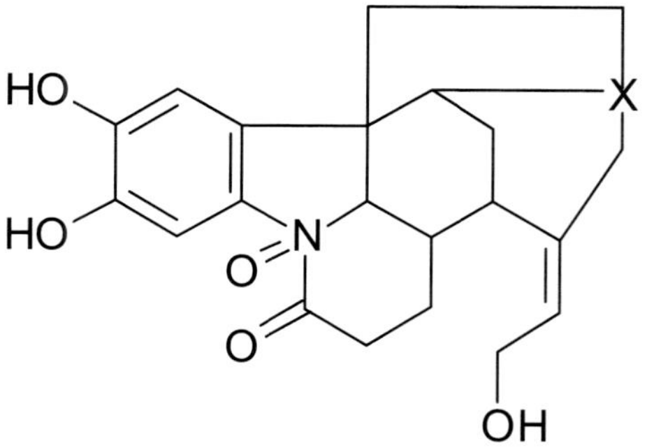

(114) Isostrychnine-N-oxide

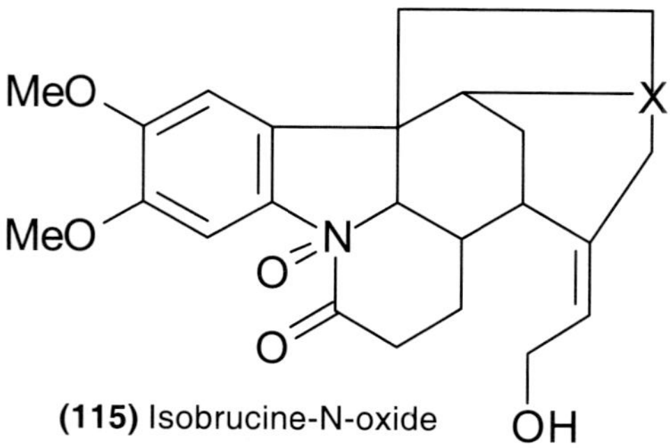

(115) Isobrucine-N-oxide

Contd...

Figure 8.1–*Contd...*

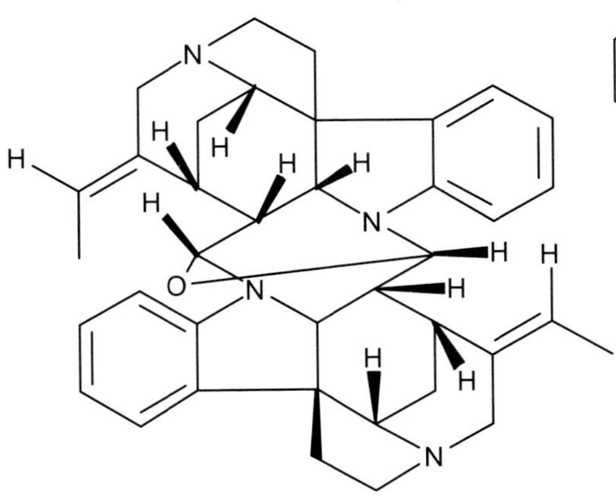

(116) Matopensine

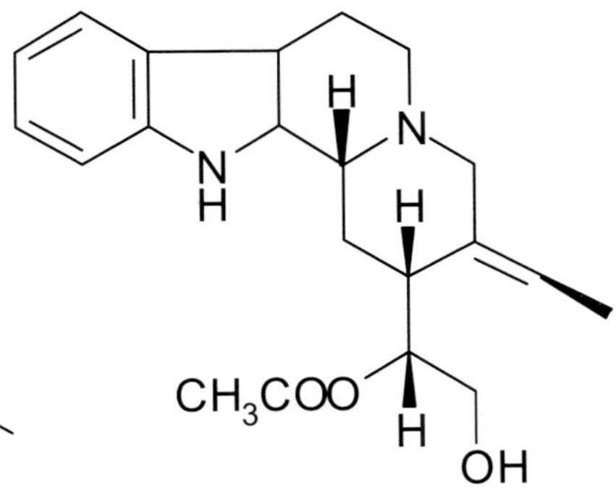

(117) 16-(S)-E-isositsirikine

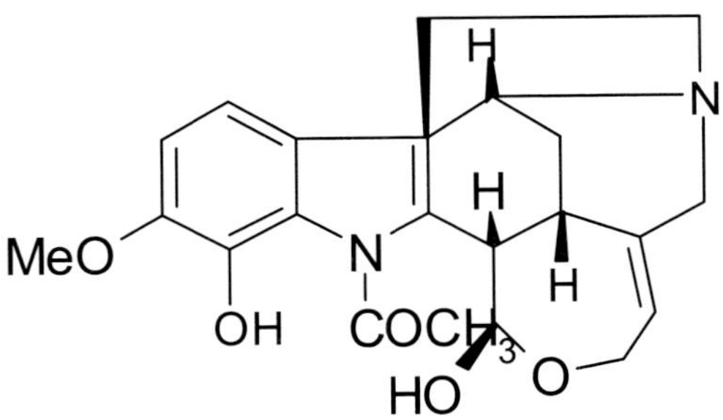

(118) 12-Hydroxy-11-methoxydiaboline

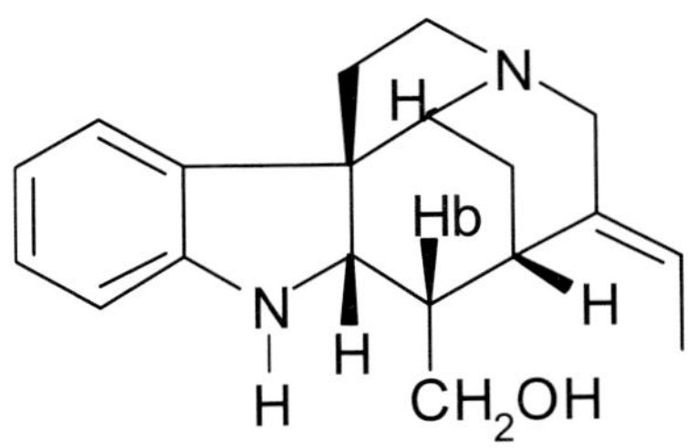

(119) N-Desacetylretuline

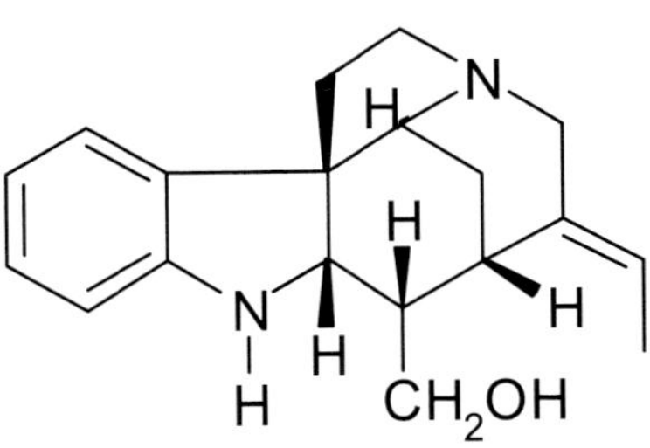

(120) N-desacetylisoretuline

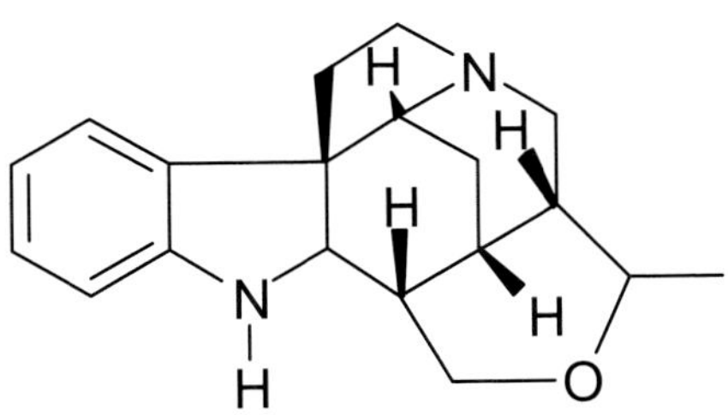

(121) N-Desacetylspermostrychnine

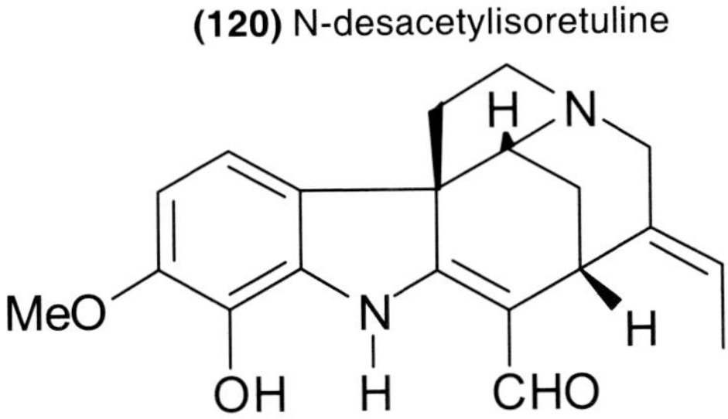

(122) 12-Hydroxy-11-methoxy-nor-C-fluorocurarine

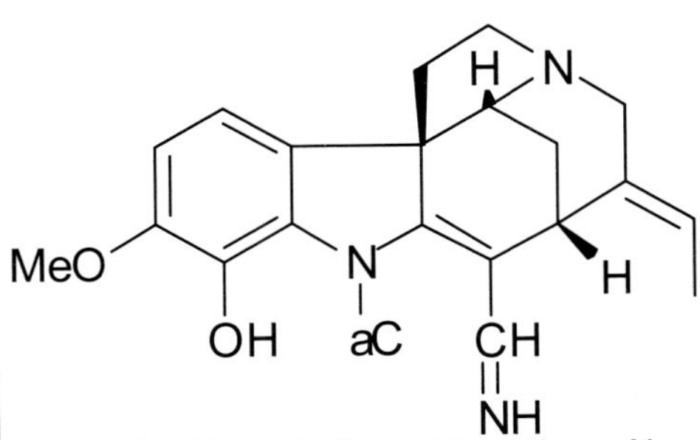

(123) 12-Hydroxy-11-methoxy-N-acetylmon-C-fluorocurarimine

Contd...

Figure 8.1–*Contd...*

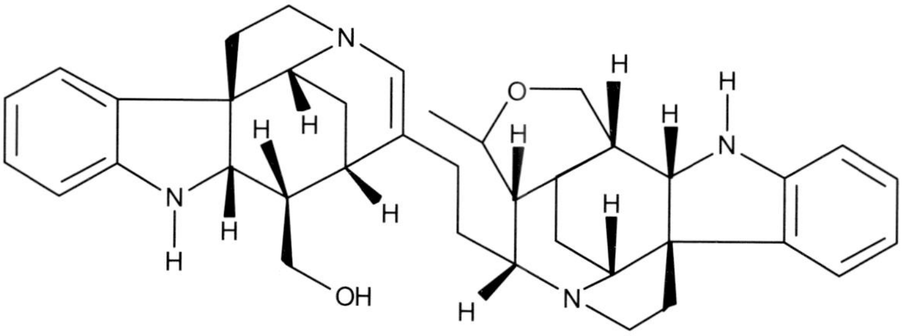

(124) Panganensines R

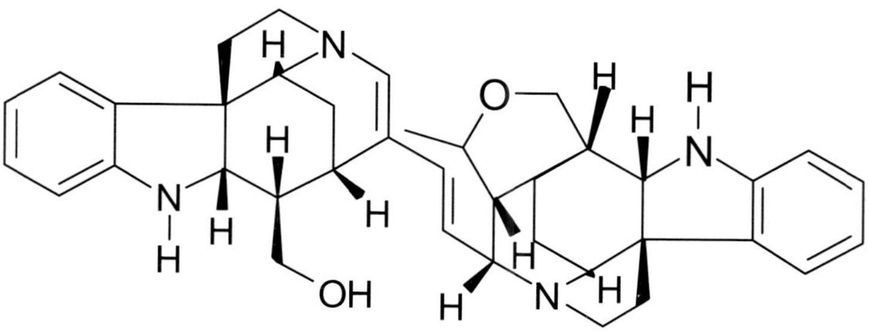

(125) Panganensines S

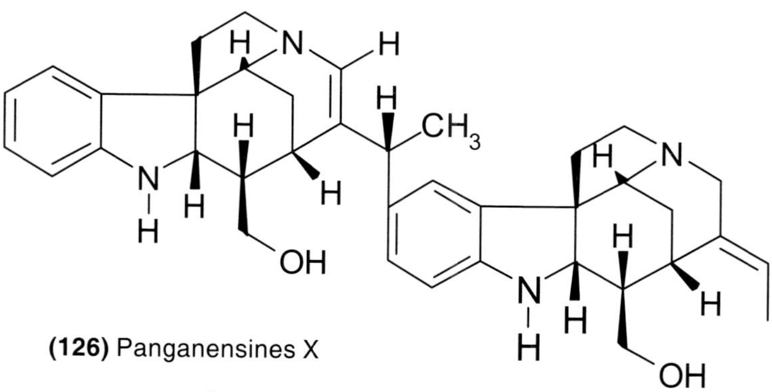

(126) Panganensines X

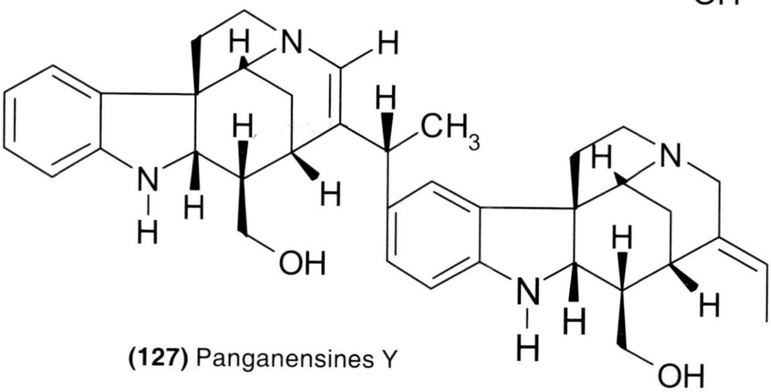

(127) Panganensines Y

Contd...

Figure 8.1–*Contd...*

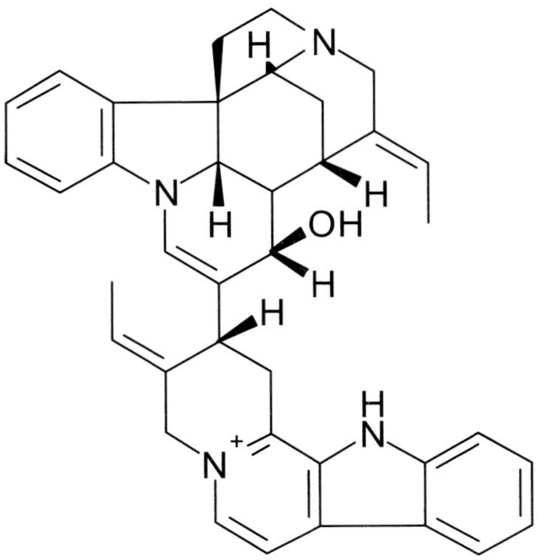

(128) 3',4',5',6'-tetradehydrolongicaudatine Y

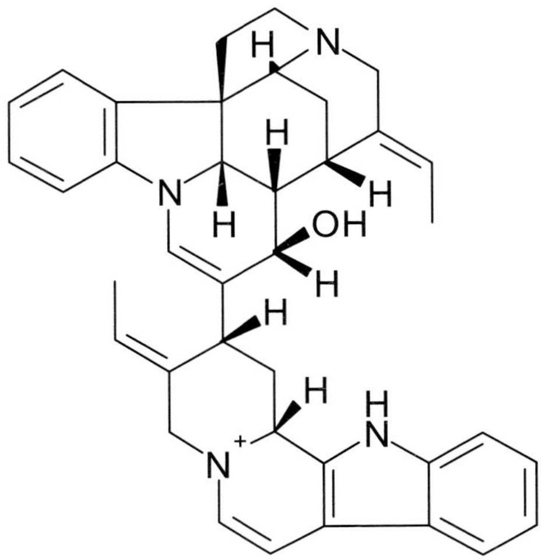

(129) Longicaudatine Y

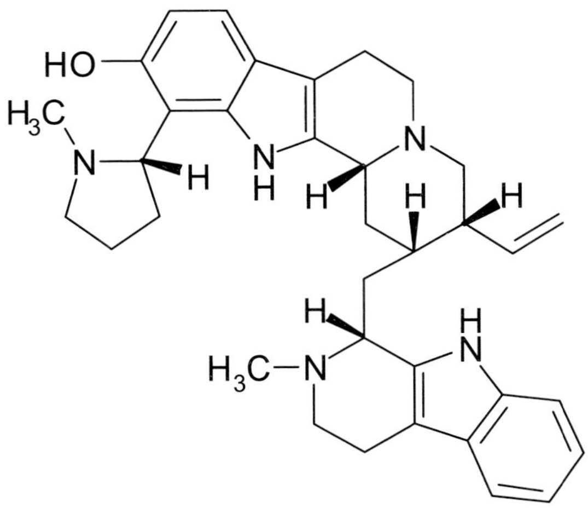

(130) Isostrychnopentamine

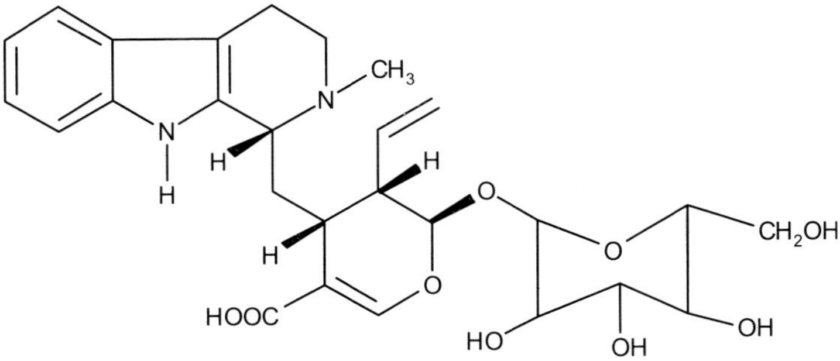

(131) 3,4-dehydropalicoside

Contd...

Figure 8.1–*Contd...*

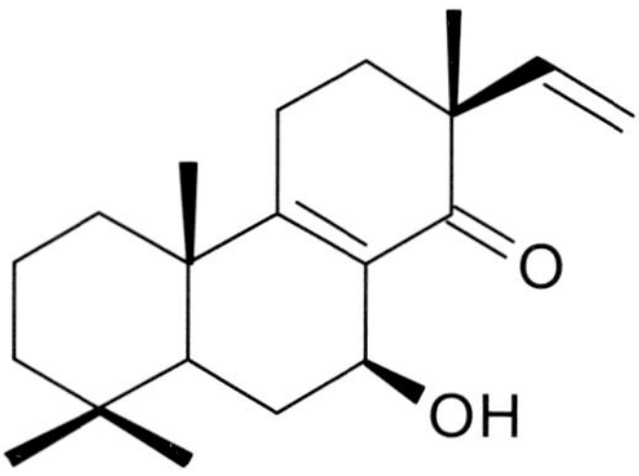

(132) 7β-hydroxypimara-8,15-dien-14-one

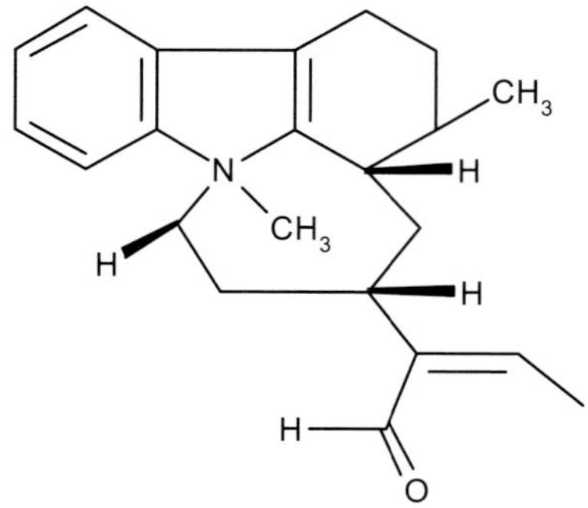

(133) 17-O-methylakagerine

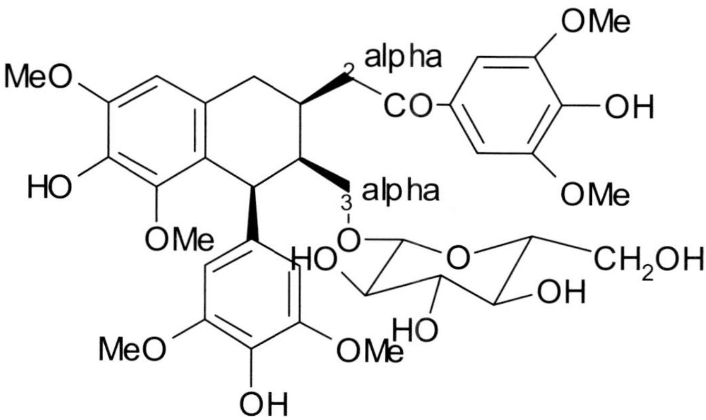

(134) Vanprukoside

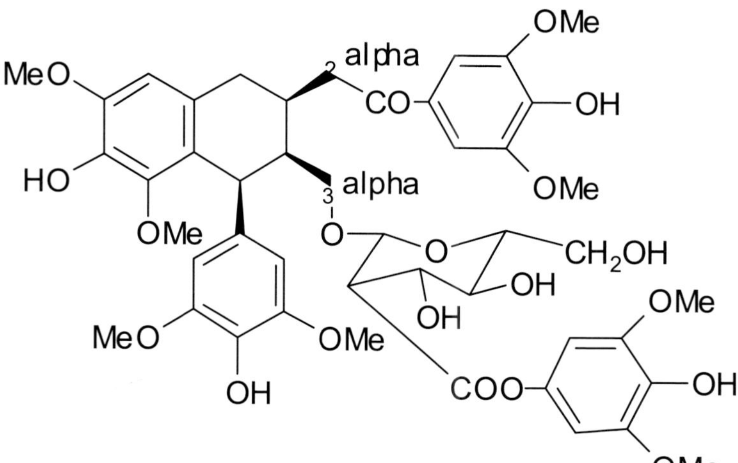

(135) Strychnoside

Contd...

Figure 8.1–*Contd...*

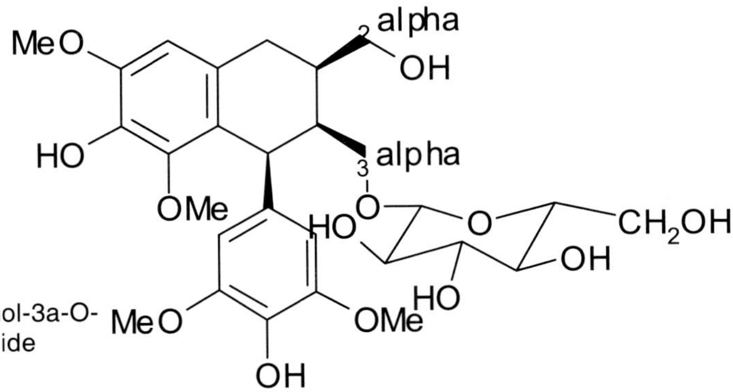

(136) (+)-lyoniresinol-3a-O-glucopyranoside

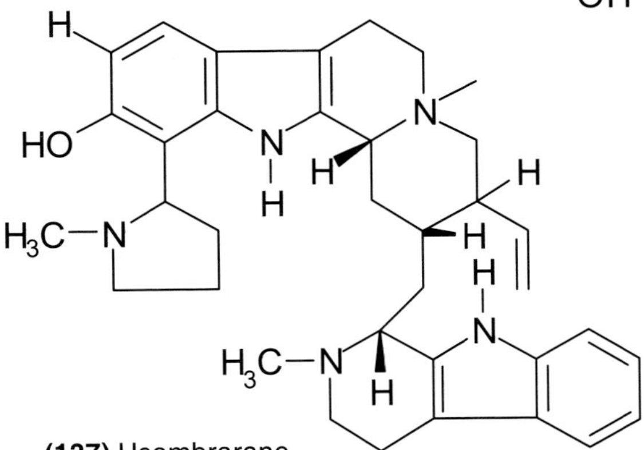

(137) Usambrarane

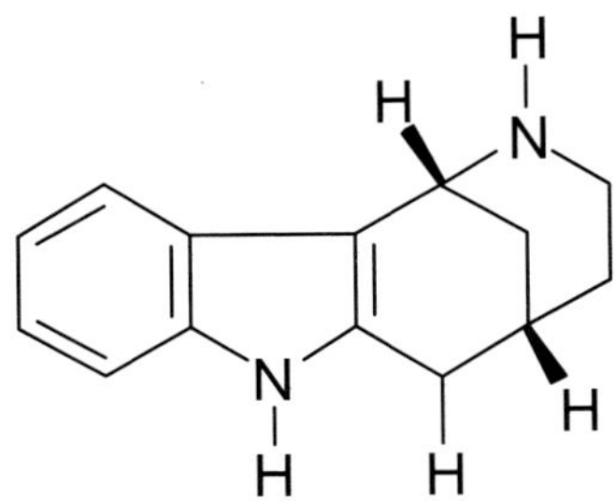

(138) Tetracyclic-1,2,3,4,5,6-hexahydro-1,5-methanoazocino(4,3-b)indole

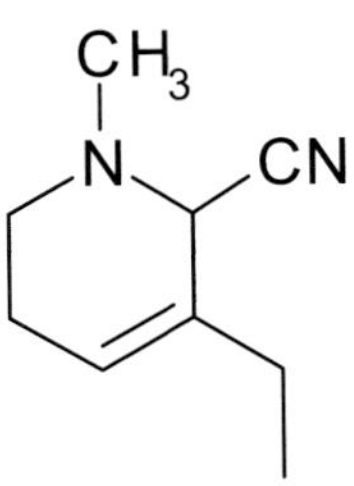

(139) 2-cyano-3-ethyl-1-methyl-1,2,3,6-tetrahydropyridine

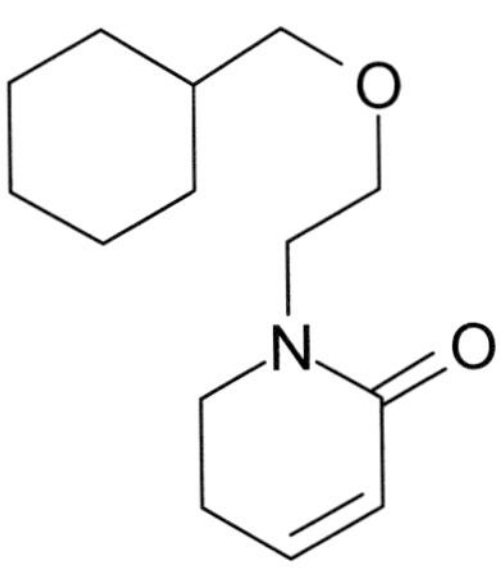

(140) N-substituted Δ^3-piperidein-2-ones

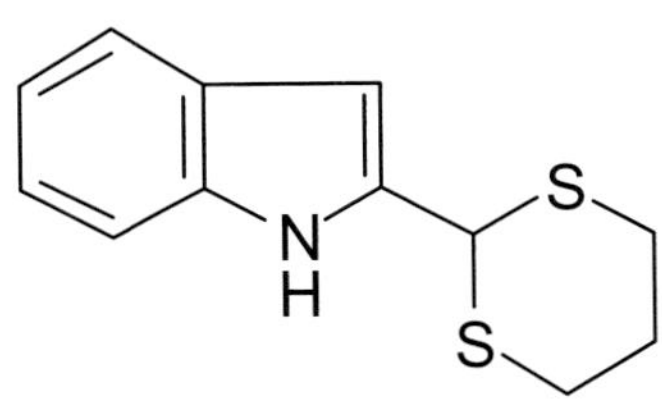

(141) 2-(1,3-dithian-2-yl)-indole

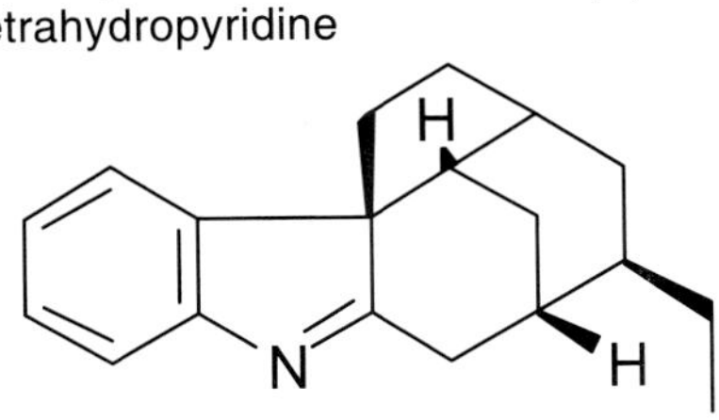

(142) (-)-Tubifoline

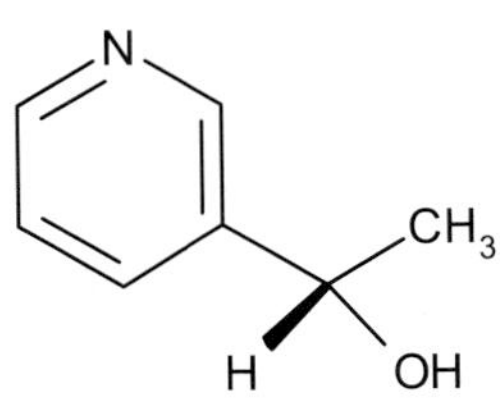

(143) 1-(3-pyridyl) ethanol

Contd...

Figure 8.1–*Contd...*

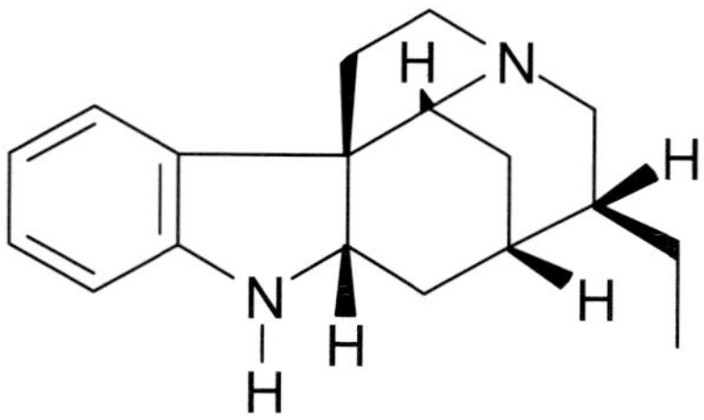

(144) (-)-tubifolidine

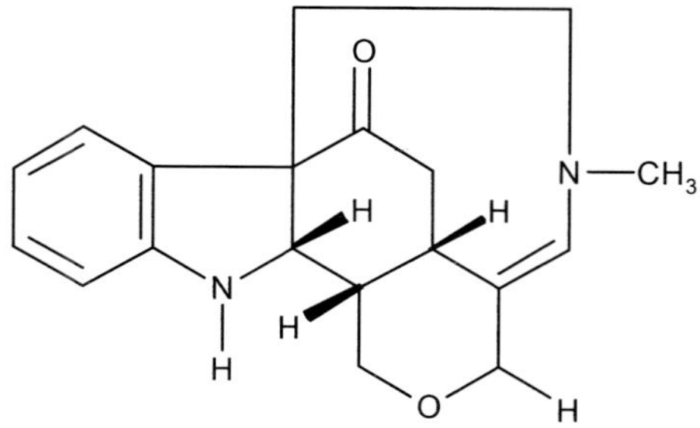

(145) N_a deacetyl-SB

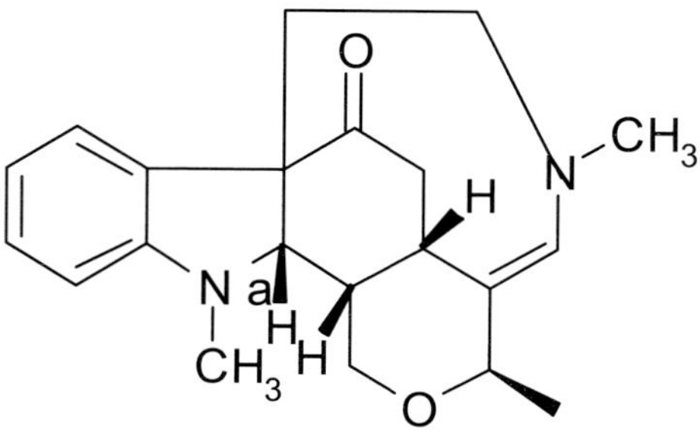

(146) N_a-deacetyl-N_a-methyl-SB

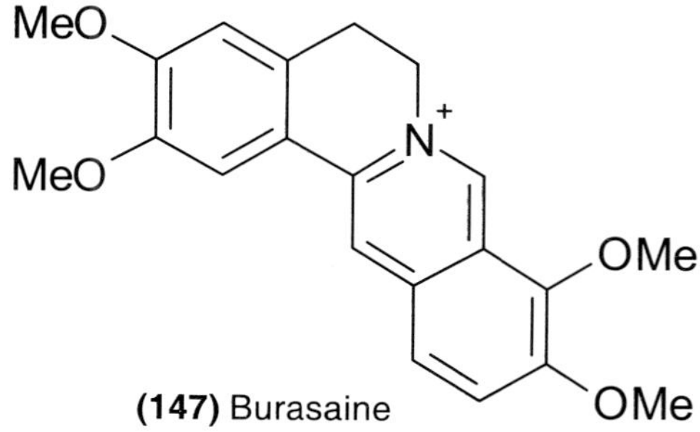

(147) Burasaine

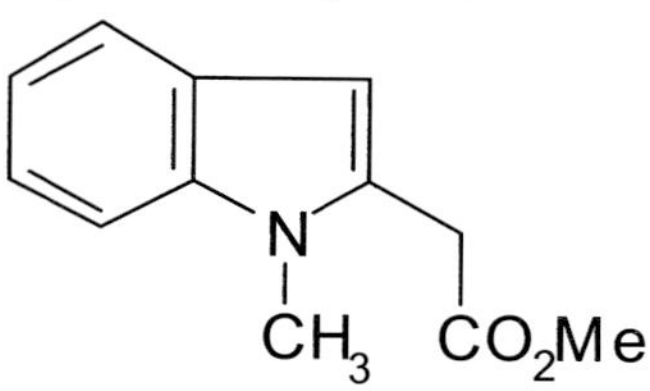

(148) 1-methyl-2-indoleacetate

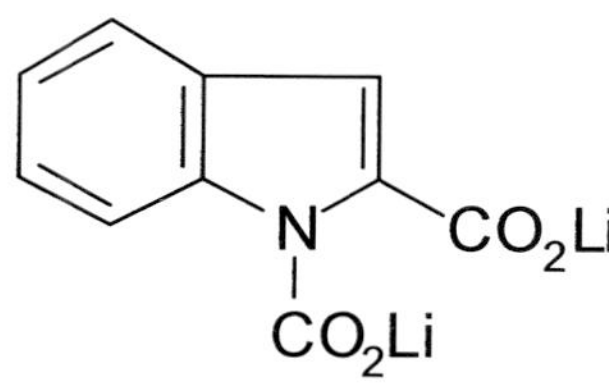

(149) Lithium-2-(lithiomethyl)indole-1-carboxylate

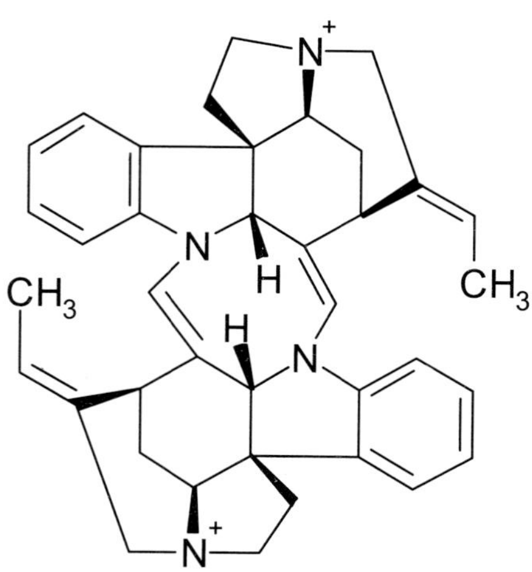

(150) C-Dihydrotoxiferine

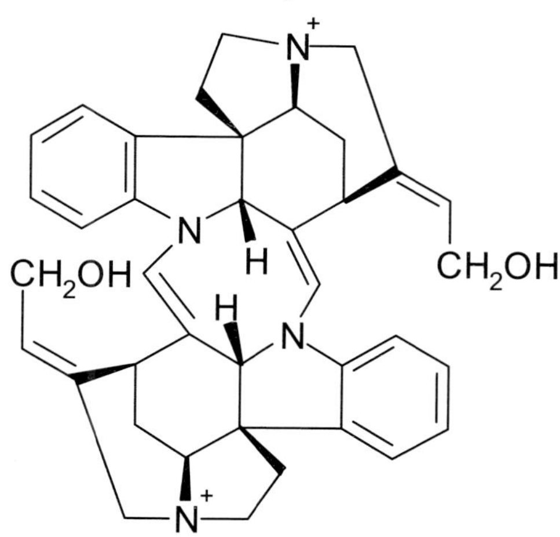

(151) C-Toxiferine

Contd...

Figure 8.1–*Contd...*

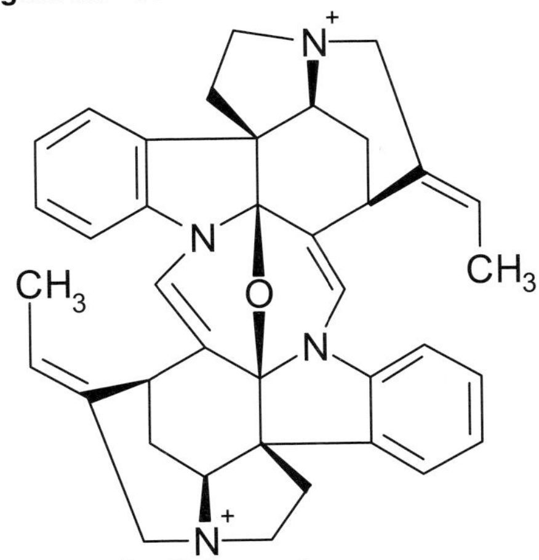

(152) C-curarine

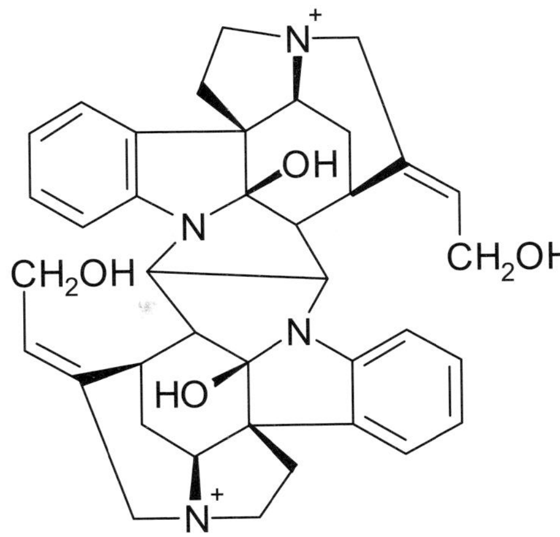

(153) C-Alkaloid A

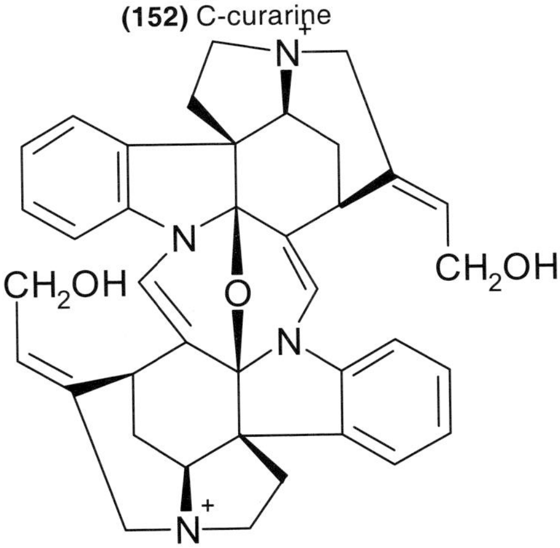

(154) C-Alkaloid E

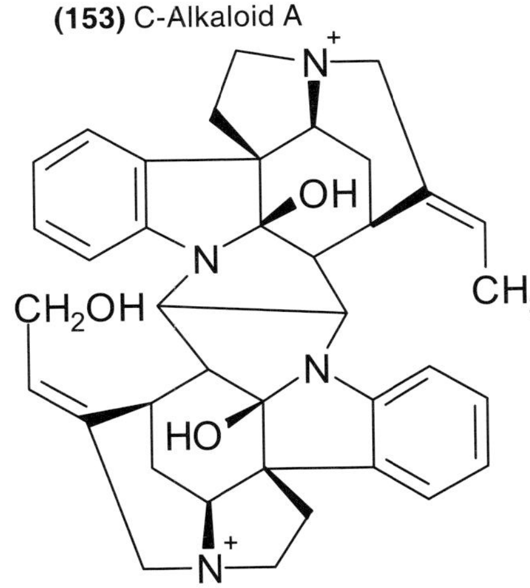

(155) C-Alkaloid F

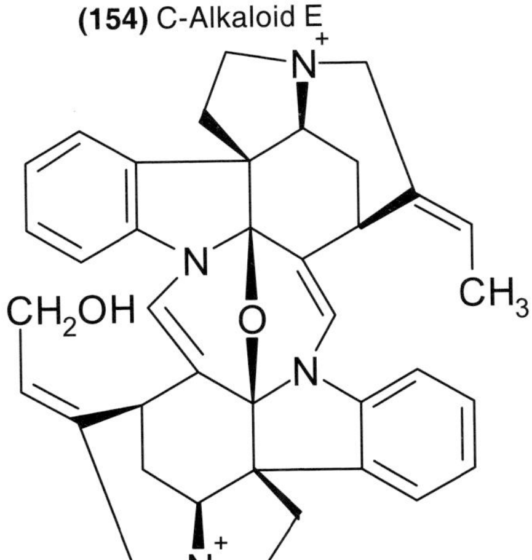

(156) C-Alkaloid G

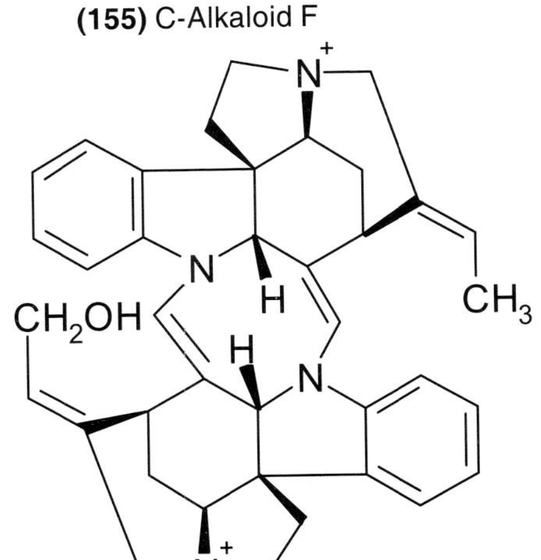

(157) C-Alkaloid H

Contd...

Figure 8.1–*Contd...*

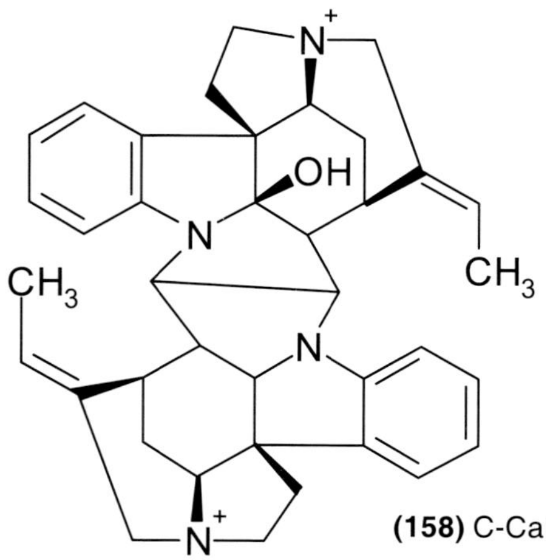

(158) C-Calebassine

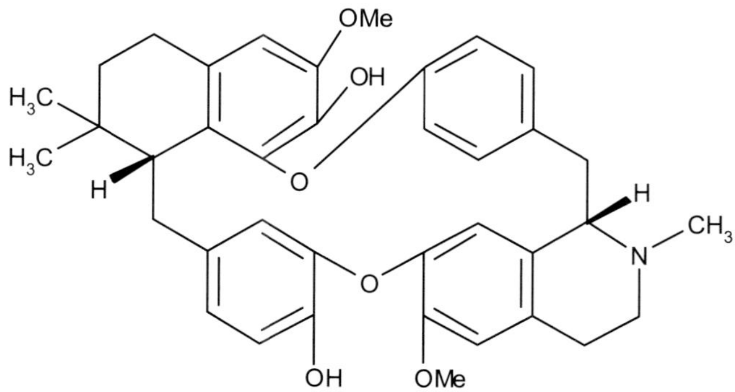

(159) (+)-Tubocurarine

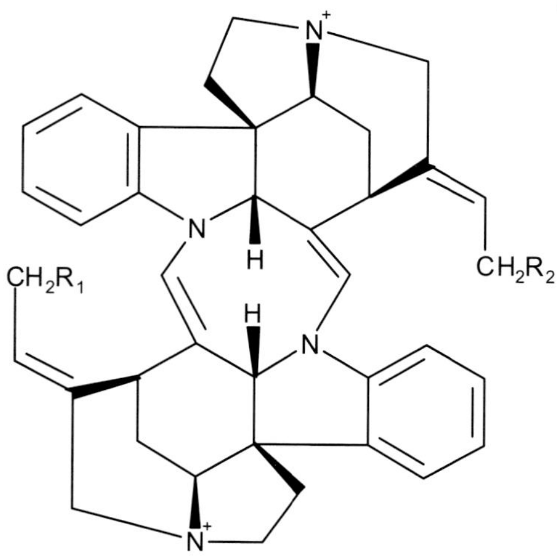

(160) N,N-diallyltoxiferine
(Alcuronium)

Contd...

Figure 8.1–*Contd...*

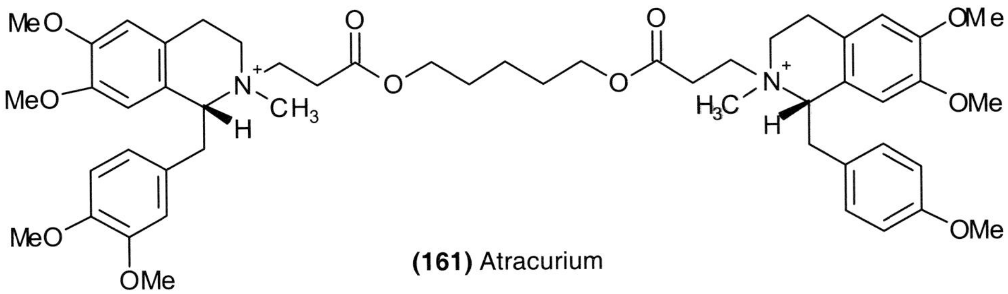

(161) Atracurium

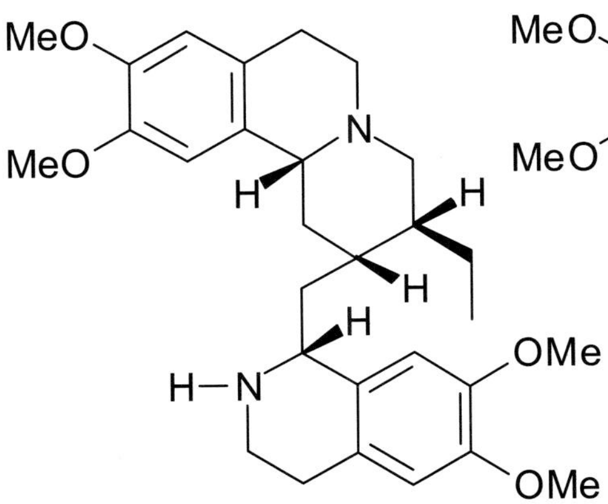

(162) Emetine

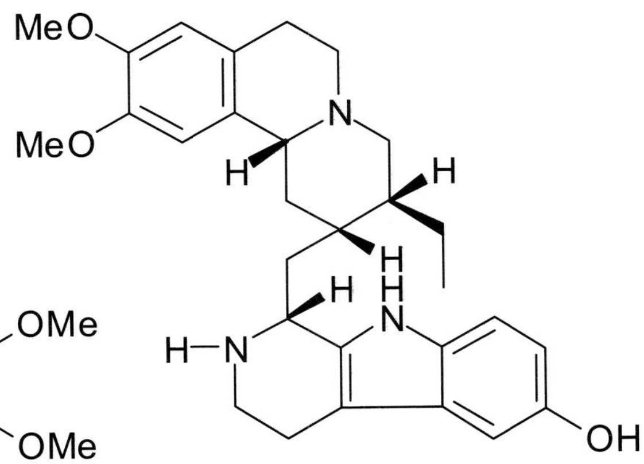

(163) Tubulosine

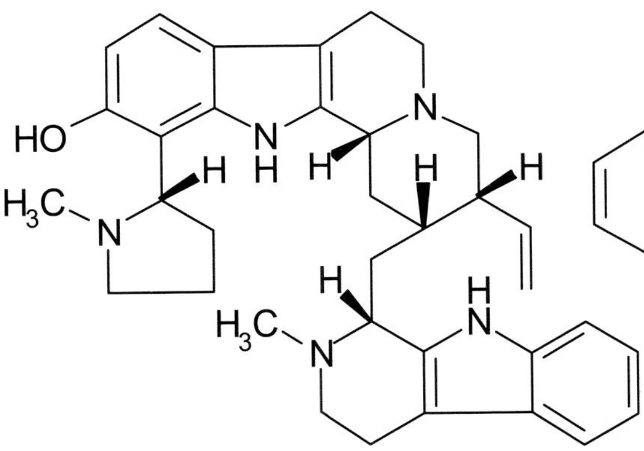

(164) Strychnopentamine

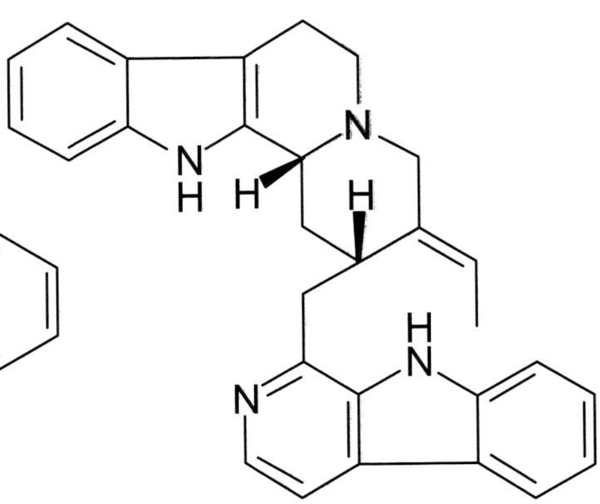

(165) Usambarensine

Contd...

Figure 8.1–*Contd...*

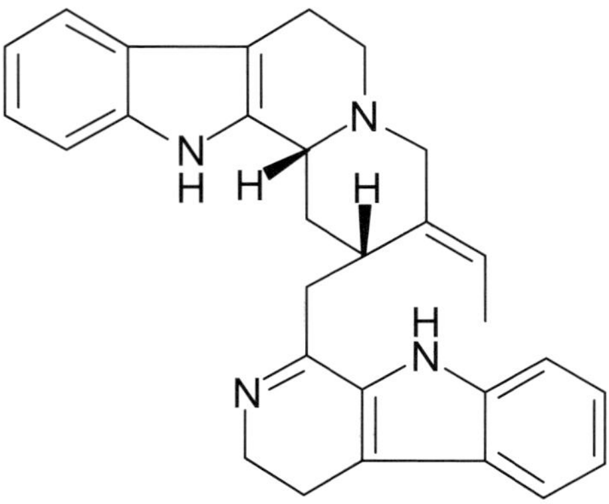

(166) Dihydrousambarensine

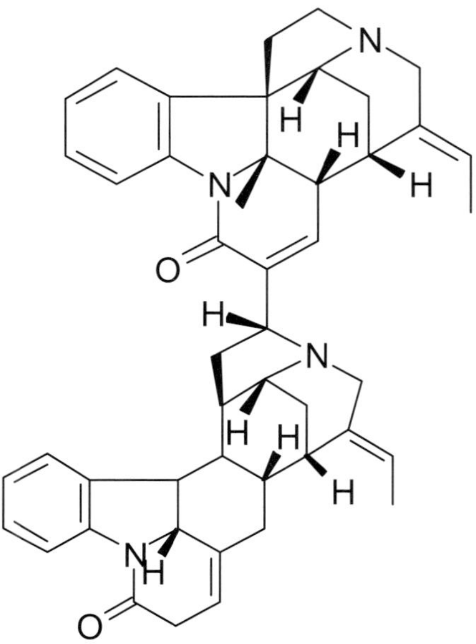

(167) Isosungucine

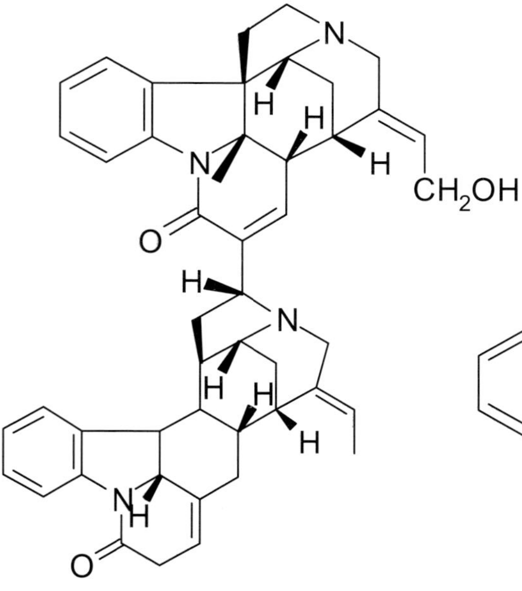

(168) 18-hydroxyisosungucine

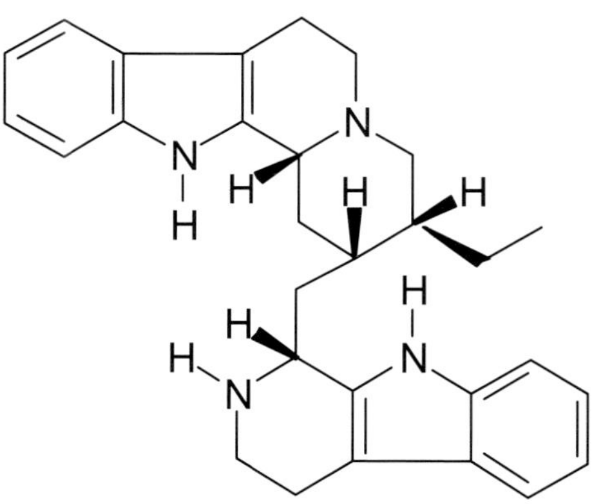

(169) Ochrolifuanine A

Contd...

Figure 8.1–*Contd...*

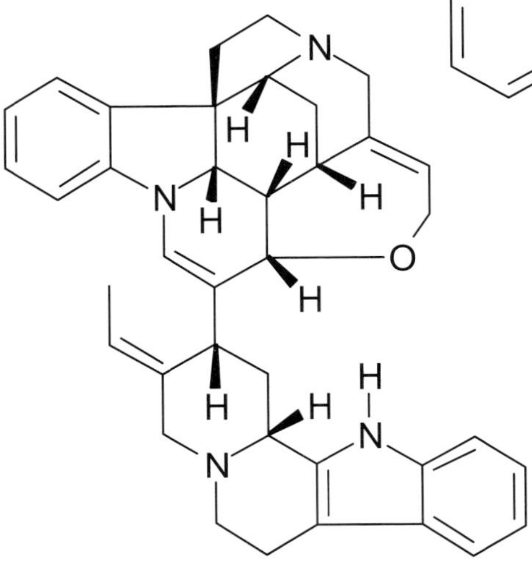

(170) Longicaudatine

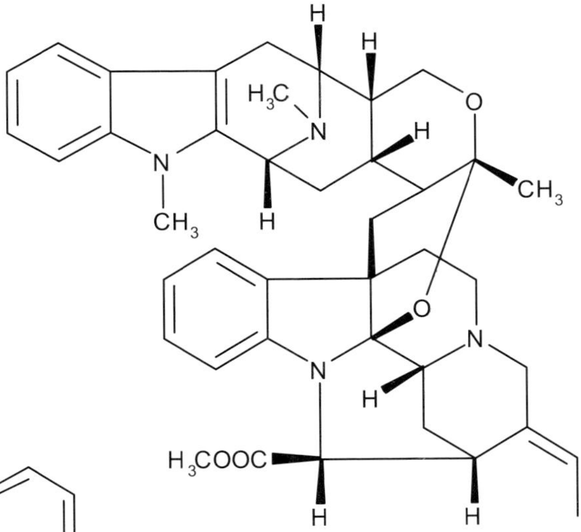

(171) Villalstonine

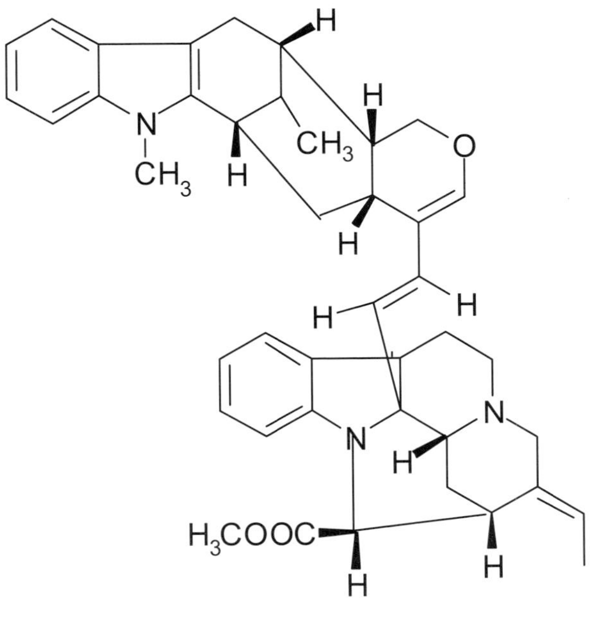

(172) Macrocarpamine

Contd...

Figure 8.1–*Contd...*

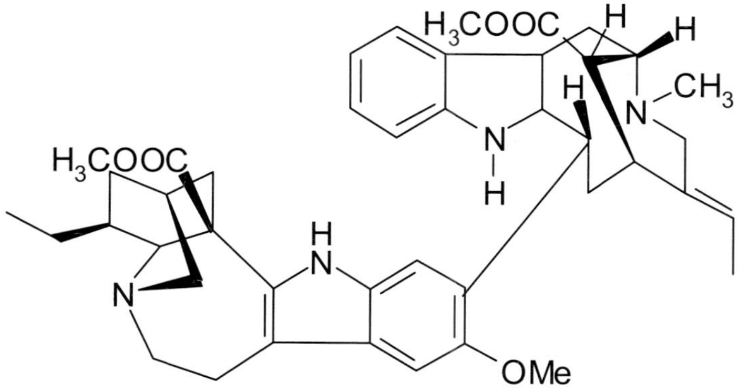

(173) Voacamine

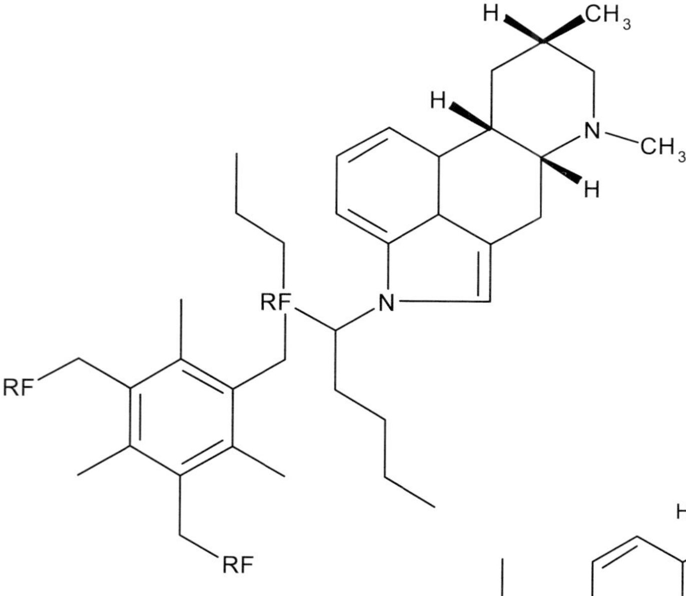

(174) Festuclavine

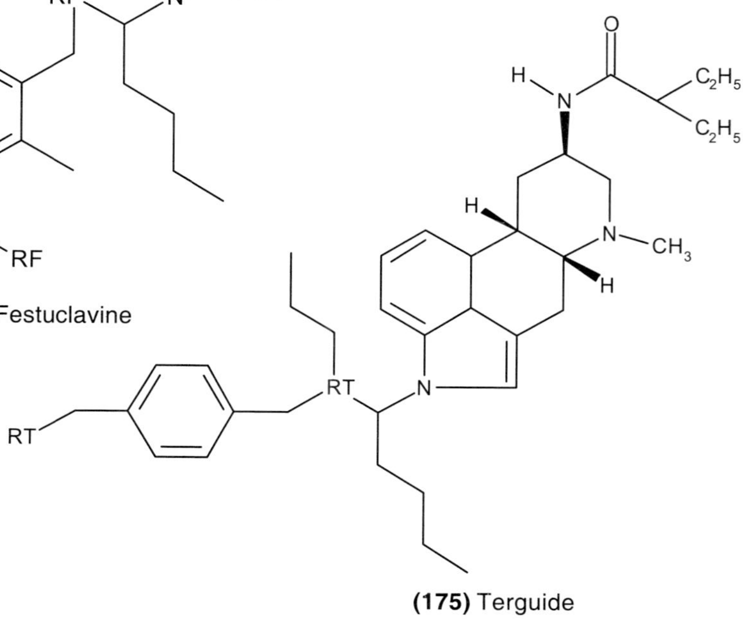

(175) Terguide

Contd...

Figure 8.1–*Contd...*

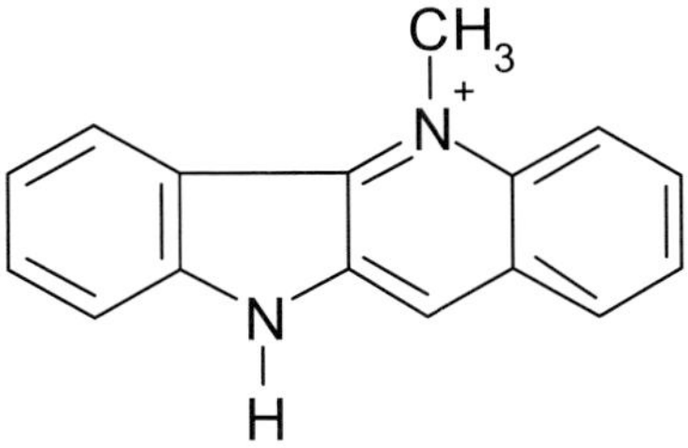

(176) Cryptolepine

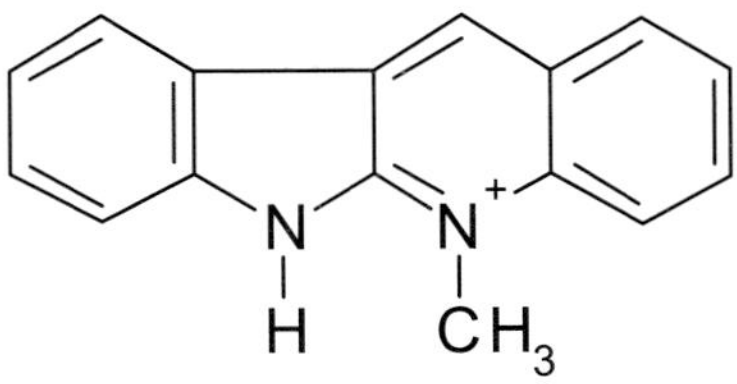

(177) Neocryptolepine

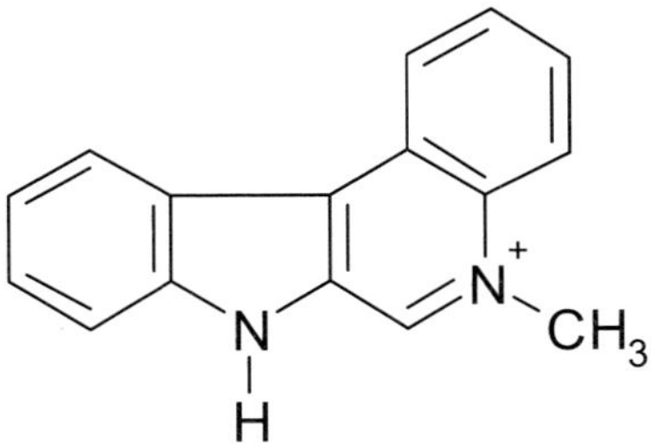

(178) Isoneocryptolepine

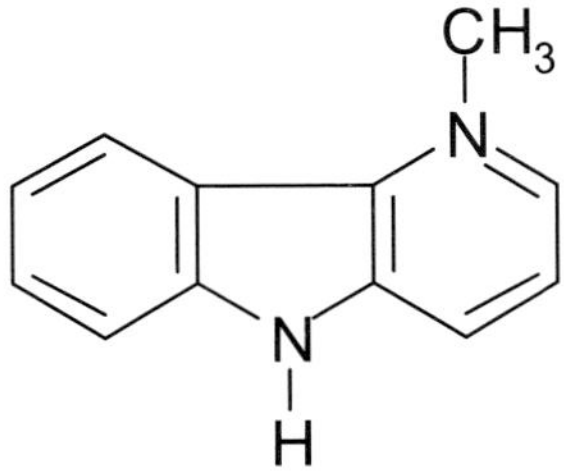

(179) N1-methyl-δ-carboline

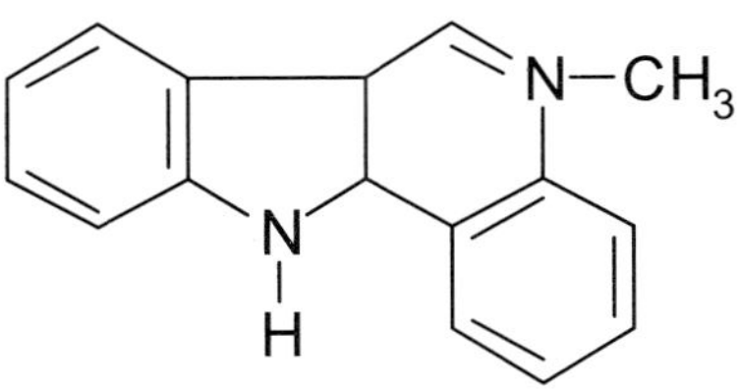

(180) Isocryptolepine

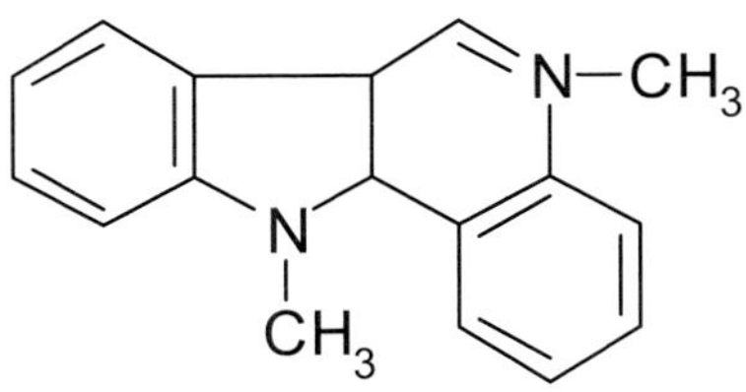

(181) N-methylisocryptolepinium

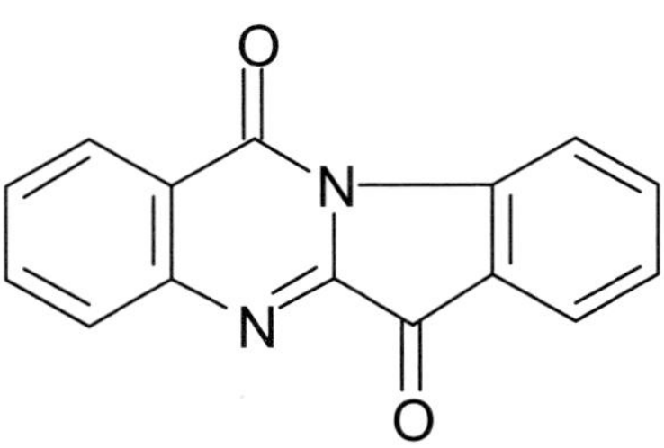

(182) Tryptothrine

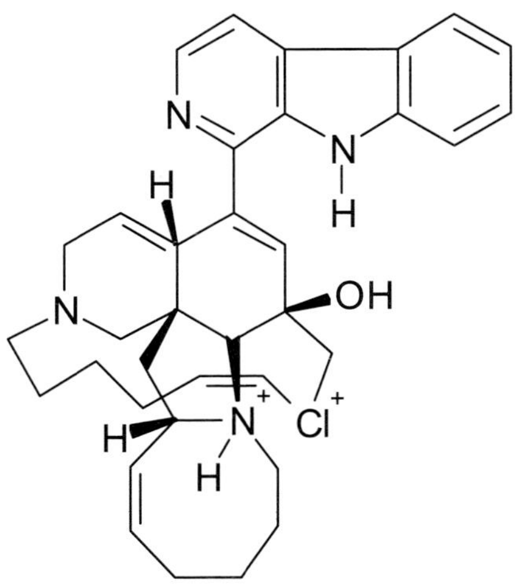

(183) Manzamine A

Contd...

Figure 8.1–*Contd...*

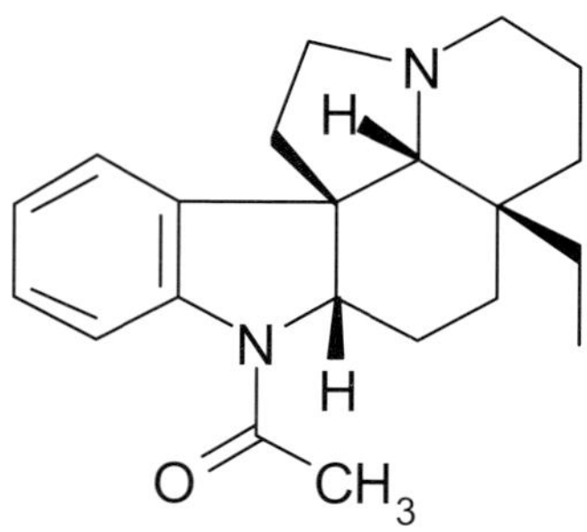

(184) N-formyl-asidospermidine

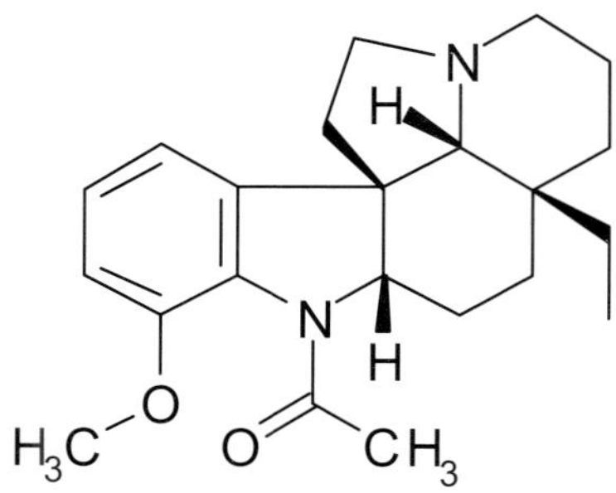

(185) Asidospermine

Strychnos innocua

The coagulant properties of the polysaccharide fractions such as galactomannan **(70)** and a galactan **(71)** were isolated from the *Strychnos innocua* by using TLC (Silica gel), column chromatography (Supelco SP 2330, Capillary column), HPLC (LiChrospher column) using acetonitrile with water as solvent systems; GLC-MS (Supelco SP 2330, Capillary column) and characterized through NMR studies (Matteo Adinolfi *et al.*, 1994).

The chemical composition of polysaccharides fractions such as 2,3,4,6-Tetra-O-methylgalactopyranose **(72)**, 2,3,6-Tri-O-methylmannopyranose **(73)** and 2,3-Di-O-methylmannopyranose **(74)** were isolated from the seeds of *S. innocua* was reported by using TLC fractionation (Silica gel) on various solvents such as ether, methanol and ethyl acetate; they were characterized through NMR studies (Corsaro *et al.*, 1995).

Strychnos johnsonii

A full account of the first chiral synthesis of normalindine **(75)** and an indolopyridonaphthyridine alkaloid isolated from *Strychnos johnsonii* was reported (Masashi Ohba *et al.*, 2000).

Strychnos lucida

A new quinic acid ester, 4-O-(3,5-dimethoxy-4-hydroxybenzoyl) quinic acid **(76)** was isolated from methanolic extract of dried barks and woods of *Strychnos lucida* and subsequentially characterized by mass spectroscopy and NMR studies (Itoh Atsuko *et al.*, 2006)

Strychnos mellodora

Two new N_b-methylated β-carbolinium glucoalkaloids such as 3,4,5,6-tetradehydropalicoside **(77)** and 3,4,5,6-tetradehydrodolichantoside **(78)**, together with the known β-carboline derivative *viz.*, desoxycordifoline **(79)** known as (β-carboline 3-carboxylate glucoalkaloid) and melinonine F **(80)** called as (N_b-methylated harmanium cation), were isolated and characterized on the basis of chromatographic studies such as TLC (Silica gel) using methanol and ammonium nitrate; MPLC using methanol in Me_2CO as gradient; HPLC (Stationary phase, LiChrosorb RP8 Select B column) using hepanesufonic acid and acetonitrile; also characterized through UV, MS and NMR from crude ethanolic extract of *Strychnos mellodora* stem bark (Viviane Brandt *et al.*, 1999).

A stable compound, strictosidine β-glucosidase **(81)** was isolated along with dolichantoside **(82)**, palicoside **(83)** from dried powdered material of *S. mellodora* by using HPLC (LiChrospher 60RP Select B column) (Viviane Brandt, 2000).

The enzymatic glucose cleavage of palicoside **(83)** revealed the biosynthetic pathway to akagerine **(84)**, whereas the conversion of dolichantoside **(82)** led to a new quaternary heteroyohimbine alkaloid N_b-methyl-21-β-hydroxy-mayumbine **(85)** (Viviane Brandt, 2001).

Strychnos minfiensine

Thermolysis of several imidofuranyl carbamate products derived from an intramolecular [4+2]-cycloaddition reaction; the ortho-azido aryl carbamate **(86)** has been used in electrocyclization with a nitrene intermediate and produced 3-substituted indole. Also the study has been revealed that following compounds minfiensine **(87)**, 9a,4a-iminoethano-carbazole **(88)** from *Strychnos minfiensine* (Drew R. Bobeck *et al.*, 2009).

Strychnos moandaensis

Moandaensine **(89)**, a novel dimeric indole alkaloid has been isolated from the *Strychnos moandaensis* De Wild. characterized through UV, 1D and 2D NMR studies (Robert Verpoorte *et al.*, 2010).

Strychnos myrtoides

Two major alkaloids, *viz.*, strychnobrasiline **(90)** and malagashanine **(91)**, four minor alkaloids, *viz.*, malagashanol **(92)**, acetylmalagashanol **(93)**, 12-hydroxymalagashanine **(94)**, 12-hydroxy-19-*epi*-malagashanine **(95)**, myrtoidine **(39)** and 11-demethoxymyrtoidine **(40)** were isolated from the stem bark of *Strychnos myrtoides* and their structures were established by 2D NMR analysis (Marie Therese Martin *et al.*, 1999).

Three new N_b, C(21)-secocuran alkaloids, *viz.*, 3-*epi*-myrtoidine **(36)**, 11-demethoxy-3-*epi*-myrtoidine **(37)**, 11-demethoxy-12-hydroxy-3-*epi*-myrtoidine **(38)** and two known compounds such as myrtoidine **(39)** and 11-demethoxymyrtoidine **(40)** were isolated from the *S. myrtoides* characterized through NMR studies (Philippe Rasoanaivo *et al.*, 2001).

Malagashanine **(91)** was isolated from Madagascan *S. myrtoides* by using HPLC analysis (Gibco, RPMI 1640 column) (David Ramanitrahasimbola *et al.*, 2006).

Strychnos nux-vomica

The only quaternary base known so far the monomeric C-mavacurine **(96)** was isolated from root bark of the Asian *Strychnos nux-vomica* by using HPLC analysis (Marini Bettolo *et al.*, 1972).

The coagulant properties of the polysaccharide fractions such as galactomannan **(70)** and a galactan **(71)** were isolated from the *S. nux-vomica* by TLC (Silica gel F_{254}) with 2-propanol and water as mobile phase, GC-MS (Supelco SP-2330, Capplliary column), GLC-MS, HPLC (LiChrospher column) using ammonia, acetonitrile with water and characterized through NMR studies (Matteo Adinolfi *et al.*, 1994).

The chemical composition of polysaccharide fractions such as 2,3,4,6-Tetra-O-methylgalactopyranose **(72)**, 2,3,6-Tri-O-methylmannopyranose **(73)**, 2,3-Di-O-methylmannopyrannose **(74)** have been isolated from the seeds of *S. nux-vomica* by using GC-MS (Supelco capillary column SP-2330) on methylated alditol acetates and NMR studies was reported (Corsaro *et al.*, 1995).

Cis-3a-(O-Nitrophenyl) hexahydroindol-4-one **(97)** promoted by ethyl ether cyclization resulted propargylic silane **(98)** afforded the tricyclic vinylidene ketone **(99)**, the process known as Michael addition; which was further converted to the *Strychnos* alkaloids tubifolidine **(100)**, akuammicine **(101)** and 19, 20-dihydroakuammicine **(102)** (Daniel Sole *et al.*, 1996).

Solutions of *S. nux-vomica* by both oral and I.P. routes prepared with 90 per cent ethanol, were investigated for their effect on alcohol-induced sleep time in mice. The solution prepared with *S. nux-vomica* 90 per cent ethanol was effective in reducing the sleep time in mice. The study has been reported the specificity of the *S. nux-vomica* at ultra high dilution and effect mediated through oral receptors (Sukul *et al.*, 1999).

The aqueous and methanolic extract of *S. nux-vomica* root bark has been reported to possess antidiarrhoeal potential in the order of methanolic>aqueous against castor-oil induced diarrhoea in mice (Gricilda Shoba *et al.*, 2001).

The analgesic and anti-inflammatory properties has been reported for the presence of strychnine **(7)**, brucine **(58)**, strychnine N-oxide **(103)** and brucine N-oxide **(104)** which was isolated from the seed extract of *S. nux-vomica*. It was further reported that the plant extracts having significant analgesic and anti-inflammatory activity (Wu Yin *et al.*, 2003).

Three iridoids, 3′-O-acetylloganic acid **(105)**, 4′-O-acetylloganic acid **(106)** and 6′-O-acetylloganic acid **(107)** were isolated together with two known iridoid glucosides such as loganic acid **(20)** and 7-O-acetylloganic acid **(108)** from seeds of *S. nux-vomica* was isolated and their structures were established by ESI-MS (Electrospray MS), 1D and 2D NMR spectroscopic methods (Xiaozhe Zhang *et al.*, 2003).

The sweeping-micellar electrokinetic chromatography (MEKC) method has been successfully applied to the quantitative analysis of strychnine **(29)** and brucine **(58)** present in *S. nux-vomica* L. and its Chinese medicinal preparations. The compound berberine **(109)** was used as the internal standard for the improvement of the experimental reproducibility. The detection limits (S/N=3:1) for strychnine **(29)** and brucine **(58)** were 0.05 and 0.07 gmL^{-1} respectively (Chun Wang *et al.*, 2006).

Strychnine **(29)** and brucine **(58)** of *S. nux-vomica* exhibited significant pharmacological activity on several neurotransmitter receptors, including some members of the super family of ligand-gated ion channels. Quaternization of strychnine

(29) and brucine **(58)** with subsequent substitution significantly eliminated the activity at the glycine receptors (Anders *et al.*, 2006).

A validated versatile method on fast, sensitive and quantitative determination of strychnine **(29)** at lower dose in urine by LC-MS/MS from *S. nux-vomica* has been reported (Van Eanoo *et al.*, 2006).

An easy, rapid method for simultaneous determination of strychnine **(29)** and brucine **(58)** from *S. nux-vomica* L. and its preparation by using non-aqueous capillary electrophoresis (NACE) without pretreatment was developed and reported (Yuqin Li *et al.*, 2006).

The strychnine **(29)**, colubrine **(57)**, brucine **(58)**, pseudostrychnine **(59)**, pseudobrucine **(60)**, icajine **(62)**, vomicine **(63)**, novacine **(64)**, strychnine N-oxide **(103)**, brucine N-oxide **(104)**, 16-hydroxy-α-colubring **(110)**, 2-hydroxy-3-methoxystrychnine **(111)**, isostrychnine **(112)**, isobrucine **(113)**, isostrychnine-N-oxide **(114)** and isobrucine-N-oxide **(115)** were the alkaloids identified from the crude *S. nux-vomica* seeds by matrix assisted laser desorption/ionization time of flight mass spectroscopy was reported by MALDI-TOFMS as a flight mass spectroscopy (Wei Wu *et al.*, 2007).

The alkaloids *viz.*, strychnine **(29)**, brucine **(58)**, brucine-N-oxide **(104)** and isostrychnine **(112)** were isolated by using NMR and anti-tumor activity was reported using HepG2 cells on seed of the *S. nux-vomica*. (Xu-Kun Deng *et al.*, 2006)

The methaonlic extracts of *S. nux-vomica* showed xanthine oxidase inhibitory activity and significant reduction in serum urate level was reported (Muthusamy Umamaheshwari *et al.*, 2007)

The cytotoxicity of four alkaloids *viz.*, strychnine **(29)**, brucine **(58)**, brucine N-oxide **(104)** and isostrychnine **(112)** from *S. nux-vomica* on human hepatoma cell lines (SMMC 7721) cells along with their possible mechanism. The seed extract of *S. nux-vomica* reported to possess significant effective against SMMC-7721 cells proliferation (Wu Yin *et al.*, 2007).

The anti-proliferative and cytotoxic activity of strychnine **(29)** and brucine **(58)** has been isolated from root extract of *S. nux-vomica* by using LC-MS and significant activity on human multiple myeloma cell line RPMI-8226 was reported (Pasupuleti sreenivasa rao *et al.*, 2009).

The antioxidant potential in non-enzymatic and enzymatic anti-oxidant variations in tender and mature leaves of *S. nux-vomica* was reported to possess significant radical scavenging ability (Remya Vijayakumar *et al.*, 2009).

Strychnos panganensis

Twelve alkaloids, seven of which are new, have been isolated from the root bark of chloroform extract of *Strychnos panganensis* by using TLC (Whatman PK6 F_{254}) with different solvents namely chloroform, methanol, ammonium hydroxide; UV and H^1 NMR. The known alkaloids are matopensine **(116)**, 16-(S)-E-isositsirikine **(117)**, 12-hydroxy-11-methoxydiaboline **(118)**, N-desacetylretuline **(119)**, N-desacetylisoretuline

(120). The novel alkaloids are N-desacetylspermostrychnine **(121)**, 12-hydroxy-11-methoxy-nor-C-fluorocurarine **(122)**, 12-hydroxy-11-methoxy-N-acetylmon-C-fluorocurarimine **(123)** and four dimeric alkaloids, panganensines R**(124)**, S **(125)**, X **(126)** and Y **(127)** (Jean Marc *et al.*, 1996).

Strychnos potatorum

The composition of the coagulant polysaccharide fraction such as 1:1.7 mixtures of a galactomannan **(115)** and a galactan **(116)** were isolated from the *Strychnos potatorum* seeds by using TLC (Silica gel F_{254}) on 2-propanol with water, GC, GLC-MS (Supelco SP 2330, Capillary colunn), HPLC (LiChrospher) using ammonia, acetonitrile with water used as a mobile phase and characterized through NMR studies (Matteo Adinolfi *et al.*, 1994).

The chemical composition of polysaccharide fractions such as 2,3,4,6-Tetra-O-methylgalactopyranose **(72)**, 2,3,6-Tri-O-methylmannopyranose **(73)** and 2,3-Di-O-methylmannopyrannose **(74)** has been isolated from the seeds *S. potatorum* by using GC-MS (Supelco SP-2330, Capillary column) and characterized through NMR studies was reported (Corsaro *et al.*, 1995).

The seeds of methanolic extract of *S. potatorum* were reported to possess significant diuretic activity (Biswas *et al.*, 2001).

The anti-diarrhoeal activity in caster oil induced diarrhoea in rats were evaluated with the methanolic extract of the dried seeds of *S. potatorum* and the study has possess significant activity (Biswas *et al.*, 2002).

Aqueous extract of seeds of *S. potatorum* was reported to possess hepatoprotective and antioxidant activities in CCl_4 induced acute hepatic injury. Enzymatic and nonenzymatic antioxidant levels and lipid peroxide levels were restored to normal by administration of aqueous extract of *S. potatorum* was reported (Sanmugapriya *et al.*, 2006).

The antiulcerogenic potential of *S. potatorum* seeds on aspirin plus pyloric ligation induced gastric ulcer model and prevents the ulcer formation by decreasing acid secretion activity and increasing the mucin level in rats. It is further evidenced through histopathological studies of stomach mucosa (Sanmugapriya *et al.*, 2007).

Aqueous solution of *S. potatorum* seed powder has been reported to possess Pb(II) removing efficiency and further confirmed by FT-IR studies (Jayaram *et al.*, 2009).

Strychnos pseudoquina

Antimalarial activity of ethanolic extract of *Strychnos pseudoquina* bark has been reported and possesses significant inhibition against pathogenesis. (Andrade-Neto *et al.*, 2003)

The genotoxic potential was reported on crude extracts of the leaves of *S. pseudoquina*, on *Salmonella typhimurium* in micronucleus test of peripheral blood cells of mice also its proved that significant activity against TA98 (-S9) and TA100 (+S9, -S9) strains of *Salmonella typhimurium* (Santos *et al.*, 2006).

Strychnos spinosa

In-vitro antitrypanosomal activity of methylene chloride, methanol and aqueous extracts of the leaves and twigs of *Strychnos spinosa* was reported (Sara Hoet *et al.*, 2004).

Strychnos trinervis

The bisnordihydrotoxiferine **(68)** has been isolated from the root bark of the *Strychnos trinervis* by using TLC. The isolated compound was reported to possess antimicrobial and cytotoxic activities (Margareth De F.F. Melo *et al.*, 1987).

Strychnos usambarensis

Four alkaloids namely guianensine **(41)**, isoretuline **(54)**, 3',4',5',6'-tetradehydrolongicaudatine Y **(128)** and Longicaudatine Y **(129)** were isolated from the stem bark of *Strychnos usambarensis* was reported by using TLC, LC and NMR (Michel Frederich *et al.*, 1998).

An usambarine type alkaloid named isostrychnopentamine **(130)**, have also been isolated from *S. usambarensis* Gilg., it is the main ingredient of an African curarising arrow poison. The *in-vitro* and *in vivo* antimalarial properties of isostrychnopentamine **(130)** have been reported (Frederich *et al.*, 2004).

Strychnos vanprukii

A gluco-indole alkaloid, 3,4-dehydropalicoside **(131)** and a pimarane diterpenoid, 7β-hydroxypimara-8,15-dien-14-one **(132)**, was isolated along with four known alkaloids scuh as 3,4,5,6-tetradehydropalicoside **(77)**, palicoside **(83)**, akagerine **(84)** and 17-O-methylakagerine **(133)** from the hexane extract of *Strychnos vanprukii* by spectroscopic evidence such as ES-MS-MS using silica gel column eluting with chloroform and hexane used as mobile phase; FT-IR and their characterization through NMR studies were reported (Piyanuch Thongphasuk, 2003).

Two new lignan glucosides, vanprukoside **(134)** and strychnoside **(135)**, were isolated together with the known lignan glucoside, (+)-lyoniresinol-3a-O-glucopyranoside **(136)** from the stem of *S. vanprukii* by using TLC, UV and NMR. The structures of these compounds were elucidated on the basis of their spectroscopic data. All three compounds were reported to possess antioxidant activity (Piyanuch Thongphasuk *et al.*, 2004).

Strychnos species

The potential cytotoxic activities of *Strychnos* species were reported on different cancer and normal cells cultured *in-vitro* method and simple micro test reported that the good reproducibility. Most of the active compounds belong to the usambrarane **(137)** skeleton has been reported (Joelle Leclercq *et al.*, 1986).

The synthesis of tetracyclic-1,2,3,4,5,6-hexahydro-1,5-methanoazocino(4,3-b)indole **(138)** as *Strychnos* indole alkaloids has been reported (Mercedes Alvarez *et al.*, 1987).

A new and versatile synthesis of three tetracyclic compounds presenting the ABED ring system from *Strychnos* alkaloids was reported. The intermediate tetrahydropyridinium compounds namely 2-cyano-3ethyl-1-methyl-1,2,3,6-tetrahydropyridine **(139)**, N-substituted Δ^3-piperidein-2-ones **(140)** salts and 2-(1,3-dithian-2-yl)-indole **(141)** were isolated (Anna Diez *et al.*, 1994).

The 19,20-Dihydroakuammicine **(102)** was isolated from the *Strychnos* spcies, by flash chromatography and characterized through mass spectroscopy, IR and NMR studies (Mercedes Amat *et al.*, 1995).

An enantioselective synthesis of the alkaloid (-)-tubifoline **(142)**, involving the kinetic resolution of racemic 1-(3-pyridyl) ethanol **(143)** from the *Strychnos* species by using NMR (Mercedes Amat *et al.*, 1996).

Three different alkaloids such as 19,20-dihydroakuammicine **(102)**, (-)-tubifoline **(142)** and (-)-tubifolidine **(144)** were isolated from *Strychnos* species by using flash chromatography (Silica gel 60) using SDS and SiO_2, HPLC (Chiral column OB) using isopropanol with hexane; and characterized through NMR studies (Mercedes Amat *et al.*, 1997).

Malagashanine **(91)** is the parent compound of a new type of indole alkaloid, the N_b-C (21)-secocuran, isolated from the Malagasy *Strychnos* species traditionally used as chloroquine adjuvants in the treatment of chronic malaria. Especially, strychnobrasiline **(90)**, malgashanine **(91)**, N_a-deacetyl-SB **(145)**, N_a deacetyl-N_a-methyl-SB **(146)** and burasaine **(147)** alkaloids has been isolated from the *Strychnos* species by using HPLC and characterized through NMR studies (Herintsoa Rafatro *et al.*, 2000).

In addition to the enolate of methyl such as 1-methyl-2-indoleacetate **(148)** and lithium 2-(lithiomethyl) indole-1-carboxylate **(149)** to pyridines and N-alkylpyridinium salts bearing a chiral auxiliary at the 3-position (tolysufinyl, acyl iron complexes, bornane-10,2-sultam), with subsequent acid cyclization of the resulting dihydropyridines, from *Strychnos* species by using NMR study was reported (Mercedes Amat *et al.*, 2003).

Strychnine **(29)**, diaboline **(30)**, guiachrysine **(44)**, guiaflavine **(50)**, brucine **(58)**, pseudostrychnine **(59)**, icajine **(62)**, sungucine **(65)**, strychnohexamine **(67)**, C-dihydrotoxiferine **(150)**, C-toxiferine **(151)**, C-curarine **(152)** C-alkaloid A **(153)**, C-alkaloid E **(154)**, C-alkaloid F **(155)**, C-alkaloid G **(156)**, C-alkaloid H **(157)**, C-calebassine **(158)**, (+)-tubocurarine **(159)**, N, N-dioallyltoxiferine (alcuronium) **(160)** and atracurium **(161)** were the alkaloids has been reported in *Strychnos* species (Genevieve Philippe *et al.*, 2004).

^{1}H Nuclear magnetic resonance spectrometry and multivariate analysis techniques were reported in the metabolic profiling of three *Strychnos* species: *Strychnos nux-vomica* (seeds, stem bark, root bark), *Strychnos ignatii* (seeds), and *Strychnos icaja* (leaves, stem bark, root bark, collar bark). The principal component analysis (PCA) of the ^{1}H NMR spectra showed that brucine **(58)**, loganin, fatty acids and *S. icaja* alkaloids such as icajine **(62)** and sungucine **(65)**. (Michel Frederich, 2004).

The toxicity of many *Strychnos* species has been used as arrow poisons or ordeals. Two completely different types of toxic mechanisms were associated with the *Strychnos* species: a tetanising activity caused by strychnine **(29)** and some of its monomeric derivatives and a paralyzing action due to a series of quaternary alkaloids included in curare poisons. (Genevieve Philippe, 2005).

The anti-plasmodial activity of crude extracts of 19 species such as *S. aculeate, S. angolensis, S. brasiliensis, S. cocculoids, S. diplotricha, S. gossweileri, S. henningsii, S. ignatii, S. innocua, S. johnsonii, S. lucens, S. mellodora, S. mitis, S. nux-vomica, S. phaeotricha, S. potatorum, S. pungens, S. spinosa and S. variabilis* by an *in-vitro* assay against a chloroquine-susceptible strain of *Plasmodium falciparum* was reported (Genevieve Philippe *et al.*, 2005a).

Isoretuline **(54)**, icajine **(62)**, sungucine **(65)**, strychnobrasiline **(90)**, malagashanine **(91)**, strychnogucine B **(66)**, isostrychnopentamine **(130)**, emetine **(162)**, tubulosine **(163)**, strychnopentamine **(164)**, usambarensine **(165)**, dihydrousambarensine **(166)**, isosungucine **(167)**, 18-hydroisosungucine **(168)**, ochrolifuanine A **(169)**, longicaudatine **(170)**, villalstonine **(171)**, macrocarpamine **(172)**, voacamine **(173)**, trimeric derivative of festuclavine **(174)** and the dimeric derivative of terguride **(175)**, crptolepine **(176)**, neocryptolepine **(177)**, isoneocryptolepine **(178)**, N1-methyl-δ-carboline **(179)**, isocryptolepine **(180)**, N-methylisocryptolepinium **(181)**, tryptanthrine **(182)**, manzamine A **(183)**, N-formyl-aspidospermidine **(184)** and aspidospermine **(185)** were reported from various species *viz., S. diplotricha, S. henningsii, S. mostueoides, S. myrtoides, S. usambarensis* and *S. variabilis* (Michel Frederich *et al.*, 2008).

Conclusions

In summary the isolation methodology in precise along with the structures of 185 chemical compounds of the *Strychnos* genus; three secocuran alkaloids, a new zwitterionic alkaloid, a new tertiary alkdaloid, two new quarternary alkaloids, two new quaternary indole alkaloids, two new N_b-methylated β-carbolinium gulcoalkaloids, a new dimeric indole alkaloid, three new N_b-C(21)-secocuran alkaloids, two new lignan glucosides, a new indole alkaloid has been found that newer chemical compounds.

References

Anders A. Jensen., Parviz Gharagozloo., Nigel J.M. Birdsall., and Darius P. Zlotos. (2006). Pharmacological characterization of strychnine and brucine analogues at glycine and α7 nicotinic acetylcholine receptors. *European Journal of Pharmacology*, **539**: 27–33.

Andrade-Neto, V.F., Brandao, M.G.L., Stehmann, J.R., Oliveira, L.A., Krettli, A.U. (2003). Antimalarial activity of *Cinchona* like plants used to treat fever and malaria in Brazil. *Journal of Ethnopharmacology*, **87**: 253-256.

Anna Diex., Josep Castells., Pilar Forns., Mario Rubiralta., David S. Grierson., Henri Philippe Husson., Xavier Soians., and Merce Font-Bardia. (1994). Synthetic applications of 2-(1,3-Dithian-2-yl) indoles. IV. One New synthesis of the tetracyclic ABED ring system of *Strychnos* alkaloids. *Tetrahedron,* **50(22)**: 6585-6602.

Atsuko Itoh, Tanaka Yasuhiro, Nagakura naotaka, Nishi Toyoyuki, Tanahashi, Takao. (2006). A quinic acid ester from *Strychnos lucida. Journal of natural Medicines,* **60(2)**: 146-148.

Atsuko Itoh., Yasuhiro Tanaka., Naotaka Nagakura., Toru Akita., and Toyoyuki Nishi., Takao Tanahashi. (2008). Phenolic and iridoid glycosides from *Strychnos axillaris*. *Phytochemist*ry, **69**: 1208-1214.

Biswas, S., Murugesan, T., Maiti, K., Ghosh, L., Pal, M., and Saha, B.P. (2001). Study on the diuretic activity of *Strychnos potatorum* Linn. Seed extract in albino rats. *Phytomedicine,* 8**(6)**: 469-471.

Biswas, S., Murugesan, T., Sanghamitra, S., Maiti, K., Jiaur Rahaman, G., Pal, M., Saha, B.P. (2002). Anti-diarrhoeal activity of *Strychnos potatorum* seed extract in rats. *Fitoterapia,* **73**: 43-47.

Chun Wang., Dandan Han., Zhi Wang., Xiaohuan Zang., and Qiuhua Wu. (2006). Analysis of *Strychnos* alkaloids in traditional Chinese medicines with improved sensitivity by sweeping micellar electrokinetic chromatography. *Analytica Chimica Acta*. **572**: 190–196.

Corsaro, M.M., Giudicianni, I., Lanzetta, R., Marciano, C.E., Monaco, P., and Parrilli. M. (1995). Polysaccharides from seeds of *Strychnos* species. *Phytochemistry,* **39(6)**: 1377-1380.

Daniel Sole., Josep Bonjoch., Silvina Garcia-Rubio., Ramon Suriol., and Joan Bosch.A (1996). New Solution for the Construction of the Piperidine Ring of *Strychnos* Alkaloids from 3a-(o-Nitrophenyl) hexahydroindol-4-ones. Total Syntheses of (+)-Tubifolidine, (+)-Dihydroakuammicine, and (+)-Akuammicine. *Tetrahedron Letters,* **37(29)**: 5213-5216.

David Ramanitrahasimbola., Philippe Rasoanaivo., Suzanne Ratsimamanga., and Henri Vial. (2006). Malagashanine potentiates chloroquine antimalarial activity in drug resistant *Plasmodium* malaria by modifying both its efflux and influx. *Molecular and Biochemical Parasitology,* **146**: 58–67.

Drew R. Bobeck, Stefan France., Carolyn A. Leverett., Fernando Sanchez-Cantalejo., Albert Padwa. (2009). Cycloaddition studies directed toward the *Strychnos* alkaloid minfiensine. *Tetrahedron Letters,* **50**: 3145-3147.

Frederich, M., Tits, M., Goffin, E., Philippe, G., Grellier, P., De Mol, P., Hayette, M.P., Angenot, L. (2004). *In-vitro* and *in vivo* antimalarial properties of isostrychnopentamine, an indolomonoterpenic alkaloid from *Strychnos usambarensis*. *Planta Medica,* **70**: 520–525.

Frederich, M., De Pauw, M.C., Prosperi, C., Tits, M., Brandt, V., Penelle, J., Hayette, M.P., De Mol, P., Angenot, L. (2001). Strychnogucines A and B, two new antiplasmodial bisindole alkaloids from *Strychnos icaja*. *Journal of Natural Products,* **64**: 12–16.

Genevieve Philippe, Geneviève Philippe, Laurent Nguyen, Luc Angenot, Michel rédérich, Gustave Moonen, Monique Tits, Jean-Michel Rigo. (2006). Study of the interaction of antiplasmodial strychnine derivatives with the glycine receptor. *European Journal of Pharmacology*, **530**: 15-22.

Genevieve Philippe., Elise Prost., Jean-Marc Nuzillard., Monique Zeches-Hanrot., Monique Tits., Luc Angenot., and Michel Frederich. (2002). Strychnoshexamine from *Strychnos icaja*, a naturally occurring trimeric idolomonoterpenic alkaloid. *Journal of Tetrahedron letters*, **43**: 3387-3390.

Genevieve Philippe., Luc Angenot., Monique Tits., and Michel Frederich. (2004). About the toxicity of some *Strychnos* species and their alkaloids. *Toxicon*, **44**: 405-416.

Genevieve Philippe., and Luc Angenot. (2005). Recent developments in the field of arrow and dart poisons. *Journal of Ethnopharmacology*. **100**: 85-91.

Genevieve Philippe., Luc Angenot., Patrick De Mol., Eric Goffin., Marie-Pierre Hayette., Monique Tits., and Michel Frederich. (2005a). *In-vitro* screening of some *Strychnos* species for antiplasmodial activity. *Journal of Ethnopharmacology*, **97**: 535-539.

Gricilda Shoba, F., and Molly Thomas. (2001). Study of antidiarrhoeal activity of four medicinal plants in castor-oil induced diarrhoea. *Journal of Ethnopharmacology*, **76**: 73–76.

Helene mavar manga., Joelle quetin leclercq., Gabriel llabres., Maria lucia belem pinheiro., Arnaldo F. imbiriba Da Rocha., and Luc Angenot. (1996). 9-Methoxygeissoschizol, An alkaloid from bark of *Strychnos guianensis*. *Phytochemistry*, **43(5)**: 1125-1127.

Herintsoa rafatro., David ramanitrahasimbola., Philippe rasoanaivo., Suzanne ratsimamanga urverg., Albert rakoto ratsimamanga., and Francois frappier. (2000). Reversal activity of the naturally occurring chemosensitizer malagashanine in *Plasmodium malaria*. *Biochemical Pharmacology*, **59**: 1053-1061.

Jacques penelle., M onique Tits., Philippe Christen., Jordi Molgo., Viviane brandt., Michel frederich., and Luc angenot. (2000). Quaternary indole alkaloids from the stem bark of *S. guianensis*. *Phytochemistry*, **53**: 1057-1066.

Jacques Penelle., Philippe Christen., jordi Molgo., Monique tits., Viviane Brandt., Michel Frederich., and Luc Angenot. (2001). 5′6′-Dehydroguiachrysine and 5′,6′-dehydroguiaflavine, two curarizing quaternary indole alkaloids from the stem bark of *Strychnos guianensis*. *Phytochemistry*, **58**: 619-626.

Jayaram, K., Murthy, I.Y.L.N., Lalhruaitluanga, H., and Prasad. M.N.V. (2009). Biosorption of lead from aqueous solution by seed powder of *Strychnos potatorum* L. *Journal Colloids and Surfaces B: Biointerfaces*, **71**: 248–254.

Jean Marc Nuzillard., Philippe Thepenier., Marie Joase Jacquier., Georges Massiot., Louisette Le Men-Olivier., and Clement Delaude. (1996). Alkaloids from root bark of *Strychnos panganensis*. *Phytochemistry*, **43(4)**: 897-902.

Joelle Leclercq., Marie Claire De Pauw Gillet., Roger Gassleer., and Luc Angenot. (1986). Screening of cytotoxic activities of *Strychnos* alkaloids. *Journal of Ethnopharmacology*, **15**: 305-316.

Joelle Quetin Leclerc., Luc Angenot., and Norman G. Bisset.(1986). South American *Strychnos* species ethnobotany (except curare) and Alkaloid screening. *Journal of Ethnopharmacology,* **28**: 1-52.

Lusakibanza, M., Mesia, G., Tona, G., Karemere, S., Lukuka, A., Tits, M., Angenot, L., and Frederich, M. (2010). *In-vitro* and *in vivo* antimarlarial and cytotoxic activity of the five plants used in Congolese traditional medicine. *Journal of Ethnopharmacology,* **129(3)**: 398-402.

Margareth de F.F. Melo., CID A. de M. Santos., Alda de A. Chiappeta., Jose F. de mello., and Rabindranath mukherjee. (1987). Chemistry and pharmacology of a tertiary alkaloid from *Stychnos trinervis* root bark. *Journal of Ethnopharmacology,* **19**: 319-325.

Marie Therese Martin., Philippe Rasoanaivo., Giovanna Palazzino., Corrado Galeffi., Marcello Nicoletti., Francois Trigalo., Francois Frappier. (1999). Minor N_b-C (21)-secocuran alkaloids of *Strychnos myrtoides. Phytochemistry,* **51**: 479-486.

Marini bettolo, G.B., Ciasca, M.A., and Galeffi. C. (1972). The occurrence of Strychnine and Brucine in an American species of *Strychnos. Phytochemistry,* **11**: 381-384.

Masashi ohba, Hiroyuki kubo and Hiroyuki ishibashi. (2000). A chiral synthesis of the Strychnos and ophiorrhiza alkaloid Noramlindine. *Tetrahedron,* **56**: 7751-7761.

Matteo adinolfi., Maria michela corsaro., Rosa Lanzetta., Michelangelo Parrilli, Geoff folkard, Willaim Grant, John Sutherland. (1994). Composition of the coagulant polysaccharide fraction from *Strychnos potatorum* seeds. *Carbohydrate research,* **263**: 103-110.

Mercedes Alvarez., Rodolfo Lavilla., Cristina Roure., Eulalia Cabot., and Joan Bosch. (1987). Studies on the *Strychnos* indole alklaoids. Introduction of the functionalized one-carbon substituent at C-16[1-2]. *Tetrahedron,* **43(11)**: 2513-2522.

Mercedes amat., Ma dolors coll., and Joan bosch. (1995). Enantiopure intermediates for the synthesis of *Strychnos* alkaloids. *Tetrahedron,* **51(39)**: 10759-10770.

Mercedes Amat., Ma Dolors Coll., Daniele Passarella., and Joan Bosch. (1996). An enantioselective synthesis of the synthesis alkaloid (-)-Tubifoline. *Tetrahedron,* **7(10)**: 2775-2778.

Mercedes Amat., Ma dolors Coll., Joan Bosch., Enric Espinosa and Elies Molins. (1997). Total synthesis of the *Strychnos* indole alkaloids (-)-tubifoline, (-)-tubifolidine and 19,20-dihydroakuammicine. *Tetrahedron,* **8(6)**: 935-948.

Mercedes Amat., Dolors Coll, Nuria Llor, M., Carmen Escolano., Elies Molins., Carles Miravitlles., and Joan Bosch. (2003). Asymmetric synthesis of tetracyclic substructures of *Strychnos* indole alkaloids. *Tetrahedron: asymmetry,* **14**: 1691-1699.

Michel Frederich., Joelle Quetin Leclercq., Rose Gadi Biala., Viviane Brandt., Jacques Penelle., Monique Tits., and Luc Angenot. (1998). 3',4',5',6' tetradehydrolongicaudatine Y, an anhydronium base from *Strychnos usambarensis. Phytochemistry,* **48(7)**: 1263-1266.

Michel frederich., Young Hae Choi., Luc angenotGoetz Harnischfeger., Alfons W.M. Lefeber., and Robert verpoorte. (2004). Metabolomic analysis of *Strychnos nux-vomica, Strychnos icaja* and *Strychnos ignatii* extracts by ^{1}H nuclear magnetic resonance spectrometry and multivariate analysis techniques. *Phytochemistry,* **65**: 1993–2001.

Michel Frederich., Monique Tits., and Luc Angenot. (2008) Potential antimalarial activity of indole alkaloids. *Transactions of the Royal Society of Tropical Medicine and Hygiene,* **102**: 11-19.

Monique Tits., Jacques Damas., Joele Quetin Leclercq., and Luc Angenot. (1991). From the ethnobotanical uses of *Strychnos henningsii* to anti-inflammatory, analgesics and antispasmodics. *Ethnophamacology,* **34**: 261-267.

Muthusamy Umamaheshwari., Kuppusamy Ashok kumar., Arumugam Somasundaram., Thirumalaisamy Sivashanmugam., Varadharajan Subhadradevi., and Thenvungal Kochupapy Ravi. (2007). Xanthine oxidase inhibitory activity of some Indian medical plants. *Journal of Ethnopharmacology,* **109**: 547-551.

Ohiri, F.C., Verpoorte, R. and Baerheim Svendsen, A. (1983). The African *Strychnos* species and their alkaloids: A review. *Journal of Ethnopharmacology,* **9**: 167-223.

Pasupuleti Sreenivasa Rao., Madduri Ramanadham., and Majeti Narasimha Vara Prasad. (2009). Anti-proliferative and cytotoxic effects of *Strychnos nux-vomica* root extract on human multiple myeloma cell line – RPMI 8226. *Food and Chemical Toxicology,* **47**: 283-288.

Pellicciari, R., Delle Monach, F., Lozano Reyes, N., Casinovi, C.G. and Marini Bettolo, G.B. (1966). Ricerche Sugli alaloidi delle *Strychnos*. Nota XV. Gli alcaloidi della *Strychnos diaboli. Annali dell' Instituto Superiore Di Sanita,* **2**: 411-413.

Philippe rasoanaivo., Giovanna palazzino., Marcello nicoletti., and Corrado galeffi. (2001). The co-occurrence of C (3) epimer N_b, C (21)-secocuran alkaloids in *Strychnos diplotricha* and *Strychnos myrtoides. Phytochemistry,* **56**: 863-867.

Piyanuch thongphasuk., Rutt suttisri., Rapepol bavovada., and Robert verpoorte. (2003). Alkaloids and a pimarane diterpenoid from *Strychnos vanprukii. Phytochemistry,* **64**: 897-901.

Piyanuch Thongphasuk., Rutt Suttisri., Rapepol Bavovada., and Robert Verpoorte. (2004). Antioxidant lignin glucosides from *Strychnos vanprukii. Fitoterapia,* **75**: 623-628.

Quetin leclercq, J., Llabres, G., Varin, R., Belem Pinheiro, M.L., Mavar Manga, H., and Angenot, L. (1995). Gianensine A zwitterionic alkaloid from *Strychnosguianensis. phytochemistry,* **40(5)**: 1557-1560.

Rajesh, P., Latha, S., Selvamani, P., Saraswathy, A., and Rajesh Kannan. V. (2009). Role of *Strychnosbicirohssa* Benth. On anti-inflammatory activity in experimental model by using wistar rats. *Current biotica,* **3(2)**: 171-181.

Remya Vijayakumar., Chang Xing Zhao., Rengasamy Gopal., and C. Abdul Jaleel. (2009). Non-enzymatic and enzymatic anti-oxidant variations in tender and mature leaves of *S. nuxvomica* L. (Family: Loganiaceae). *Comptes rendus Biologies,* **332**: 52-57.

Robert verpoorte., Michel frederich., Clement delaude., Luc Angenot., Georges Dive., Philippe., Thepenier., Marie Jose Jacquier., Monique zecheds Hanrot., Catherine Lavaud., and Jean-Marc Nuzillard. (2010). Moandaensine, A dimeric indole alkaloid from *Strychnos moandaensis* (*Logninaceae*). *Phytochemistry letters.* (Issue is now online).

Sanmugapriya, E., and Venkataraman, S. (2006). Studies on hepatoprotective and antioxidant actions of *Strychnos potatorum* Linn. Seeds on CCl_4-induced acute hepatic injury in experimental rats. *Journal of Ethnopharmacology,* **105**: 154–160.

Sanmugapriya, E., and Venkataraman, S. (2007). Antiulcerogenic potential of *Strychnos potatorum* Linn. seeds on Aspirin plus pyloric ligation-induced ulcers in experimental rats. *Phytomedicine,* **14**: 360–365.

Santos, F.V., Colus, I.M.S., Silva, M.A., Vilegas, W., and Varanda. E.A. (2006). Assessment of DNA damage by extracts and fractions of *Strychnos pseudoquina*, a Brazilian medicinal plant with antiulcerogenic activity. *Food and Chemical Toxicology,* **44**: 1585–1589.

Sara Hoet., Frederik Opperdoes., Reto Brun., Victor Adjakidje., and Joelle Quetin Leclercq. (2004). *In-vitro* antitrypanosomal activity of ethnophamacologically selected Beninese plants. *Journal of Ethnopharmacology,* **91**: 37-42.

Sukul, A., Sinhabau, S.P., and Sukul, N.C. (1999). Reduction of alcohol induced sleep time in albino mice by potentized *Nux-vomica* prepared with 90 per cent ethanol. *British Homeopathic Journal,* **88**: 58-61.

Van Eanoo, P., Deventer, K., Roels, K., and Delbeke, F.T. (2006). Quantitative LC–MS determination of strychnine in urine after ingestion of a *Strychnos nux-vomica* preparation and its consequences in doping control. *Forensic Science International,* **164**: 159–163.

Viviane Brandt., Monique tits., Arjan geerlings., Michel frederich., Jacques penelle., Clement delaude., Robert Verpoorte., and Luc Angenot. (1999). β-carboline glucoalkaloids from *Strychnos mellodora. Phytochemistry,* **51**: 1171-1176.

Viviane Brandt., Arjan Geerlings., Monique Tits., Clement Delaude., Robert Van Der Heijden., Robert verpoorte., and Luc angenot. (2000). New strictosidine β-glucosidase from *Strychnos mellodora. Plant Physiol Biochem.,* **38**: 187-192.

Viviane brandt., Monique Tits., Jacques Penelle., Michel Frederich., and Luc Angenot. (2001). Main glucosidase conversion products of the gluco-alkaloids dolichantoside and palicoside. *Phytochemistry,* **57**: 653-659.

Wei Wu., Chunfeng Qiao., Zhitao Liang., Hongxi Xu., Zhongzhen Zhao., and Zongwei Cai. (2007). Alkaloid profiling in crude and processed *Strychno nux-vomica* seeds by matrix-assisted laser desorption/ionization-time of flight mass spectroscopy. *Pharmaceutical and Biomedical analysis,* **45**: 430-436.

Wu Yin., Tian-Shan wang., Fang-Zhou Yin., and Bao-Chang Cai. (2003). Analgesic and anti-inflammatory properties of brucine and brucine N-oxide extracted from the seeds of *Strychnos nux-vomica*. *Journal of Ethnopharmacology,* **88**: 205-214.

Wu Yin., Xu-Kun Deng., Fang-Zhou Yin., Xiao-Chun Zhang., and Bao-Chang Cai. (2007). The cytotoxicity induced by brucine from the seed of *Strychnos nux-vomica* proceeds via apoptosis and is mediated by cyclooxygenase 2 and caspase 3 in SMMC 7221 cells. *Food and chemical toxicology,* **45**: 1700-1708.

Xiaozhe Zhang., Qing Xu., Hongbin Xiao., and Xinmiao Liang. (2003). Iridoid glucosides from *Strychnos nux-vomica*. *Phytochemistry,* **64**: 1341-1344.

Xu-Kun Deng., Wu Yin., Wei-Dong Li., Fang-Zhou Yin., Xiao-Yu Lu., Xiao-Chun Zhang., Zi-Chun Hua., and Bao-Chang Cai. (2006). The anti-tumor effects of alkaloids from the seeds of *Strychnos nux-vomica* on HepG2 cells and its possible mechanism. *Journal of Ethnopharmacology,* **106**: 179-186.

Yuqin Li., Xiaojun He., Shengda Qi., Wenhua Gao., Xingguo Chen., and Zhide Hu. (2006). Seperation and determination of strychnine and brucine in *Strychnos nux-vomica* L. and its preparation by non-aqueous capillary electrophoresis. *Pharmaceutical and Biomedical analysis,* **41**: 400-407.

Bioactive Phytochemicals: Perspectives for Modern Medicine Vol. 1 (2012) *Pages* **331–380**
Editor: **V.K. Gupta**
Published by: **DAYA PUBLISHING HOUSE, NEW DELHI**

9

Phytochemicals as Natural Antimicrobials: Prospects and Challenges

Sujogya K. Panda [1] and Chandi C. Rath[2*]

ABSTRACT

Development of multiple drug resistance among pathogens is of global concern today. It is mainly due to non-target use of drugs (poultry, aquaculture, veterinary), over or under use of drugs, prolonged use of an antibiotic or chemotherapeutic agent, use of an antibiotic without the knowledge of the antibiogram pattern of pathogens, and non-completion of drug doses prescribed. Further, it may be due to pre-existing factors in the microorganisms or may be due to some acquired factors resistance is developed amongst the microorganisms towards the drugs and after resistance is acquired, it can spread in the community and among themselves though horizontal gene transfer. It has renewed the interest of researchers and academicians for the development of plant based medicines or more precisely herbal medicines, from medicinal and aromatic plants, as the plant products are without any side effects, do not add any physiological pressure on the pathogens for the development of drug resistance, easily degradable, non accumulative in the environment, do not cause environmental pollution too. However, the development and use of herbal drugs are lagged behind due to several factors. In this present review, we have made an attempt to discuss various plant derived compounds used as phyto-medicines, their extraction procedures, different screening techniques used to evaluate their potency as antimicrobial compounds with their limitations. Special effort is made to enlist different antimicrobial activity of plant derived drugs described by several workers from time to time in literature. The basic drawbacks of this traditional system are also discussed.

Keywords: Medicinal plants, Phytochemicals, Antimicrobial activity, Test procedures, Herbal drugs.

1 Department of Biotechnology, North Orissa University, Baripada, India.

2 P.G. Department of Botany, North Orissa University, Baripada – 757 003, India.

* *Corresponding author*: E-mail: chandicharanrath@yahoo.com

Introduction

Infectious diseases are world's leading killers after cardiovascular diseases as they account for death of 13.3 million people globally (25 per cent of total global deaths, WHO, 2000). Microorganism's *viz.*, bacteria, fungi, viruses and protozoa which have the capacity to cause disease are referred to as pathogenic or infectious microorganisms. Pathogenic or infectious microorganisms can be killed or inhibited by agents of biological or non-biological origin commonly referred as antimicrobials. Antimicrobials are used in therapeutically to treat infections.

Drug-resistant infectious microorganisms are those, which are not killed or inhibited by antimicrobial compounds. The increasing incidences of drug resistance and emergence and reemergence of deadly microorganisms are posing a great threat to the society. Drug resistance and emergence of new infectious microorganisms is a set of complex problems driven by a variety of factors ranging from miss use of antimicrobials, interactions of prescriber's and patients, economic incentives, characteristics of a country's health system, and the regulatory environment. Patient's perception of a new drug in the market to be more effective than older drugs leads to self-medication. Prescriber's perceptions regarding patient expectations and demands substantially influences prescribing practice. Physicians can be pressured by patient expectations to prescribe antimicrobials even in the absence of appropriate indications. Patient compliance with recommended treatment is another major problem. Patients forget to take medication, interrupt their treatment when they begin to feel better, or may be unable to afford a full course, thereby creating an ideal environment for microbes to adapt rather than be killed. Hospitals, worldwide are major contributors of the problem of antimicrobial resistance. The combination of highly susceptible patients, intensive and prolonged antimicrobial use and cross-infection have resulted in nosocomial infections with highly resistant bacterial pathogens. Resistant hospital-acquired infections are expensive to control and extremely difficult to eradicate. Around the world, as much as 60 per cent of hospital-acquired infections are caused by drug-resistant microorganisms (World Chiropractic Alliance, 2000). In a nutshell development of drug resistance among pathogens can be attributable to: (*i*) Indiscriminate use of antibiotics and chemotherapeutic agent, (*ii*) Prolonged use of a particular antibiotic, (*iii*) Application of broad spectrum antibiotic without prior knowledge of the antibiogram patterns of the pathogens, (*iv*) Failure of the complete course of antibiotic, (*v*) Use of sub optional antibiotics. Further, application of chemotherapeutic agent in poultry and dairy is another major cause of development of drug resistance among pathogens. Furthermore, use of various chemicals in modern aging culture adds a physiological pressure for development of resistance to these compounds.

Developing countries especially, Africa and India suffer significant population losses each year from infectious and parasitic diseases. Approximately 2 million people in India die each year because of these diseases. Thus Africa and India together account for 70 per cent of deaths due to infectious diseases worldwide. Today, 20-50 per cent of *Streptococcus pneumoniae* are resistant to widely available antibiotics such as Penicillin, Erythromycin and Sulfamethoxazole. In Vietnam, the majority of

Salmonella typhi are resistant to all first line antibiotics *e.g.*, Ampicillin, Chloroamphenicol and Sulfamethoxazle. Some microorganisms are showing resistance to second and third line antibiotics as well. In some countries up to 80 per cent of hospital acquired *Staphylococcus aureus* infections are methicillin resistant (MRSA) (WHO, 2002). In India, *S. aureus*, *Enterococcus faecalis*, *Mycobacterium tuberculosis* and *Pseudomonas aeruginosa* have already evaded every antibiotic in the clinician's armamentarium, a stockpile of more than 100 drugs (The Hindu, 2001). Once drug resistance is acquired by the pathogens it can transmit or spread among other pathogens through horizontal gene transfer (Transformation, Transduction and Conjugation). Beside these pathogens more specially bacteria develop drug resistance through either of the routes a) the organism may lack the structure of the antibiotics inhibit, for instance, some bacteria such as *Mycoplasma* lack a typical bacterial cell wall and are resistant to penicillin; b) the organism may be impermeable to antibiotics *e.g.*, most Gm-ve bacteria are impermeable to Penicillin; c) the organism may be able to alter the antibiotic to an inactive form such as *Staphylococci* contain ß-lactamase that cleave the ß-lactum ring of most of the Penicillin; d) the organism may be able to pump out an antibiotic entering the wall; e) the organism may modify the target of the antibiotic; f) by genetic change alteration may occur in a metabolic pathway that the antimicrobial agents blocks beside the antibiotics and chemotheraptic agents produce a numbers of side effects inside human body. Of the many hundreds of the antibiotics discovered only, few are of wide application in medicine. Prolonged use may weak the body's natural defense against invading germs and may have undesirable side effects. Few examples are quoted here. Excessive doses damage the kidney in case of Streptomycin, some times causing complete and permanent deafness, large doses of Penicillin and Streptomycin have a neurotoxic action. Tetracycline affects the lever, Chloromycetin has toxic effects on haematopoietic (blood cell forming) organs and Chlorotetracycline and Oxytetracycline upon intravenous injection may lead to collapse with lethal outcome. Many times allergic reaction arising during local application of antibiotics too.

Treating resistant infections often requires the use of more expensive or more toxic drugs and can result in longer hospital stays for infected patients and thus impose higher healthcare costs. WHO (2000) in its annual report on infectious diseases, "Overcoming Antimicrobial Resistance", quotes that people throughout the world "may only have a decade or two to make use of many of the medicines presently available to stop infectious diseases". Susceptible microorganisms can replace resistant microorganisms by removing selection pressure. Proposed solutions outlined by the Centre for Disease Control (CDC), USA and World Health Organization (WHO) as a multi-pronged approach includes: prevention, (such as vaccination); improved monitoring; and the development of new treatments. It is the last solution that would encompass the development of new antimicrobials to combat the problems posed by increasing drug resistance as well as emergence and reemergence of deadly infectious diseases (Fauci, 1998). Therefore, the human race in a dive need of an alternate. Amongst all medicinal and aromatic plant products are the foremost choice. As plants are in use for the treatment of various infections since time immemorial.

Secondly the products are nature based biodegradable, don't accumulate in the ecosystem causing biomagnification or do not cause any environmental pollution as compared to costly harmful antibiotics and chemotheraptic agents. Most significantly plants have co-evolved in nature along with various pathogens, implies for synthesis of various chemical compounds namely secondary metabolites against these pathogens for self defense.

It is estimated that plant materials are present in, or have provided the models for 50 per cent Western drugs (Robbers, 1996). Many commercially proven drugs used in modern medicine were initially used in crude form in traditional or folk healing practices, or for other purposes that suggested potentially useful biological activity. The primary benefits of using plant derived medicines are that they are relatively safer than synthetic alternatives, offering profound therapeutic benefits and more affordable treatment. There are essentially two routes of drug discovery, the first one pertains to synthesizing entirely new chemicals and evaluating them for a particular pharmaceutical use and the other approach is identifying the chemical of biological origin (natural product chemistry) and evaluate it for direct or indirect use as a template for development of new drug. 19th century was marked as the golden era for development of synthetic drugs. More and more people became interested in synthetic drugs because of their quick action as compared to traditional medicines and secondly because of their bulk production in industries. Since, 1970's almost 75 per cent of all standard medicines are of synthetic origin or the product of fermentation. The emerging number of incidences of resistance of microbes towards synthetic drugs and antibiotics of microbial origin has turned the attention of scientists, towards traditional medicines especially herbal drugs or drugs of plant origin.

Plant Derived Antimicrobials

The search for antimicrobial agents has mainly been concentrated on lower plants, fungi and bacteria as sources. Much less research has been conducted on antimicrobials from higher plants (Iwu *et al.*, 1999). Since the advent of antibiotics, in the 1950s, the use of plant derivatives as antimicrobials has been virtually nonexistent. The interest in using plant extracts for treatment of microbial infections has increased in the late 1990s as conventional antibiotics become ineffective (Cowan, 1999). For example, none of the conventional antifungal drugs used to date seems to be ideal in efficacy, safety and antifungal spectrum (Ablordeppey *et al.*, 1999). In addition, many of the antimicrobial drugs in use have undesirable effects or are very toxic, produce recurrence, show drug-drug interactions or lead to the development of resistance (White *et al.*, 1998). Although some new drugs have emerged for the treatment of obstinate fungal infections, such as Allylamines and Caspofungine (Vincent *et al.*, 2003), and combination therapy is sometimes used to make the treatment more effective, there is a real need for a next generation of safer and more potent antifungal drugs (Bartoli *et al.*, 1998). Also, it is increasingly difficult to deliver new antibacterial leads by modifying known antibacterial compounds. Therefore, the focus on much antibacterial research has moved to the identification of new chemical classes and many smaller pharmaceutical companies have taken up this challenge (Boggs and Miller, 2004). Antimicrobial compounds from plants may inhibit bacteria or fungi through different mechanisms than conventional antibiotics, and could therefore be of clinical value in the treatment of resistant microbes (Eloff, 1998). Phytomedicines derived from plants have shown great promise in the treatment of infectious diseases including opportunistic AIDS infections (Iwu *et al.*, 1999). Investigations on plants used in traditional medicine for skin afflictions might provide new topical antiseptics urgently needed in the third world countries (Taylor *et al.*, 2001). Rapid extinction of some habitats and plant species due to deforestation, especially in the tropical parts of the world, lead to a loss of valuable antimicrobial chemicals (Lewis and Elwin-Lewis, 1995). Thus, many pharmaceutical companies are now intensifying their screening programs on medicinal plants.

Defence Chemicals Produced by Plants

Higher plants produce a great diversity of chemicals that have antimicrobial activity *in vitro* (Van-Etten *et al.*, 1994). Most of these defence molecules are secondary metabolites, of which at least 12, 000 have been isolated (Schultes, 1978). There are two broad categories of plant produced antimicrobials (*i*) Phytoalexins and (*ii*) Phytoanticipins. Phytoalexins are low molecular compounds which are produced in response to microbial, herbivorous or environmental stimuli (Van-Etten *et al.*, 1994). These compounds are synthesized *de novo*, and thus require activation of certain genes and enzymes required for their synthesis. Phytoalexins are chemically diverse and include simple phenyl propanoid derivates, flavonoids, isoflavonoids, terpenes and polyketides (Bailey and Mansfield, 1982; Dixon, 1986; Greayer and Harborne, 1994). Phytoanticipins are low molecular compounds which are present in plants before the challenge by microorganisms or are produced from pre-existing constituents after infection (Van-Etten *et al.*, 1994). These phytoanticipin toxins, *e.g.* phenolic and iridoid glycosides, glucosinolates and saponins are normally stored as less toxic glycosides in the vacuoles of plant cells. If the integrity of the cell is broken when penetrated by the microbe, the glycoside comes into contact with hydrolyzing enzymes present in other compartments of the cell, releasing the toxic aglycone (Osbourn, 1996). There is no sharp boundary between phytoalexins and phytoanticipins, and in one plant species a certain chemical can function as a phytoalexin, whereas, it has the function of a phytoanticipin in another species (McMurchy and Higgins, 1984; Higgins and Smith, 1972). The rich diversity of secondary metabolites in plants has partly arisen because of selection for improved defence mechanisms against a broad array of microbes, insects and other plants. Related plant families often make use of similar secondary compounds for defence purposes (isoflavonoids in Leguminosae; sesquiterpenes in Solanaceae). Most antimicrobial secondary metabolites have relatively broad spectrum of activity. The specificity is determined to whether the pathogen has the enzymes necessary to detoxify a particular host product (Van-Etten *et al.*, 1994).

Plant Derived Individual Compounds with Antimicrobial Effects

Phenolic Compounds

Some of the simplest bioactive phytochemicals consist of a single substituted phenolic ring. Cinnamic and caffeic acids are common representatives of a wide group of phenylpropane-derived compounds which are in the highest oxidation state, known to possess antimicrobial effects (Brantner *et al.,* 1996). Catechol and pyrogallol both are hydroxylated phenols shown to be toxic against micro organisms. Increased hydroxylation of the phenol group has been found to result in increased toxicity to microorganisms (Geissman, 1963). The site(s) and number of hydroxyl groups on the phenol group are thought to be related to their relative toxicity to microorganisms, with evidence that increased hydroxylation results in increased toxicity (Geissman, 1963). On the contrary, it has in some cases been found that highly oxidized phenols are inhibitory (Scalbert, 1991). Phenolic compounds are thought to inhibit microbial enzymes possibly through reaction with sulfohydryl groups (the oxidized phenols) or through non-specific interactions with the proteins (Mason and Wasserman, 1987).

Quinones

The potential range of quinone antimicrobial effects seems to be great. Probable targets for the quinones in the microbial cell are the surface exposed adhesins, cell wall polypeptides and enzymes bound to the membranes. Quinones are known to complex irreversibly with nucleophilic amino acids in proteins (Stern *et al.,* 1996) thus leading to inactivation of the protein and loss of its function. It is also possible that quinones render substrates unavailable to the microorganism (Cowan, 1999). Anthraquinones, the largest group of quinones (Harborne *et al.,* 1999), have been found to possess antibacterial effects by inhibiting nucleic acid synthesis, at least in *Bacillus subtilis* (Levin *et al.,* 1988).

Stilbenoids

Stilbenoids are composed of two benzene rings separated with an ethane or ethene bridge, called bibenzyls and stilbenes, respectively. Phenanthrenes are biosynthetically derived from the bibenzyls and stilbenes. Stilbenes occur as aglycones or glycosides, and sometimes as polymers. Many higher plant families are known to produce stilbenes. Bibenzyls and their derivatives are rare in higher plants but occur in some families including Orchidaceae, Combretaceae and Dioscoreaceae, often alongside the corresponding phenanthrene or stilbene derivates. Many stilbenoids are known for their antifungal and antibacterial properties (Bruneton, 1999). Eloff *et al.* (2005) have found that leaves of the South African *Combretum woodii* contain high concentrations of the antimicrobially active bibenzyl, combretastatin B5.

Flavonoids

Flavonoids are constitutive compounds but are also synthesized by plants in response to microbial infection (Dixon *et al.,* 1983). Nearly half of the 200 phytoalexins characterized up to now belong to the flavonoids (Harborne, 1988). Flavonoids have been found to show *in vitro* antimicrobial activity against a wide range of microorganisms, some showing potent activity against MRSA (Iinuma *et al.,* 1994). Their activity has been attributed to their ability to complex with extracellular and soluble proteins and to complex with bacterial cell walls (Cowan, 1999). Lipophilic flavonoids may also disrupt microbial membranes (Tsuchiya *et al.,* 1996). There are conflicting findings on the kind of molecular substitutions needed for a flavonoid in order to recognize antimicrobial activity. Some authors have found that flavonoids lacking hydroxyl groups on their β-rings are more active against microorganisms than flavonoids containing these groups and this finding supports the idea that their microbial target is the membrane specific (Chabot *et al.*, 1992). Several authors have, however, also found the opposite effect; the more hydroxyl groups the greater antimicrobial activity (Sato *et al.*, 1996). The low toxic potential of flavonoids makes them ideal as antimicrobial medicines (Cowan, 1999).

Tannins

Tannins are a large group of polyphenolic compounds which have received attention in recent years due to their claimed ability to cure a variety of diseases (Serafini *et al.*, 1994). Tannins are subdivided into two groups: hydrolysable tannins and proantocyanidins (condensed tannins). Hydrolysable tannins are gallic acid and ellagic acid esters of core molecules that consist of polyols such as sugars. Proantohocyanidins are polymers of flavan-3-ols (for example catechin) and flavan-3, 4-diols linked through an interflavan bond that is not susceptible to hydrolysis (Haslam, 1989). A wide range of anti-infective actions have been assigned to tannins (Haslam, 1996). Tannins have the ability to complex with proteins through nonspecific forces such as hydrogen bonding and hydrophobic effects and also through covalent binding (Stern *et al.*, 1996). The antimicrobial mode of action for tannins may thus be related to their ability to inactivate microbial adhesins, enzymes, cell envelope transport proteins, etc. (Cowan, 1999). There is also evidence that tannins directly inactivate microorganisms, because already low concentrations of tannin (0.063 mg/ml) modify the morphology of germ tubes of *Crinipellis perniciosa* (Brownlee *et al.*, 1990). Tannins have also been found to induce changes in the morphology of several species of ruminal bacteria (Jones *et al.*, 1994). Due to their ability to bind to proteins and metals, tannins also inhibit the growth of microorganisms through substrate and metal ion deprivation (Scalbert, 1991). Hydrolysable and condensed tannins have been found to possess similar antifungal (filamentous fungi) and antibacterial potency, but the hydrolysable tannins were found to be more effective against yeasts (Cowan, 1999). Latté and Kolodziej (2000) found that a panel of different hydrolysable tannins had low antibacterial effects, but that they possessed fairly high anticryptococcal effects. Some research has been performed on the relationship between tannin structure and antimicrobial activity. The presence of a hexahydroxydiphenoyl moiety or its oxidatively modified entities was an important feature for the anticryptococcal activity of the ellagitannins corilagin, pelargoniin B and phyllanthusiin (Latté and Kolodziej, 2000). The pattern of B-ring hydroxylation of monomeric flavonols in condensed tannins has been shown to affect the level of growth inihibition of *Streptococcus sobrinus* and *Streptococcus mutans* (Sakanaka *et al.*, 1989), *Clostridium botulinum* (Hara and Watanabe, 1989), *Proteus vulgaris* and *Staphylococcus* sp. (Mori *et al.*, 1987), and in all cases gallocatechins were inhibitorier than their catechin counterparts. The toxicity of tannins and lower molecular weight phenols has been discussed also in relation to their oxidation state; catechin was found to be devoid of any toxicity against methanogenic bacteria, whereas if oxidized it strongly reduced methane production (Field *et al.*, 1989). The synthesis of red beet β-glucan synthase was found to be strongly inhibited by various oxidized phenols, but the effect of oxidation was less marked for tannic acid (hydrolysable tannin) than for smaller phenols (Mason *et al.*, 1987). It has also been proposed that tannin toxicity would be related to molecular size since the larger the molecule the more effectively it binds to proteins. This has been observed in many cases; dimeric ellagitannins have been found to be more adstringent than related monomers (McManus *et al.*, 1985). On the other hand, in some cases the toxicity of tannins was found to be no higher than that of catechins (Siwaswamy *et al.*, 1986), although catechins have very poor affinity to proteins. Kakiuchi *et al.* (1986) found that adding BSA to a glucosyl transferase solution before addition of gallotannins failed to remove the inhibition of the enzyme by the tannins and they concluded that inhibition of the enzyme is not necessarily due to the nonspecific binding of tannins to it. In their study of an array of different tannins and their effects on ligand binding to various enzyme receptors. Zhu *et al.* (1997) found that some of the tannins inhibited ligand binding to specific receptors. Thus, this study shows that tannins have specific activity at the receptor level, and that these effects cannot solely be explained in terms of protein binding.

Coumarins

Coumarins are phenolic substances made of fused benzene and a-pyrone rings (O'Kennedy and Thornes, 1997). They are responsible for the characteristic odor of food. As of 1996, at least 1,300 had been identified (Hoult and Paya, 1996). Coumarin was found *in vitro* to inhibit *Candida albicans*. Hydroxycinnamic acids, related to coumarins, seem to be inhibitory to Gram-positive bacteria (Fernandez *et al.*, 1996). Also, phytoalexins, which are hydroxylated derivatives of coumarins, are produced in carrots in response to fungal infection and can be presumed to have antifungal activity (Hoult and Paya, 1996). General antimicrobial activity was documented in *Galium odoratum* extracts (Thomson, 1978). How ever, data about specific antibiotic properties of coumarins are scarce, although many reports give reason to believe that some utility may reside in these phytochemicals (Hamburger and Hostettmann, 1991; Scheel, 1972). Recently, Smyth *et al.* (2008) studied the antimicrobial activities of 43 naturally occurring and synthetic coumarins using a microtitre assay against both Gram-positive and Gram-negative bacteria, including a hospital isolate of methicillin-resistant *Staphylococcus aureus* (MRSA) and result showed the coumarins exhibiting good bioactivity against clinically isolated MRSA strains.

Terpenoids and Essential Oils

Terpenes are a large group of compounds responsible for the fragrance of plants and comprise the so called essential oil fraction. They are synthesized from isoprenoid units, and share origins with fatty acids. They differ from fatty acids in that they are branched and cyclized. Their general chemical structure is $C_{10}H_{16}$ and occur as diterpenes, triterpenes, and tetraterpenes (C_{20}, C_{30}, and C_{40}), as well as hemiterpenes (C_5) and sesquiterpenes (C_{15}). When the compounds contain additional elements, usually oxygen, they are termed terpenoids (Cowan, 1999). Terpenoids are synthesized from acetate units, and as such they share their origins with fatty acids. They differ from fatty acids in that they contain extensive branching and are cyclized. Examples of common terpenoids are methanol and camphor (monoterpenes) and farnesol and artemisin (sesquiterpenoids). Terpenes and terpenoids have been found to possess antibacterial activity (Ahmad *et al.*, 1993; Amaral *et al.*, 1998; Barre *et al.*, 1997; Himejima *et al.*, 1992; Mendoza *et al.*, 1997; Scortichini and Rossi, 1991; Tassou *et al.*, 1995; Taylor *et al.*, 1996), fungi (Ayafor *et al.*, 1994; Hasegawa *et al.*, 1994; Kubo *et al.*, 1993; Rana *et al.*, 1997; Rao *et al.*, 1993; Suresh *et al.*, 1997; Taylor *et al.*, 1996), viruses (Fujioka and Kashiwada, 1994; Hasegawa *et al.*, 1994; Pengsuparp *et al.*, 1994; Sun *et al.*, 1996; Xu *et al.*, 1996), and protozoa (Ghoshal *et al.*, 1996; Viswakarma, 1990). In 1977, it was reported that 60 per cent of essential oil derivatives examined to date were inhibitory to fungi while 30 per cent inhibited bacteria (Chaurasia and Vyas, 1977). The mechanism of action of terpenes is not fully understood but is speculated to involve membrane disruption by the lipophilic compounds. Mendoza *et al.* (1997) found that increasing the hydrophilicity of kaurene diterpenoids by addition of a methyl group drastically reduced their antimicrobial activity. Cichewicz and Thorpe (1996) found that capsaicin might enhance the growth of *Candida albicans* but that it clearly inhibited various bacteria to differing extents. Two diterpenes isolated by Batista *et al.* (1994) were found to be more democratic; they worked well against *S. aureus*, *V. cholerae*, *P. aeruginosa*, and *Candida* species.

Alkaloids

Heterocyclic nitrogen compounds are called alkaloids. The first medically useful example of an alkaloid was morphine, isolated in 1805 from the opium poppy *Papaver somniferum*. Diterpenoid alkaloids, commonly isolated from the plants of the Ranunculaceae family (Atta-ur-Rahman and Chaudhary, 1995), are commonly found to have antimicrobial properties (Omulokoli *et al.*, 1997). Solamargine, a glycoalkaloid from the berries of *Solanum khasianum*, and other alkaloids may be useful against HIV infection (McMahon *et al.*, 1995; Sethi, 1979) as well as intestinal infections associated with AIDS (McDevitt *et al.*, 1996). Szlavik *et al.*(2004) reported that lycorine, homolycorine, and acetyllycorine hemanthamine isolated from *Leucojum vernum* possessed high antiretroviral activities with low therapeutic indices, while drymaritin isolated from *Drymaria diandra* had anti-HIV activity (Hsieh *et al.*, 2004). Interestingly the whole extract and harman alkaloid fraction of *Ophiorrhiza nicobarica*, a folklore plant of the little Andaman Islands, completely inhibited the plaque formation and delayed the eclipse phase of HSV replication (Chattopadhyay *et al.*, 2006).

Lectins and Polypeptides

Peptides which are inhibitory to microorganisms were first reported by Balls *et al.* (1942). They are often positively charged and contain disulfide bonds and their mechanism of action may be the formation of ion channels in the microbial membrane (Terras *et al.*, 1993; Zhang *et al.*, 1997) or competitive inhibition of adhesion of microbial proteins to host polysaccharide receptors (Sharon and Ofek, 1986). Recent interest has been focused mostly on studying anti-HIV peptides and lectins, but the inhibition of bacteria and fungi by these macromolecules, such as that from the herbaceous *Amaranthus* sps, has long been known (De Bolle *et al.*, 1996). Thionins are peptides commonly found in barley and wheat and consist of 47 amino acid residues and they are toxic to yeasts and Gram-negative and Gram-positive bacteria (Fernandes de Caleya *et al.*, 1972). Fabatin, a newly identified 47- residue peptide from fava beans, appears to be structurally related to g-thionins from grains and inhibits *E. coli*,

P. aeruginosa, and *Enterococcus hirae* but not yeats (Zhang and Lewis, 1997). The larger lectin molecules, which include mannose specific lectins are reported from several plants (Balzarin *et al.*, 1991), MAP30 from bitter melon (Lee-Haung *et al.*, 1995), and jacalin (Favero *et al.*, 1993), are inhibitory to viral proliferation (HIV, Cytomegalovirus), probably by inhibiting viral interaction with critical host cell components. It is worth emphasizing that molecules and compounds such as these whose mode of action may be to act synergistically.

Other Compounds

Many phytochemicals not mentioned above have been found to exert antimicrobial properties. This review has attempted to focus on reports of chemicals which are found in multiple instances to be active. It should be mentioned, however, that there are reports of antimicrobial properties associated with polyamines (in particular spermidine) (Flayeh and Sulayamen, 1987), isothiocyanates (Donberger *et al.*, 1975, Iwu *et al.*, 1991), thiosulfinates (Tada *et al.*, 1988), and glucosides (Rucker *et al.*, 1992). Polyacetylenes deserve special mention. Estevez-Braun*et al.* (1994) isolated a C17polyacetylene compound from *Bupleurum salicifolium*, a plant native to the Canary Islands. The compound, 8S-heptadeca-2(Z), 9(Z)-diene-4,6-diyne-1,8-diol, was inhibitory to *S. aureus* and *B. subtilis* but not to Gram-negative bacteria or yeasts (Esteevez-Braun *et al.*, 1994). Acetylene compounds and flavonoids from plants traditionally used in Brazil for treatment of malaria fever and liver disorders have also been associated with antimalarial activity (Brandao *et al.*, 1997). Much has been written about the antimicrobial effects of cranberry juice. Historically, women have been told to drink the juice in order to prevent and even cure urinary tract infections.

An Overview of the Analytical Methods

Nowadays, the interest in study of natural products is growing rapidly, especially as part of drug discovery programs. There are various methods available for the extraction of secondary metabolites from plants.

Extraction Techniques

Solvent Extraction

Solvent extraction is widely used and long-standing methods in studies of natural products.

Maceration

This is simple, and still widely used, procedure involves leaving the pulverized plant to soak in suitable solvent in a closed container at room temperature. To increase the speed of extraction, occasional or constant stirring is added. However, this method also has limitations. Its main disadvantage is a time consumption process. Besides that, to extract exhaustively, a large volume of solvent is used. In addition, some compounds are not extracted effectively because of insolubility at room temperature.

Percolation

The powdered material is soaked initially in a solvent in a percolator. Additional solvent is then poured on top of the material and allowed to percolate slowly out of the bottom of the percolator. As maceration, it also takes time and volumes of solvents.

Soxhlet Extraction

This method is convenient and widely used for extraction because of its continuous process, less time and solvent-consumption than maceration and percolation. The powdered plant is placed in a Soxhlet apparatus, which is on top of a collecting flask beneath a reflux condenser. A suitable solvent is added to flask and the set up is heated under reflux. The steam of the solvent, which contacts with material will dissolve metabolites and brings back to flask. Because of the boiling point of the solvent used, the heat may damage the metabolites.

Refluxing Extraction

Material is inundated in solvent in a round bottomed flask, which is connected to a condenser. The solvent is heated until it reaches its boiling point. As the vapor is condensed, the solvent is recycled to the flask. The metabolites may a little damage.

Supercritical Fluid Extraction

SFE (Supercritical Fluid Extraction) has long used in industries for extraction of various commercial natural products *viz.*, coffee, hops, spices, flavors and vegetables oils but still it has a limit in natural products extraction. Supercritical fluids (SCFs) are increasingly replacing organic solvents because of a solvent free and environment friendly method of extraction has become the method of choice. The critical point of a pure substance is defined as the highest temperature and pressure, which the substance can exist in vapor-liquid equilibrium. Above this point, a supercritical fluid is formed. It is heavy like a liquid and has the penetration of gas. These qualities make SCFs effective. The choice of the SFE solvent is similar to the regular extraction. Principle considerations are the followings:

- ☆ Good solvent properties
- ☆ Inert to the product
- ☆ Easy separation from the product
- ☆ Among solvents, *e.g.*, ethane, butane, pentane, N_2O, CHF_3, water and Carbon dioxide is the most commonly used SCF, due primarily to its low critical parameters (31.1°C, 73.8 bar), low cost and non toxicity. However, several other SCFs have been used in both commercial and new processes.

Advantages

- ☆ Dissolving power of the SCF is controlled by pressure and/or temperature.
- ☆ SCF is easily recoverable from the extract due to its volatility.
- ☆ Non toxic solvents leave no harmful residue.
- ☆ High boiling components are extracted at relatively low temperatures.
- ☆ Separations not possible by processes that are more traditional can sometimes are effected.

- Thermally labile compounds can be extracted with minimal damage as low temperatures can be employed by the extraction.

Disadvantages

- Elevated pressure required.
- Compression of solvent requires elaborate recycling measures to reduce energy costs.
- High capital investment for equipment.

Chromatographic Methods

Chromatography is the method of choice in separating the problem of isolation of a compound of interest from a complex natural mixture. There are various methods from basic to advance just supporting for isolation and separation compounds effectively.

Thin Layer Chromatography (TLC)

TLC is an easy, cheap, rapid, and basic method for the analysis and isolation of organic natural and synthetic compounds. TLC involves the use of a particulate sorbent spread on an inert sheet of glass, plastic, or metal as a stationary phase. The mobile phase is allowed to travel up the plate carrying the sample that was initially spotted on the sorbent just above the solvent. Depending on the nature of the stationary phase, the separation can be either partition (C18 reversed phase) or adsorption chromatography (Silica gel, alumina, cellulose, and polyamide). The advantage of TLC is that the samples do not have to undergo the extensive cleanup steps, and the ability to detect a wide range of compounds, using reactive spray reagents. Non-destructive detection (fluorescent indicators in the plates, examination under a UV lamp) also makes it possible for purified samples to be scraped off the plate and be analyzed by other techniques.

Preparative TLC (PTLC)

Preparative TLC has long been a popular method as a primary or final purification step in an isolation procedure. Separation can be effected rapidly and the amount of material isolated is from 1mg to 1g. The sorbent thickness of PTLC is 0.5-4 mm is compared with analytical TLC (0.1-0.2mm sorbent thickness). In commercial available PTLC plates, sorbents silica, alumina, C18 and cellulose are usually of thickness 0.5, 1.0, and 2.0 mm. Nevertheless, there are also having advantages and disadvantages.

Advantages

- Simple technique.
- Low cost than the others instrument, for example, HPLC or CC.
- Isolate compounds quickly from milligram to gram.
- Almost any separation can be achieved with the correct stationary phase and mobile phase.

Disadvantages

- ☆ Poor control of detection and elution compared to HPLC.
- ☆ Manual operation.

TLC Bioassays

In addition, the simplicity, and the ability of TLC to separate mixtures quickly with little expense, it can be readily used to detect biological activity of separated components. Currently, TLC bioassays are used more and more widely. TLC bioassays against fungi and bacteria have proved exceptionally popular owing to their ease of use, low cost, rapidity and ability to be scaled up to assess antimicrobial activity of a large number of samples. Generally, TLC plates are running and then the microorganism is applied to the plate, as a spray (in case of direct bioautography) or plate is cover with a growth medium containing the microorganism in dish or tray (overlay assay). These simple bioassays will continue to prove useful in antimicrobial activity of natural product extracts.

Column Chromatography (CC)

Column chromatography consists of a column of particulate material such as silica or alumina that has a solvent passed through it at atmospheric, medium, or low pressure. The separation can be liquid/solid (adsorption) or liquid/liquid (partition). Most systems rely on gravity to push the solvent through, but medium pressure pumps are commonly used in flash CC. The sample is dissolved in a solvent and applied to the front of the column (wet packing), or alternatively adsorbed on a coarse silica gel (dry packing). The solvent elutes the sample through the column, allowing the components to separate. Normally, the solvent is non-polar and the surface polar, although there are a wide range of packing including chemically bound phase systems. The solvent is usually changed stepwise, and fractions are collected according to the separation required, with the eluting products usually monitored by TLC. The solvent system is developed using TLC. The technique is not efficient, with relatively large volumes of solvent being used, and particle size is constrained by the need to have a flow of several ml/min. The advantage is that no expensive equipment is required, and the technique can be scaled up to handle sample sizes approaching gram amounts.

Gas Chromatography (GC)

This is very useful to analysis volatile compounds in natural products. The mobile phase in GC is a carrier gas to convey the sample in a vapor state through stationary phase. The columns of stationary phase are capillary or packed of silica. Nevertheless, capillary column is more used. The column is installed in an oven that has temperature control, and the column can be slowly heated up to 350-450°C starting from ambient temperature to provide separation of a wide range of compounds. The carrier gas is usually hydrogen or helium under pressure, and the eluting compounds can be detected in several ways (*a*) "universal" including flames (flame ionization detector-FID), (*b*) by mass spectrometry (MS), (*c*) by changes in properties of the carrier (thermal conductivity detector-TCD). Among them, FID and MS is very common applied in organic compounds and is the appropriate tool to investigate essential oils, the other is only used to analysis gases; b) "selective" (Electron Capture (ECD), Nitrogen-Phosphorus (NPD), FID etc.) detection for substances which are having negative electric atoms or function groups, such as Halogen, N, P, etc.

Advantages

- ☆ Low viscosity of gas allows for the use of long columns (up to 60m).
- ☆ Requires thermally stable compounds that are also volatile (B.P. < 300°C). If a compound does not have these attributes it may be possible to derivative it to a compound that does.
- ☆ High gas flow rate allows for fast analysis and can be automated.
- ☆ Many different detection methods allow for analysis of molecules containing specific functional groups *e.g.*, halogens or nitrogen.

Disadvantages

- ☆ Not applicable to non volatile compounds.
- ☆ Requires the use of relatively expensive equipment.
- ☆ Requires skilled operators.

High Pressure Liquid Chromatography (HPLC)

Currently, HPLC plays an important role not only in science research field but also in many application areas such as the pharmaceutical industry. HPLC is a development of column chromatography. To improve resolution, HPLC columns are packed with small sized particles (3, 5, 10μm) with a narrow size distribution. Flow rate and column dimensions can be adjusted to minimize band broadening. The required pressures are supplied by pumps that could withstand the involved chemicals. The selection of solvents and eluent condition (gradient or isocratic) are upon to the mixture components and the interested compounds. The commonly used detector in HPLC systems are Ultraviolet/Visible (UV/Vis), Refractive index (RI), Evaporative light scattering (ELS), MS, and Fluorescence detector.

Ultraviolet detectors are not only places constraints on the solvents that can be used but also is limited to absorbing compounds. RI detectors considered as universal but cannot easily be used with solvent gradients. However, recently, the ELS have emerged as a universal detector. ELS works by passing the eluate through a heated nebulizer to volatilize the eluate and evaporate the solvent. The solvent is carried away as a gas but the solute form is a stream of fine particles, which passes between a light source and detector and scatters the light. The detector measures this scattering effect. The advantages of ELS that it is applied for detection of non volatile and semi-volatile samples and the unprocessed of chromophore compounds. In addition, it can be used with both the isocratic and gradient eluent conditions. But this type of detector can be used for all solutes having a lower volatility than the mobile phase. If any compounds are having the boiling point close to mobile phase, they cannot be detected because of the misapprehension to the background.

Analytical HPLC is used just for separation and identification of a small amount mixture of samples but the pure isolated compounds cannot be collected. However, crude extracts consist of a mixture of numerous components. Therefore, to isolate or purify fast and efficiently a large amount, preparative HPLC is developed. Preparative HPLC uses one of these kinds: normal phase, reversed phase, gel permeation, and ion exchange chromatography. Nevertheless, reversed phase with C8 and C18 is preferred for isolation most classes of natural products.

Spectroscopic Techniques

Nuclear Magnetic Resonance Spectroscopy (NMR)

NMR has become a very important spectroscopic method and the premier organic spectroscopy available to chemists to determine the detailed chemical structure of the compounds they were isolated from natural products. NMR spectroscopy is routinely used by chemists to study chemical structure of simple molecules using simple one dimensional techniques (1D-NMR). Two-dimensional techniques (2D-NMR) are used to determine the structure of more complicated molecules.

Mass Spectrometry (MS)

Mass spectrometry is an analytical technique used to measure the mass-to-charge ratio of ions. This is a powerful, sensitive, and highly selective method to identify compounds. It provides both molecular weight and fragmentation pattern of the compound. It relies of production of ions from a parent compound and the subsequent characterization of the pattern that are produced. Mass spectrometers can be divided into three fundamental parts, namely the ionization source, the analyzer, and the detector. The sample has to be introduced into the ionization source of the instrument. Once inside the ionization source, the parent compound is bombarded by high energy electrons stream then converted to ions, because ions are easier to manipulate than neutral molecules. These ions are extracted into the analyzer region of the mass spectrometer where they are separated according to their mass-to-charge ratios (m/z) in a magnetic or electric field. The separated ions are detected by a detector and this signal sent to a data system where the m/z ratios are stored together with their relative abundance for presentation in the format of an m/z spectrum.

Antibacterial Assays

Perhaps the most common *in vitro* assay used for plant extracts is the assessment of antibacterial activity, with the majority of researchers using one of the three following assays: disk diffusion, agar dilution, or broth dilution or micro dilution. These methods are based on those described for standardized testing of antibiotics (Andrew, 2001a; 2001b; 2004; 2005; 2006; 2007; Brown, 2001; King and Brown, 2001; Livermore *et al.*, 2001; Livermore and Brown, 2001; MacGowan and Wise, 2001; Wheat, 2001), however several factors may affect the suitability of these methods for use with plant extracts. These factors include the type of organism being tested, concentration of inoculum, type of media and nature of the extract being tested (pH, solubility etc.) (Griffin, 2000; Hood *et al.*, 2004). The methods can be used to simply determine whether or not antibacterial activity is present or can be used to calculate a minimum inhibitory concentration (MIC). Table 9.1 summarizes the limitations and advantages of these various methods. All these methods are those most widely used for *in vitro* testing of plant extracts for antibacterial activity, while some other methods are also have been used. For example, Garedew *et al.* (2004) report on the use of a flow calorimetric

Table 9.1: Comparison of strengths and limitations of various assays for antimicrobial activity.

Method	Strength	Limitation
Disk well diffusion	☆ Low cost ☆ Results available within 1–2 days. ☆ Does not require specialized laboratory facilities. ☆ Uses equipment and reagents readily available in a microbiology laboratory. ☆ Can be performed by most laboratory staff. ☆ Data is only collected at one or two time points. ☆ Large numbers of samples can be screened. ☆ Results are quantifiable and can be compared statistically.	☆ Differential diffusion of extract components due to partitioning in the aqueous media. ☆ Inoculum size, presence of solubilizing agents, and incubation temperature can affect zone of inhibition. ☆ Volatile compounds can affect bacterial and fungal growth in closed environments.
Agar dilution	☆ Low cost ☆ Does not require specialized laboratory facilities. ☆ Uses equipment and reagents readily available in a microbiology laboratory. ☆ Can be performed by most laboratory staff.	☆ Hydrophobic extracts may separate out from the agar. ☆ Inoculum size, presence of solubilizing agents and incubation temperature can affect zone of inhibition. ☆ Volatile compounds can affect bacterial and fungal growth in closed environments. ☆ Data is only collected at one or two time points. ☆ Use of scoring systems is open to subjectivity of the observer. ☆ Some fungi are very slow growing.
Broth dilution	☆ Allows monitoring of activity over the duration. ☆ More accurate representation of antibacterial activity. ☆ Micro-broth methods can be used to screen large numbers of samples in a cost-effective manner.	☆ Essential oils may not remain in solution for the duration of the assay, emulsifier and solvent may interfere with accuracy of results. ☆ Labor and time intensive if serial dilution are used to determine cell count ☆ Highly colored extracts can interfere with colorimetric endpoints in micro broth methods.
TLC bioautograpy	P Simultaneously fractionation and determination of bioactivity.	☆ Unsuitable where activity is due to component synergy ☆ Dependent on the extraction methods and TLC solvent used.

Contd...

Table 9.1–*Contd...*

Method	*Strength*	*Limitation*
Antiviral assay	☆ Allow simultaneously assessment of cell toxicity with antiviral assay. ☆ Few methods available therefore comparability across studies is high.	☆ Labor, time and cost intensive. ☆ Requires access to cell culture and viral containment facility. ☆ Essential oils may not remain in the solution for the duration of the assay.
Antiparasitic assay	☆ Methods are well documented. ☆ Some assay, allow simultaneously assessment of cell toxicity.	☆ Labor, time and cost intensive. ☆ May require access to cell culture facility. ☆ Essential oils may not remain in the solution for the duration of the assay.

method to assess antibacterial activity of honey and demonstrated better sensitivity than other methods and Pitner *et al.* (2000) propose the use of high throughput systems that measure bacterial respiration via a fluorescent signal. However, the practicality of these methods for screening of plant extracts is yet to be determined. An additional method TLC–bioautography allows for identification of bioactive fractions of extracts within a single assay.

Disk Diffusion Method

The disk diffusion method (also known the zone of inhibition method) is probably the most widely of all methods used for testing antibacterial activity. It uses only small amounts of the test substance (10–30 µL), can be completed by research staff with minimal training, and as such may be useful in field situations. The method involves the preparation of a Petri dish containing 15–25 mL agar, bacteria at a known concentration are then spread across the agar surface and allowed to establish. A paper disk (6 or 8 mm) containing a known volume of the test substance is then placed in the center of the agar and the dish incubated for 24 h or more. At this time the "cleared" zone (zone of inhibition) surrounding the disk is measured and compared with zones for standard antibiotics or literature values of isolated chemicals or similar extracts. Where the extract is viscous or a semi-solid (*e.g.* honey) a well can be created in the agar and the substance allowed diffusing out of the well rather than away from a disk. Data from these assays are typically presented as mean size of zone of inhibition (with or without standard deviation), although some authors employ a ranking system of "+", "++", and "+++" to indicate levels of activity. Few authors provide statistical analysis of their data and levels of activity (slight, moderate, strong) are used without any reference to standardized criteria.

One of the major criticisms of this method is that it relies on the ability of the extract to diffuse through agar and any component of the extract that does diffuse away from the disk will create a concentration gradient, potentially creating a gradient of active antibacterial compound. All of the antibacterial testing methods use an aqueous base for dispersion of the test substance, either via diffusion in agar or dispersion within nutrient broth, consequently assays using extracts with limited solubility in aqueous media (*e.g.*, essential oils) may not reflect the true antibacterial activity. There is also no consensus on the best agar to use for these assays. A further limitation that has not been directly addressed in the literature, but for which evidence exists, is inference in the assay from vapours liberated from the extract during incubation. This is unlikely to be a major consideration in aqueous or solvent extracts but may be a significant confounder in assays of essential oils.

Agar Dilution Method

The agar dilution method is another relatively quick method that does not involve the use of sophisticated equipment. Any laboratory with facilities for basic microbiological work can use this method. In this method the test substance is incorporated at known concentrations into the agar and, once set, bacteria are applied to its surface. Replicate dishes can be set up with a range of concentrations of the test substance and by dividing the surface of the agar into wedges or squares, a number of bacterial species may be applied to a single dish. In this way, a large number of bacteria may be screened within a single assay run. The dishes are incubated for 24 h or more and the growth of the bacteria on the extract/agar mix is scored either as present/absent or a proportion of the control (*e.g.*, 0, 25 per cent, 50 per cent, 75 per cent, 100 per cent). A criticism of this method is that when a scoring system is used it is difficult to guarantee objectivity and to therefore, compare one set of results with another. This method suffers from several other limitations, including many that have been discussed previously: (a) use of larger volumes of test substance than in other methods, (b) confounding antibacterial actions from volatiles, (c) difficulty of achieving stable emulsions of essential oils in agar and (d) restriction on the maximum concentration that can be used before the agar becomes too dilute to solidify properly. Perhaps the most frustrating of these is the difficulty of stably incorporating essential oils and other hydrophobic extracts into aqueous environments. This problem occurs not just in agar dilution assays but also in broth dilution and other antimicrobial assays. Many researchers has thought they had incorporated their essential oil into nutrient broth or other media only to find that, on return to the experiment after an hour or so, the oil had separated out and was floating on top of the media. Griffin (2000) in their work on tea tree oil found that at concentrations above 2 per cent v/v the oil separated from the agar substrate and was seen as droplets on the agar surface. The most commonly utilized method to overcome this problem is the use of surfactants such as Tween-20, Tween-80, and alkyl dimethyl betaine (ADB). Several authors have described the use of these products and the effect on antibacterial activity. The results of their studies show that surfactants can interfere with calculation of MIC values and the growth of some test organisms (Hammer *et al.*, 1999) however it has also been demonstrated that it is possible to use very small quantities of Tween (<0.5 per cent v/v) to emulsify the essential oil in media and thus avoid the effects on organism growth (Griffin, 2000; Hood *et al.*, 2004). Hammer *et al.* (1999) also showed that inclusion of organic matter such as bovine serum albumin in the agar also affected the antibacterial activity of tea tree oil.

Broth Dilution Method

Difficulties with partitioning of hydrophobic compounds in agar and a desire to more accurately monitor antibacterial activity over time has resulted in a move to broth dilution method for testing of plant extracts. In this method, bacteria are grown in test-tubes in a liquid medium in the presence of the test substance. At regular time intervals (*e.g.*, every 10 min or every hour) a sample is removed and the bacterial count determined by serial dilution of the sample, subsequent incubation on agar and counting of colony forming units (CFU). In contrast to the single data point (*e.g.*, 24 h incubation) utilized in disk diffusion and agar dilution assays, the broth dilution method allows much finer evaluation of the antibacterial events over time and features such as recovery from the effects of the test substance and proportion of organisms killed at a given time point can be determined. However, the method is also time and resource intensive and can be impractical where very large numbers of test substances are to be screened. As with other testing methods incorporation of hydrophobic compounds and essential oils into the aqueous media is problematic, and as there is no solid phase to trap these compounds they rapidly separate from the media and form a layer across the surface of the media. For organisms sensitive to oxygen tension in the media this can present an additional problem as the oil can inhibit gaseous exchange. Tween or ethanol may be used to enhance incorporation into the aqueous media, however as previously discussed these compounds may interfere with the assay results.

Micro broth dilution method have also been developed, which utilize microtiter plates, thus reducing the volume of extract needed, and have end points that can be determined spectrophotmetrically, either a measure of turbidity or use of a cell viability indicator (*e.g.*, resazurin, methylthiazoldiphenyltetrazolium (MTT)) (Mann and Markham, 1998). They also propose that the cell viability indicator is the best method of endpoint determination for essential oils as the oil/water interface may interfere with turbidity measures. While these micro-broth methods generally work well for plant extracts, problems arise when the extract is heavily colored as this can interfere with the measurement of the indicator chemical. Further, as these methods use plastic microtiter plates, essential oils that have a solvent action on plastics (*e.g.*, *Letospermum petersonii*, *Backhousia citriodora*) cannot be used. Also the addition of essential oils to media, changes its pH and this might be expected to be more significant in small volumes, like the micro broth method (Hood *et al.*, 2004). Whether other plant extracts will also have the effect is unknown. Micro broth methods are also less time and resource intensive than other broth methods as the need for multiple serial dilutions to determine bacterial count is eliminated.

TLC-Bioautography

While the methods above are used to test whole extracts or extracts fractionated at another time there is an increasing interest in bioassay guided fractionation, where the separation of extracts into fractions is completed simultaneously with identification of bioactivity. In this method TLC is performed using crude extracts, extract fractions, or whole essential oils. The developed TLC plate is then sprayed with, or dipped into, a bacterial or fungal suspension (direct bioautography) or overlain with agar and the agar seeded with the microorganism (overlay bioautography) (Hamburger and Cordell, 1987; Homans and Fuchs, 1970; Rahalison *et al.*, 1991). The later method has been particularly used for determining the activity of extract against yeasts such as *Candida albicans*, however Masoko and Eloff (2005), suggested that use of fresh cultures of yeasts and shorter incubation times eliminated the previously reported difficulties of using the direct method with yeasts. This method has been used to screen a range of crude and solvent prepared extracts with the activity observed dependent on both the method of extraction and solvents used in the TLC process (Diallo *et al.*, 2001; Nakamura *et al.*, 1999; Nostro *et al.*, 2000; Sridhar *et al.*, 2003). While this method has the advantage of combining both separation of extract constituents and simultaneous identification of those fractions with bioactivity, it is not a suitable method for detecting activity that is a product of synergy between two or more compounds. Further, the results will be affected by the breakdown or alteration of compounds during the fractionation phase.

Antifungal Assays

Antifungal assays are regularly used to determine whether plant extracts will have potential to treat human fungal infections (*e.g.*, tinea) or have use in agricultural/

horticultural applications. In general these assays are quick, low cost, and do not involve access to specialized equipments. Activity of plant extracts against the yeast *Candida* is typically assessed using the disk or well diffusion method described above, and many studies report anti-candidal activity with antibacterial activity rather than with activity against fungi for this reason (Haraguchi *et al.*, 1999; Iskan *et al.*, 2002; Rahua *et al.*, 2000; Wilkinson and Cavanagh, 2005). Activity against filamentous fungi can be evaluated in well diffusion, agar dilution, and broth/microbroth methods with many of the same limitations and advantages as previously discussed for antibacterial assays (Inouye *et al.*, 2001). When the well diffusion and disk diffusion techniques are used, fungal plugs are removed from an actively growing colony and placed at a predetermined distance (typically 2 cm) from the centre of an agar dish. A well is then bored in the centre of the agar and test substance added to the well, or the test substance is added to a paper disk and the disk placed in the centre of the agar (The specific agar to be used, and temperature and time of incubation, will be determined by the fungi to be used). The growth of the fungi is monitored and any inhibition of mycelia growth noted. This inhibition of growth is then expressed as a percentage of the growth of control colonies. In the agar dilution method (also known as the poison food technique) the test substance is incorporated into the agar substrate and then a sample of actively growing fungus is placed at the centre of the plate. The radial growth of the fungus after an appropriate time, depending on the growth characteristics of the fungus, is then measured and compared with control samples. Sridhar *et al.* (2003) used this method to show the activity of essential oils against a range of fungi of agricultural and medical importance. Alternatively, a fungal cell suspension may be inoculated onto the plate and the MIC determined by the lowest concentration of test substance that prevents visible fungal growth de Aquino Lemos *et al.* (2005). Antisporulation activity can be assessed by using scanning electron microscopy (Inouye *et al.*, 1999), while effects on conidium germination can be evaluated by exposing the conidia to the test substance and subsequently counting the number of conidia with germ tubes equal to 1-1.5 times conidium length (Antonov *et al.*, 1997). Additional observations of germinated conidia over a set period will also allow evaluation of the effect of the plant extract on germ tube growth. All the methods have their own advantages and disadvantages as describe above in testing of antibacterial activity. In addition to these Inouye *et al.* (2001) showed that the inclusion of Tween-80 resulted in weaker bioactivity in agar dilution assays and the size of the original fungal inoculum had a significant effect with larger inoculums being more resistant to antifungal effects. Shahi *et al.* (1999) in their study of the antifungal activity of essential oils found that the antifungal response was altered by modifying the pH of the fungal growth media. As the media pH become more alkaline the eucalyptus essential oils had a greater inhibitory effect on the fungi (*Trichophyton* spp., *Microsporum* spp., and *Epidermophyton* spp.).

In vivo Assessment of Antibacterial and Antifungal Activity

The preceding discussion clearly demonstrates the similarity in methods used for *in vitro* antibacterial and antifungal assays of plant extracts and there are many papers in the literature using one or more of the methods. A smaller number of research groups have moved beyond the *in vitro* environment and are investigating the *in vivo* efficacy of those extracts that show promise in the laboratory. This is a more complex and costly activity as not only does the activity against the microorganisms need to be evaluated, there must also be consideration of mammalian cell toxicity and allergic reactions (Matura *et al.*, 2005). To date most *in vivo* testing of plant extracts has involved the use of essential oils against human skin infections, particularly fungal infections, and testing of extracts follow standard clinical trial protocols. Perhaps the plant extracts best known for its *in vivo* antibacterial activity is honey, with a large number of studies demonstrating *in vivo* activity (Dunford *et al.*, 2000; Moore *et al.*, 2001). It is important to note here that demonstrated activity *in vitro* does not always translate to activity *in vivo*. The best example of this is tea tree oil, which has been shown to have excellent activity *in vitro* against the fungi responsible for various tinea's (MIC 0.004–0.06 per cent) (Hammer *et al.*, 2002) yet the results from clinical trials have been far from conclusive (Satchell *et al.*, 2000). This illustrates the caution with which researchers should view results from *in vitro* assays and reinforces the need for clinical trials of plant extracts that show therapeutic promise.

Methods for Assessing Antiviral Activity

In addition to antibacterial and antifungal activities, researchers are also investigating the use of plant extracts for antiviral activities; of particular interest is activity against herpes simplex virus (HSV), human immunodeficiency virus (HIV), and hepatitis C virus (HCV). Standard cytopathic assays are used to determine antiviral activity with activity both pre- and post-infection evaluated. As these assays are performed in an aqueous environment the problems of solubility that have been discussed at length previously are also an issue in these assays. These assays also require expertise in cell culture and appropriate laboratory containment facilities for working with viruses; these two features make these assays more expensive and labor intensive than other assays. However, as viruses require a cell host this assay has the added benefit of being able to assess cell toxicity of the test substance as part of the antiviral assay protocol. This means that those extracts with significant cell toxicity, and therefore little potential for use, can be eliminated from investigations prior to *in vivo* testing. Abad *et al.* (2000) tested 10 extracts (both aqueous and ethanol) and demonstrated that aqueous extracts of five plants showed activity against HSV-1 and vesicular stomatitis virus (VSV) with one extract showing activity against poliovirus. These authors suggest that antiviral activity is more likely to be found in aqueous rather than ethanol extracts; this is in contrast to antibacterial and antifungal assays where activity is more commonly seen in solvent extracts and essential oils. However, other studies have identified activity in both aqueous and solvent (ethanol or methanol) extracts of a wide range of plants against the hepatitis C virus (Hussain *et al.*, 2000), VSV (Abad *et al.*, 1999) and human parainfluenza virus type 2 (HPIV-2) (Karagaz *et al.*, 2003). Few plant extracts/essential oils have been shown to demonstrate antiviral activity *in vivo* (Abad *et al.*, 1999). With work by Nawawi *et al.* (1999) demonstrated that, as with other *in vitro* assays, activity *in vitro* is not always matched by a similar level of activity *in vivo*.

Table 9.2: Antimicrobial screening of different plants.

Sl.No.	Plant	Family	Part*	Activity Against**	References
1.	*Abrus precatorius* L.	Fabaceae	Lf	Sa	Valsaraj *et al.*, 1997
2.	*Acacia catechu* Willd.	Mimosaceae	St	Bs Ec Pa Sa An Ca	Valsaraj *et al.*, 1997
3.	*Achillea millefolium* L.	Compositae	Ap Rh	Bc Sa	Kokoska *et al.*, 2002
4.	*Achyranthes aspera* L.	Amaranthaceae	Lf St	Bs Sa	Valsaraj *et al.*, 1997
5.	*Acorus calamus* L.	Araceae	Rh Rt	Bs Sa	Mc Gaw *et al.*, 2000; Valsaraj *et al.*, 1997
6.	*Adhatoda vasica* Ness	Acanthaceae	Lf	Bs Pa Sa	Valsaraj *et al.*, 1997
7.	*Aegle marmelos* (L.) Corr.	Rutaceae	Rt	Bs Ec Sa Samr Stf Pa Par Mp	Taylor *et al.*, 1996; Valsaraj *et al.*, 1997
8.	*Aframomum melegueta* K. Schum.	Zingiberaceae	Sd	Bs Ec Pa Sa An Ca	Konning *et al.*, 2004
9.	*Ageratum conyzoides* L.	Asteraceae	Wp	Bc Pa	Wiart *et al.*, 2004
10.	*Alangium salviifolium* Wang.	Alangiaceae	Rt	Bs Ec Pa Sa An Ca	Valsaraj *et al.*, 1997
11.	*Allium cepa* L.	Alliaceae	Lf	Bs Ec Ml Se	Rauha *et al.*, 2000
12.	*Aloe vera* L.	Liliaeeae	Lf	Sa	Martinez *et al.*, 1996
13.	*Alstonia scholaris* R. Br.	Apocynaceae	Rb	Bs Ec Pa Sa	Valsaraj *et al.*, 1997
14.	*Amaranthus blitum* L.	Amaranthaceae	Wp	Bc	Wiart *et al.*, 2004
15.	*Anchusa strigosa* Lab.	Boranginaceae	Rt	Sa Pv Ca	Ali-shtayeh *et al.*, 1998
16.	*Andrographis paniculata* Ness	Acanthaceae	Rt	Bs Ec Pa Sa	Valsaraj *et al.*, 1997
17.	*Anisomeles malabarica* (Linn.) R. Br. ex Sims	Lamiaceae	Lf	Bs Ec Pa Sa	Valsaraj *et al.*, 1997
18.	*Artemisia vulgaris* L.	Asteraceae	Lf	Bs Ec Pa Sa	Valsaraj *et al.*, 1997
19.	*Asphodeline lutea* (L.) Rehb.	Liliaceae	Wp	Ec Kp Pa Pv Sa Ca	Ali-shtayeh *et al.*, 1998
20.	*Asteracantha longifolia* L.	Acanthaceae	Lf	Ea Bp Sa	PerumalSamy, 2005
21.	*Avena sativa* L.	Poaceae	Lf	Bs Ec Ml Sa Se An Ca	Rauha *et al.*, 2000

Contd...

Table 9.2–*Contd...*

Sl.No.	*Plant*	*Family*	*Part**	*Activity Against***	*References*
22.	*Baccharis glutinosa* Pers	Compositiae	Wp	Mc Mg Tt Ef Ss Na Nb Sd Cf Ya Lm Pv Cp	Verastegui *et al.*, 1996
23.	*Bauhinia vahlii* Wight and Arnott	Fabaceae	Rt	Bs Samr Sf Pa Par Mp	Taylor *et al.*, 1996
24.	*Boswellia ameero* Balf. f.	Burseraceae	Bk	Bc Mf Sa Se Sh Sa-NGR	Mothana *et al.*, 2005
25.	*Boswellia elongata* Balf. f.	Burseraceae	Bk	Bc Mf Sa Se Sh Sa-NGR	Mothana *et al.*, 2005
26.	*Brassaiopsis palmata* Kurz	Araliaceae	Lf Bk	Bc Ca Ec Sa	Wiart *et al.*, 2004
27.	*Buxus hildebrandtii* Baill.	Buxaceae	Lf	Bc Mf Sa Se Sh Sa-NGR	Mothana *et al.*, 2005
28.	*Calluna vulgaris* L. Hull	Ericaceae	Lf NM	Bs Ml Se Sa Sh	KumarSamy *et al.*, 2002; Rauha *et al.*, 2000
29.	*Calophyllum inophyllum* L.	Clusiaceae	Sb Lf	Bs Ec Pa Sa	Valsaraj *et al.*, 1997
30.	*Calotropis gigantea* L.	Asclepiadaceae	Lf	Bs Ec Pa Sa	Valsaraj *et al.*, 1997
31.	*Capparis spinosa* L.	Capparidaceae	Rt Fl Fr	Pv Sa	Ali-shtayeh *et al.*, 1998
32.	*Cardiospermum halicacabum*	Sapindaceae	Lf St	Bs Ec Pa Sa	Valsaraj *et al.*, 1997
33.	*Carica papaya* L.	Caesalpiniaceae	Sd	Bs Sa	Valsaraj *et al.*, 1997
34.	*Cassia tora* L.	Rubiaceae	Lf	Bc Mf Sa Se Sh Sa-NGR	Mothana *et al.*, 2005
35.	*Cassia fistula* L.	Caesalpiniaceae	Sd	Bs Ec Pa Sa An	Valsaraj *et al.*, 1997
36.	*Carphalea obovata* (Balf. f.) Verdcourt	Caesalpiniaceae	Rt	Bs Ec Pa Sa	Valsaraj *et al.*, 1997
37.	*Catha edulis* (Vahl.) Endl.	Celastraceae	Bk	Bs Sa	Mc Gaw *et al.*, 2000
38.	*Celosia argentea* L.	Celastraceae	Rt	Bs Sa	Mc Gaw *et al.*, 2000
39.	*Centaurea appendicigera* L.	Amaranthaceae	Wp	Bc Ca Ec Pa Sa	Wiart *et al.*, 2004
40.	*Centaurium erythraea* Rafn	Asteraceae	NM	Sa Samr Sh	KumarSamy *et al.*, 2002
41.	*Centella asiatica Urban*	Apiaceae	Wp	Bs Sa	Valsaraj *et al.*, 1997
42.	*Chelidonium majus* L.	Papaveraceae	Ap Rt	Bc Ca Sa	Kokoska *et al.*, 2002

Contd...

Table 9.2–*Contd...*

Sl.No.	Plant	Family	Part*	Activity Against**	References
43.	*Cichorium intybus* L.	Compositae	Ap Rt	Bc Sa	Kokoska *et al.*, 2002
44.	*Cinnamomum iners* Reinw. Ex B.	Lauraceae	Lf	Bc Ca Ec Pa	Wiart *et al.*, 2004
45.	*Cissampelos pareira* L.	Menispermaceae	Lf St	Bs Ec Pa Sa	Valsaraj *et al.*, 1997
46.	*Cissus quandrangularis* L.	Vitaceae	Rt St	Bc Bcg Bmt Bp Bst Bs Ssp Sb Sf Sa Se St Sp	Lin *et al.*, 1999
47.	*Citrus acida* Roxb. Hook. f.	Rutaceae	Lf	Bp Sa	PerumalSamy, 2005
48.	*Citrus aurantifolia* (Chrism.) Swingle	Rutaceae	Fr	Af Ag Bc Bco Bs Ec Ml Mp Mr Mro Ms Pf Pv Sa Sm	Melendez *et al.*, 2006
49.	*Citrus aurantium* L.	Rutaceae	Fr	Af Ag Bc Bco Bs Ec Ml Mp Mro Ms Pf Pv Sa Sm	Melendez *et al.*, 2006
50.	*Clausena excavata* Burm. f.	Rutaceae	Lf Bk	Bc Bs Sa	Wiart *et al.*, 2004
51.	*Clematis cirrhosa* L.	Ranunculaceae	Ap	Ec Kp Pa Pv	Ali-shtayeh *et al.*, 1998
52.	*Cleome socotrana* Balf. f.	Capparaceae	Lf	Bc Mf Sa Se Sh Sa NGR	Mothana *et al.*, 2005
53.	*Clerodendrum indicum* (L.) Kuntze.	Verbenaceae	Ap	Bs Samr Sf Pa Par Mp	Taylor *et al.*, 1996
54.	*Clerodendrum infortunatum* L.	Verbenaceae	Lf Rt	Bs Ec Pa Sa	Valsaraj *et al.*, 1997
55.	*Clerodendrum serratum* (L.) Moon	Verbenaceae	Lf	Bs Ec Pa Sa	Valsaraj *et al.*, 1997
56.	*Clidemia hirta* (L.) D. Don	Melastomataceae	Lf	Ec Ml Mp Mro Ms Pf Pv Sa	Melendez *et al.*, 2006
57.	*Cola greenwayi* Brenan	Staphyleaceae	Lf Tw	Bs Ec Kp Sa	Reid *et al.*, 2005
58.	*Combretum apiculatum* Loefl.	Combretaceae	Lf	Bs Sa	Mc Gaw *et al.*, 2000
59.	*Commelina communis* L.	Commelinaceae	Wp	Ca	Wiart *et al.*, 2004
60.	*Commiphora parvifolia* Engl.	Burseraceae	Bk	Bc Mf Sa Se Sh Sa NGR	Mothana *et al.*, 2005
61.	*Crescentia cujete* L.	Bignoniaceae	Lf	Af Ag Bc Bco Bs Mp Mr Mro Ms Pf Sa	Melendez *et al.*, 2006

Contd...

Table 9.2–*Contd...*

Sl.No.	*Plant*	*Family*	*Part**	*Activity Against***	*References*
62.	*Crithmum maritimum* L.	Apiaceae	NM	Bc Ec	KumarSamy *et al.*, 2002
63.	*Croton hirtus* L Her	Euphorbiaceae	Wp	Bc Bs Sa	Wiart *et al.*, 2004
64.	*Curtisia dentata* (Burm.f.) C.A.Sm.	Coranaceae	Bk	Bs	Mc Gaw *et al.*, 2000
65.	*Cuscuta reftexa* Roxb.	Convolvulaceae	Wp	Bs Ec Pa Sa	Valsaraj *et al.*, 1997
66.	*Cussonia spicata* Thunb.	Araliacae	Lf	Bs Ec Kp Sa	Mc Gaw *et al.*, 2000
67.	*Cyclea pehata* Hook. f. et Thorns;	Menispermaceae	Rt	Bs Pa Sa	Valsaraj *et al.*, 1997
68.	*Cyperus rotundus* L.	Cyperaceae	Rt Bb	Bs Ec Pa Sa	Valsaraj *et al.*, 1997
69.	*Cyphostemma flaviflorum* (Sprague) Descoings	Vitaceae	Lf Rt St	Af Bcg Bmt Bp Bst Bs Ca Kp Ml Pm Pmg Ps Psr Sf Sa Se Sf Sp	Lin *et al.*, 1999
70.	*Cyphostemma lanigerum* (Harv.) Descoings ex Wild and Drum	Vitaceae	Lf Rt St	Af Bcg Bmt Bp Bst Bs Ca Kp Ml mp Ms Pm Pmg Pv Ps Psr Sa Se St Sp	Lin *et al.*, 1999
71.	*Cyphostemma natalitium* (Szyszyl.) J.V.D. Merwe	Vitaceae	Lf Rt St	Af Bc Bcg Bmt Bp Bst Bs Ca Ea Kp Ml Mp Ms Pm Pmg Pv Ps Psr Ssp Sb Sf Sa Se St Sp	Lin *et al.*, 1999
72.	*Cyphostemma* sp.	Vitaceae	Lf Rt St	Bc Bp Bst Bs Ca Kp Ml Ms Ps Psr Sc S Sb	Lin *et al.*, 1999
73.	*Cystostemon socotranus* Balf. f.	Boraginaceae	Lf	Bc Mf Sa Se Sh Sa-NGR	Mothana *et al.*, 2005
74.	*Datura stramonium* L.	Solanaceae	Sd	Ec Sa	Uzum *et al.*, 2004
75.	*Daucus carota* L.	Apiaceae	NM	Bc	KumarSamy *et al.*, 2002
76.	*Delphinium formosum*	Ranunculaceae	Lf Fl	Bc Bs Hp Sa Tr	Buruk *et al.*, 2006
77.	*Desmos dumosus* (Roxburgh) Safford	Annonaceae	Lf Bk	Bc BsSa	Wiart *et al.*, 2004
78.	*Didymocarpus crinita* Jack	Gesneriaceae	Wp	Bc	Wiart *et al.*, 2004

Contd...

Table 9.2–*Contd...*

Sl.No.	*Plant*	*Family*	*Part**	*Activity Against***	*References*
79.	*Dillenia suffruticosa* (Griff.) Martelli	Dilleniaceae	Lf	Bc Bs Ca Pa	Wiart *et al.*, 2004
80.	*Dombeya burgessiae* Gerr. ex Harv.	Sterculiaceae	Lf	Bs Ec Kp Sa	Reid *et al.*, 2005
81.	*Dombeya cymosa*	Sterculiaceae	Lf Tw	Bs Ec Kp Sa	Reid *et al.*, 2005
82.	*Dombeya rotundifolia* (Hochst.) Planch.	Sterculiaceae	Lf	Bs Sa	Mc Gaw *et al.*, 2000
83.	*Drynaria quercifolia* (L.) Sm.	Polypodiaceae	Wp	Bs Pa Sa	Valsaraj *et al.*, 1997
84.	*Eclipta alba* Hassk.	Asteraceae	Lf	Bs Ec Pa Sa Ca	Valsaraj *et al.*, 1997
85.	*Eclipta prostrata* L.	Asteraceae	Wp	Bc Bs Ca Sa	Wiart *et al.*, 2004
86.	*Elaeocarpus tuberculatus* Roxb.	Elaeocarpaceae	Sb	Bs Ec Pa Sa	Valsaraj *et al.*, 1997
87.	*Elaeodendron transvaalense* (Burtt Davy) R.H. Archer	Celastraceae	NM	Bc Bp Bs Sa	Tshikalange *et al.*, 2005
88.	*Elephantopus scaber* L.	Asteraceae	Lf St Wp	Bc Bs Ec Pa Sa	Valsaraj *et al.*, 1997; Wiart *et al.*, 2004
89.	*Elephantorrhiza burkei* Benth.	Fabaceae	NM	Bp Bs Sa	Tshikalange *et al.*, 2005
90.	*Eleusine indica* Gaertn.	Poaceae	Wp	Ca	Wiart *et al.*, 2004
91.	*Emilia sonchifolia* L. DC	Asteraceae	Wp	Bc	Wiart *et al.*, 2004
92.	*Empetrum nigrum* L.	Ericales	Lf	Bs Ml	Rauha *et al.*, 2000
93.	*Enicostema littorale* Blume	Gentianaceae	Lf	Bs Sa	Valsaraj *et al.*, 1997
94.	*Epilobium angustifolium* L.	Onagraceae	Lf	Bs Ec Ml Sa Se	Rauha *et al.*, 2000
95.	*Equisetum telmateia* Ehrh.	Equisetaceae	Ap	Ec Sa Ca	Uzum *et al.*, 2004
96.	*Eryngium creticum* Lam.	Umbilliferae	Lf St Rt	Kp Pa Pv	Ali-shtayeh *et al.*, 1998
97.	*Erythrophleum lasianthum* Corbishley	Fabaceae	Lf	Bs	Mc Gaw *et al.*, 2000
98.	*Eupatorium odoratum* L.	Asteraceae	Ap	Bs Sams Samr	Taylor *et al.*, 1996
99.	*Euphorbia hirta* L.	Euphorbiaceae	Wp	Bc Bs Ca Sa	Wiart *et al.*, 2004

Contd...

Table 9.2–*Contd...*

Sl.No.	*Plant*	*Family*	*Part**	*Activity Against***	*References*
100.	*Euryops arabicus* Steud.ex Jaub.&Spach	Asteraceae	Lf	Sa-NGR	Mothana *et al.*, 2005
101.	*Fagonia luntii* Baker	Zygophyllaceae	Lf	Bc Mf Sa	Mothana *et al.*, 2005
102.	*Ficus benghalensis* L.	Moraceae	Ap	Bs Sa	Valsaraj *et al.*, 1997
103.	*Ficus religiosa* L.	Moraceae	Lf	Bs Ec Pa Sa	Valsaraj *et al.*, 1997
104.	*Filipendula ulmaria* (L.) Maxim.	Rosaceae	Lf	Bs Ec Ml Sa Se	Rauha *et al.*, 2000
105.	*Geranium asphodeloides* Burm. f.	Geraniaceae	Ap	Sa Se	Uzum *et al.*, 2004
106.	*Glycyrrhiza uralensis* Fischer	Leguminosae	Ap Rt	Bc Sa	Kokoska *et al.*, 2002
107.	*Gunnera perpensa* L.	Gunneraceae	Rt Rh	Sa	Mc Gaw *et al.*, 2000
108.	*Gymnantes lucida* Sw.	Euphorbiaceae	Lf	Bs Sa	Martinez *et al.*, 1996
109.	*Harpephyllum caffrum* Bernh.	Anacardiaceae	Bk	Bs Ec Kp Sa	Mc Gaw *et al.*, 2000
110.	*Hedyotis capitellata* Wall. ex G. Don	Rubiaceae	Lf Bk	Bs Ca	Wiart *et al.*, 2004
111.	*Hedyotis congesta* Wall	Rubiaceae	Lf Bk	Ca Pa	Wiart *et al.*, 2004
112.	*Hemidesmus indicus* R. Br.	Asclepiadaceae	Lf Rt	Bs Ec Pa Sa	Valsaraj *et al.*, 1997
113.	*Heracleum platytaenium*	Umbelliferae	Lf Fl	Bc Bs Hp Sa Ca Tr	Buruk *et al.*, 2006
114.	*Heteromorpha trifoliata* (Spreng.) Cham. and Schltdl.	Apiaceae	Lf	Bs	Mc Gaw *et al.*, 2000
115.	*Hippophae rhamnoides* L.	Elaeagnaceae	Lf Rt Fr	Bc Ca Pa Sa	Kokoska *et al.*, 2002
116.	*Holarrhena antidysenterica* Wall.	Apocynaceae	Rb	Bs Ec Pa Sa	Valsaraj *et al.*, 1997
117.	*Hyptis suaveolens* Poit.	Lamiaceae	Wp	Ca	Wiart *et al.*, 2004
118.	*Inula viscosa* (L.) Ait.	Compositae	Wp	Kp Pa Pv Sa	Ali-shtayeh *et al.*, 1998
119.	*Jatropha unicostata* Balf. f.	Euphorbiaceae	Bk Lf	Bc Mf Sa Se Sh Sa-NGR	Mothana *et al.*, 2005
120.	*Juglans regia* L.	Juglandaceae	Fl Fr	Kp Pa Pv Sa	Ali-shtayeh *et al.*, 1998

Contd...

Table 9.2–*Contd...*

Sl.No.	*Plant*	*Family*	*Part**	*Activity Against***	*References*
121.	*Juniperus lucayana* (L) Britt.	Cupressaceae	St Br	Sa	Martinez *et al.*, 1996
122.	*Kalanchoe farinacea* Balf. f.	Crassulaceae	Lf Fr	Bc Mf Sa Se Sh Sa-NGR	Mothana *et al.*, 2005
123.	*Kalanchoe pinnata* Pers.	Crassulaceae	Lf	Bc Bs	Wiart *et al.*, 2004
124.	*Knema malayana* Warb.	Myristicaceae	Lf Bk	Bc Bs Ca Pa Sa	Wiart *et al.*, 2004
125.	*Lagerstroemia speciosa* (L.) Pers.	Lythraceae	Lf	Bs Sa	Melendez *et al.*, 2006
126.	*Lamium album* L.	Labiatae	Ap Rh	Bc Sa	Kokoska *et al.*, 2002
127.	*Lantana camara* L.	Verbenaceae	lf	Bs Ec Pa Sa	Valsaraj *et al.*, 1997
128.	*Larrea tridentata* (DC.)Cov.	Zygophyllaceae	Wp	Mc Mg Tt Ef S Na Nb Sd Lm Cp Pv	Verastegui *et al.*, 1996
129.	*Leucas aspera* Link	Lamiaceae	Lf	Bs Sa	Valsaraj *et al.*, 1997
130.	*Lippia nodiflora* (L.) Riche.	Verbenaceae	Ap	Bs Samr Sf Pa Par Mp	Taylor *et al.*, 1996
131.	*Lithraea molleoides* Hook et Arn.	Anacardiaceae	NM	Bs Ml Msp Sa	Penna *et al.*, 2001
132.	*Lycium europeum* L.	Solanaceae	Wp	Kp Pa Pv Sa	Ali-shtayeh *et al.*, 1998
133.	*Lycopodium cernuum* L.	Lycopodaceae	Wp	Bc Ca	Wiart *et al.*, 2004
134.	*Lythrum salicaria* L.	Lythraceae	Lf	Bs Ec Ca Ml Se	Rauha *et al.*, 2000
135.	*Mallotus phillppensis* (Lam.) Muell.-Arg.	Euphorbiaceae	Bk	Bs Sams Mp	Taylor *et al.*, 1996
136.	*Malva moschata* L.	Malvaceae	NM	Sa Se Ec Pm	KumarSamy *et al.*, 2002
137.	*Mangifera indica* L.	Anacardiaceae	Sb	Sa	Valsaraj *et al.*, 1997
138.	*Mapania cuspidata* (Miq) Uitt	Cyperaceae	Rt Bk Lf	Bc Pa	Wiart *et al.*, 2004
139.	*Maranta arundinaceae* L.	Marantaceae	Rt	Bs Ec Pa Sa	Valsaraj *et al.*, 1997
140.	*Matricaria chamomilla*	Compositae	Lf	Bs Ec Ml Se	Rauha *et al.*, 2000
141.	*Melastoma malabathricum* L.	Melastomataceae	Lf	Bs	Wiart *et al.*, 2004

Contd...

Table 9.2–*Contd...*

Sl.No.	Plant	Family	Part*	Activity Against**	References
142.	*Melicoccus bijugatus* Jacq.	Sapindaceae	Lf	Af Ag Bc Bs Ml Mp Pv Sa	Melendez *et al.*, 2006
143.	*Memecylon excelsum* Bl.	Melastomataceae	Lf Bk	Bc Bs Sa	Wiart *et al.*, 2004
144.	*Micromeria nervosa* (Desf.) Benth.	Labiatae	Lf	Ec Kp Pa Pv Sa Ca	Ali-shtayeh *et al.*, 1998
145.	*Millettia extensa* (Bentham) Baker	Fabaceae	Rt	Mp	Taylor *et al.*, 1996
146.	*Mimosa pigra* L.	Mimosaceae	Lf	Bs Sa	Martinez *et al.*, 1996
147.	*Momordica charantia* L.	Cucurbitaceae	Lf	Sa	Martinez *et al.*, 1996
148.	*Monochordia vaginalis* (Burm. f.) Prels.	Pontideraceae	Wp	Bc Bs Sa	Wiart *et al.*, 2004
149.	*Moringa oleifera* Lam.	Moringaceae	Sb	Bs Pa Sa	Valsaraj *et al.*, 1997
150.	*Murraya exotica* L.	Rutaceae	Lf	Bs Ec Pa Sa	Valsaraj *et al.*, 1997
151.	*Murraya koenigii* Spreng.	Rutaceae	Lf	Bs Ec Pa Sa	Valsaraj *et al.*, 1997
152.	*Myrcianthes cisplatensis* (Camb.) Berg	Myrtaceae	NM	Sa	Penna *et al.*, 2001
153.	*Neonauclea pallida* (Reinw. ex Havil.) Bakh. f.	Rubiaceae	Lf Bk	Bs Ca	Wiart *et al.*, 2004
154.	*Ocimum sanctum* L.	Lamiaceae	Wp	Pa Sa	Wiart *et al.*, 2004
155.	*Oldenlandia corymbosa* L.	Rubiaceae	Wp	Bs Ec Pa Sa	Valsaraj *et al.*, 1997
156.	*Onobrychis armena* L.	Labiatae	Lf	Bc Bs Sa Tr	Buruk *et al.*, 2006
157.	*Oroxylum indicum* Kurz	Bignoniaceae	Fr	Bs Ec Pa Sa	Valsaraj *et al.*, 1997
158.	*Oxalis corniculata* L.	Oxalidaceae	Lf	Bs Ec Pa Sa	Valsaraj *et al.*, 1997
159.	*Papaver lateritium* K. Koch	Papaveraceae	Lf Fl	Bc Bs Hp Sa Tr	Buruk *et al.*, 2006
160.	*Parietaria diffusa* (Mert. & Koch)	Urticacaceae	Ap	Ec Kp Pa Pv Sa Ca	Ali-shtayeh *et al.*, 1998
161.	*Pergularia daemia* Chiov.	Asclepiadaceae	Lf St	Bs Ec Pa Sa	Valsaraj *et al.*, 1997
162.	*Peristrophe tinctoria* Nees	Acanthaceae	Wp	Bc Bs Ca Ec Pa Sa	Wiart *et al.*, 2004

Contd...

Table 9.2–*Contd...*

Sl.No.	*Plant*	*Family*	*Part**	*Activity Against***	*References*
163.	*Petitia domingensis* Jacq.	Verbenaceae	Lf	Af Ag Bc Bco Bs Ec Ml Mp Mro Ms Pf Pv Sa Sm	Melendez *et al.*, 2006
164.	*Phaganalon rupestre* (L.) DC.	Compositae)	Wp	Ec Kp Pa Pv Sa	Ali-shtayeh *et al.*, 1998
165.	*Phyllanthus acidus* (L.) Skeels	Euphorbiaceae	Fr	Af Ag Bc Bco Bs Ec Ml Mp Mr Mro Ms Pf Pv Sa Sm	Melendez *et al.*, 2006
166.	*Phyllanthus emblica* L.	Euphorbiaceae	Fr	Bs Ec Pa Sa	Valsaraj *et al.*, 1997
167.	*Picea abies* (L.) H. Karst.	Pinaceae	Lf	Bs Ml Se	Rauha *et al.*, 2000
168.	*Pinus sylvestris* L.	Pinaceae	Lf	Bs Ml Sa Se	Rauha *et al.*, 2000
169.	*Piper guineense* L.	Piperaceae	Sd	Bs Ec Pa Sa An Ca	Konning *et al.*, 2004
170.	*Piper longum* L.	Piperaceae	Fl	Bs Ec Pa Sa	Valsaraj *et al.*, 1997
171.	*Piper nigrum* L.	Piperaceae	Lf	Bs Pa Sa	Valsaraj *et al.*, 1997
172.	*Piper porphyrophyllum* N E Br	Piperaceae	Wp	Ca	Wiart *et al.*, 2004
173.	*Piper stylosum* Miq	Piperaceae	Wp	Bc Bs Ca Sa	Wiart *et al.*, 2004
174.	*Pistacia lentiscus* L.	Anacardiaceae	Lf	Ec Kp Pa Pv Sa Ca	Ali-shtayeh *et al.*, 1998
175.	*Pittosporum viridiflorum* Sims	Pittosporaceae	Bk	Bs Sa	Mc Gaw *et al.*, 2000
176.	*Plantago intermedia* L.	Plantaginaceae	Lf	Ec	Uzum *et al.*, 2004
177.	*Plumbago indica* L.	Plumbaginaceae	Lf	Bs Ec Pa Sa An Ca	Valsaraj *et al.*, 1997
178.	*Podocarpus* sp.	Podoearpaceae	Lf	Bs Sa	Martinez *et al.*, 1996
179.	*Polyalthia lateriflora* King	Annonaceae	Lf	Bc Bs Ca Pa Sa	Wiart *et al.*, 2004
180.	*Polyalthia longijblia* Thw.	Annonaceae	Lf	Bs Ec Pa Sa	Valsaraj *et al.*, 1997
181.	*Polygonum punctatum* Elliot var. aquatile (Martins)	Polygonaceae	NM	Bs Ml Msp Sa An	Penna *et al.*, 2001
182.	*Primula longipes*	Primulaceae	Lf Fl Fr	Bc Bs Hp Sa Ca Tr	Buruk *et al.*, 2006

Contd...

Table 9.2–*Contd...*

Sl.No.	*Plant*	*Family*	*Part**	*Activity Against***	*References*
183.	*Prunus padus* L.	Rosaceae	NM	Sa Samr Sh Lp Pm	KumarSamy *et al.*, 2002
184.	*Psoralea corylifolia* L.	Fabaceae	Sd	Bs Pa Sa	Valsaraj *et al.*, 1997
185.	*Psychotria capensis* (Eckl.) Vatke	Rubiaceae	Rt	Sa	Mc Gaw *et al.*, 2000
186.	*Psychotria nervosa* Sw.	Rubiaceae	Lf	Ag Bc Ml Mp Mro Ms Pf Pv Sa	Melendez *et al.*, 2006
187.	*Pulicaria stephanocarpa* Balf. f	Asteraceae	Lf	Bc Mf Sa Se Sh Sa-NGR	Mothana *et al.*, 2005
188.	*Punica granatum* L.	Punicaceae	Lf	Af Ag Bc Bco Bs Ec Ml Mp Mr Mro Pf Pv Sa Sm	Melendez *et al.*, 2006
189.	*Punica protopunica* Balf. f	Punicaceae	Lf	Bc Mf Sa Se Sh Sa-NGR	Mothana *et al.*, 2005
190.	*Quercus macranthera* sp. *syspirensis*	Fagaceae	Lf Fl	Bc Bs Hp Sa Tr	Buruk *et al.*, 2006
191.	*Quercus pontica*	Fagaceae	Lf	Bc Bs Hp Sa Tr	Buruk *et al.*, 2006
192.	*Rafflesia hasseltii* Suring	Rafflesiaceae	Wp	Bc Bs Pa Sa	Wiart *et al.*, 2004
193.	*Randia spinosa* Poir.	Rubiaceae	Fr	Bs Pa Sa	Valsaraj *et al.*, 1997
194.	*Rauvolfia caffra*	Apocynaceae	Lf	Sa	Mc Gaw *et al.*, 2000
195.	*Rauvolfia caffra* Sond.	Apocynaceae	NM	Ecl	Tshikalange *et al.*, 2005
196.	*Reseda lutea* L.	Resedaceae	NM	Sa Se Sh Sm	KumarSamy *et al.*, 2002
197.	*Rhaponticum carthamoides* (Willd.) Iljin	Compositae	Ap Rt	Bc Sa	Kokoska *et al.*, 2002
198.	*Rhodamnia cinerea* Jack	Myrtaceae	Lf	Bc Bs Sa	Wiart *et al.*, 2004
199.	*Rhododendron ponticum* sp. *ponticum* var. *heterophyllum*	Ericaceae	Lf Fl	Bc Bs Hp Sa Tr	Buruk *et al.*, 2006
200.	*Rhoicissus digitata* (L.F.) Gilg and Brandt	Vitaceae	Lf Rt St	Af Bc Bcg Bmt Bp Bst Bs Ca Kp Ml Mp Ms Pm Pmg Pv Ps Psr Ssp Sf Sa Se St Sp	Lin *et al.*, 1999

Contd...

Table 9.2–*Contd...*

Sl.No.	Plant	Family	Part*	Activity Against**	References
201.	*Rhoicissus rhomboidea* (E. Mey. Ex Harv.) Planch	Vitaceae	Lf Rt St	Af Bc Bcg Bmt Bp Bst Bs Ca Ea Kp Ml Mp Ms Pm Pmg Pv Ps Psr Sc Ssp Sb Sa Se St Sp	Lin *et al.*, 1999
202.	*Rhoicissus tomentosa* (Lam.) Wild and Drum	Vitaceae	Lf Rt St	Af Bc Bcg Bmt Bp Bst Bs Ca Kp Ml mp Ms Pm Pmg Pv Ps Psr Sc Ssp Sa Se St Sp	Lin *et al.*, 1999
203.	*Rhoicissus tridentata* (L.F.) Wild and Drum	Vitaceae	Lf Rt St	Af Bc Bcg Bp Bst Ca Ml Ms Pm Pmg Sb Pv Ps Psr Ssp Sa Se St Sp	Lin *et al.*, 1999
204.	*Rhoicissus tridentata* (L.F.) Wild and Drum subsp. *cuneifolia* (Eckl. and Zeyh.) N.R. Urton	Vitaceae	Rt	Af Bc Bcg Bp Bst Ml Ms Pm Pmg Pv Ps Psr Ssp Sa Se St sp	Lin *et al.*, 1999
205.	*Ribes nigrum* L.	Grossulariaceae	Lf	Ml	Rauha *et al.*, 2000
206.	*Rosa canina* L.	Rosaceae	NM	Ec	KumarSamy *et al.*, 2002
207.	*Rosa pisiformis*	Rosaceae	Lf	Bc Bs Hp Sa Ca Tr	Buruk *et al.*, 2006
208.	*Rosmarinus officinalis* L.	Lamiaceae	Lf	Af Ag Bco Ml Mp Mr Mro Ms Pf Sa	Melendez *et al.*, 2006
209.	*Rubus chamaemorusa*	Rosaceae	Be Lf	Bs Ec Ml Se	Rauha *et al.*, 2000
210.	*Rubus idaeus*	Rosaceae	Lf	Bs	Rauha *et al.*, 2000
211.	*Rumex hastatus* D. Don	Polygonaceae	Rt	Bs Samr Sf Pa Par Mp	Taylor *et al.*, 1996
212.	*Rungia parviflora* (Retz.) Nees	Acanthaceae	Ap	Mp	Taylor *et al.*, 1996
213.	*Ruscus aculeatus* L.	Liliaceae	Rt	Ec Pa Pv Sa Ca	Ali-shtayeh *et al.*, 1998
214.	*Ruta chalepensis* L.	Rutaceae	Wp	Ec Kp Pv Sa Ca	Ali-shtayeh *et al.*, 1998
215.	*Ruta graveolens* L.	Rutaceae	Lf	Bs Pa Sa	Valsaraj *et al.*, 1997
216.	*Salacia microsperma* L.	Acanthaceae	Lf	Bp Sa Pv	perumalSamy, 2005

Contd...

Table 9.2–*Contd...*

Sl.No.	*Plant*	*Family*	*Part**	*Activity Against***	*References*
217.	*Salix caprea*	Silicaceae	Lf	Bs Ml Se	Rauha *et al.*, 2000
218.	*Salix rizeensis*	Salicaceae	Lf Fr	Bc Bs Hp Sa Tr	Buruk *et al.*, 2006
219.	*Salvia fruticosa* (L.) Mill.	Labiateae	Lf	Kp Pa Pv Sa Ca	Ali-shtayeh *et al.*, 1998
220.	*Sanguisorba officinalis* L.	Rosaceae	Ap Rh	Bc Ca Ec Pa Sa	Kokoska *et al.*, 2002
221.	*Sansevieria hyacinthoides* Thunb	Ruscaceae	Lf	Bs	Mc Gaw *et al.*, 2000
222.	*Sarcopoterium spinosum* (L.) Spach	Rasaceae	Lf St Fr	Ec Kp Pa Pv Sa Ca	Ali-shtayeh *et al.*, 1998
223.	*Schefflera heterophylla* Harms	Araliaceae	Wp	Bc Bs Ca Sa	Wiart *et al.*, 2004
224.	*Schefflera oxyphylla* Miq. Vig.	Araliaceae	Lf Bk	Bc Bs	Wiart *et al.*, 2004
225.	*Schinus terebinthifolius* Raddi	Anacardiaceae	Lf	Bs Ec Pa Sa	Martinez *et al.*, 1996
226.	*Schotia brachypetala* Sond.	Fabaceae	Lf	Bs Sa	Mc Gaw *et al.*, 2000
227.	*Scindapsus officinals* (Roxb.) Schott	Araceae	Fr	Tm	Taylor *et al.*, 1996
228.	*Sclerocarya birrea* (A. Rich.) Hochst.	Anacardiaceae	Bk	Bs Sa	Mc Gaw *et al.*, 2000
229.	*Sebastiania brasiliensis* Spreng.	Euphorbiaceae	NM	Ml Msp Sa	Penna *et al.*, 2001
230.	*Sebastiania klotszchiana* Muell. Arg.	Euphorbiaceae	NM	Msp Sa	Penna *et al.*, 2001
231.	*Secale cereale* M. Biebe	Poaceae	Lf	Bs Ml Se	Rauha *et al.*, 2000
232.	*Senecio vulgaris* L.	Asteraceae	Rt	Ec	Uzum *et al.*, 2004
233.	*Sennapetersiana* (Bolle) Lock	Fabaceae	NM	Bc Bp Bs Ecl Sa Sm	Tshikalange *et al.*, 2005
234.	*Sida cordata* (Bruin. f.) Borss.	Malvaceae	Rt	Mp	Taylor *et al.*, 1996
235.	*Sida shomibtia* L.	Malvaceae	Sb	Bs Ec Sa	Valsaraj *et al.*, 1997
236.	*Smila leucophylla* Bl.	Smilacaceae	Lf	Bc	Wiart *et al.*, 2004
237.	*Solanum torvum* Sw.	Solanaceae	Lf	Bs Ec Pa Sa An	Valsaraj *et al.*, 1997

Contd...

Table 9.2–*Contd...*

Sl.No.	*Plant*	*Family*	*Part**	*Activity Against***	*References*
238.	*Solanum torvum* Swartz	Solanaceae	Lf	Bc Bs Ca Pa Sa	Wiart *et al.*, 2004
239.	*Solanum tuberosum* L.	Solanaceae	Lf	Bs Ml Sa Se	Rauha *et al.*, 2000
240.	*Sonerila begoniaefolia* Ridl.	Melastomataceae	Lf	Ca Sa	Wiart *et al.*, 2004
241.	*Spirostachys africana* Sond.	Euphorbiaceae	Rt St	Sa	Mc Gaw *et al.*, 2000
242.	*Spondias pinnata* Kurz	Anacardiaceae	Rb	Pa Sa	Valsaraj *et al.*, 1997
243.	*Stachytarpheta indica* L. Vahl	Verbinaceae	Wp	Pa	Wiart *et al.*, 2004
244.	*Stellaria holostea*	Caryophyllaceae	NM	Pa	KumarSamy *et al.*, 2002
245.	*Tachyspermum ammi* L.	Apiaceae	Fr	Bs Ec Pa Sa An Ca	Valsaraj *et al.*, 1997
246.	*Tamarindus indica* L.	Caesalpiniaceae	Lf	Af Ag Bc Bco Bs Ml Mr Mp Ms Pf Sa	Melendez *et al.*, 2006
247.	*Tecomaria capensis* Cape Honeysuckle	Bignoniaceae	Bk	Sa	Mc Gaw *et al.*, 2000
248.	*Terminalia alata* Heyne ex Roth	Combretaceae	Bk	Samr Sf Pa Par Mp	Taylor *et al.*, 1996
249.	*Terminalia bellerica* Roxb.	Combretaceae	Ec	Bs Ec Pa Sa An Ca	Valsaraj *et al.*, 1997
250.	*Terminalia catappa* L.	Combretaceae	Lf	Bco Bs Ea Ml Ms Pf Pv Sa	Melendez *et al.*, 2006
251.	*Terminalia chebula* Retz.	Combretaceae	Ec	Bs Ec Pa Sa	Valsaraj *et al.*, 1997
252.	*Terminalia sericea* Burch. ex DC.	Combretaceae	NM	Bc Bp Bs Sa	Tshikalange *et al.*, 2005
253.	*Thespesia lampas* Dalz.	Malvaceae	Lf Sb	Bs Sa	Valsaraj *et al.*, 1997
254.	*Thespesia populnea*	Malvaceae	Sb	Ec Pa Sa	Valsaraj *et al.*, 1997
255.	*Thottea siliquosa* Lam.	Aristolochiaceae	Rt	Bs Ec Pa Sa	Valsaraj *et al.*, 1997
256.	*Thymus vulgaris*	Lameaceae	Lf	Bs Ec Ml Se	Rauha *et al.*, 2000
257.	*Tinospora cordifolia* (Willd.) Hook. f. et Thomas	Menispermaceae	St Br	Bp Ea Pv Sa	PerumalSamy, 2005

Contd...

Table 9.2–*Contd...*

Sl.No.	*Plant*	*Family*	*Part**	*Activity Against***	*References*
258.	*Tinospora cordifolia* Miers.	Menispermaceae	L St	Bs Ec Pa Sa	Valsaraj *et al.*, 1997
259.	*Trachystemon orientalis* (L.) G. Don.	Boraginaceae	Wp	Ec	Uzum *et al.*, 2004
260.	*Trevesia burckii* Boerlage	Araliaceae	Lf Bk	Bc Ca Sa	Wiart *et al.*, 2004
261.	*Trichocalyx obovatus* Balf. f.	Acanthaceae	Lf Fr	Se Sa NGR	Mothana *et al.*, 2005
262.	*Trichopus zeylanicus* Gaertn.	Dioscoreaceae	Lf	Bs Sa	Valsaraj *et al.*, 1997
263.	*Tussilago farfara* L.	Compositae	Ap Rh	Bc Sa	Kokoska *et al.*, 2002
264.	*Typha capensis* (Rohrb.) N.E.Br.	Typhaceae	Rh	Bs	Mc Gaw *et al.*, 2000
265.	*Urena lobata* L. ssp. *lobata*	Malvaceae	Lf	Sa	Melendez *et al.*, 2006
266.	*Vaccinium myrtillus* L.	Ericaceae	Lf	Ml Ec Pa	Rauha *et al.*, 2000; Valsaraj *et al.*, 1997
267.	*Vaccinium oxycoccus*	Ericaceae	Lf	Ec Sa	Rauha *et al.*, 2000
268.	*Verbascum varians var. trapezunticum*	Scrophulariaceae	Lf St	Bc Ca Tr	Buruk *et al.*, 2006
269.	*Vernonia cinerea* Less.	Asteraceae	Lf St	Bs Ec Pa Sa	Valsaraj *et al.*, 1997
270.	*Vitex leucoxyhm* Schau.	Verbenaceae	Sb	Bs Ec Pa Sa	Valsaraj *et al.*, 1997
271.	*Vitex negundo* L.	Verbenaceae	Lf	Bs Ec Pa Sa	Valsaraj *et al.*, 1997
272.	*Withania adunensis* Vierh	Solanaceae	Lf	Bc Mf Sa Se Sh Sa-NGR	Mothana *et al.*, 2005
273.	*Withania riebeckii* Schweinf.ex Balf.f.	Solanaceae	Lf	Bc Mf Sa Se Sh Sa-NGR	Mothana *et al.*, 2005
274.	*Woodfordia fruticosa* Kurz	Lythraceae	Fl	Bs Ec Pa Sa An	Valsaraj *et al.*, 1997
275.	*Xylopia aethiopica* (Dun.) A. Rich.	Annonaceae	Fr	Bs Ec Pa Sa An Ca	Konning *et al.*, 2004
276.	*Zingiber officinale* L.	Zingiberaceae	Rh	Bs Ec Pa Sa An Ca	Konning *et al.*, 2004
277.	*Zingiber officinale* Rosc.	Zingiberaceae	Rh	Bp Ea Sa	PerumalSamy, 2005

Contd...

Table 9.2–*Contd...*

Sl.No.	*Plant*	*Family*	*Part**	*Activity Against***	*References*
278.	*Zizyphus jujuba* Lam.	Rhamnaceae	Fr	Bs Ec Pa Sa	Valsaraj *et al.*, 1997
279.	*Zizyphus spinachristi*	Rhamnaceae	Wp	Pa	Ali-shtayeh *et al.*, 1998
280.	*Zygophyllum quatarense* M. N. Hadidi	Zygophyllaceae	Lf	Bc Mf Sa	Mothana *et al.*, 2005

***Parts used:** Ar: Aerial root; Bb: Bulb; Ec: Exocarp; Fl: Flower; Fr: Fruit; Lf: Leaf; Rb: Root bark; Rt: Root; Rz: Rhizome; Sb: Stem bark; Sd: Seeds; St: Stem; Wp: Whole plant.

** **Activity Against-Bacteria:** Af: *A. Faecalis;* Bcl: *Bacillus coagulens;* Bp: *B. Pumilus;* Bce: *Bacillus cereus;* Bcc: *Branhamella catarrhalis* ATCC 25238; Kp: *Klebesiella pneumoniae;* Lp: *Lactobacillus plantarum;* MSA: multiresistant *Staphylococcus aureus*; MSE: multiresistant *Staphylococcus epidermidis*; Mrsh-multiresistant *Staphylococcus haemolyticus*; Mp: *Mycobacterium phlei*; Sa NGR: *Staphylococcus aureus North German reference strain*, Pm: *Proteus mirabilis;* Pmg: *Proteus morganii;* Pv: *Proteus vulgaris;* Pa: *Pseudomonas aeruginosa;* Ps: *Pseudomonas solanaceaeum;* Psr: *Pseudomonas syringae;* Sc: *Saccharomyces cervisiae;* Sm: *Salmonella marcescens;* Ss: *Salmonella sps.;* St: *Salmonella typhimurium;* Smr: *Serratia marcescens;* Sb: *Shigella boydii;* Sf: *Shigella flexneri;* Samr: *Staphylococcus aureus-methicilin* resistant, Sams: *Staphylococcus aureus-methicilin sensitive;* Sh: *Staphylococcus hominis;* Sf: *Streptococcus faecalis;* Sp: *Streptococcus pyrogenes.*

Fungi: An: *Aspergillus niger;* Ca: *Candida albicans;* Cab: *Cryptococcus albidus;* Ck: *Candida krusei;* Cl: *Cryptococcus laurenti;* Cm: *Candida maltosa* SBUG; Cn: *Cryptococcus neoformans;* Cr: *Candida rugosa;* Ef: *Epidermophyton floccosum;* Hp: *Helicobacter pylori ATCC 49503;* Mc: *Microsporum canis;* Mg: *Microsporum gypseum;* Msp: *Mucor sp.;* Sch: *Sporotrix schenckii;* Tm: *Trichophyton mentagrophytes;* Tr: *Trichophyton rubrum.*

Screening of Plant Extracts for Antiparasitic Activity

Parasitic infections are a major public health issue in many parts of the world, causing significant morbidity and mortality, and increasing resistance to the standard treatments for these infections, has led to interest in the identification of plant extracts with antiparasitic activity (Rossignol, 1998; Upcroft and Upcroft, 2001). Upcroft and Upcroft, (2001) described the main drug susceptibility methods: essentially the parasite is incubated in the presence of test substance in either a test tube or microtiter plate and cell counts determined at preset time intervals. Results are then reported as 50 per cent inhibitory concentration (IC50), minimum lethal concentration (MLC), or graphed as a percentage of controls over the length of the incubation period. As with other antimicrobial assays the aqueous environment used in assays for antiparasitic activity can pose difficulties and the need for repeated cell counts makes the assay labour intensive. Microtiter plate methods are less time consuming but have high variability in terms of the gaseous environment in each well, important for anaerobic protozoa, and they cannot be used with essential oils that "eat" plastic. Evaluation of extracts against intracellular parasites (*e.g.*, *Leishmania* and *Plasmodium*) also requires access to an appropriate host cell line, cell culture facilities, and staff with expertise in cell culture. Despite these difficulties, a large number of plant extracts have been tested against *Leishmania*, *Giardia lamblia*, *Trypanosoma* sp., and *Plasmodium* species (Asres *et al.*, 2001; Tripathi *et al.*, 1999; Waechter *et al.*, 1999). Interestingly, most of the work on antiparasitic activity of plant extracts, and also antiviral activity, has used aqueous and ethanol/methanol extracts of plant parts, with few studies involving essential oils. Why this is the case is unknown, but it may be related to difficulties associated with solubility or to the types of plant products traditionally used for parasitic and viral infections. Perhaps this traditional use reflects the fact that viral and parasitic infections tend to be internal and therefore require an ingestible, easily produced remedy (essential oils are rarely used internally due to toxicity and are produced via steam distillation).

Antimicrobial Effects of Plant Extracts

In traditional and alternative medicine it is common to use medicinal plants as such, without isolating the active ingredients from them. Using crude extracts might be a more important way to use medicinal plants than has been realized in Western medicine, since plants contain numerous secondary metabolites, and pathogens in nature interact with many chemicals simultaneously (Izhaki, 2002). Traditional plant remedies or phytomedicines, include crude vegetable drugs (herbs) as well as galenical preparations (extracts, fluids, tinctures, infusions) prepared from them. Although a number of studies of the antimicrobial effects of plant extracts have been performed, many plants used in different traditional medicinal systems have never been evaluated for their antimicrobial effects. For example, in Africa, over 5000 plants are known to be used for medicinal purposes, but only a small percentage have been described or studied scientifically, and different combinations of plant species used in traditional medicines have been studied even to a lesser extent (Taylor *et al.*, 2001). The major problem in investigations on the biological activities of plant extracts and phytomedicines lies in the fact that a variety of plants may be used in a single traditional medicine preparation, and in the possibility of synergistic effects resulting from the interactions of the compounds in the extract. This can even result in a loss of activity as the extract is purified (Couzinier and Mamatas, 1986). Eloff and McGaw (2006) pointed out that biologically active extracts can be extremely useful in their entirety, taking into account synergistic and other effects, and according to them an approval of standardized and formulated plant extracts as drugs might be the starting point in developing countries for a successful pharmaceutical industry to be able to compete with Western pharmaceutical companies.

Conclusions

Herbal medicines make an enormous contribution to primary health care and have shown great potential in modern phytomedicine against numerous ailments and the complex diseases of the modern world. Scientists from divergent fields are investigating plants with an eye to their antimicrobial utility. All over the world thousands of phytochemicals have found which have inhibitory effects on all types of microorganisms *in vitro*. There is still a need for more scientific evaluation of Asian herbal medicines including their active constituents, synergistic interactions, formulation strategies, herb drug interactions,standardization, pharmacological and clinical evaluation, toxicity, safety and efficacy evaluation and quality assurance. Furthermore, more of these compounds should be subjected to animal and human studies to determine their effectiveness in whole organism systems, including in particular toxicity studies as well as an examination of their effects on beneficial normal microbiota. It would be advantageous to standardize methods of extraction and *in vitro* testing so that the search could be more systematic and interpretation of results would be facilitated. Also, alternative mechanisms of infection prevention and treatment should be included in initial activity screenings. Attention to these issues could accompany in a poorly needed new era of chemotherapeutic treatment of infection by using plant derived principles.

This review outliners the main methods used in the evaluation of antimicrobial activity of plant extracts; each method has advantages and limitations and all have been widely cited in the literature. The question of which is the best one to use is essentially unanswerable as preferred methods depend on a variety of factors including access to specialized equipment and facilities, the number of samples to be screened and the nature of the plant extract (*e.g.*, volume, extract versus essential oil, chemical composition). For large-scale screening of extracts for antibacterial and antifungal activities disk and agar diffusion methods offer a fast, cost effective, low tech, and generally reliable method of sorting those extracts worthy of further investigation from those unlikely to be of value. Broth dilution methods provide more information but are more time and labour intensive and are best used as a follow up to a large scale screening of plant extracts. Antiviral and antiparasitic assays are the most time and labour intensive of the *in vitro* antimicrobial testing methods and often require access to cell culture or other specialized laboratory facilities. These are used less frequently than antibacterial and antifungal assays. Despite the limitations of many of the assay techniques, there is a vast amount of good data demonstrating that some plant extracts possess strong to excellent antimicrobial activity. The next step is to continue this work into the *in vivo* environment and to evaluate the activity of these extracts in the treatment of infectious disease.

References

Abad, M.J., Bermejo, P., Palomino, S.S., Chiriboga, X., and Carrasco, L. (1999). Antiviral activity of some South American medicinal plants. *Phytotherapy Research*, **13**: 142-146.

Abad, M.J., Guerra, J.A., Bermejo, P., Irurzun, A., and Carrasco L. (2000). Search for antiviral activity in higher plant extracts. *Phytotherapy Research*, **14**: 604-607.

Ablordeppey, S., Fan, P., Ablordeppey, J. H., and Mardenborough, L. (1999). Systemic antifungal agents against AIDS-related opportunistic infections: current status and emerging drugs in development. *Current Medicinal Chemistry*, **6**: 1151-1195.

Ahmed, A.A., Mahmoud, A.A., Williams, H.J., Scott, A.I., Reibenspies, J.H., and Mabry, T.J. (1993). New sesquiterpene a-methylene lactones from the Egyptian plant *Jasonia candicans*. *Journal of Natural Products*, **56**: 1276-1280.

Ali-Shtayeh, M.S., Yaghmour, R.M.R., Faidi, Y.R., Salem, K.H., and Al-Nuri, M.A. (1998). Antimicrobial activity of twenty medicinal plants used in folkloric medicine in the Palestinian area. *Journal of Ethno-pharmacology*, **60**: 265-271.

Amaral, J.A., Ekins, A., Richards, S.R., and Knowles, R. (1998). Effect of selected monoterpenes on methane oxidation, denitrification, and aerobic metabolism by bacteria in pure culture. *Applied and Environmental Microbiology*, **64**: 520-525.

Andrews, J.M. (2001a). Determination of minimum inhibitory concentrations. *Journal of Antimicrobial Chemotherapy*, **48**: 5-16.

Andrews, J.M. (2001b). The development of the BSAC standardized method of disc diffusion testing. *Journal of Antimicrobial Chemotherapy*, **48**: 29-42.

Andrews, J.M. (2004). BSAC standardized disc susceptibility testing method (version 3). *Journal of Antimicrobial Chemotherapy*, **53**: 713-28.

Andrews, J.M. (2005). BSAC standardized disc susceptibility testing method (version 4). *Journal of Antimicrobial Chemotherapy*, **56**: 60-76.

Andrews, J.M. (2007). BSAC standardized disc susceptibility testing method (version 6). *Journal of Antimicrobial Chemotherapy*, **60**: 20-41.

Antonov, A., Stewart, A., Walter, M. (1997). Inhibition of condium germination and mycelial growth of *Botrytis cinerea* by natural products. *In:* 50th Conference Proceeding of the New Zealand Plant Protection Society, pp. 159-164.

Aquino Lemos, A., de Rosario Rodrigues Silva, M. (2005). Antifungal activity from *Ocimum gratissimum L.* towards *Cryptococcus neoformans*. *Memorias do Instituto Oswaldo Cruz.*, **100**: 55-58.

Asres, A., Bucar, F., Knauder, E., Yardley, V., Kendrick, H., and Croft, S.L. (2001). *In vitro* antiprotozoal activity of extract and compounds from the stem bark of *Combretum molle*. *Phytotherapy Research*, **15**: 613-617.

Atta-ur-Rahman and Choudhary, M.I. (1995). Diterpenoid and steroidal alkaloids. *Natural Products Rep.*, **12**: 361-379.

Ayafor, J.F., Tchuendem, M.H.K. and Nyasse, B. (1994). Novel bioactivediterpenoids from *Aframomum aulacocarpos*. *Journal of Natural Products*, **57**: 917-923.

Bailey, J. A., Mansfield, J. W. (1982). Phytoalexins. Glasgow Blackie (Eds) pp: 334

Balls, A.K., Hale, W.S., and Harris T.H. (1942). A crystalline protein obtained from a lipoprotein of wheat flour. *Cereal Chemistry*, **19**: 279-288.

Balzarini, J., Schols, D., Neyts, J., Van Damme, E., Peumans, W., and De-Clercq, E. (1991). a-(1,3)- and a-(1,6)-D-mannose-specific plant lectins are markedly inhibitory to human immunodeficiency virus and cytomegalovirus infections *in vitro*. *Antimicrobial Agents and Chemotherapy*, **35**: 410-416

Barre, J.T., Bowden, B.F., Coll, J.C., Jesus, J., Fuente, V.E., Janairo, G.C., and Ragasa, C.Y. (1997). A bioactive triterpene from *Lantana camara*. *Phytochemistry*, **45**: 321-324.

Bartoli, J., Turmo, E., Alguero, M., Boncompte, E., Vericat, M., Conte, L., Ramis, J., Merlos, M., Garcia- Rafanell, J., and Forn, J. (1998). New azole antifungals Synthesis and antifungal activity of 3-substituted- 4(3H)-quinazolinone derivatives of 3-amino-2-aryl-1-azolyl-2-butanol. *Journal of Medicinal Chemistry*, **41**: 1869-1882.

Batista, O., Duarte, A., Nascimento, J. and Simones, M.F. (1994).Structure and antimicrobial activity of diterpenes from the roots of *Plectranthus hereroensis*. *Journal of Natural Products*, **57**: 858-861.

Boggs, A.F., and Miller, G.H. (2004). Antibacterial drug discovery: is small pharma the solution? *Clinical Microbiology Infection*, **10**: 32-36.

Brandao, M.G.L., Krettli, A.U., Soares, L.S.R., Nery, C.G.C., and Marinuzzi, H.C. (1997). Antimalarial activity of extracts and fractions from *Bidens pilosa* and other *Bidens* species (Asteraceae) correlated with the presence of acetylene and flavonoid compounds. *Journal of Ethnopharmacology*, **57**: 131-138.

Brantner, A.Z., Males, S., Pepeljnak, S., and Antolic, A. (1996). Antimicrobial activity of *Paliurus spina-christi* Mill. *Journal of Ethnopharmacology*, **52**: 119-122.

Brown, D.F.J. (2001). Detection of methicillin/oxacillin resistance in *Staphylococci*. *Journal of Antimicrobial Chemotherapy*, **48**: 65-70.

Brownlee, H.E., McEuen, A.R., Hedger, J., and Scott, I.M. (1990). *Physiological and Molecular Plant Pathology*, **36**: 39-48.

Chattopadhyay, D., Arunachalam, G., Mandal A.B., and Bhattacharya, S.K. (2006). *Chemotherapy*, **52(3)**: 151-157.

Chaurasia, S. C., and Vyas. K.K. (1977). *In vitro* effect of some volatile oil against *Phytophthora parasitica* var. *piperina*. *Journal of Research in Indian Medicine Yoga and Homeopathy*, **1**: 24-26.

Cichewicz, R.H., and Thorpe, P.A. (1996). The antimicrobial properties of chile peppers (*Capsicum* species) and their uses in Mayan medicine. *Journal of Ethnopharmacology*, **52**: 61-70.

Couzinier, J.P., and Mamatas, S. (1986). Basic and applied research in the pharmaceutical industry into natural substances. *In:* Advances in Medical Phytochemistry. Ed. By Barton, D., and Ollis, W.D., Proceedings of the International Symposium of medicinal Phytochemistry, Morocco, London. John Libbey & Co., pp. 57-61.

Cowan, M.M. (1999). Plant products as antimicrobial agents. *Clinical Microbiology Reviews*, 12: 564-582.

De Bolle, M.F., Osborn, R.W., Goderis, I.J., Noe, L., Acland, D., Hart, C.A., Torrekens, S., Van Leuven, F. and Broekart, N.F. (1996). Antimicrobial properties from *Mirablis jalapa* and *Amaranthus caudalus*: expression, pro-cussing, localization and biological activity in transgenic tobacco. *Plant Molecular Biology*, **1**: 993-1008.

Diallo, D., Marston, A., Terreaux, C., Toure, Y., Smestad Paulsen, B., and Hostettmann, K. (2001). Screening of Malian medicinal plants for antifungal, larvicidal, molluscicidal, antioxidant and radical scavenging activities. *Phytotherapy Research*, **15**: 401-406.

Dixon, R.A. (1986). The phytoalexin response: elicitation, signaling and control of host gene expression. *Biology Reviews*, **61**: 239-291.

Dornberger, K., Bockel, V., Heyer, J., Schonfeld, C., Tonew, M. and Tonew. E. (1975). Studies on the isothiocyanates erysolin and sulforaphan from *Cardaria draba*. *Pharmazie*, **30**: 792-796.

Dunford, C., Cooper, R., Molan, P., White, R. (2000). The use of honey in wound management. *Nursing Standard*, **15**: 63-68.

Eloff, J.N. (1998). A sensitive and quick microplate method to determine the minimal inhibitory concentration of plant extracts for bacteria. *Planta Medica*, **64**: 711-713.

Eloff, J.N., and McGaw, L.J. (2006). Plant Extracts Used to Manage Bacterial, Fungal and Parasitic Infections in Southern Africa. *In:* Modern Phytomedicine. Turning Medicinal Plants into Drugs, Ed. By Ahmad, I., Aqil, F., and Owais, M., Wiley-WCH verlag, Weinheim. pp. 97-121

Estevez-Braun, A., Estevez-Reyes, R., Moujir, L.M., Ravelo, A.G. and Gonzalez, A.G. (1994). Antibiotic activity and absolute configuration of 8 *S*-heptadeca-2(Z),9(Z)-diene-4,6-diyne-1,8-diol from *Bupleurum salicifolium*. *Journal of Natural Products*, **57**: 1178-1182.

Fauci, A.S. (2003). HIV and AIDS: 20 Years of Science. *Nature Medicine*, **9**: 839-843.

Favero, J., Corbeau, P., Nicolas, M., Benkirane, M., Trave, G., Dixon, J.F.P., Aucouturier, P. Rasheed, S., and Parker, J.W. (1993). Inhibition of human immuno-deficiency virus infection by the lectin jacalin and by a derived peptide showing a sequence similarity with GP120. *Europian Journal Immunology*, **23**: 179-185.

Fernandes de Caleya, R., Gonzalez-Pascual, B., Garcia-Olmedo, F. and Carbonero, P. (1972). Susceptibility of phytopathogenic bacteria to wheat pu-rothionins *in vitro*. *Applied Microbiology*, **23**: 998-1000.

Fernandez, M. A., Garcia, M.D., and Saenz, M.T. (1996). Antibacterial activity of the phenolic acids fraction of *Scrophularia frutescens* and *Scrophularia sambucifolia*. *Journal of Ethno-pharmacology*, **53**: 11-14.

Field, J.A., Kortekaas, S., and Lettinga, G., (1989). The tannin theory of methanogenic toxocity. *Biology Wastes*, **29**: 241-262.

Flayeh, K.A., and Sulayman, K.D. (1987). Antimicrobial activity of the amine fraction of cucumber (*Cucumis sativus*) extract. *Journal Applied Microbiology*, **3**: 275-279.

Fujioka, T., and Kashiwada, Y. (1994). Anti-AIDS agents. 11- Betulinic acid and platanic acid as anti-HIV principles from *Syzigium claviflorum*, and the anti-HIV activity of structurally related triterpenoids. *Journal of Natural Products*, **57**: 243-247.

Garedew, A., Schnmolz, E., Lamprecht, I. (2004). Microbiological and calorimetric investiga-tions on the antimicrobial actions of different propolis extracts: an *in vitro* approach. *Thermochimica Acta.*, **41(5)**: 99-106.

Geissman, T.A. (1963). Flavonoid compounds, tannins, lignins and related compounds, *In:* Pyrrole pigments, isoprenoid compounds and phenolic plant constituents, vol. 9. Ed. By Florkin, M. and Stotz E.H., Elsevier, New York, N.Y. p. 265.

Ghoshal, S., Krishna Prasad, B.N., and Lakshmi, V. (1996). Antiamoebic activity of *Piper longum* fruits against *Entamoeba histolytica in vitro* and *in vivo*. *Journal of Ethno-pharmacology*, **50**: 167-170.

Grayer, R.J., and Harborne, J.B., (1994). A survey of antifungal compounds from plants, 1982-1993. *Phytochemistry*, **37**: 19-42.

Griffin, S. (2000) Aspects of antimicrobial activity of terpenoids and the relationship to their molecular structure. Ph.D thesis, University of Western Sydney, Sydney,Australia.

Hamburger, H., and Hostettmann, K. (1991). The link between phytochemistry and medicine. *Phytochemistry*, **30**: 3864-3874.

Hammer, K.A., Carson, C.F. and Riley, T.V. (1999). Influence of organic matter, cations and surfactants on the antimicrobial activity of *Melaleuca alternifolia* (tea tree) oil *in vitro*. *Journal of Applied Microbiology*, **86(3)**: 446-452.

Hara, Y., and Watanabe, M. (1989). Antibacterial activity of tea polyphenols against *Clostridium botulinum*. *Journal of Japanese Society of Food Science and Technology*, **36**: 951-955.

Haraguchi, H., Kataoka, S., Okamoto, S., Hanafi, M., and Shibata, K. (1999). Antimicrobial triterpenes from *Ilex integra* and the mechanism of antifungal action. *Phytotherapy Research*, **13**: 151-156.

Harbone, J.B. (1973). Phytochemical Methods, Chapman and Hill, London.

Harborne J.B. (1988). The flavonoids: recent advances. *In:* Plant Pigments. Ed. By Goodwin, T.W., London, England: Academic Press, pp. 299-343.

Harborne, J.B., Baxter, H., and Moss, G.P. (1999). Phytochemical Dictionary-A hand book of bioactive compounds from plants, 2nd Edition, Taylor & Francis Ltd, London, p.528.

Hasegawa, H., Matsumiya, S., Murakami, C., Kurokawa, T, Kasai, R., Ishibashi, S. and Yamasaki, K. (1994). Interactions of ginseng extract, ginseng separated fractions, and some triterpenoid saponins with glucose transporters in sheep erythrocytes. *Planta Medica,* **60**(2): 153-7.

Higgins, V. J., and Smith, D.G. (1972). Separation and identification of two pterocarpanoid phytoalexins produced by red clover leaves. *Phytopathology,* **62**: 235-238.

Himejima, M., Hobson, K.R., Otsuka, T., Wood, D.L., and Kubo, I. (1992). Antimicrobial terpenes from oleoresin of ponderosa pine tree *Pinus ponderosa*: a defense mechanism against microbial invasion. *Journal of Chemistry and Ecology,* **18**: 1809-1818.

Homans, A.L., and Fuchs, A. (1970). Direct bioautographic on thin-layer chromatograms as a method for detecting fungitoxic substances. *Journal of Chromatography,* **51**: 327.

Hood, J.R., Cavanagh, H.M.A., and Wilkinson, J.M. (2004). Effects of essential oil concentration of the pH of nutrient and Iso-sensitest broth. *Phytotherapy Research,* **18**: 947-949.

Hoult, J.R.S., and Paya, M. (1996). Pharmacological and biochemical actions of simple coumarins: natural products with therapeutic potential. *General Pharmacology,* **27**: 713-722.

Hsieh, P.W., Chang, F.R., Lee, K. H., Hwang, T.L., Chang, S.M., and Wu, Y.C. (2004). *Journal of Natural Products,* **67**: 1175-1177.

Hussein, G., Miyashiro, H., Nakamura, N., Hattori, M., Kakiuchi, N., Shimotohno, K. (2000). Inhibitory effects of Sudanese medicinal plant extracts on hepatitis C virus (HCV) protease. *Phytotherapy Research,* **14**: 510-516.

Inouye, S., Tsuruoka, T., Uchida, K. and Yamaguchi, H. (2001). Effect of sealing and Tween 80 on the antifungal susceptibility testing of essential oils. *Microbiology and Immunol ogy,* **45**: 201-208.

Inouye, S., Watanabe, M., Nishiyama, Y., Takeo, K., Akao, M. and Yamaguchi, H. (1998). Antisporulating and respiration-inhibitory effects of essential oils on filamentous fungi. *Mycoses,* **41**: 403-410.

Iscan, G., Kirimer, N., Kurkcuoglu, M., Husnu Can Baser, K., and Demirci, F. (2002). Antimicrobial screening of mentha piperita essential oils. *Journal of Agricultural Food Chemistry,* **50**: 3943-3946.

Iwu, M.M., Unaeze, N.C., Okunji, C.O., Corley, D.J., Sanson, D.R. and Tempesta, M.S. (1991). Antibacterial aromatic isothiocyanates from the essential oil of *Hippocratea welwitschii* roots. *International Journal of Pharmacognosy,* **29**: 154-158.

Iwu, M.M., Duncan, A.R. and Okunji, C.O. (1999). New antimicrobials of plant origin. *In:* Perspectives on new crops and new uses. Ed. By Janick, J., ASHS Press, Alexandria, VA. pp. 457-462.

Izhaki, I., (2002). Emodin- a secondary metabolite with multiple ecological functions in higher plants. *New Phytologist*, **155**: 205-217.

Kakiuchi, N., Hattori, M., Nishizawa, (1986). Studies on dental caries prevention by traditional medicines. VIII. Inhibitory effects of various tannins on glucan synthesis by glucosyltransferase from *Streptococcus mutans*. *Chemical and Pharmaceutical Bulletin*, **34**: 720-725.

Karagoz, A., Onay, E., Arda, N., Kuru, A. (2003). Antiviral potency of mistletoe (*Viscum album* ssp. *album*) extracts against human parainfluenza virus type 2 in Vero cells. *Phytotherapy Research*, **17**: 560-562.

King, A., and Brown, D.F.J. (2001). Quality assurance of antimicrobial susceptibility testing by disc diffusion *Journal of Antimicrobial Chemotherapy*, **48**: 71-76.

Kokoska, L., Polesny, Z., Rada, V., Nepovim, A. and Vanek, T. (2002). Screening of some Siberian medicinal plants for antimicrobial activity. *Journal of Ethnopharmacology*, **82**(1): 51-53.

Konning, G.H., Agyare, C. and Ennison, B. (2004). Antimicrobial activity of some medicinal plants from Ghana. *Fitoterapia*, **75(1)**: 65-67.

Kubo, I., Muroi, H. and Himejima, M. (1993). Combination effects of antifungal agilactones against *Candida albicans* and two other fungi with phenylpropanoids. *Journal of Natural Products*, **56**: 220-226.

Rahalison, L., Hamburger, M., Hostettmann, K., Monod, M. and Frenk, E. (1991). A bioautographic agar overlay method for the detection of antifungal compounds from higher plants. *Phytochemistry Anals*, **2**: 199-203.

Lee-Huang, S., Huang, P.L., Chen, H.C., Huang, P.L., Bourinbaiar, A., Huang, H.I. and Kung, H.F. (1995). Anti-HIV and anti-tumor activities of recombinant MAP30 from bitter melon. *Gene*, (Amsterdam) **161**: 151-156.

Levin, H., Hazenfrantz, R., Friedman, J., and Perl, M. (1988). Partial purification and some properties of the antibacterial compounds from *Aloe vera*. *Phytotherapy Research*, **1**: 1-3.

Lewis, W.H., and Elvin-Lewis, L.W. (1995). Medicinal plants as sources of new therapeutics. *Annals Molecular Botanical Garden*, **82**: 16-24.

Lin, J., Opoku, A.R., Geheeb-Keller, M., Hutchings, A.D., Terblanche, S.E., Jager, A. K. and van Staden, J. (1999). Preliminary screening of some traditional Zulu medicinal plants for anti-inflammatory and anti-microbial activities. *Journal of Ethnopharmacology*, **68(1-3)**: 267-274.

Livermore, D.M., Winstanley, T.J. and Shannon, K. (2001). Interpretative reading: recognizing the unusual and inferring resistance mechanisms from resistance phenotypes. *Journal of Antimicrobial Chemotherapy*, **48**: 87-102.

Hamburger, M.O. and Cordell, A.G. (1987). Direct bioautographic TLC assay for compounds possessing antibacterial activity. *Journal of Natural Products*, **50**: 19-22.

MacGowan, A. P. and Wise, R. (2001). Establishing MIC breakpoints and the interpretation of *in vitro* susceptibility tests. *Journal of Antimicrobials Chemotherapy*, **48**: 17-28

Mann, C.M., and Markham, J.L. (1998). A new method for determining the minimum inhibitory concentration of essential oils. *Journal of Applied Microbiology*, **84**: 538-544.

Martinez, H., Ryan, G.W., Guiscafre, H., and Gutierrez, G. (1998). An intercultural comparison of home case management of acute diarrhoea in Mexico: implications for program planners. *Archieves Medical Research*, **29**: 351-360.

Masoko, P., and Eloff, J.N. (2005). Bioautography indicates the multiplicity of antifungal compounds from twenty-four southern African *Combretum* species (Combretaceae). *African Journal of Biotechnology*, **4**: 1425-1431.

Mason, T.L., and Wasserman, B.P. (1987). Inactivation of red beet â-glucan synthase by native and oxidized phenolic compounds. *Phytochemistry*, **26**: 2197-2202.

Matura, M., Slkold, M., Borje, A., Andersen, K.E., Bruze, M., Frosch, P., Goosssens, A., Johansen, J.D., Svedman, C., White, I.R., and Karlberg, A. (2005). *Contact Dermatitis*, **52**: 320-328.

McDevitt, J.T., Schneider, D.M., Katiyar, S.K., and Edlind, T.D. (1996). Berberine: a candidate for the treatment of diarrhea in AIDS patients, *In:* Program and Abstracts of the 36th Interscience Conference on Antimicrobial Agents and Chemotherapy. American Society for Microbiology, Washington, D.C.

McGaw, L.J., Jager, A.K., and van Staden, J. (2000). Antibacterial, antihelminthic and anti-amoebic activity in South African medicinal plants. *Journal of Ethno-pharmacology*, **72(1-2)**: 247-263.

McMahon, J.B., Currens, M.J., Gulakowski, R.J., Buckheit, R.W.J., Lackman-Smith, C., Hallock, Y.F., and Boyd, M.R. (1995). Michellamine B, a novel plant alkaloid, inhibits human immunodeficiency virus-induced cell killing by at least two distinct mechanisms. *Antimicrobial Agents Chemotherapy*, **39**: 484-488.

McManus, J.P., Davis, K.G., Beart, J.E., Gaffney, S.H., Lilley, T.H., and Haslam, E. (1985). Polyphenol interactions-Part1. Introduction: Some observations on the reversible complexation of polyphenols with proteins and polysackarides. *Journal of Chemical Society Perkin Trans* II, **9**: 1429-1438.

McMurchy, R.A., and Higgins, V.J. (1984). Trifolirhizin and maackiain in red clover: Changes in *Fusarium roseum* "Avenaceum"-infected roots and *in vitro* effects on the pathogen. *Physiology Plant Pathology*, **25**: 229-238.

Mendoza, L., Wilkens, M. and Urzua, A. (1997). Antimicrobial study of the resinous exudates and of diterpenoids and flavonoids isolated from some Chilean *Pseudognaphalium* (Asteraceae). *Journal of Ethno-pharmacology*, **58**: 85-88.

Moore, O.A., Smith, L.A., Campbell, F., Seers, K., McQuay, H.J., and Moore, R.A. (2001). Systematic review of the use of honey as a wound dressing. *BMC Complementary Alternative Medicine*, **1**: 2.

Mori, A., Nishino, C., Enoki, N., Tawata, S. (1987). Antibacterial activity and mode of action of plant flavonoids against *Proteus vulgaris* and *Staphylococcus aureus*. *Phytochemistry*, **26**: 2231-2234.

Nakamura, C.V., Ueda-Nakamura, T., Bando, E., Melo, A.F.N., Cortez, D.A.G., Filho, B.P.D. (1999). Antibacterial activity of *Ocimum gratissimum* L. essential oil. *Mem. Inst. Oswaldo Cruz, Rio de Janeiro*, **94**: 675-678.

Nawawi, A., Nakamura, N., Hattori, M., Kurokawa, M., Shiraki, K. (1999). Inhibitory effects of Indonesian medicinal plants on the infection of herpes simplex virus type 1. *Phytotherapy Research*, **13**: 37-41.

Nostro, A., Germano, M.P., D'Angelo, V., Marino, A., and Cannatelli, M.A. (2000). Extraction methods and bioautography for evaluation of medicinal plant antimicrobial activity. *Letters in Applied Microbiology*, **30**: 379-384.

O'Kennedy, R., and Thornes, R.D. (1997). Coumarins: biology, applications and mode of action. John Wiley & Sons, Inc., New York, N.Y.

Omulokoli, E., Khan, B., and Chhabra, S.C. (1997). Antiplasmodial activity of four Kenyan medicinal plants. *Journal of Ethno-pharmacology*, **56**: 133-137.

Osbourn, A.E., (1996). Preformed antimicrobial compounds and plant defense against fungal attack. *The Plant Cell*, **8**: 1821-1831.

Pengsuparp, T., Cai, L., Fong, H.H.S., Kinghorn, A.D., Pezzuto, J.M., Wani, M.C. and Wall, M.E. (1994). Pentacyclic triterpenes derived from *Maprounea africana* are potent inhibitors of HIV-1 reverse transcriptase. *Journal of Natural Products*, **57**: 415-418.

PerumalSamy, R. (2005). Antimicrobial activity of some medicinal plants from India *Fitoterapia*, **76(7-8)**: 697-699.

Pitner, J.B., Timmins, M.R., Kashdan, M., Nagar, M. Stitt, D.T. (2004). High-throughputs assay system for the discovery of antibacterial drugs, AAPS. *Planta Medica*, **70**: 871-873.

Rana, B.K., Singh, U.P. and Taneja, V. (1997). Antifungal activity and kinetics of inhibition by essential oil isolated from leaves of *Aegle marmelos*. *Journal of Ethno-pharmacology*, **57**: 29-34.

Rao, K.V., Sreeramulu, K., Gunasekar, D., and Ramesh, D. (1993). Two new sesquiterpene lactones from *Ceiba pentandra*. *Journal of Natural Products*, **56**: 2041-2045.

Rauha, J.P., Remes, S., Heinonen, M., Hopia, A., Kahkonen, M., Kujala, T., Pihlaja, K., Vuorela, H., Vuorela, P. (2000). Antimicrobial effects of Finnish plant extracts containing flavonoids and other phenolic compounds. *International Journal of Food Microbiology*, **56**: 3-12.

Robbers, J., Speedie, M., and Tyler, V. (1996). Pharmacognosy and pharmacobiotechnology. Williams and Wilkins, Baltimore. pp. 1-14.

Wheat, F. P. (2001). History and development of antimicrobial susceptibility testing methodology. *Journal of Antimicrobial Chemotherapy*, **48**: 1-4

White, T., Marr, K., Bowden, R.(1998). Clinical, cellular and molecular factors that contribute to antifungal drug resistance. *Clinical Microbiology Reviews*, **11**: 382-402.

WHO (2000). The WHO Recommended Classification of Pesticides by Hazard and Guidelines to Classification 2000-2202 (WHO/PCS/01.5). International Programme on Chemical Safety, World Health Organization, Geneva.

WHO (2002). General Guidelines for Methodologies on Research and Evaluation of Traditional Medicine. World Health Organization, Geneva.

Wiart, C., Mogana Khalifah, S., Mahan, M., Ismail, S., Buckle, M., Narayana, A.K. and Sulaiman, M. (2004). Antimicrobial screening of plants used for traditional medicine in the state of Perak, Peninsular Malaysia. *Fitoterapia*, **75**(1): 68-73.

Wiart, C., Mogana Khalifah, S., Mahan, M., Ismail, S., Buckle, M., Narayana, A.K. and Sulaiman, M. (2004). Antimicrobial screening of plants used for traditional medicine in the state of Perak, Peninsular Malaysia. *Fitoterapia*, **75**(1): 68-73.

Wilkinson, J.M., Cavanagh, H.M.A.(2005). Antibacterial activity of essential oils from Australian native plants. *Phytotherapy Research*, **19**: 643-646.

World Chiropractic Alliance (2000). http: //www.worldchiropracticalliance.org

Xu, H. X., F. Q. Zeng, M. Wan, and K. Y. Sim. 1996. Anti-HIV triterpene acids from *Geum japonicum*. *Journal of Natural Products*, **59**: 643-645.

Zhang, Y., and K. Lewis. 1997. Fabatins: new antimicrobial plant peptides. *FEMS Microbiology Letters*, **149**: 59-64.

Zhu, M., Phillipson, D., Greengrass, P. M., Bowery, N. E., Cai, Y.(1997) Plant polyphenols: biologically active compounds or non-selective binders to protein? *Phytochemistry*, **44 (3)**: 441-447.

Bioactive Phytochemicals: Perspectives for Modern Medicine Vol. 1 (2012)
Editor: **V.K. Gupta**
Published by: **DAYA PUBLISHING HOUSE, NEW DELHI**

Pages **381–393**

10

Biomedical Potentials of Filamentous Marine Cyanobacterial Natural Products

Lik Tong Tan[1]* and Ashootosh Tripathi[1]

ABSTRACT

Filamentous marine cyanobacteria produce a wide range of biologically active secondary metabolites with therapeutic applications. A majority of these compounds are nitrogen-containing biosynthesized by hybrid modular polyketide synthase and non-ribosomal polypeptide synthetase enzymes, resulting in highly functionalized chemical structures. A number of potent cytotoxic compounds exert their activity by interfering with the dynamic of microtubule and actin filaments, making these compounds an attractive source of potential anticancer drugs. Within the past three years, natural products research on marine cyanobacteria has uncovered these microbes to be a potential source of novel neurotoxins as well as antiprotozoal compounds. The present review highlights the importance of marine cyanobacteria as a source of potential therapeutic agents.

Keywords: Marine cyanobacteria, Natural products, Drug discovery, Anticancer, Neurotoxins, Antimalarial.

Introduction

The prokaryotic filamentous marine cyanobacteria have been shown to be a prolific producer of biologically unique secondary metabolites. Natural products research on this group of marine microorganisms started in the early 1970s by the late Professor Richard Moore from the University of Hawaii. Since then, other research

1 Natural Sciences and Science Education, National Institute of Education, Nanyang Technological University, 1 Nanyang Walk, Singapore 637616.

* *Corresponding author*: E-mail: liktong.tan@nie.edu.sg

groups, including Professor William Gerwick's research group at the Scripps Institution of Oceanography at San Diego, have contributed significantly to the scientific literature on the reports of novel marine cyanobacterial metabolites. To date, more than 320 nitrogen-containing compounds have been reported mainly from *Lyngbya*, *Symploca*, and *Oscillatoria* genera. These compounds are structurally diverse with a majority belonging to the hybrid polyketide-polypeptide structural class. These compounds are usually highly functionalized with the occurrence of unique structural moieties, including aromatic heterocycles (*e.g.*, thiazole and oxazole), β-amino/hydroxy acids, high degree of *N*-methylations, and polypeptide chains with unusual methylation patterns.

Associated with the diverse chemical structures of marine cyanobacterial compounds are the potent biological activities reported for some of these molecules, including anticancer, antimicrobial, and neurotoxic properties. In recent years, a growing number of marine cyanobacterial compounds have been shown to exhibit significant antiprotozoal activities, particularly as antimalarial agents. In the area of cancer research, many marine cyanobacterial compounds exert their cytotoxic activity by interfering with the dynamics of microtubule and actin filaments. This makes cyanobacterial compounds an attractive source of therapeutic agents for the treatment of various cancer diseases. For instance, the linear depsipeptides, dolastatins 10 and 15, were in clinical testings as potential anticancer drugs. Furthermore, a number of synthetic analogs, such as TZT-1027 and ILX651, based on the structural templates of dolastatins 10 and 15 are currently in various phases of clinical trials for the treatment of different cancer forms. The biological activities of these natural and synthetic compounds have been thoroughly reviewed by several authors, including those by Gerwick *et al.* (2001), Tan (2007), and Tan (2010). The present chapter on marine cyanobacterial compounds therefore serves to highlight recent discoveries of notable compounds having significant biological activities, particularly as anticancer, neurotoxic, and antiprotozoal agents.

Biology of Cyanobacteria

Cyanobacteria, also known as blue-green algae or Cyanophyta, are a phylum of bacteria that obtain their energy through photosynthesis. They were originally considered as algae because of their microscopic morphology, pigmentation, and possession of oxygen evolving photosystems, PS I and PS II. Their genomic size, representative of all major taxonomic groups, lies in the range of 1.6×10^9 to 8.6×10^9 Da which is comparable to that of bacteria (1.0 to 3.6×10^9 Da) (Herdman *et al.*, 1979). Cyanobacteria are the pioneer oxygenic phototrophs on earth whose distribution around the world is surpassed only by bacteria (Adams, 2000). Fossil evidence points to their presence in geographically diverse regions during the Precambrian more than 3.5 billion years ago.

Colonial cyanobacteria often occur with their cells arranged in chains or in hairlike filaments, sometimes appearing as mats in nature. *Coccoid* species occur in irregular, spherical or plate like colonies wherein cell numbers may range from few to many and the individual cells being held together by the gelatinous sheaths which varies in appearance, pigmentation, consistency, and thickness. Filamentous forms produce a row of cells, referred to as trichome. Trichomes may be simple straight, and/or permanently spirally coiled. Some filamentous species are also characterized by true cell differentiation, forming larger, colorless, nitrogen-fixing cells called heterocysts. Members of the genera *Nostoc* and *Anabaena* may produce thick walled cells called akinetes, which can resist freezing and other adverse conditions (Thajuddin *et al.*, 2005).

Cyanobacteria are ubiquitous and are common in temporary pools or ditches, particularly if the water is polluted. They are found abundantly at rocky shores (*e.g.*, *Oscillatoria nigroviridis*, *Lyngbya confervoides*, and *Lyngbya majuscula*), hypersaline (*e.g.*, *Lyngbya aestuarii*), brackish waters, fresh water (*e.g.*, *Nostoc*, *Oscillatoria*, *Lyngbya*, and *Microcystis*), paddy fields (*e.g.*, *Anabaena*, *Aulosira*, and *Calothrix*), hot springs (*e.g.*, *Phormidium tenue* and *Mastigocoleus laminosus*), and polar regions (*e.g.* *Anabaena*, *Calothrix*, *Lyngbya*, *Oscillatoria*, *Plectonema*, and *Scytonema*) (Broady *et al.*, 1996). In many environments, cyanobacteria are the primary producers at the base of a food web of the ecosystem. Certain marine cyanobacterial strains are also found in symbiosis with other marine micro or macroorganisms, such as tunicates, sponges, echiuroid worms, and dinoflagellates (Carpenter and Foster, 2002).

Biologically Active Marine Cyanobacterial Secondary Metabolites

Anticancer Agents

A large proportion of marine cyanobacterial compounds are found to be cytotoxic with activities ranging from micromolar to nanomolar range. Among the cytotoxic compounds, many were found to be either microtubule disruptors (*e.g.*, dolastatins 10 and analogs and curacin A) or actin disruptors (*e.g.*, dolastatin 11 and analogs and lyngbyabellins/hectochlorin) (Tan, 2010). Due to their potent activities, several marine cyanobacterial compounds, such as dolastatins 10 and 15, have been in clinical testings, and currently a number of their synthetic derivatives (*e.g.*, TZT-1027 in Phase III and ILX651 in Phase II) are at various stages of clinical trials for the treatment of different cancer forms (Mayer *et al.*, 2010; Tan, 2010).

In recent years, one of the more exciting cytotoxic marine cyanobacterial compounds is the discovery of largazole (**1**) (Figure 10.1) in 2008 by the laboratory of Dr. Luesch (Taori *et al.*, 2008). This molecule was isolated from the Floridian marine cyanobacterium, *Symploca* sp., and was later found to be a potent class I histone deacetylase inhibitor. Due to its exceptional biological activity, several research groups reported the total synthesis of this molecule as well as its analogs for further SAR studies. This has been reviewed recently by Tan (2010) and will not be covered in this chapter. Largazole was recently screened in the NCI's 60 cancer cell lines and showed that it was preferentially active against colon cancer cell types (Liu *et al.*, 2010). Furthermore, it was found that largazole stimulated histone hyperacetylation in tumor tissue, based on an *in vivo* system using a human HCT116 xenograft mouse model, resulting in the inhibition of tumor growth and induction of apoptosis of tumor cells (Liu *et al.*, 2010).

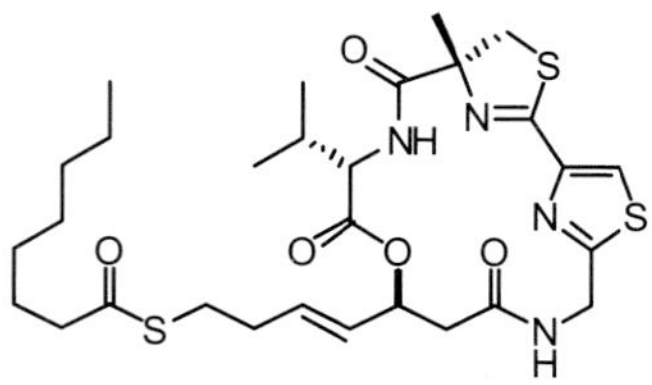

Largazole (**1**)

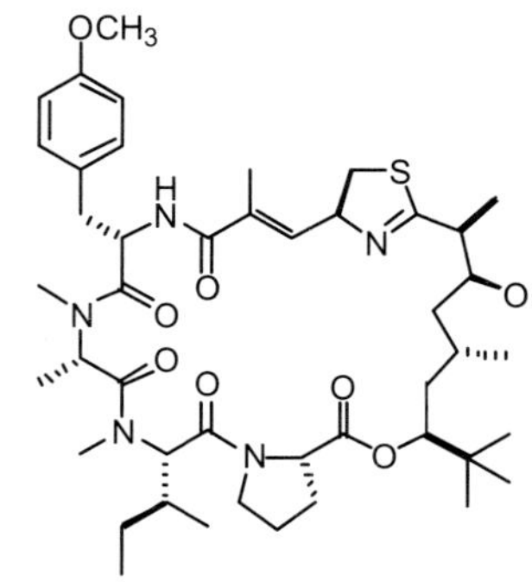

Apratoxin A (**2**)

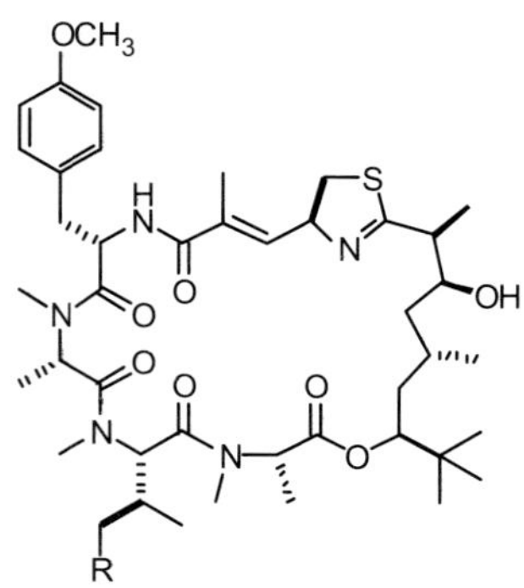

Apratoxin F (**3**): R = CH_3
Apratoxin G (**4**): R = H

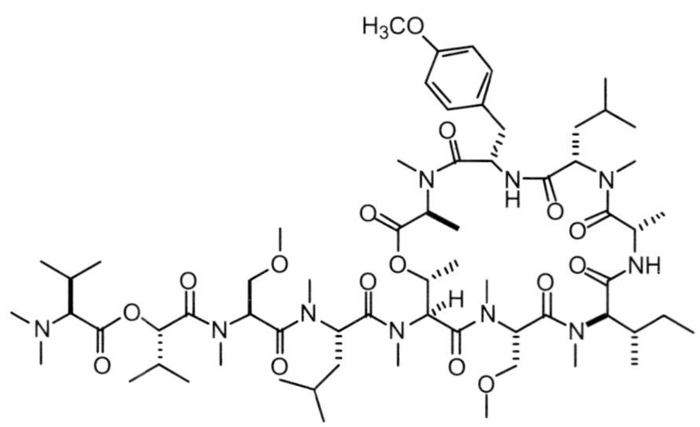

Coibamide A (**5**)

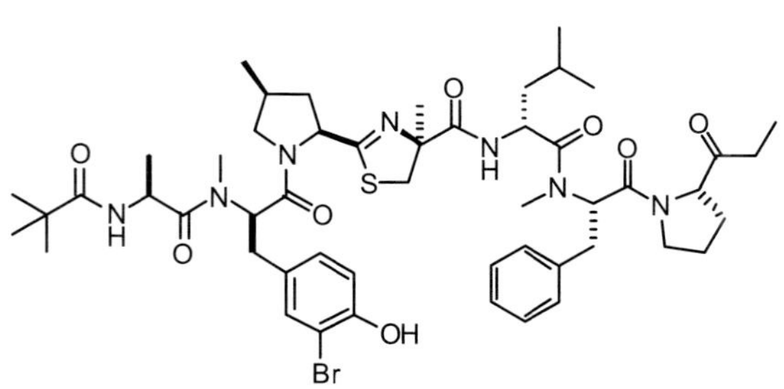

Bisebromoamide (**6**)

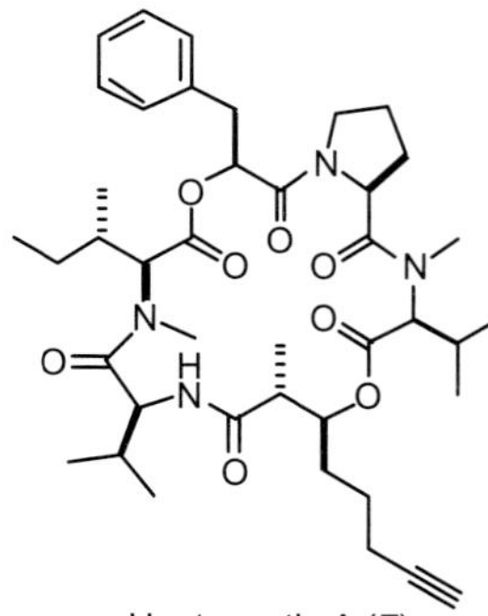

Hantupeptin A (**7**)

Figure 10.1: Recent cytotoxic marine cyanobacterial natural products.

The apratoxin class of molecules is a series of marine cyanobacterial cyclic depsipeptides with potent cytotoxic activities usually in the nanomolar range. The first compound of this series, apratoxin A (**2**) (Figure 10.1), was discovered in 2001 from the marine cyanobacterium, *Lyngbya majuscula*, and displayed subnanomolar *in vitro* cytototoxcity against several cancer cell lines (Luesch *et al.*, 2001). The structures and biological activities of apratoxins A to E have been reviewed recently by Tan (2010). Since the publication of that review, two additional apratoxin-analogs, apratoxins F (**3**) and G (**4**) (Figure 10.1), have been reported from a Palmyra collection of *Lyngbya bouillonii* (Tidgwell *et al.*, 2010). The main difference of these two new molecules is the presence of a *N*-methyl Ala unit in place of a Pro unit in apratoxins A – E. In spite of this difference, apratoxins F and G still displayed potent cytotoxicity against H-460 cancer cells with IC_{50} values of 2 and 14 nM, respectively.

Other recently reported marine cyanobacterial compounds having significant cytotoxic properties include coibamide A (**5**), bisebromoamide (**6**), and hantupeptin A (**7**). Coibamide A (**5**) (Figure 10.1) is a potent antiproliferative lariat-type cyclic depsipeptide, isolated from the Panamanian marine cyanobacterium, *Leptolyngbya* sp. (Medina *et al.*, 2008). This compound was isolated as part of an International Cooperative Biodiversity Groups program (ICBG), between research groups in the US and Panama, to screen and identify bioactive compounds from natural sources in the later country. This molecule possesses a high degree of *N*-methylation with eight out of 11 amino acid residues being *N*-methylated. The chemical structure of compound **5** was established by extensive 2D NMR spectroscopic experiments (*e.g.*, COSY, TOCSY, multiplicity-edited HSQS, HSQC-TOCSY, HMBC, H2BC, ^{1}H-^{15}N gHMBC, and ROESY) as well as mass spectroscopic analysis. The absolute stereochemistry of the **5** was determined by Marfey's method as well as chiral HPLC analysis. Coibamide A displayed potent cytotoxicity against NCI-H460 lung cancer cells and mouse neuro-2a cells, with LC_{50}s less than 23 nM. In addition, the compound was evaluated in the NCI's panel of 60 cancer cell lines and it exhibited significant activities against MDA-MB-231, LOX IMVI, HL-60(TB), and SNB-75 at 2.8 nM, 7.4 nM, 7.4 nM, and 7.6 nM, respectively. COMPARE analysis indicated that coibamide A could inhibit cancer cell proliferation via a novel mechanism (Medina *et al.*, 2008).

Bisebromoamide (**6**) (Figure 10.1) is a cytotoxic linear peptide isolated recently from an Okinawan strain of the filamentous marine cyanobacterium, *Lyngbya* sp. (Teruya *et al.*, 2009). Its planar structure was determined by 1D and 2D NMR experiments and its complete stereochemistry was established using chemical manipulation and chiral HPLC analysis. This novel compound contained a unique *N*-methyl-3-bromotyrosine, a modified 4-methylproline, a 2-(1-oxo-propyl)pyrrolidine as well as a *N*-pivalamide unit. Bisebromoamide possessed cytotoxic property against HeLa S_3 cells with an IC_{50} value at 0.04 μg/mL. When tested against a panel of 39 human cancer cell lines, bisebromoamide gave an average GI_{50} value of 40 nM. In addition, a series of biochemical experiments suggested that the ERK (extracellular signal regulated protein kinase) signaling pathways could potentially be a target for this compound.

Hantupeptin A (**7**) (Figure 10.1), a cyclic depsipeptide, is a potent cytotoxic molecule isolated from a persistent strain of *Lyngbya majuscula* found at the western lagoon of Pulau Hantu, Singapore (Tripathi *et al.*, 2009). This molecule consisted of four α-amino acids, one α-hydroxy acid, and a PKS-derived β-hydroxy acid residue and its complete structure was determined by extensive NMR experiments and MS data. Hantupeptin A is an example of a hybrid polyketide-polypeptide synthetase class of molecule. The presence of the PKS-derived unit of 3-hydroxy-2-methyloctynoic acid residue in **7** appears to be widespread in marine cyanobacterial cyclic depsipeptides. More than 60 cyclic depsipeptides from marine cyanobacteria contain such a PKS derived unit, usually in the form of β-hydroxy acid or β-amino acid residue (Gerwick *et al.*, 2001; Tan, 2007). In all cases, chain extension occurs at the C-2 position and either single methylation or dimethylation is observed at the C-1 position of the β-hydroxy acid or β-amino acid unit. Such structural feature is a hallmark of marine cyanobacterial natural products and together with the different combination of α-amino/hydroxy acids, emphasize the amazing combinatorial biosynthetic capacity of marine cyanobacteria. Hantupeptin A has been reported to display significant cytotoxic activity against the MOLT-4 leukemia cell line with IC_{50} of 32 nM.

Neurotoxins

Neurotoxins are a growing class of bioactive marine cyanobacterial natural products. A number of these compounds were shown to act either as activators (*e.g.*, antillatoxin) or blockers (*e.g.*, kalkitoxin and jamaicamide A) of the mammalian voltage-gated sodium channels (VGSCs) (Araoz *et al.*, 2010). VGSCs are important for the generation as well as the propagation of electrical signals in neuronal cells. Compounds that potently modulate the functions of VGSCs have therapeutic value for the treatment of neurological disorders, such as epilepsy, neuropathic pain, stroke, and heart failure (Clare *et al.*, 2000).

In recent years a number of novel polyketide-polypeptide type neurotoxins have been reported from filamentous strains of marine cyanobacteria. One of these neurotoxins is hoiamide A (**8**) (Figure 10.2) isolated from an assemblage of two cyanobacteria *Lyngbya majuscula* and *Phormidium gracile* obtained from Hoia Bay, Papua New Guinea (Pereira *et al.*, 2009). Hoiamide A consists of a number of unique structural features, including an acetate extended isoleucine-derived unit, two methylated thiazoline units, a thiazole unit, and a highly methylated and oxygenated polyketide-derived moiety. Its structure was determined by extensive NMR and chemical manipulation methods. Using neurochemical and pharmacological methods, it was shown that hoiamide A is a potent inhibitor of [3H]batrachotoxin binding to VGSCs and it activates sodium influx with IC_{50} and EC_{50} values of 92.8 nM and 2.31 μM, respectively. Since its first discovery in 2009, two more analogs, hoiamides B (**9**) and C (**10**) (Figure 10.2), have been isolated from various marine cyanobacteria samples from Papua New Guinea (Choi *et al.*, 2010). When tested on neocortical neural cells, hoiamide B (**9**) promote sodium influx but reduced spontaneous Ca^{2+} oscillations with EC_{50} values at 3.9 μM and 79.8 nM, respectively.

Alotamide A (**11**) and palmyrolide A (**12**) (Figure 10.2) are two new neurotoxins isolated from marine cyanobacteria from Milne Bay, Papua New Guinea and Palmyra Atoll, respectively (Soria Mercado *et al.*, 2009; Pereira *et al.*, 2010). These molecules are structurally unique consisting of extensive polyketide portion linking with peptidic residues. The polyketide portion of alotamide A (**11**) (Figure 10.2), obtained from the marine cyanobacterium *Lyngbya bouillonii*, consists of seven acetate units as part of the macrocyclic ring structure (Soria-Mercado *et al.*, 2009). Three other peptidic

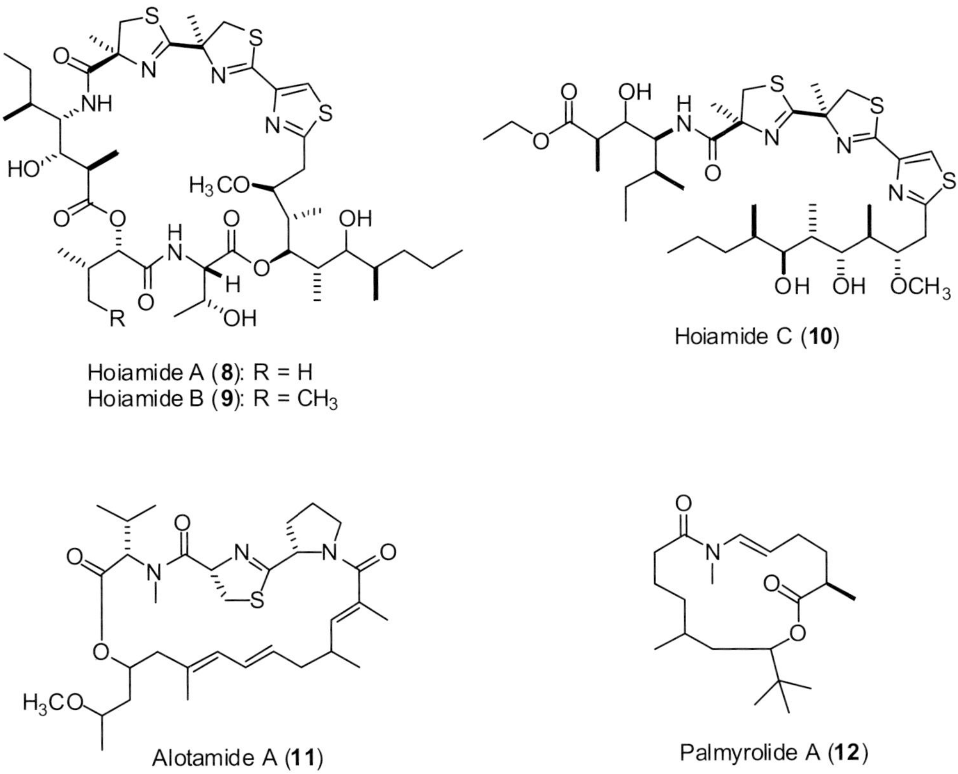

Figure 10.2: Recent neurotoxins from marine cyanobacteria.

residues, an *N*-Me-Val, a cysteine-derived thiazoline unit and Pro, are linked to the polyketide unit completing the overall macrocyclic structure of the molecule. When tested on murine cerebrocortical neurons, alotamide A showed unusual Ca^{2+} influx activation profile with EC_{50} of 4.18 µM. Palmyrolide A (**12**) (Figure 10.2) was isolated from a marine cyanobacterial consortium of *Leptolyngbya cf.* and *Oscillatoria* sp. (Pereira *et al.*, 2010). This molecule is structurally related to the laingolides by featuring a *tert*-butyl group possibly deriving from malonyl-CoA with the methyl groups contributed by *S*-adenosyl-L-methionine (SAM). Palmyrolide A was found to suppressed calcium influx in cerebrocortical neurons with IC_{50} of 3.7 µM. In addition, it possesses moderate sodium channel blocking activity in neuro-2a cells with IC_{50} of 5.2 µM.

Marine Cyanobacterial Compounds Active Against Tropical Diseases

In recent years, a number of marine cyanobacterial compounds having antiprotozoal activities have been reported in the literature. The discovery of these compounds stemmed from natural products research initiated by the Panamanian International Cooperative Biodiversity Group (ICBG) program. One of the aims of this NIH-funded program is to screen terrestrial and marine samples from Panama for compounds against tropical diseases, such as malaria, schistosomiasis, leishmaniasis, and chagas.

One of the early reports of antimalarial cyanobacterial compounds were venturamides A (**13**) and B (**14**) (Figure 10.3) isolated from *Oscillatoria* sp. collected from Buenaventura Bay located at the Portobelo National Marine Park, Panama (Linington *et al.*, 2007). The chemical structures of these modified cyclic hexapeptides were deduced based on extensive 1D and 2D NMR experiments as well as data comparison with the literature. Venturamide A, in particular, showed preferential *in vitro* activity against the W2 chloroquine-resistant strain of the malaria parasite, *Plasmodium falciparum*, with IC_{50} at 8.2 µM over mammalian Vero cells. Both compounds showed mild activity when tested against other tropical parasites such as *Trypanosoma cruzi* and *Leishmania donovani*.

In addition to cyclic peptides, a number of linear lipopeptides have been reported to exhibit significant antiprotozoal properties. The linear lipodepsipeptides, viridamides A (**15**) and B (**16**) (Figure 10.3), are antiprotozoal compounds isolated from the marine cyanobacterium, *Oscillatoria nigroviridis*, cultured from an assemblage of *Lyngbya majuscula* from Curacao (Simmons *et al.*, 2008). The structures of viridamides A and B consisted of six *N*-methylated amino acids, hydroxy acids as well as an unusual 5-methoxydec-9-ynoic acid residue. The planar and absolute structural elucidations of these compounds were achieved through NMR and mass spectroscopic methods as well as chemical manipulation involving Marfey's method and chiral HPLC analysis, respectively. Viridamide A (**15**) showed promising activities against three parasitic protozoa, namely *Trypanosoma cruzi*, *Leishmania mexicana*, and *Plasmodium flaciparum*, with IC_{50} values ranging from 1.1 to 5.8 µM.

Gallinamide A (**17**) (Figure 10.3) is a highly functionalized linear lipodepsipeptide containing a methylmethoxypyrrolinone moiety (Linnington *et al.*, 2009). This unusual molecule was isolated from the red-tipped *Schizothrix* sp. obtained from the Portobelo National Marine Park, Panama and exhibited moderate *in vitro* activity against *Plasmodium falciparum* with IC_{50} value of 8.4 µM. In addition, it showed moderate activities against mammalian Vero cells (TC_{50} of 10.4 µM) and *Leishmania donovani* (IC_{50} of 9.3 µM). It was further observed by Linington and co-workers (Linnington *et al.*, 2009) that linear peptides having either terminal *N,N*-dimethylvaline or *N,N*-dimethylisoleucine moieties are a potential class of compounds that possess antiparasitic and anticancer properties. Gallinamide A is structurally related to the highly potent dolastatins 10 and 15. Unlike dolastatins 10 and 15, gallinamide A showed moderate cytotoxicity when tested against Vero cells and no *in vitro* cytotoxicity when tested against NCI-H460 human lung tumor and neuro-2 mouse neuroblastoma cell lines.

Almiramides A (**18**) – C (**20**) (Figure 10.3) were recently reported to possess significant antileishmanial property, representing a new class of leishmaniasis lead compounds (Sanchez *et al.*, 2010). These compounds are highly N-methylated linear lipopeptides isolated from *Lyngbya majuscula* from the Bocas del Toro Marine Park, Panama. The chemical structures of almiramides were established by NMR, MS, as well as chemical manipulations, including Marfey's analysis to determine their

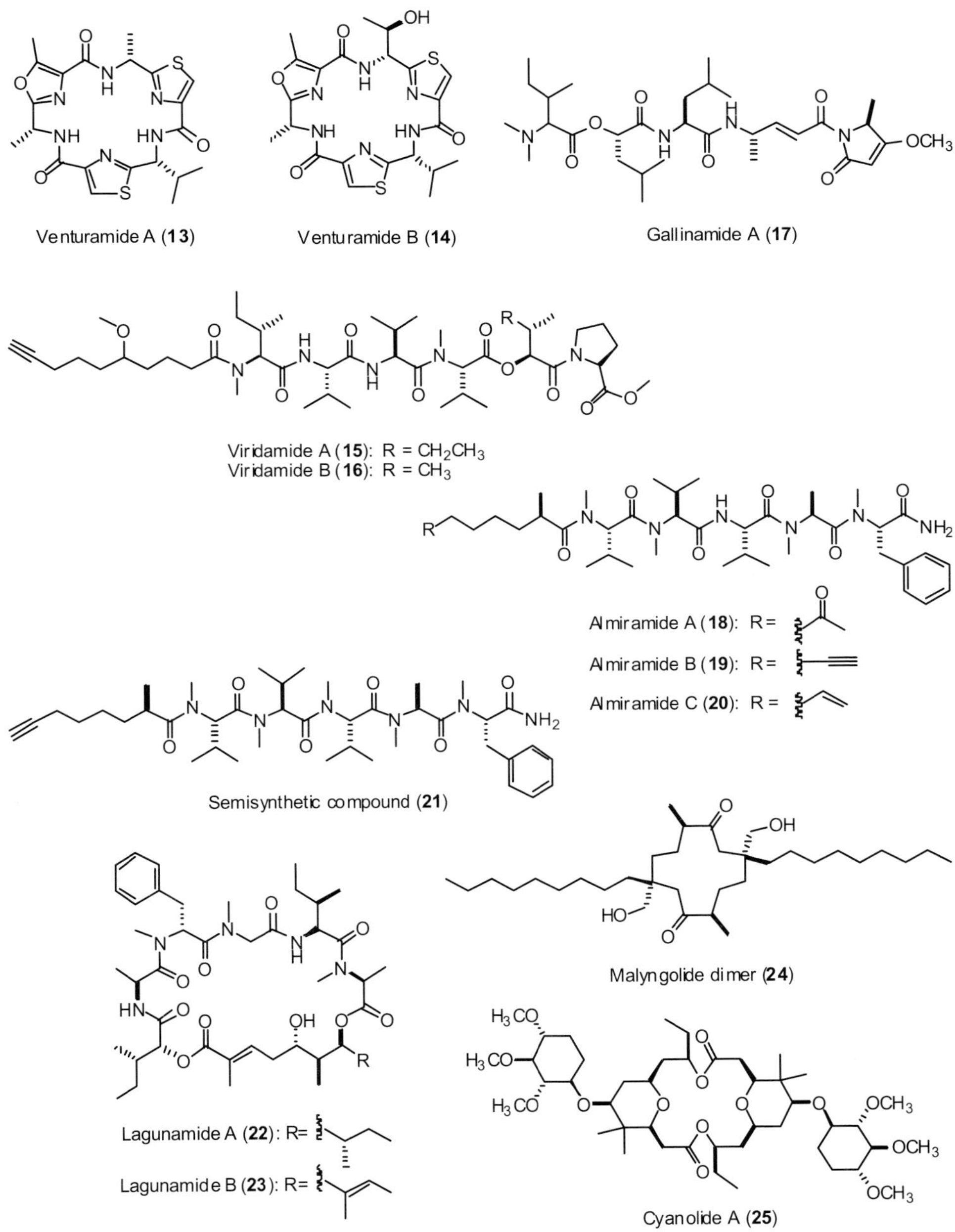

Figure 10.3: Recent marine cyanobacterial compounds active against tropical diseases.

absolute stereochemistry. Almiramides B (**19**) and C (**20**) were reported to exhibit significant *in vitro* antileishmanial activity against *L. donovani* with IC_{50} values at 2.4 and 1.9 μM, respectively. In addition to the natural compounds, a number of semisynthetic derivatives were synthesized using solid phase peptide synthesis method and provided compound **21** (Figure 10.3) having superior *in vitro* activity with IC_{50} value at 1.6 µM when tested against *L. donovani*. The almiramides are structurally related to other marine cyanobacterial compounds, such as carmabin A, dragomabin, and the dragonamides. Inspite of their structural similarities with the almiramides, these related compounds were inactive against *L. donovani* when tested at 10 µg/mL. Antimalarial activity were instead reported for carmabin A (IC_{50} value at 4.3 µM), dragomabin (IC_{50} value at 6.0 µM), and dragonamide A (IC_{50} value at 7.7 µM) when tested against the W2 chloroquine-resistant malaria strain (McPhail *et al.*, 2007).

Recently from our laboratory, we isolated a series of aurilide-related compounds, lagunamides A (**22**) and B (**23**) (Figure 10.3), from a collection of *Lyngbya majuscula* from Pulau Hantu, Singapore (Tripathi *et al.*, 2010). The chemical structures of these new compounds were established by NMR techniques, HR-MS data, as well as Mosher's and Advanced Marfey's methods. In addition to its exquisite nanomolar cytotoxicity against P388 murine leukemia cell lines, the lagunamides A and B displayed significant antimalarial properties when tested against *Plasmodium falciparum* with IC_{50} values of 0.19 µM and 0.91 µM, respectively. Furthermore, these cyanobacterial compounds exhibited moderate anti-swarming activities when tested against *Pseudomonas aeruginosa* PA01.

Majority of the marine cyanobacterial compounds active against various tropical diseases are of the polyketide-polypeptide class. To date, only two macrolides, a malyngolide dimmer (**24**) and cyanolide A (**25**) (Figure 10.3), have been reported to have either antiprotozoal or antimolluscicidal (based on the bioassay using the snail vector *Biomphalaria glabrata*) activity. The malyngolide dimer (**24**) is a symmetric cyclodepside isolated from a Panamanian marine cyanobacterium *Lyngbya majuscula* (Gutierrez *et al.*, 2010). The structure of this dimer was established by NMR and HRESI-TOFMS data coupled with chemical degradation, chiral GC-MS analysis, and data comparison with malyngolide seco-acid. This molecule showed moderate *in vitro* antimalarial activity with IC_{50} of 19 µM when tested against the chloroquine-resistant *Plasmodium falciparum*.

Using a simple molluscicidal bioassay based on the snail, *Biomphalaria glabrata*, Gerwick and co-worker (Pereira *et al.*, 2010) isolated the glycosidic macrolide, cyanolide A (**25**) (Figure 10.3), with potent antimolluscicidal activity. *Biomphalaria glabrata* is a vector that carries the protozoa, *Schistosoma* sp., known to cause schistosomiasis. Cyanolide A, a symmetrical dimer, is possibly the first glycosidic macrolide having potent antimolluscicidal property with LC_{50} of 1.2 µM. It has been speculated that the ecological function of cyanolide A serves to deter predation by herbivorous mollusks. The biosynthesis of the aglycone portion of the monomeric portion could derive from five acetate units as well as methylation by SAM. Its total synthesis and confirmation of its absolute stereochemistry was recently reported by Kim and Hong (2010).

Conclusion

This review presented about two dozen marine cyanobacterial compounds with significant activities, including anticancer, neurotoxicity, and antiprotozoal activities, recently published in the literature. A large number of these bioactive compounds, particularly antimalarial compounds, were isolated as part of the ICBG program between US and Panama. A majority of these molecules are biosynthesized by hybrid polyketide synthase and the non-ribosomal polypeptide synthetase enzymatic systems. Together with other tailoring enzymes, this result in the formation of diverse structural types, often time with novel carbon skeletons. The reports of these recent bioactive marine cyanobacterial compounds demonstrate the prolific nature of these prokaryotes as a source of novel pharmaceuticals.

References

Adams, D.G. (2000). Cyanobacterial phylogeny and development: questions and challenges. *In* Prokaryotic Development, Ed. by Brun, Y.V. and Shimkets, L.J., Washington D.C.: ASM Press, pp. 51-81.

Araoz, R., Molgo, J., and Tandeau de Marsac, N. (2010). Neurotoxic cyanobacterial toxins. *Toxicon*, **56**: 813-828.

Broady, P.A., Garrick, R., and Anderson, G.M. (1996). Diversity, distribution and dispersal of Antarctic terrestrial algae. *Biodiversity Conservation*, **5**: 1307-1335.

Carpenter, E.J., and Foster, R.A. (2002). Marine cyanobacterial symbioses. *In* Cyanobacteria in Symbiosis, Ed. By Rai, A.N., Bergman, B., Rasmussen, U., The Netherlands: Kluwer Academic Press, pp. 11-18.

Choi, H., Pereira, A.R., Cao, Z., Shuman, C.F., Engene, N., Byrum, T., Matainaho, T., Murray, T.F., Mangoni, A., and Gerwick, W.H. (2010). The hoiamides, structurally intriguing neurotoxic lipopeptides from Papua New Giunea marine cyanobacteria. *Journal of Natural Products*, **73**: 1411-1421.

Clare, J.J., Tate, S.N., Nobbs, M., and Romanos, M.A. (2000). Voltage-gated sodium channels as therapeutic agents. *Drug Discovery Today*, **5**: 506-520.

Gerwick, W.H., Tan, L.T., and Sitachitta, N. (2001). Nitrogen-containing metabolites from marine cyanobacteria. *In:* The Alkaloids: Chemistry and Biology, Vol. 57, Ed. by Cordell, G.A., San Diego: Academic Press, pp. 75-184.

Gutierrez, M., Tidgewell, K., Capson, T.L., Engene, N., Almanza, A., Schemies, J., Jung, M., and Gerwick, W.H. (2010). Malyngolide dimer, a bioactive symmetric cyclodepside from the Panamanian marine cyanobacterium *Lyngbya majuscula*. *Journal of Natural Products*, **73**: 709-711.

Herdman, M., Janvier, M., Rippka, R., and Stanley, R.Y. (1979). Genome size of cyanobacteria. *Journal of General Microbiology*, **111**: 73-85.

Kim, H., and Hong, J. (2010). Total synthesis of cyanolide A and confirmation of its absolute configuration. *Organic Letters*, **12**: 2880-2883.

Linington, R.G., Gonzalez, J., Urena, L.-D., Romero, L.I., Ortega-Barria, E., and Gerwick, W.H. (2007). Venturamides A and B: antimalarial constituents of the Panamanian marine cyanobacterium *Oscillatoria* sp. *Journal of Natural Products*, **70**: 397-401.

Linington, R.G., Clark, B.R., Trimble, E.E., Almanza, A., Urena, L.-D., Kyle, D.E., and Gerwick, W.H. (2009). Antimalarial peptides from marine cyanobacteria: Isolation and structural elucidation of gallinamide A. *Journal of Natural Products*, **72**: 14-17.

Liu, Y., Salvador, L.A., Byeon, S., Ying, Y., Kwan, J.C., Law, B.K., Hong, J., and Luesch, H. (2010). Anti-colon cancer activity of largazole, a marine-derived tunable histone deacetylase inhibitor. *Journal of Pharmacology and Experimental Therapeutics*, In press.

Luesch, H., Yoshida, W.Y., Moore, R.E., Paul, V.J., and Corbett, T.H. (2001). Total structure determination of apratoxin A, a potent novel cytotoxin from the marine cyanobacterium *Lyngbya majuscula*. *Journal of the American Chemical Society*, **123**: 5418-5423.

Mayer, A.M., Glaser, K.B., Cuevas, C., Jacobs, R.S., Kem, W., Little, R.D., McIntosh, J.M., Newman, D.J., Potts, B.C., and Shuster, D.E. (2010). The odyssey of marine pharmaceuticals: a current perspective. *Trends in Pharmacological Sciences*, **31**: 255-265.

McPhail, K.L., Correa, J., Linington, R.G., Gonzalez, J., Ortega-Barrie, E., Capson, T.L., and Gerwick, W.H. (2007). Antimalarial linear lipopeptides from a Panamanian strain of the marine cyanobacterium *Lyngbya majuscula*. *Journal of Natural Products*, **70**: 984-988.

Pereira, A.R., Cao, Z., Murray, T.F., and Gerwick, W.H. (2009). Hoiamide A, a sodium channel activator of unusual architecture from a consortium of two Papua New Guinea cyanobacteria. *Chemistry and Biology*, **16**: 893-906.

Pereira, A.R., Cao, Z., Shuman, C.F., Engene, N., Soria-Mercado, *I.E.*, Murray, T.F.,and Gerwick, W.H. (2010). Palmyrolide A, an unusually stablilized neuroactive macrolide from Palmyra Atoll cyanobacteria. *Organic Letters*, In press.

Pereira, A.R., McCue, C.F., and Gerwick, W.H. (2010). Cyanolide A, a glycosidic macrolide with potent molluscicidal activity from the Papua New Guinea cyanobacterium *Lyngbya bouillonii*. *Journal of Natural Products*, **73**: 217-220.

Sanchez, L.M., Lopez, D., Vesely, B.A., Togna, G.D., Gerwick, W.H., Kyle, D.E., and Linington, R.G. (2010). Almiramides A-C: Discovery and development of a new class of leishmaniasis lead compounds. *Journal of Medicinal Chemistry*, **53**: 4187-4197.

Simmons, T.L., Engene, N., Urena, L.-D., Romero, L.I., Ortega-Barria, E., Gerwick, L., and Gerwick, W.H. (2008). Viridamides A and B, lipodepsipeptides with antiprotozoal activity from the marine cyanobacterium *Oscillatoria nigro-viridis*. *Journal of Natural Products*, **71**: 1544-1550.

Soria-Mercado, IE., Pereira, A.R., Cao, Z., Murray, T.F., and Gerwick, W.H. (2009). Alotamide A, a novel neuropharmacological agent from the marine cyanobacterium *Lyngbya bouillonii*. *Organic Letters*, **11**: 4704-4707.

Tan, L.T. (2007). Bioactive natural products from marine cyanobacteria for drug discovery. *Phytochemistry*, **68**: 954-979.

Tan, L.T. (2010). Filamentous tropical marine cyanobacteria: a rich source of natural products for anticancer drug discovery. *Journal of Applied Phycology*, **22**: 659-676.

Taori, K., Paul, V.J., and Luesch, H. (2008). Structure and activity of largazole, a potent antiproliferative agent from the Floridian marine cyanobacterium *Symploca* sp. *Journal of the American Chemical Society*, **130**: 1806-1807.

Teruya, T., Sasaki, H., Fukazawa, H., and Suenaga, K. (2009). Bisebromoamide, a potent cytotoxic peptide from the marine cyanobacterium *Lyngbya* sp.: isolation, stereostructure, and biological activity. *Organic Letters*, **11**: 5062-5065.

Thajuddin, N., and Subramanium, G. (2005). Cyanobacterial biodiversity and potential applications in biotechnology. *Current Science*, **89**: 47-57.

Tidgewell, K., Engene, N., Byrum, T., Media, J., Doi, T., Valeriote, F.A., and Gerwick, W.H. (2010). Evolved diversification of a modular natural product pathway: apratoxins F and G, two cytotoxic cyclic depsipeptides from a Palmyra collection of *Lyngbya bouillonii*. *ChemBioChem*, **11**: 1458-1466.

Tripathi, A., Puddick, J., Prinsep, M.R., Lee, P.P.F., and Tan, L.T. (2009). Hantupeptin A, a cytotoxic cyclic depsipeptide from a Singapore collection of *Lyngbya majuscula*. *Journal Natural Product*, **72**: 29-32.

Tripathi, A., Puddick, J., Prinsep, M.R., Rottmann, M., and Tan, L.T. (2010). Lagunamides A and B: cytotoxic and antimalarial cyclodepsipeptides from the marine cyanobacterium *Lyngbya majuscula*. *Journal of Natural Products*, In press.

Bioactive Phytochemicals: Perspectives for Modern Medicine Vol. 1 (2012) *Pages* **395–412**
Editor: **V.K. Gupta**
Published by: **DAYA PUBLISHING HOUSE, NEW DELHI**

11

Natural Bioactive Compound from Marine Plants with Anticancer Potential: A Review

S. Arif Nisha[1], R. Sakthivel[1], S. Karutha Pandian[1] and K. Pandima Devi[1*]

ABSTRACT

Cancer is a multifactorial disease, which affects people of all ages. Chemotherapy and radiation therapy remains the most widely adopted approach against a large variety of cancers. These therapeutic methods often cause negative consequences like chemotoxicity and radiation toxicity, which ultimately results in the severe damage of vital organs. Therefore identification of natural compounds with lesser side effects and with greater therapeutic potentials is crucial. In recent years, marine natural products have become a boon to the field of cancer therapy with enormous bioactive potentials. The current research in cancer therapeutics is mainly focused on developing drugs or vaccines to target key molecules for combating tumor cell growth, metastasis and proliferation. Studies on a large spectrum of marine natural products show that these marine sources can act as potent anti-inflammatory, antioxidant and anticancer agents. Moreover, a vast structural diversity of marine natural compounds has been extensively studied and it serves as lead compounds for the improvement of therapeutic potential against cancer. Additionally, semi-synthesis processes of new compounds, obtained by molecular modification of the functional groups of lead compounds, are able to generate structural analogues with greater pharmacological properties. Recent technological advances in structure elucidation, organic synthesis, and biological assay have resulted in the rapid isolation and evaluation of prospective and novel anticancer agents from marine flora. This

1 Department of Biotechnology, Alagappa University, Karaikudi – 630 003, Tamil Nadu, India.

* *Corresponding author*: E-mail: devikasi@yahoo.com

review highlights the bioactive potential of several marine natural products and their synthetic derivatives isolated from marine plants as excellent anticancer drugs.

Keywords: Cancer, Marine natural compounds, Antioxidant, Anticancer, Apoptosis, Immunomodulation.

Introduction

Ocean cover more than 70 per cent of our planet's surface and life on Earth has its origin in the sea. In certain marine ecosystems, such as coral reefs or the deep sea floor, experts estimate that the biological diversity is higher than in tropical rain forests (Haefner, 2003). This intense concentration of species coexisting in these limited extent habitats makes them highly competitive and complex. As a result of this intense competition, a high percentage of species have evolved chemical means to defend against its harmful environment. These chemical adaptations generally take the form called secondary metabolites, which includes the chemical classes like terpenoids, alkaloids, peptides, polyketides, steroids and sugars (Simmons *et al.*, 2005). During the past 20 years, thousands of novel compounds and their metabolites with diverse biological activities ranging from antiviral to anticancer have been isolated from various marine sources. Earlier reports reveal that approximately 150 compounds were found to be cytotoxic against the tumor cells (Arif *et al.*, 2004). Previous evidences suggest that around 35 compounds have known mechanisms of action for their antitumor effect, while 124 marine compounds yet to be studied for their detailed mechanism of action (Mayer and Gustafson, 2003; Haefner, 2003; Mayer and Lehmann, 2001). Compared with the study of terrestrial natural products, the study of marine natural products is still in its infancy. A 2006 report revealed that over the past few decades, during which the study of marine natural products has begun in earnest, approximately 16,000 novel marine natural products have been discovered. In 2006, it has been reported that 67 per cent of cancer chemotherapeutic agents on the market were natural products or small molecules based upon natural product leads (Donnelly, 2010).

Cancer and its Progression

Cancer is the second leading cause of death world wide, characterized by uncontrolled proliferation of cells. In the year 2007, cancer claimed the lives of around 7.6 million people in the world. There are over 100 different types of cancer, and are classified by the type of the cell that is initially affected. These cancer cells divides to form lumps or masses of tissue called tumors (except in leukemia, where the abnormal cell division occurs in the blood stream). Tumors can grow and interfere with the digestive, nervous, and circulatory systems and they can release hormones that alter body function. Tumors that stay in one spot and demonstrate limited growth are generally considered to be benign. Malignant tumors are the ones, which move throughout the body using the blood or lymphatic systems destroying the healthy tissues of other parts of the body, a process called metastasis. Several lines of evidence suggests that tumorigenesis in humans is a multistep process, which involves the genetic alterations that drives the progressive transformation of normal human cells into highly malignant derivatives (Hanahan and Weinberg, 2000). In general, tumor consists of intricate network of cell types, including endothelial cells that comprise blood vessels and the stromal pericytes that stabilize the developing tumour vasculature. Many other cell types, including stromal cells and immune cells, also surround the cancer cells and influence their development. Anticancer agents are being developed against many of these cell types. Combination therapies that target more than one cell type might be particularly effective.

In addition to transcription factors, many signalling pathways are involved in tumor cell development. In recent years, it has been demonstrated that the interaction between growth factors and its receptors plays a vital role in the initiation and progression of cancer and they have become potential target for the action of lead drug compounds. These combinations include receptor tyrosine kinases (RTKs) such as human epidermal growth factor receptors (HER and EGFR family members) and their ligands, as well as insulin-like growth factor (IGF) and IGF1R. Two of the most important pathways in tumour development involve RAS and phosphatidylinositol-3-kinase (PI3K)-mediated signalling. Many therapeutic agents have been developed to disrupt these pathways, including RAF and MEK inhibitors, which block cancer cell proliferation. PI3K inhibitors promote apoptosis in two ways. First, they lead to the nuclear translocation of the FKHR transcription factor, which activates transcription of genes that encode pro-apoptotic factors such as BIM and FAS ligand. Second, AKT signalling regulates the activity of mitochondrial proteins such as BAD, which promotes apoptosis. Hence, inhibition of key molecules in signaling pathways retards the cancer cell protein translation and thereby results in cell death.

In general, marine-derived anticancer therapeutics exhibits their activity through several mechanisms of action on a diverse range of biological targets. The common anticancer targets include signal transduction, angiogenesis, apoptosis, cell cycle, DNA synthesis, mitochondrial respiration, mitosis and multidrug efflux (Donnelly, 2010).

Seaweeds and its Antitumor Properties

Seaweeds or marine algae have provided a great biological diversity for sampling in the phase of drug discovery and development. Marine organisms in general have been an important source of compounds with potential anticancer activity. They are not only significant sources of essential proteins, vitamins, and minerals, but several species of algae also produce or contain secondary metabolites, polysaccharides, and glycoproteins with anti-tumor and immuno-stimulatory activity. Marine algae contain large amounts of characteristic bioactive molecules like polysaccharides, sterols, terpenoids and fatty acids with potential therapeutic activities (Choi *et al.*, 2009). Previously, it has been shown that oxygenated desmosterols (a kind of sterol), isolated from *Galaxaura marginata* have been shown to possess significant cytotoxic effects against several types of cancer cells (Sheu *et al.*, 1996). Palmitic acid (a most common saturated fatty acid) isolated from *Colpomenia sinuosa* have been shown to possess anti-tumor activity (Kwon and Nam, 2007).

Role of Sulfated Polysaccharides from Seaweeds in Cancer Inhibition

Polysaccharides such as alginate, fucoidan, carrageenan and agarose represents a very interesting class of macromolecules that are widespread in nature and have recently attracted more attention in the biochemical and medical areas due to their immunomodulatory and anti-cancer effects (Ooi and Liu, 2000). The seaweeds are a great source of sulfated polysaccharides with cytotoxic, antitumor, antimetastatic, antiangiogenesis and immunostimulating properties. In recent studies, several natural products, including the polysaccharides, have been investigated for their anti-tumor activities both *in vitro* and *in vivo* (Kwon and Nam, 2007). *Champia feldmannii* (Diaz-Pifferer, 1977) is a red alga from the family Lomentariaceae, found on the coast of Brazil, from which a sulfated polysaccharide (Cf-PLS) has been recently isolated. This *C. feldmannii* sulfated polysaccharide (Cf-PLS) showed inhibitory activity against Sarcoma 180 tumor growth in mice. Moreover, when the tumor-bearing animals were treated simultaneously with both the sulfated polysaccharide and the chemotherapeutic agent, 5-fluorouracil (5-FU), a significant inhibition in tumor was observed. These results pave the way to improve the current anticancer therapy through the development of combinatorial drugs with greater efficacy and less side effects (Lins *et al.*, 2008). In one way, these findings will facilitate in improving the efficacy of current anticancer therapy through the development of various combinatorial approaches. Previous evidences suggest that sulfated polysaccharides like heparin, fucoidan, Carrageenan lambda exhibits significant inhibitory activity against lung metastasis (Coombe *et al.*, 1987). Reports also show that the polysaccharide fractions from eight different seaweeds (*Laminaria angustata, Laminaria angustata* var. *longissima, Laminaria japonica* var. *ochoten, Ecklonia cava, Eisenia bicyclis, Laminaria religiosa, Undaria pinnatifida, Monostroma nitidum*) showed effective *in vivo* inhibition of the growth of tumor cells, which are implanted through sub-cutaneous injection into mice (Yamamoto *et al.*, 1986). Reports also demonstrate that Ulvans, a new source of green seaweed sulfated polysaccharide from *Ulva lactuca* showed cytotoxic and cytostatic activity against colonic cancerous epithelial cells (Kaeffer *et al.*, 1999).

Apoptosis Inducing Activity of Seaweeds Polysaccharides

Apoptosis is an energy-dependent, tightly regulated and selective physiologic process that governs the removal of supernumerary or defective cells. Apoptosis plays an important role in oncogenesis. Extrinsic and intrinsic pathways are the two different pathways through which the programmed cell death occurs (Philchenkov *et al.*, 2004). The receptor triggered or extrinsic apoptotic pathway involves the death receptors such as Fas (fibroblast associated antigen, also called Apo-1 or CD95) and tumour necrosis factor receptor (TNFR) 1; they belong to TNF-R family and contain a cytosolic death domain (DD). Ligation of death receptor causes formation of death inducing signalling complex (DISC) in which the adaptor proteins FADD and/or TRADD bind with their death domain (DD) to a DD in the cytoplasmic region of the receptors.

Activated caspase-8 then directly cleaves pro-caspase-3 or other executioner caspases, eventually leading to the apoptosis.

The intrinsic or mitochondrial pathway is activated by a variety of extra- and intracellular stresses, including oxidative stress, irradiation, and treatment with cytotoxic drugs. Unlike the death receptor dependent pathway, the mitochondria dependent pathway is mediated by Bax/Bak insertion into mitochondrial membrane, and subsequent release of Cytochrome c from the mitochondrial inter-membrane space into the cytosol. Anti-apoptotic Bcl-2 family members, such as Bcl- 2 and Bcl-XL, prevent Cytochrome c release, presumably by binding and inhibition of Bax and Bak. BH3-only proteins, such as Bid and Bim, contribute to the pro-apoptotic function of Bax or Bak by inducing homo-oligomerisation of these proteins. Cytochrome c then binds to the Apaf1 and together with ATP causes recruitment of pro-caspase-9 to the complex. The formed multi-protein complex is called apoptosome, which contains several units of Apaf1 and other above molecules. The activated caspase-9 in turn activates caspase-3 and initiates the proteolytic cascade. In addition to Cytochrome c, mitochondria release a large number of other polypeptides, including AIF, Endo G, second mitochondrial activator of caspases (Smac/DIABLO) and HtrA2/Omi from the inter-membrane space. Smac/Diablo and Omi/HtrA2 promote caspase activation through neutralizing the inhibitory effects of inhibitor of apoptosis proteins (IAPs), while AIF and endonuclease G cause DNA damage and condensation (Ghavami *et al.,* 2009).

Earlier it has been reported that the dysregulation of intrinsic apoptotic program is common in cancer cells. The resulting impaired removal of mutated cells is important for tumor progression due to one of the following reasons. (1) Increased probability of preserving and propagating the mutations and other genetic abnormalities, ultimately resulting in large scale genomic instability. (2) Abolition of cell cycle check points that result in occurrence of DNA lesions. (3) Escape of malignant tumour cells from immune effector cells. (4) Ability to acquire resistance to chemotherapeutic drugs (Philchenkov *et al.,* 2004).

Recently, it has been demonstrated that fucoidan, derived from *Fucus evanescens* and *Cladosiphon okamuranusa* (brown seaweeds) exhibited anti-proliferative effect by inducing apoptosis of cancer cells through caspase-3 and 7 activation-dependent pathway (Figure 11.1) (Aisa *et al.,* 2005, Philchenkov *et al.,* 2007; Teruya *et al.,* 2007). It has been suggested that the treatment of oversulfated fucoidan caused an excellent activation of caspase-3 and -7 in a time- and dose-dependent manner in U937 cells when compared to native fucoidan (Teruya *et al.,* 2007). Fucoidan is a sulfated polysaccharide found in the cell-wall matrix of brown algae. The major constituents of fucoidan include L-fucose and sulfate but the composition varies in small proportions of D-galactose, D-mannose, D-xylose and uronic acid with the species (Teruya *et al.,* 2007). Hyun *et al.* (2009) demonstrated the anti-tumor activity of fucoidan obtained from the brown algae *Fucus vesiculosus* using HCT-15 colon cancer cell lines. This fucoidan has been found to inhibit the proliferation of the cancer cells in a dose-dependent manner. HCT-15 colon cancer cell lines, upon treatment with fucoidan reduce the level of Bcl-2, an anti-apoptotic protein. The findings also suggest that fucoidan obtained from *F. vesiculosus* activates caspase-9 which in turn results in the

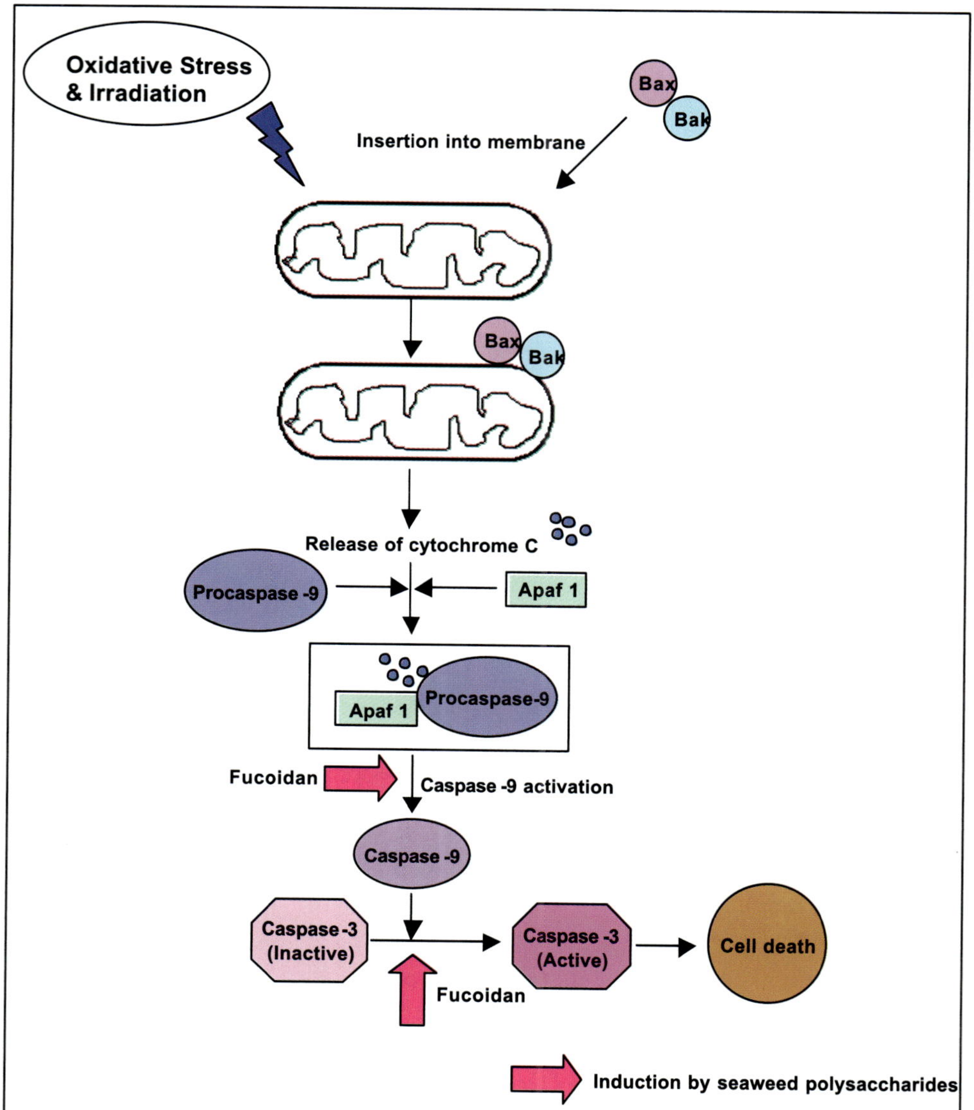

Figure 11.1: Mechanism of apoptosis induction by seaweed polysaccharides in cancer cells.

activation of caspase-3 (through the cleavage of PARP, a nuclear enzyme that is involved in DNA repair in response to various stress) finally leading to apoptosis.

Effect of Seaweed Polysaccharides on Cancer Provoking Altered Signaling Pathways

Mitogen-activated protein kinase (MAPK) pathways are evolutionarily conserved kinase modules that link extracellular signals to the machinery that controls fundamental cellular processes such as growth, proliferation, differentiation, migration and apoptosis. To date six distinct groups of MAPKs have been characterized in mammals; extracellular signal-regulated kinase ERK 1/2, ERK 3/4, ERK5, ERK7/8, Jun N-terminal kinase (JNK) 1/2/3 and the p38 isoforms α/β/γ (ERK6)/δ. The ERK pathway is the best studied of the mammalian MAPK pathways, and is deregulated in approximately, one-third of all human cancers. Active ERKs phosphorylate numerous cytoplasmic and nuclear targets, including kinases, phosphatases, transcription factors and cytoskeletal proteins. ERK signalling regulates processes such as proliferation, differentiation, survival, migration, angiogenesis and chromatin remodeling. Because of its importance in cancer the ERK pathway has been a focus for drug discovery for almost 15 years with Ras, Raf and MEK as the main targets (Dhillon *et al.*, 2007). Aisa *et al.* (2005) demonstrated that fucoidan; a sulfated polysaccharide obtained from *Fucus vesiculosus* possesses anti-cancer effect by modulating the ERK signalling pathways (Figure 11.2).

The type 1 insulin-like growth factor receptor (IGF-IR) plays an important role in both normal and abnormal growth. It is particularly important in anchorage independent growth. Impairment of its function causes apoptosis of tumor cells and inhibition of tumor growth in experimental animals. However, the IGF-IR can also induce differentiation, and eventually cell death, of certain types of cells. Its major substrates, IRS-1 and Shc, determine whether the IGF-IR will transform cells or will cause their differentiation (Baserga, 1999). In general, IGF-IR stimulates autophosphorylation of certain tyrosine residues on the receptor's β subunits. IRS-1, being a major substrate of IGF-IR serves as a docking protein for a variety of signaling molecules including p85 regulatory subunit of PI3K. Upon activation of PI3K, in turn it activates Akt (a downstream signalling molecule), which mediates diverse cellular processes like cell proliferation, survival, and apoptosis by activating downstream molecules. Recently, the IGF-I signalling pathway was examined in several types of transformed and cancerous cells. A reduction in IGF-I receptors was found to induce apoptosis in tumor cells, but not in untransformed cells, in which it only arrested growth. Moreover, a high level expression of this receptor has been observed in several cancer types, including breast, prostate, colon, and stomach cancer cells. Therefore, IGF-IR receptor signalling has become an important target for chemopreventative agents that control tumor cell proliferation. Previously, it has been demonstrated that polysaccharide (PS) of the marine alga *Capsosiphon fulvescens*, (Cf-PS) decreases the stimulatory effect of IGF-I on p85 recruitment to IGF-IR and IRS-1, leading to decreased PI3K/Akt activation (Figure 11.2). These results suggest that the inhibition of cell proliferation and induction of apoptosis by Cf-PS are mediated, in part, by its ability to inhibit IGF-IR signalling and the PI3K/Akt pathway in AGS gastric cancer cells (Kwon and Nam, 2007).

Immunomodulation and Anticancer Activity of Sulfated Polysaccharides

In the past decades great interests have been shown on the anticancer treatments based on exploiting the host's own antitumor defense mechanism (Ehrke, 2003). Recently, the therapeutic potentials of carrageenan with such an immunomodulatory effect have been studied in detail. Carrageenan is a collective term for a group of sulfated polysaccharides extracted from marine red algae. It consists of alternating 3-

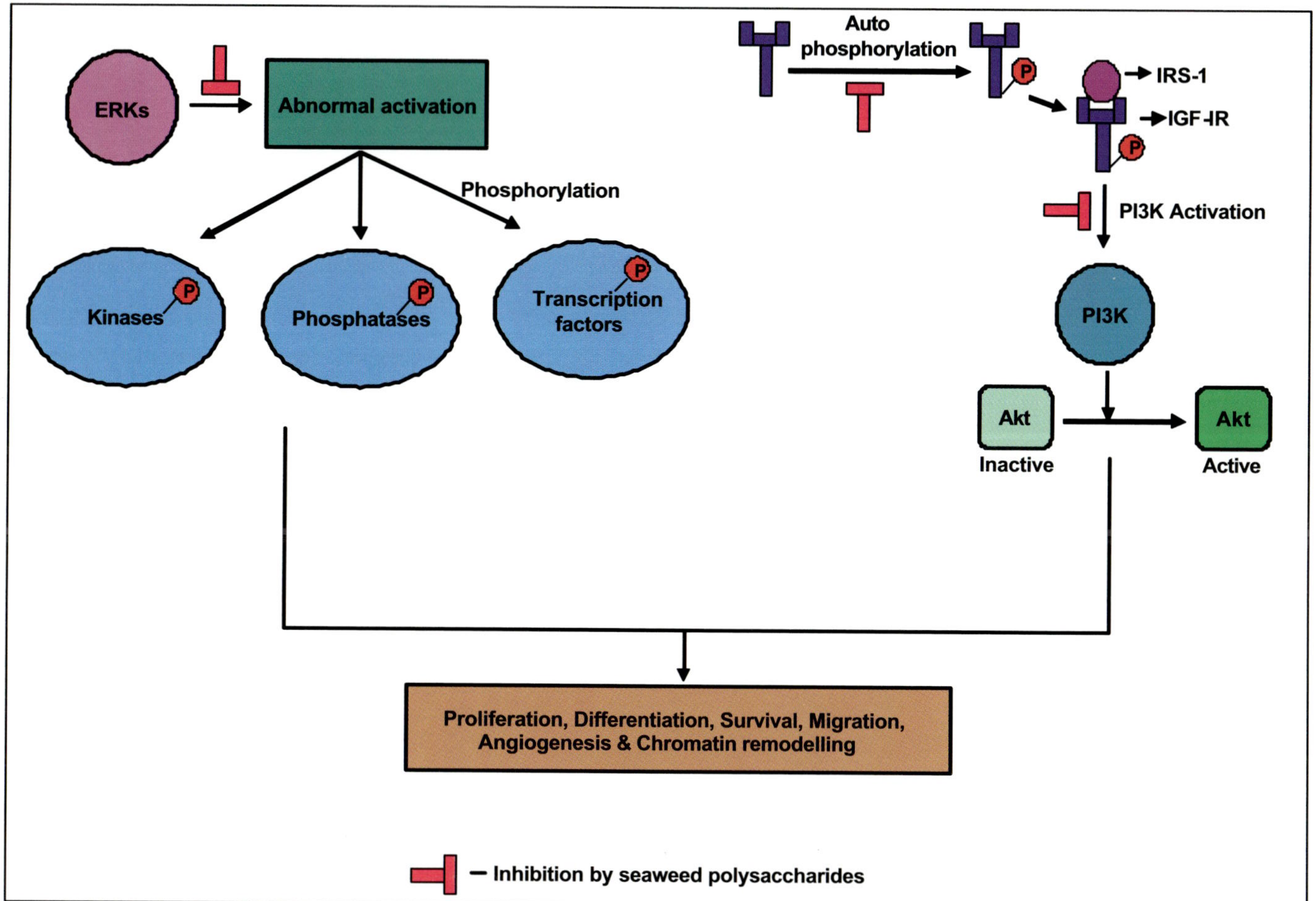

Figure 11.2: Inhibition of cancer induction by polysaccharides obtained from seaweeds (*Capsosiphon fulvescens* and *Fucus vesiculosus*).

linked β-D-galactose and 4-linked α-D-galactose or 4-linked 3, 6-anhydro-D-galactose. Yuan *et al.* (2006) demonstrated that carrageenan oligosaccharides from *Kappaphycus striatum* exhibited anticancer effect in S-180 bearing mice. In addition to that, carrageenan has shown to increase Natural Killer cells activity and also increases TNF-α production significantly (Figure 11.3), which ultimately results in the significant inhibition of the tumor growth. In general, phagocytosis is essential in host defense against microbial pathogens and in clearance of apoptotic cells (Blander and Medzhitov, 2004). Activated macrophages are considered to be one of the important components of the host defense against tumor growth and the phagocytosis plays an essential role in building and consolidating immunological defense systems of humans and animals against malignancies like cancer cell development, and numerous infectious and non-infectious factors. These oligosaccharides have shown to increase the phagocytic activity and secretion of antibodies by spleen cells, thereby activating humoral immune response. Tumor necrosis factor (TNF-α) is a cytokine, possessing antitumor and immunomodulatory properties. Once the antitumor response triggers in the body, the immunocompetent cells communicates with one another through the

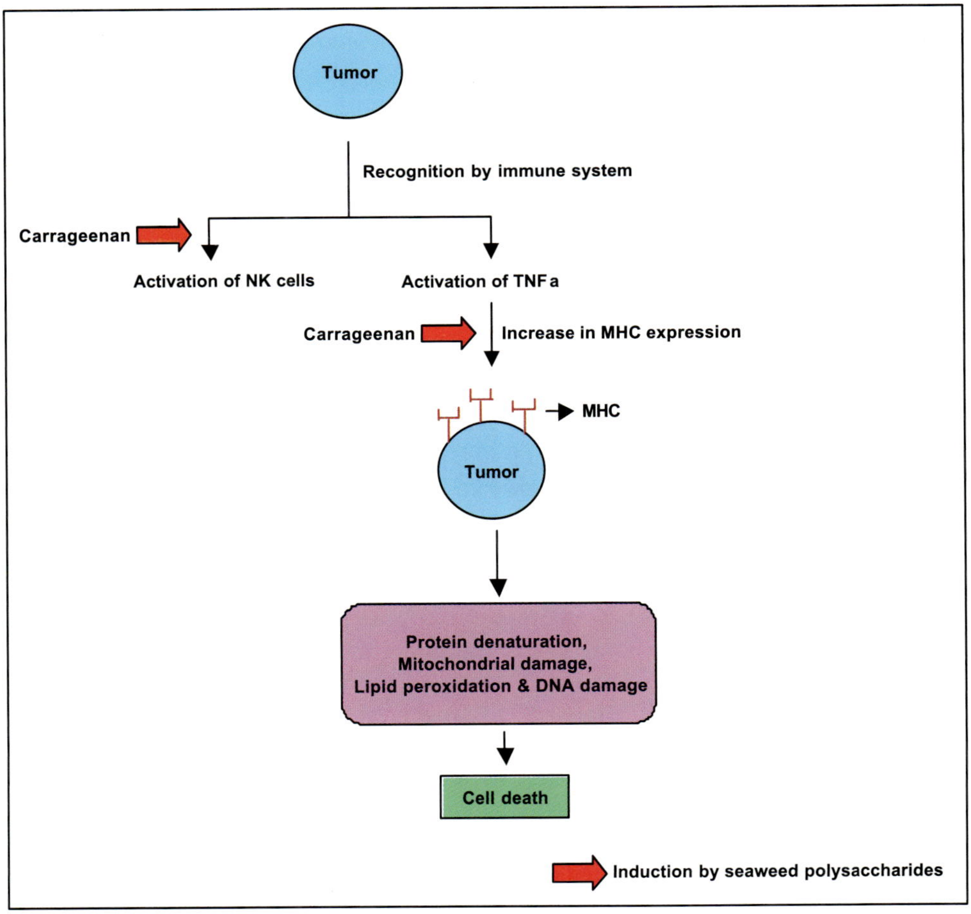

Figure 11.3: Anti-tumor immunomodulatory effect of seaweed polysaccharides.

secreted mediators called cytokines, with TNF-α, a principle component. The mechanism of antitumor action of TNF-α is complex and it includes, direct cytotoxic and cytostatic action, apoptosis induction, and indirect effect leading to the activation of immune cells as well as synthesis and release of other mediators. TNF- α also enhances the expression of MHC antigens on the tumor cells and thereby increases its immunogenicity, which ultimately results in intense antitumor immune response. Once the tumor cells were recognized by the host immune system, TNF- α stimulates the generation of active oxygen forms, which cause protein denaturation, mitochondrial damage, lipid peroxidation and DNA damage (Figure 11.3). Thus, by damaging vital structures TNF-α leads to cell death (Terlikowski, 2002). Hence, an antitumor drug that could induce the antitumor immune response will be a potential drug candidate to eliminate tumors.

Antioxidants from Marine Plants: Potential for Developing Anti-Cancer Drugs

Reactive oxygen species (ROS), which consist of free radicals such as superoxide anion ($O2^{\cdot -}$) and hydroxyl ($HO^{\cdot}$) radicals and non-free radical species such as H_2O_2 and singled oxygen ($^1O_2$), are different forms of activated oxygen (Senevirathne *et al.*, 2006). ROS are produced by all aerobic organisms and can easily react with most biological molecules including proteins, lipids, lipoproteins and DNA. ROS has both positive and negative implications towards biological systems. Generally, they are essential for biological functions. They regulate many signal transduction pathways by directly reacting with and modifying the structure of proteins, transcription factors and genes to modulate their functions. ROS are involved in signalling cell growth and differentiation, regulating the activity of enzymes (such as ribonucleotide reductase), mediating inflammation by stimulating cytokine production, and eliminating pathogens and foreign particles (Trachootham *et al.*, 2009). On the other hand, these ROS causes irreversible oxidative damage in the biomolecules, which results in a variety of pathophysiological disorders such as arthritis, diabetes, inflammation, cancer and genotoxicity (Senevirathne *et al.*, 2006). A moderate increase in ROS can promote cell proliferation and differentiation. It has also been demonstrated that an increase in ROS is associated with the disrupted redox homeostasis, which results in cancer cell growth, either due to an elevation of ROS production or to a decline of ROS-scavenging capacity, a condition known as oxidative stress (Toyokuni *et al.*, 1995). Henceforth, the ROS in cancer cells were believed to play an important part in the initiation and progression of cancer (Behrend *et al.*, 2003). In addition to this, ROS can modulate the activities and expression of many transcription factors and signalling proteins that are involved in the stress response and cell survival through multiple mechanisms (Trachootham *et al.*, 2008). As the tumor progresses, the cells generally exhibit genetic instability and shows a significant increase in ROS generation, which induces gene mutations leading to further metabolic malfunction and ROS generation (Trachootham *et al.*, 2009). Therefore, a compound that possesses antioxidant activity can inhibit mutation and cancer because they scavenge free radicals or induce antioxidant enzymes. In the past decades, it has been demonstrated that marine plants secretes large number of secondary metabolites with potential antioxidant properties. The major component of secondary metabolites is the polyphenols, with proved antioxidant properties. Hence, major research is being carried on delineating the therapeutic properties of these potential natural products.

Seaweeds

Several studies have been reported on the antioxidant potential of seaweeds. Je *et al.* (2009) demonstrated that the enzymatically hydrolyzed water-soluble extracts of *Undaria pinnatifida*, exhibited potential antioxidant activity, when checked through ESR spectroscopy. Another study shows that methanolic extracts of *Padina antillarum* (previously known as *Padina tetrastromatica*), a brown algae exhibited antioxidant property, which was verified through various *in vitro* antioxidant systems (Chew *et al.*, 2008). The antioxidant capability of *Laminaria* sp. and *Porphyra* sp. were evaluated by various groups and found that the aqueous and organic extracts obtained from them possess significant antioxidant potentials (Escrig *et al.*, 2001; Ismail and Hong, 2002). Kumar *et al.* (2008) screened the various solvent extracts of *Kappaphycus alvarezii* for *in vitro* antioxidant activity. The extracts showed excellent radical scavenging activity and reducing power potentials when verified through FRAP and DPPH radical scavenging assays. The free radical scavenging activity of DMSO and methanolic extracts was evaluated through various radical scavenging assays and found that both the extracts showed significant antioxidant potential (Lekameera *et al.*, 2008). Antioxidant activity of crude extract and ethyl acetate soluble fractions of the red alga, *Polysiphonia urceolata*, were evaluated by Duan *et al.* (2006). The ethyl acetate soluble fractions were found to possess the highest antioxidant activity, when checked through various antioxidant systems like β-carotene–linoleate assay system and DPPH radical assays. In India, Chandini *et al.* (2008) assessed the antioxidant properties of various solvent extracts of brown seaweeds (*Sargassum marginatum*, *Padina tetrastomatica* and *Turbinaria conoides*). All the three seaweeds exhibited reducing power activity in a dose dependent manner and the Ethyl Acetate fraction of *S. marginatum* exhibited higher total antioxidant activity. Research from our group have also demonstrated the antioxidant activities of methanolic extracts of ten seaweeds, which includes *Gelidiella acerosa* (Rhodophyta), *Gracilaria edulis* (Rhodophyta), *Turbinaria conoides* (Phaeophyta), *Padina gymnospora* (Phaeophyta), *Chondrococcus hornemanni* (Rhodophyta), *Hypnea pannosa* (Rhodophyta), *Dictyota dichotoma* (Phaeophyta), *Jania rubens* (Rhodophyta), *Sargassum wightii* (Phaeophyta) and *Haligra* sp. The results suggest that among all the seaweeds evaluated *G. acerosa* found to possess highest antioxidant activity (Devi *et al.*, 2008). In addition to that the antioxidant potential of various solvent extracts of *G. acerosa* were evaluated and found that benzene and dichloromethane extract showed excellent antioxidant activity, when verified in various *in vitro* antioxidant systems (Suganthy *et al.*, 2010).

Mangroves

Mangrove forest is considered to be one of the highly endangered ecosystems and uninterrupted man-made disturbances ranging from deforestation to pollution threatens their survival throughout the world. Mangrove plants require specific conditions to grow, thus restricting their geographic range. Plants that live in mangrove ecosystem are adopted to encounter high salinity, tidal extremes and heavy winds. Mangroves occur in 121 countries covering 15 million ha worldwide. Asia harbors the largest mangroves in the world and India alone contributes for 3 per cent of the global mangrove habitat. Mangrove plants are great resource for tannin and the timbers, which are of great value. They are highly rich in polyphenols like tannins, which has been reported to hold various therapeutic applications for a wide range of disorders. Mangrove plants like *Bruguiera cylindrica, Rhizophora apiculata, Rhizophora lamarkii* and *Rhizophora mucronata* have been reported as rich sources of polyphenols (Agoramoorthy, 2008).

Previous findings suggest that pyroligneous acid from *Rhizophora apiculata*, a dark liquid produced through the natural act of carbonization possess potential antioxidant activity, when checked in various oxidative systems. Syringol, catechol and 3-methoxycatechol have been isolated from the mangrove and they have been checked for their antioxidant activity through DPPH radical scavenging activity, ABTS radical cation scavenging activity, phosphomolybdenum and ferric reducing antioxidant power (FRAP) assays. All the three compounds have been found to exhibit excellent antioxidant properties (Loo *et al.*, 2008). Berenguer *et al.* (2006) demonstrated that *Rhizophora mangle*, a red mangrove increases the activity of the antioxidant enzymes like glutathione peroxidase (GSH-Px) and superoxide dismutase (SOD) and decreases the lipid peroxidation. Previous findings suggest that tannins exhibit potential antioxidant and radical scavenging activities, and these red mangroves possess polymeric tannins (80 per cent) and hydrolysable tannins (20 per cent), which could be the possible reason for the antioxidant property of *Rhizophora mangle*. Earlier, the antioxidant capability of *Rhizophora stylosa* has been evaluated by Takara *et al.* (2008) through DPPH radical scavenging assay. The results show that the compounds isolated from this mangrove have shown significant antioxidant activity since the activity was more than the standard antioxidant L-ascorbic acid. Ellagic acid, a precursor form of ellagitannins obtained from *Excoecaria agallocha* and *Terminalia catappa* have been found to exhibit potential antioxidant activity, which was verified through various antioxidant assays like DPPH radical scavenging assay, linoleic acid oxidation assay, and oxidative cell death assay (Masuda *et al.*, 1999). Another report suggests that methanolic extracts of *Acanthus ilicifolius*, a mangrove found in western coastal area, has profound antitumor activity against DLA (Dalton's Lymphoma Ascites tumor cells). The extract also found to reduce the solid tumors induced in the mouse models (Babu *et al.*, 2002). The free radical scavenging activity of *B. cylindrica*, *C. decandra*, *R. apiculata*, *A. corniculatum*, *R. mucronata* were evaluated through DPPH assay and their IC_{50} values were found to be 42.9 µg/mL, 51.9 µg/mL, 64.9 µg/mL, 74.3 µg/mL and 79.7 µg/mL respectively (Agoramoorthy, 2008). Banerjee *et al.* (2008) demonstrated that mangroves like *Avicennia alba, Aegiceras corniculatum, Bruguiera gymnorrhiza, Ceriops decandra, Rhizophora mucronata, Sonneratia apetala* from Sundarbans were found to possess excellent antioxidant activity when checked through various *in vitro* antioxidant systems. Since the active extracts were rich in polyphenolic content and that could be the possible reason for its antioxidant potentials. Our group has also revealed the antioxidant potential of the methanolic leaf extracts of various mangrove plants, which includes *Avicennia marina, R. mucronata,*

R. apiculata, R. annamalayana, Ceriops decandra, Suaeda monica, Pruscaria celligrica, Lumnitzera racemosa. Among all the mangrove plants*R. mucronata* showed significant antioxidant activity in all the antioxidant assays employed. In addition to that a strong correlation was observed between the amount of polyphenolic content and antioxidant activity (Suganthy *et al.*, 2009).

Xylocarpus granatum Koenig, a marine mangrove plant mainly distributed along the shore of the Indian Ocean and sea shores of Southeast Asia, was one of the three species in the genus*Xylocarpus* (Meliaceae). *Xylocarpus granatum* was found to be rich in limonoids, which was a highly oxygenated nortriterpenoids with their structural features either containing or being derived from a precursor with a furanylsteroid skeleton. From 80's of 20th century, limonoids were recognized as natural compounds, which had potential biological activities. Animal experiments indicated that limonoids could inhibit the liver cancer, bowel cancer, mouth cancer and skin cancer, which were induced by chemical materials, and nontoxic to animal model. Recently, it has been verified that Gedunin, a Limonoid from *Xylocarpus granatum*, inhibits the growth of CaCo-2 Colon Cancer Cell line *in vitro* (Uddin *et al.*, 2007).

Seagrasses

Seagrasses are a group of about 60 species of marine flowering plants, belongs to the families, Hydrocharitaceae and Potamogetonaceae and they are not related to the terrestrial grasses of Poaceae (Kannan *et al.*, 2010). Seagrasses are conspicuous and wide spread in the shallow marine environment throughout the world, producing a greater amount of organic matter and serves as a good substratum for a variety of epiphytic algae including diatoms and sessile fauna. Seagrasses are rich in organic matter and nutrients, as mangrove and coral reef ecosystems are closely associated with them. Seagrass meadows are highly productive and dynamic ecosystems, which rank among the most productive ecosystems of the oceans. The true importance of seagrass meadows to the coastal marine ecosystem is not fully understood and generally under-estimated. The rapidly expanding scientific knowledge on seagrasses has led to a growing awareness that seagrasses are valuable coastal resources. Seagrasses also acts as sediment stabilizers, provide a suitable substratum for epiphytes and a good source of food for marine herbivores, as well as fodder and manure (Umamaheswari *et al.*, 2009).

In the past, seagrasses have been used for treating a variety of diseases and disorders including fever, skin diseases, muscle pains, wounds and stomach problems. Earlier reports show that seagrasses also possess antibacterial, antialgal, antifungal, antiviral, antiprotozoal, anti-inflammatory and antidiabetic activities. The phenolic compounds present in the seagrasses were found to exhibit potential free radical scavenging activity. Kannan*et al.* (2010) evaluated the antioxidant activity of the seagrasses like (*Enhalus acoroides* (L.f.) Royle, *Thalassia hemprichii* (Ehrenb.) Asch., *Syringodium isoetifolium* (Asch.) Dandy and *Halodule pinifolia* (Miki) Hartog and found to possess excellent antioxidant activites. It has also been showed that all the seagrasses used for screening were rich in polyphenols. The antioxidant potential of the seagrasses like *Cymodocea serrulata, Syringodium isoetifolium, Halophila ovalis, Halodule pinifolia, Thalassia hemprichii* was evaluated and all of them were found to possess a strong antioxidant potential. Since these seagrasses possess rich source of Vitamin A and E, that could be the possible reason for its potential antioxidant activity (Athiperumalsami *et al.*,2010). Gokcea and Haznedaroglu (2008) demonstrated the free radical scavenging activity of the extract of *Posidonia oceanica*. Since the pharmacological studies on seagrasses were very limited, further research will provide a better opportunity to explore the hidden therapeutic potentials.

Conclusions

The marine environment is an exceptional reservoir of the marine natural products, many of which exhibit structural features not found in terrestrial natural products. Every year, an increasing number of novel marine metabolites are reported in the literature indicating that the marine environment is likely to continue to be a prolific source of new natural products in years to come (Carte, 1996). Although, new biologically active compounds are being isolated from marine organisms, the potential for anyone of these metabolites to reach the clinical trials is very much dependent on the aggressiveness with which they are tested in diverse disease areas. Since the use of chemotherapeutic drugs in cancer therapy involves the risk of life threatening host toxicity, the search for the identification and development of drugs from natural products continues, which selectively act on tumour cells. The identification of medically useful compounds produced by marine organisms has led not only to vitally important drug-development opportunities but also to increased interest in preserving ocean habitats for research.

Acknowledgements

KPD wishes to thank UGC, India for the research grant. SAN wishes to thank UGC-MANF for the Junior Research Fellowship provided. The authors gratefully acknowledge the computational and bioinformatics facility provided by the Alagappa University Bioinformatics Infrastructure Facility (funded by Department of Biotechnology, Government of India vide Grant No. BT/BI/25/001/2006).

References

Agoramoorthy, G., Chen, A.N., Venkatesalu, V., Kuo, D.H., and Shea, P.C. (2008). Evaluation of antioxidant polyphenols from selected mangrove plants of India. *Asian Journal of Chemistry*, **20**: 1311-1322.

Aisa, Y., Miyakawa, Y., Nakazato, T., Shibata, H., Saito, K., Ikeda, Y., and Kizaki, M. (2005). Fucoidan induces apoptosis of human HS-Sultan cells accompanied by activation of Caspase-3 and down-regulation of ERK pathways. *American Journal of Hematology*, **78**: 7–14.

Arif, M.J., Amal, A., Al-Hazzani., Kunhi, M., and Al-Khodairy, F. (2004). Novel marine compounds: Anticancer or genotoxic? *Journal of Biomedicine and Biotechnology*, **2**: 93-98.

Athiperumalsami, T., Rajeswari, V. D., Poorna, S. H., Kumar, V., and Jesudass, L. L. (2010). Antioxidant activity of seagrasses and seaweeds. *Botanica Marina*, **53**: 251–257

Babu, B.H., Shylesh, B.S., and Padikkala, J. (2002). Tumor reducing and anti-carcinogenic activity of *Acanthus ilicifolius* in mice. *Journal of Ethnopharmacology*, **79**: 27–33.

Banerjee, D., Chakrabarti, S., Hazra, A.K., Banerjee, S., Ray, J., and Mukherjee, B. (2008). Antioxidant activity and total phenolics of some mangroves in Sundarbans. *African Journal of Biotechnology*, **7**: 805-810.

Baserga, R. (1999). The IGF-I receptor in cancer research. *Experimental Cell Research*, **253**: 1–6.

Behrend, L., Henderson, G., and Zwacka, R. M. (2003). Reactive oxygen species in oncogenic transformation. *Biochemistry Society Transactions*, **31**: 1441–1444.

Berenguer, B., S×anchez, L.M., Qu×ýlez, A., L×opez-Barreiro, M., Haro, O., G×alvez, J., and Mart×ýn M.J. (2006). Protective and antioxidant effects of *Rhizophora mangle* L. against NSAID-induced gastric ulcers. *Journal of Ethnopharmacology*, **103**: 194–200.

Blander, J.M. and Medzhitov, R. (2004). Regulation of phagosome maturation by signals from Toll-Like Receptors. *Science*, **304**: 1014-1018.

Carte, B.K. (1996). Biomedical potential of marine products. *Bioscience*, **46**: 271-286.

Chandini, S.K., Ganesan, P., Bhaskar, N. (2008). *In vitro* antioxidant activities of three selected brown seaweeds of India. *Food Chemistry*, **107**: 707–713.

Chew, Y.L., Lim, Y.Y., Omara, M., Khoo, K.S. (2008). Antioxidant activity of three edible seaweeds from two areas in South East Asia. *LWT*, **41**: 1067–1072.

Choi, E.Y., Hwang, H.J., Kim, I.H., and Nam, T.J. (2009). Protective effects of a polysaccharide from *Hizikia fusiformis* against ethanol toxicity in rats. *Food and Chemical Toxicology*, **47**: 134–139.

Coombe, D.R., Parish, C.R., Ramshaw, *I.E.*, and Snowden, J.M. (1987). Analysis of the inhibition of tumour metastasis by sulfated polysaccharides. *International Journal of Cancer*, **39**: 82–88.

Devi, K.P., Suganthy, N., Kesika, P., and Pandian, S.K. (2008). Bioprotective properties of seaweeds: *In vitro* evaluation of antioxidant activity and antimicrobial activity against food borne bacteria in relation to polyphenolic content. *BMC Complementary and Alternative Medicine*, **8**: 38-49.

Dhillon, A.S., Hagan, S., Rath, O., and Kolch, W. (2007). MAP kinase signalling pathways in cancer. *Oncogene*, **26**: 3279–3290.

Duan, X.J., Zhang, W. W., Li, X. M., and Wang, B. G. (2006). Evaluation of antioxidant property of extract and fractions obtained from a red alga, *Polysiphonia urceolata*. *Food Chemistry*, **95**: 37–43.

Ehrke, M.J. (2003). Immunomodulation in cancer therapeutics. *International Immunopharmacology*, **3**: 1105–1119.

Escrig A. J., Jime´nez I. J., Pulido, R and Calixto, F.S. (2001). Antioxidant activity of fresh and processed edible seaweeds. *Journal of the science of food and agriculture*, **81**: 530-534.

Gokce, G., and Haznedaroglu, M. Z. (2008). Evaluation of antidiabetic, antioxidant and vasoprotective effects of *Posidonia oceanica* extract. *J Ethnopharmacol.,* **115**: 122-130.

Ghavami, S., Hashemi, M., Ande, S.R., Yeganeh, B., Xiao, W., Eshraghi, M., Bus, C.J, Kadkhoda, K., Wiechec, E., Halayko, A.J., and Los, M. (2009). Apoptosis and cancer: mutations within caspase genes. *Journal of Medical Genetics,* **46**: 497–510.

Haefner, B. (2003). Drugs from the deep: marine natural products as drug candidates. *Drug Discovery Today,* **8**: 536-544.

Hanahan, D and Weinberg, R.A. (2000). The hallmarks of cancer. *Cell,* **100**: 57–70.

Ismail, A. and Hong, T. S. (2002). Antioxidant activity of selected commercial seaweeds. *Malaysian Journal of Nutrition,* **8**: 167-177.

Je, J. Y., Park, P. J., Kim, E. K., Park, J. S., Yoon H. D., Kim, K.R.,and Ahn, C.B. (2009). Antioxidant activity of enzymatic extracts from the brown seaweed *Undaria pinnatifida* by electron spin resonance spectroscopy. *LWT - Food Science and Technology,* **42**: 874–878.

Kaeffer, B., Bernard, C., Lahaye, M., Blottiere, H.M., and Cherbut, C. (1999). Biological properties of ulvan, a new source of green seaweed sulfated polisaccharides, on cultured normal and cancerous colonic epithelial cells. *Planta Medica,* **65**: 527–531.

Kannan, R. R. R., Arumugam, R., Meenakshi, S., and Anantharaman, P. (2010). Thin layer chromatography analysis of antioxidant constituents from seagrasses of Gulf of Mannar Biosphere Reserve, South India. *International Journal of ChemTech Research,* **2(3)**: 1526-1530,

Kwon, M.J. and Nam, T.J. (2007). A polysaccharide of the marine alga *Capsosiphon fulvescens* induces apoptosis in AGS gastric cancer cells via an IGF-IR-mediated PI3K/Akt pathway. *Cell Biology International,* **31**: 768-775.

Lekameera, R., Vijayabaskar, P. and Somasundaram, S. T. (2008). Evaluating antioxidant property of brown alga*Colpomenia sinuosa* (DERB. ET SOL).*African Journal of Food Science,* **2**: 126-130.

Lins, K.O.A.L., Bezerra, D.P., Alves, A.P.N.N., Alencar, N.M.N., Lima, M.W., Torres, V.M., Farias, W.R.L., Pessoa, C., Moraesa, M.O., and Costa-Lotufoa, L.V (2009). Antitumor properties of a sulfated polysaccharide from the red seaweed *Champia feldmannii* (Diaz-Pifferer). *Journal of Applied Toxicology,* **29**: 20–26.

Loo, A.Y., Jain, K., and Darah, I. (2008). Antioxidant activity of compounds isolated from the pyroligneous acid, *Rhizophora apiculata*. *Food Chemistry,* **107**: 1151–1160.

Masuda, T., Yonemori, S., Oyama, Y., Takeda, Y., Tanaka, T., Andoh, T., Shinohara, A., and Nakata, M. (1999). Evaluation of the antioxidant activity of environmental plants: Activity of the leaf extracts from seashore plants. *Journal of Agricultural and Food Chemistry,* **47**: 1749–1754.

Mayer, A.M., and Lehmann, V.K. (2001). Marine pharmacology in 1999: antitumor and cytotoxic compounds. *Anticancer Research*, **21**: 2489–2500.

Mayer A.M and Gustafson K.R. (2003). Marine pharmacology in 2000: antitumor and cytotoxic compounds. *International Journal of Cancer*, **105**: 291–299.

Ooi, C.V. and Liu, F. (2000). Immunomodulation and anti-cancer activity of polysaccharide–protein complexes. *Current Medicinal Chemistry*, **7**: 715–729.

Philchenkov, A., Zavelevich, M., Kroczak, T.J., Los, M. (2004). Caspases and cancer: Mechanisms of inactivation and new treatment modalities. *Experimental oncology*, **26**: 82-97.

Senevirathne, M., Kim, S.H., Siriwardhana, N., Ha, J.H., Lee, K.W., and Jeon, Y.J. (2006). Antioxidant potential of *Ecklonia cava* on reactive oxygen species scavenging, metal chelating, reducing power and lipid peroxidation inhibition. *Food Science and Technology International*, **12**: 27–38.

Sheu, J.H., Huang, S.Y., and Duh, C.Y. (1996). Cytotoxic oxygenated desmosterols of the red alga *Galaxaura marginata*. *Journal of Natural Products*, **59**: 23–26.

Simmons, T.L., Andrianasolo, E., McPhail, K., Flatt, P., and Gerwick, W.H. (2005). Marine natural products as anticancer drugs. *Molecular Cancer Therapeutics*, **4**: 333-342.

Suganthy, N., Kesika, P., Pandian, S. K., and Devi, K. P. (2009). Mangrove plant extracts: Radical scavenging activity and the battle against food-borne pathogens. *Forsch Komplementmed*, **16**: 41-48.

Suganthy, N., Nisha, S. A., Pandian, S. K., and Devi, K. P. (2010). Antioxidant and metal chelating potential of the solvent fractions of *Gelidiella acerosa* the red algae inhabiting South Indian coastal area. *Biomedicine and Pharmacotherapy*, (In press).

Takara, K., Kuniyoshi, A., Wada, K., Kinjyo, K., and Iwasaki, H. (2008). Antioxidative flavaon-3-ol glycosides from stems of *Rhizophora stylosa*. *Bioscience, Biotechnology, and Biochemistry*, **72**: 1-4.

Terlikowski, S.J. (2002). Local immunotherapy with rhTNF-α mutein induces strong antitumor activity without overt toxicity–a review. *Toxicology*, **174**: 143–152.

Toyokuni, S., Okamoto, K., Yodoi, J., and Hiai, H. (1995). Persistent oxidative stress in cancer. *FEBS Letters*, **358**: 1–3.

Trachootham, D., Alexandre, J., and Huang, P. (2009). Targeting cancer cells by ROS-mediated mechanisms: a radical therapeutic approach? *Nature reviews - Drug discovery*, **8**: 579-591.

Trachootham, D., Lu, W., Ogasawara, M. A., Nilsa, R. D., and Huang, P. (2008). Redox regulation of cell survival. *Antioxidants and Redox Signaling*, **10**: 1343–1374.

Uddin, S.J., Nahar, L., Shilpi, J.A., Shoeb, M., Borkowski, T., Gibbons, S., Middleton, M., Byres, M., and Sarker, S.D. (2007). Gedunin, a limonoid from *Xylocarpus granatum*, inhibits the growth of CaCo-2 colon cancer cell line *In Vitro*. *Phytotherapy Research*, **21**: 757–761.

Umamaheswari, R., Ramachandran, S., and Nobi, E. P. (2009). Mapping the extend of seagrass meadows of Gulf of Mannar Biosphere Reserve, India using IRS ID satellite imagery. *International Journal of Biodiversity and Conservation*, **1(5)**: 187-193

Yamamoto, I., Maruyama, H., Takahashi, M., and Komiyama K. (1986). The effect of dietary or intraperitoneally injected seaweed preparations on the growth of sarcoma-180 cells subcutaneously implanted in to mice. *Cancer Letters*, **30**: 125-131.

Yuan, H., Song, J., Li, X., Li, N., and Dai, J. (2006). Immunomodulation and antitumor activity of k-carrageenan oligosaccharides. *Cancer Letters*, **243**: 228–234.

http: //www.organicdivision.org/ama/orig/Fellowship/2009_2010_Awardees/Essays/Donnelly.pdf

Kannan L and Thangaradjou T - http: //ocw.unu.edu/international-network-on-water-environment-and-health/unu-inweh-course-1 mangroves/Seagrasses.pdf.

Bioactive Phytochemicals: Perspectives for Modern Medicine Vol. 1 (2012) *Pages* **413–436**
Editor: **V.K. Gupta**
Published by: **DAYA PUBLISHING HOUSE, NEW DELHI**

12

The Lauraceae Alkaloids

Dayana L. Custódio[1], Diego C. Squinello[1] and Valdir F. Veiga Junior[1]*

ABSTRACT

Lauraceae is among one of the botanical families of greatest economic importance, being widely used in the food and wood industries. The family presents a pantropical distribution with approximately 50 genus and 2,500 species. Among the genus that presents high quality wood are Ocotea, Nectandra and Aniba, which are commonly known as cinnamon, laurels or imbuia, and rosewood, respectively. Aniba also produces essential oils widely used in perfumes, such as A. rosaeodora and A. canelilla. Some Lauraceae species are also used as condiments, as Laurus nobilis (laurel), Dicypellium caryophyllaceum (false cinnamon) and Cinnamomum verum (cinnamon). There are several chemical studies concerning species of this family showing the presence of various neolignans and alkaloids. Most of these alkaloids are isoquinoline, but indole and pyridine alkaloids are also present. Among the isoquinoline alkaloids, several aporphine, benzylisoquinoline and pavine skeletons are observed. These alkaloids have several qualities already noted, such as antimicrobial, trypanossomicide, antiviral, antioxidant, antinociceptive, analeptic, depressant action on central nervous system, and others. This chapter will focus on the alkaloids present in this family and their various activities, due to it being a very important class of substance among all natural products.

Keywords: Alkaloids, Indole, Isoquinoline, Lauraceae, Pyridine, Pavine.

Introduction

Lauraceae has a tropical and subtropical distribution concentrated in Asian and American rain forests. The family includes about 50 genus and 2.500 species. In

1 Chemistry Department – Amazonas Federal University, Av. Gal. Rodrigo Octávio, 3.000, ICE, Japiim, 69077-000, Manaus – AM, Brazil.

* *Corresponding author*: E-mail: valdirveiga@ufam.edu.br

Brazil approximately 25 genus and 400 species have been observed. Lauraceae is among one of the most important families of the floristic composition in some of Brazil's forest ecosystems, being observed in Atlantic and Southern region forests and in the Amazon rainforest (Souza and Lorenzi, 2005).

Several species have been used by industry in the manufacturing of various products. However, some species have their use restricted to the traditional communities, who have empirical knowledge about the use of these plants (Marques, 2001).

The Lauraceae family has great economic value among the botanical families, as it is used in several areas, such as the food and wood industries. These include *Ocotea porosa*, the popular Imbuia, and *Ocotea odorifera*, known as Sassafras. Also, natural products observed in species, such as *Aniba rosaeodora*, achieve a high economic value in international markets. Their essential oils are composed mainly of linalool, an excellent perfume fixative (Zanin and Lordello, 2007). Many neolignans are described in this family, and these substances have been used as lead compounds for new drug development (Apers *et al.*, 2003). Besides the neolignans and essential oils, this family presents several alkaloids. Among the main alkaloid classes observed are the pyridine, indole, and isoquinoline. The aporphine and the benzyltetrahydroisoquinoline are the main skeletons (Gottlieb, 1972; Henriques *et al.*, 1999).

Isoquinoline Alkaloids

The isoquinoline alkaloids are produced by the reaction between phenylethylamines derived from tyrosine. This reaction is followed by cyclization, forming the tetrahydroisoquinoline core (1). The isoquinoline alkaloids have a great importance and several pharmacological activities have already been described. The more common skeletons are benziltetrahydroisoquinolines (2) and aporphines (3), but pavine alkaloids are also observed. They are present in various Lauraceae genus, from the widely studied *Cryptocarya* to the lesser studied *Dehaasia*. Some of them are very common and observed in species of different genus. Among these are the actinodaphnine and the laurolitsine, as well as others which will be presented in this chapter. The basic isoquinoline skeletons are pictured in Figure 12.1.

Some Lauraceae isoquinoline alkaloids stand out as they have been detected in several species. These structures are present in various plants species, such as isoboldine, laurolitsine, actinodaphnine, dicentrine, liriodenine, laurotetanine, N-methyllaurotetanine, reticuline, palidine and isocorydine (Table 12.1).

The aporphine alkaloids actinodaphnine (4), dicentrine (5), liriodenine (6), isoboldine (7), laurolitsine (8), boldine (9), laurotetanine (10), N-methyllaurotetanine (11), and reticuline (12) present differences between the substituent groups. The actinodaphnine (4), dicentrine (5) and liriodenine (6) exhibit a dioxymethylene in C-1 and C-2. The laurotetanine (10) is an oxoaporphine due to the carbonilic carbon in position 7 of the structure. The reticuline is a benzyltetrahydroisoquinoline alkaloid with two hydroxyls in C-7 and C-11, two methoxyls in C-6 and C-10, and a methyl in the nitrogen atom. The palidine (13) is a morphinone type alkaloid with one hydroxyl in C-1, two methoxyl in C-2 and C-6 and one methyl in the nitrogen atom. Among the aparphine structures, actinodaphnine (4), laurolitsine (8), boldine (9), laurotetanine

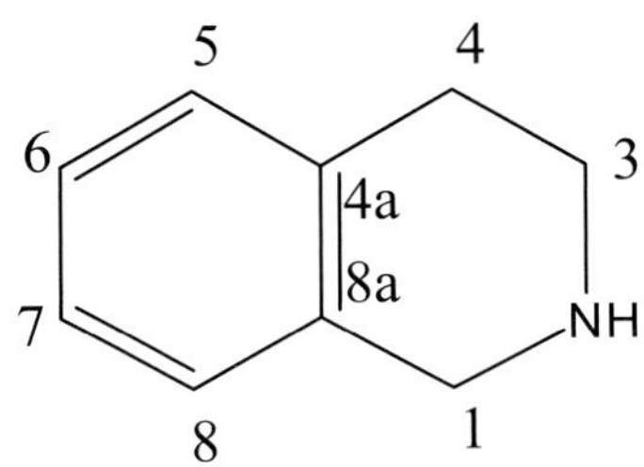

1

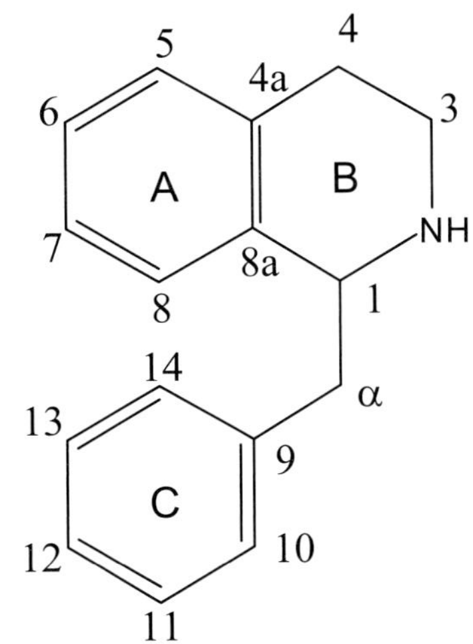

2

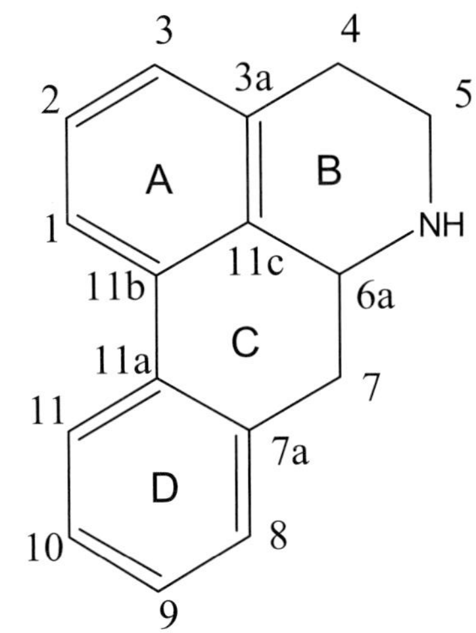

3

Figure 12.1 : Basic isoquinoline skeletons.

(10) and N-methyllaurotetanine (11) have one hydroxyl in C-9. The actinodaphnine (4), dicentrine (5), isoboldine (7), boldine (9), laurotetanine (10), N-methyllaurotetanine (11), and isocorydine (14) have a methoxyl in C-10. The laurolitsine has a methyl in the C-10, the laurolitsine (8), boldine (9), laurotetanine (7), N-methyllaurotetanine (8). Isocorydine (11) has a methoxyl in C-1 and the laurolitsine (8) and boldine (9) have a hydroxyl in C-2. Laurotetanine (7), N-methyllaurotetanine (11) and isocorydine (14) have a methoxyl in C-2. The Figure 12.2 shows these structures.

Table 12.1: Distribution of the most common isoquinoline alkaloids from Lauraceae.

Alkaloid	*Genus*	*Species*	*Part of the Plant*	*Reference*
Actinodaphnine	*Actinodaphne*	*obovata*	Leaves and branches	Uprety *et al.*, 1972
	Cassytha	*filiformis*	Aerial part	Cava and Rao, 1968; Wu *et al.*, 1997; Stévigny *et al.*, 2002; Tsu *et al.*, 2008
	Litsea	*sebifera*	Leaves and branches	Uprety *et al.*, 1972
		laurifolia	Leaves	Leboeuf *et al.*, 1979
	Neolitsea	*sericea*	Leaves	Lee *et al.*, 2007, Nakasato and Asada, 1966
		acuminatissima	Stem bark	Chang *et al.*, 2002
Dicentrine	*Actinodaphne*	*sesquipedalis*	Stem bark	Din *et al.*, 1994
	Cassytha	*filiformis*	Aerial part	Cava and Rao, 1968; Stévigny *et al.*, 2002; Tsu *et al.*, 2008
	Ocotea	*brachybotra*	Leaves	Vecchietti *et al.*, 1977
		macrophylla	Leaves	Barrera and Suárez, 2009
		vellosiana	Stem, leaves and fruits	Garcez *et al.*, 1995
Liriodenine	*Cassytha*	*filiformis*	Aerial part	Cava and Rao, 1968
	Neolitsea	*acuminatissima*	Stem bark	Chang *et al.*, 2002
	Phoebe	*chinensis*	Stem bark	Nguyen and Nguyen, 2004
		formosana	Stem bark	Lu and Su, 1973
Isoboldine	*Aniba*	*muca*	Stem bark	Bravo *et al.*, 1996
	Cassytha	*filiformis*	Aerial part	Wu *et al.*, 1997
		pubescens		Johns *et al.*, 1966
	Cryptocarya	*chinensis*	Leaves	Lin *et al.*, 2001
	Lindera	*angustifolia*	Root	Zhao *et al.*, 2005
	Neolitsea	*acuminatissima*	Stem bark	Chang *et al.*, 2002
	Sassafras	*albidum*	Root bark	Chowdhury *et al.*, 1976

Contd...

Table 12.1–*Contd...*

Alkaloid	*Genus*	*Species*	*Part of the Plant*	*Reference*
Laurolitsine (norboldine)	*Actinodaphne*	*nitida*	Stem bark	Johns *et al.*, 1969
		pruinosa	Stem bark	Rachmatiah *et al.*, 2009
	Lindera	*aggregata*	Root	Chou *et al.*, 2005
		angustifolia	Root	Zhao *et al.*, 2005
		chunii	Root	Zhang *et al.*, 2002
	Litsea	*laurifolia*	Stem bark	Leboeuf *et al.*, 1979
		wightiana	Stem bark	Uprety *et al.*, 1972
		leefeana	Leaves	Lamberton and Vashist, 1972
	Neolitsea	*acuminatissima*	Stem bark	Chang *et al.*, 2002
		sericea	Stem bark and leaves	Lee *et al.*, 2007; Nakasato and Asada, 1966
	Phoebe	*chinensis*	Stem bark	Nguyen and Nguyen, 2004
		formosana	Stem bark	Lu and Su, 1973
		grandis	Stem bark	Mukhtar *et al.*, 1997
		scortechinii	Stem bark	Mukhtar *et al.*, 2008
	Sassafras	*albidum*	Root bark	Chowdhury *et al.*, 1976
Boldine	*Actinodaphne*	*nitida*	Stem bark	Johns *et al.*, 1969
		pruinosa	Stem bark	Rachmatiah *et al.*, 2009
	Laurus	*nobilis*	Leaves	Pech and Bruneton, 1982
	Lindera	*aggregata*	Root	Chou *et al.*, 2005
		angustifolia	Root	Zhao *et al.*, 2005
	Litsea	*leefeana*	leaves	Lamberton and Vashist, 1972
		sebifera	Leaves and branches	Uprety *et al.*, 1972
		wightiana	Stem bark	Uprety *et al.*, 1972
	Neolitsea	*acuminatissima*	Stem bark	Chang *et al.*, 2002
		sericea	Stem bark and leaves	Lee *et al.*, 2007; Nakasato and Asada, 1966
	Phoebe	*grandis*	Stem bark	Mukhtar *et al.*, 1997
	Sassafras	*albidum*	Root bark	Chowdhury *et al.*, 1976
Laurotetanine	*Actinodaphne*	*obovata*	Leaves and branches	Uprety *et al.*, 1972
	Cryptocarya	*odorata*	Stem bark	Bick *et al.*, 1972
	Lindera	*angustifolia*	Root	Zhao *et al.*, 2005
		benzoin	Branches	Babcock and Segelman 1974

Contd...

Table 12.1–*Contd...*

Alkaloid	*Genus*	*Species*	*Part of the Plant*	*Reference*
	Litsea	*sebifera*	Leaves and branches	Uprety *et al.,* 1972
	Neolitsea	*sericea*	Stem bark and leaves	Lee *et al.,* 2007; Nakasato and Asada, 1966
	Phoebe	*chinensis*	Stem bark	Nguyen and Nguyen, 2004
		grandis	Stem bark	Mukhtar *et al.,* 1997
N-methillaur-	*Actinodaphne*	*obovata*	Leaves and branches	Uprety *et al.,* 1972
otetanine	*Cryptocarya*	*odorata*	Stem bark	Bick *et al.,* 1972
	Lindera	*angustifolia*	Root	Zhao *et al.,* 2005
		pipericarpa	Stem bark	Lajis *et al.,* 1992
	Litsea	*cubeba*	Stem bark	Lu and Lin, 1967
		sebifera	Leaves and branches	Uprety *et al.,* 1972
	Neolitsea	*sericea*	Stem bark and leaves	Lee *et al.,* 2007; Nakasato and Asada, 1966
Reticuline	*Aniba*	*muca*	Stem bark	Bravo *et al.,* 1996
	Cryptocarya	*odorata*	Stem bark	Bick *et al.,* 1972
	Laurus	*nobilis*	Leaves	Pech and Bruneton, 1982
	Lindera	*aggregata*	Root	Chou *et al.,* 2005
	Litsea	*laurifolia*	Leaves	Leboeuf *et al.,* 1979
		leefeana	Leaves	Lamberton and Vashist, 1972
	Neolitsea	*acuminatissima*	Stem bark	Chang *et al.,* 2002
		sericea	Leaves	Lee *et al.,* 2007
	Ocotea	*duckei*	Stem bark and leaves	Barbosa-Filho *et al.,* 1999
		vellosiana	Fruits	Garcez *et al.,* 1995
	Phoebe	*pittieri*	Stem bark	Castro *et al.,* 1985
	Sassafras	*albidum*	Stem root	Chowdhury *et al.,* 1976
Palidine	*Dehaasia*	*longipedicellata*	Leaves	Mukhtar *et al.,* 2004
	Lindera	*aggregata*	Root	Chou *et al.,* 2005
	Neolitsea	*sericea*	Leaves	Lee *et al.,* 2007
	Ocotea	*brachybotra*	Leaves	Vecchietti *et al.,* 1977
Isocorydine	*Cryptocarya*	*odorata*	Stem bark	Bick *et al.,* 1972
	Dehaasia	*triandra*	Leaves	Lu and Wang, 1977
	Lindera	*pipericarpa*	Stem bark	Lajis *et al.,* 1992
	Ocotea	*vellosiana*	Fruits	Garcez *et al.,* 1995

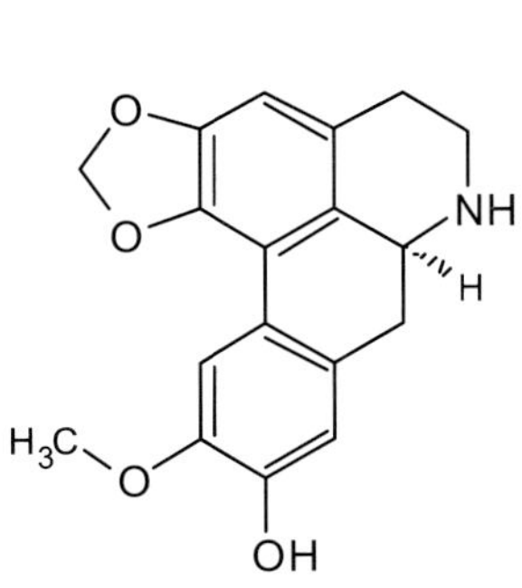

4

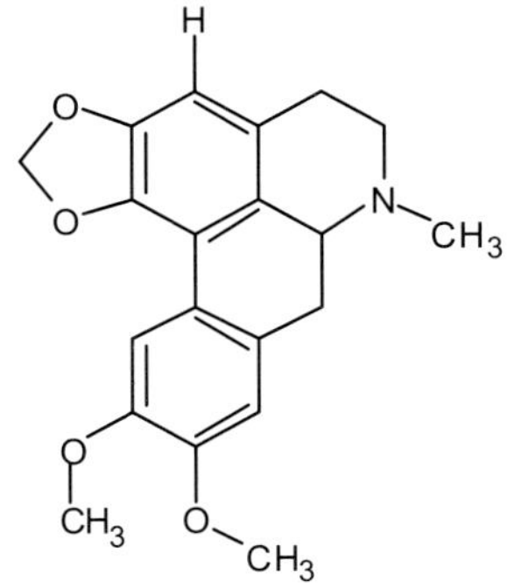

5

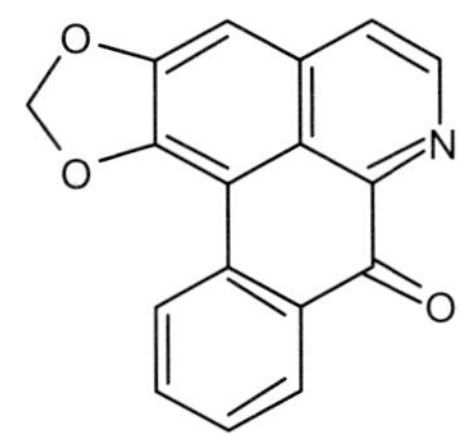

6

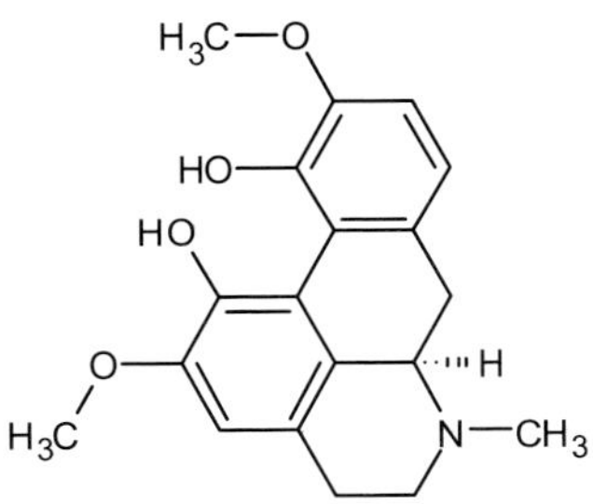

7

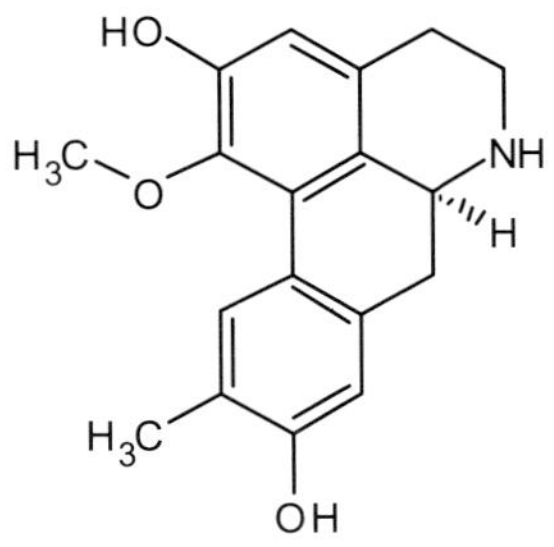

8

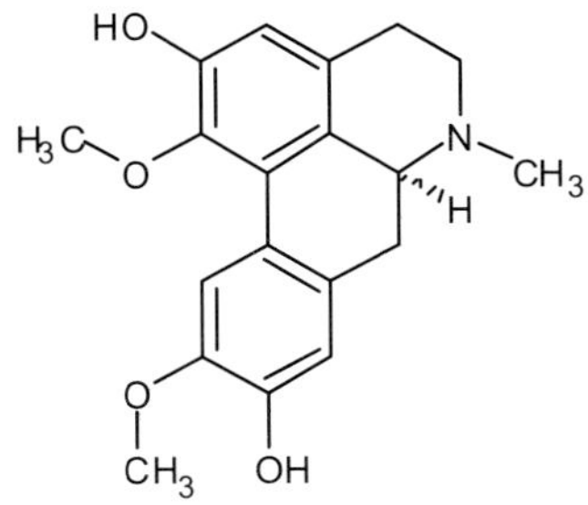

9

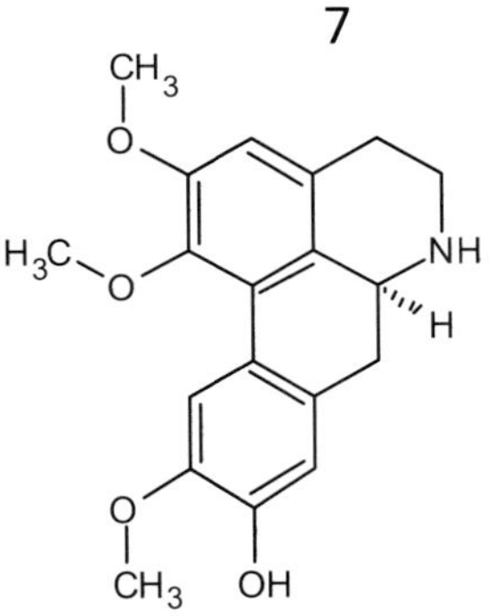

10

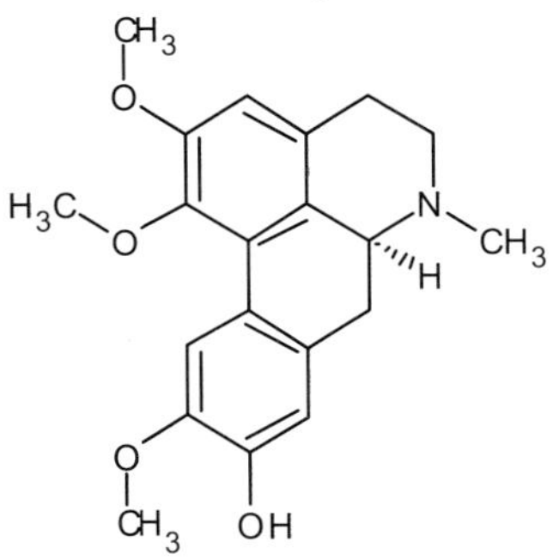

11

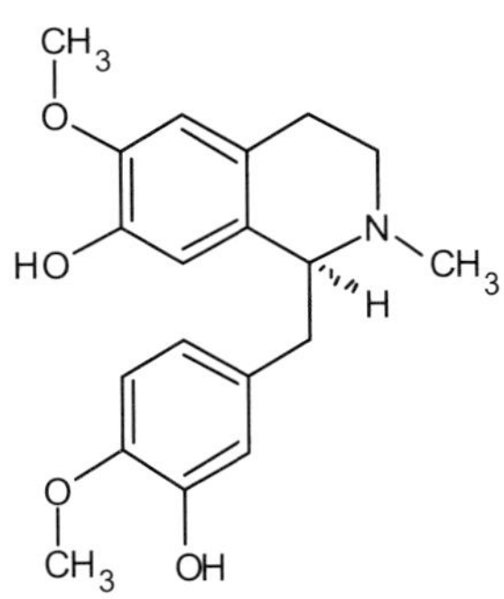

12

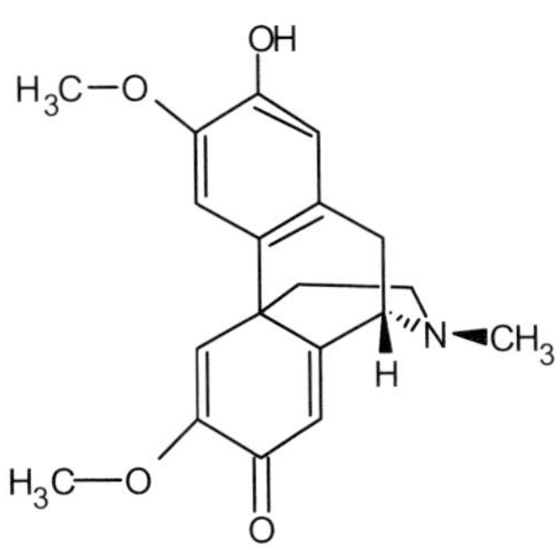

13

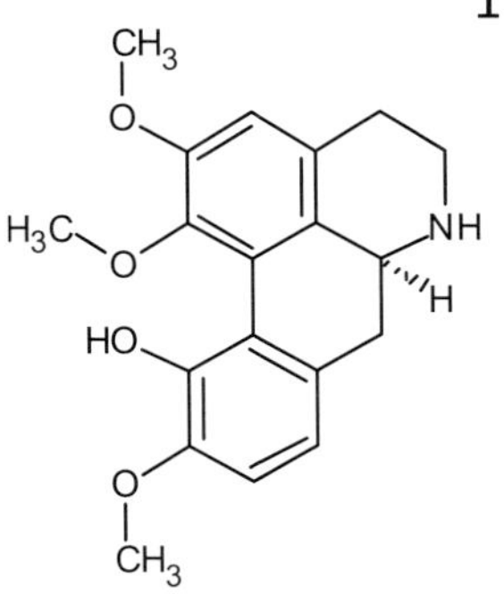

14

Figure 12.2: Most frequently lauraceae alkaloids.

Several of these alkaloids have been studied and present pharmacological activities with promising results concerning its use in different health areas. Morais *et al.* (1998) in neuropharmacological studies, carried out with reticuline in mice, observed that this alkaloid caused changes in sleep behavior, motor coordination and conditioned avoidance responses. This study suggests that reticuline possesses potent effects as a central nervous system depressant. Dias *et al.* (2004) also observed a blood pressure lowering effect in rats exposed to reticuline.

Stévigny *et al.* (2002) observed that actinodaphnine showed high activity against Mel-5 cells (IC_{50} of 25.7 μM) and HL-60 cells (IC_{50} of 15.4 μM). Boldine showed antiinflamatory activity using the model of the edema induced by carregeenin (Barbosa-Filho *et al.*, 2006). Zhao *et al.* (2005) observed that boldine also presented antinociceptive activity. Hoet *et al.* (2004) observed that dicentrine presented negative effects towards *Trypanossoma brucei* in *in vitro* assays. The similarity of the substances and the pharmacological activities already observed strongly indicates that further studies must be performed. These alkaloids are commonly obtained in very small quantities. The isolation in gram scale would allow several others pharmacological experiments.

Beyond these more ordinary structures, there are many others isoquinoline alkaloids with more restricted distribution among some genus. Bravo *et al.* (1996) related N-methylcoclaurine in *Aniba muca* stem bark. Oger *et al.* (1992) isolated from *Aniba canellila* stem bark, (R)-(+)-noranicanine (15), a trioxygenated benzilisoquinoline alkaloid. These species were related to the presence of other 11 benziltetra-hydroisoquinoline alkaloids, where four are mono substituted at ring C with an hydroxyl in C-11, (-)-norcanelilline (16), (+)-canelilline (17), anicanine (18) and canelillinoxine (19); two mono substituted in C-9 of ring D, (-) -anibacanine (20) and (+)-manibacanine (21); two mono substituted in C-11 of ring D (-)-pseudoanibacanine (22) and (+)-pseudoanibacanine (23); and three alkaloids with the same substitution pattern at rings A and B with a methyl substitute in positions 8α and 8β, (-)-α-8-methylpseudoanibacanine (24), (-)-β-8-methylpseudoanibacanine (25) and (-)-α-8-methylanibacanine (26) (Oger *et al.*, 1993). Some *Aniba* isoquinoline alkaloids can be observed in Figure 12.3.

Various alkaloids are described for the species *Cassytha filiformis*, such as cassifiline (=cassitine) (27) (Kava and Rao, 1968; Wu *et al.*, 1997; Stévigny *et al.*, 2002; Tsai *et al.*, 2008); O-methylcassifiline (28) (=O-methylcassitine), cassitidine (29) (Cava and Rao, 1968; Tsai *et al.*, 2008); cassamedine (30) and cassameridine (31) (Cava and Rao, 1968; Wu *et al.*, 1997); launobine (32), bulbocapnine (33), (+)-nornuciferine (34), (+)-nuciferine (35), aterospermidine (36) and O-methylateroline (37) (Cava and Rao, 1968); catafiline, cataformine and lisicamine (Wu *et al.*, 1997); isofiformine, cassythic acid, norpredicentrine, (-)-O-methylflavinatine, (-)-salutaridine and 1,7-methylenedioxy-3,10,11-trimethoxyaporphine (Tsai *et al.*, 2008). Figure 12.4 presents some of these compounds. Cassythine showed high activity against Mel-5 cells (IC_{50} at 24.3 μM) and HL-60 cells (IC_{50} at 19.9 μM), and was active against *Trypanossoma brucei* in *in vitro* assays (Hoet *et al.*, 2004). Stévigny *et al.* (2002) observed cytotoxicity activity of neolitsine against tumor cells HeLa and 3T3 with IC_{50} at 21.6 μM at 21.4 μM respectively.

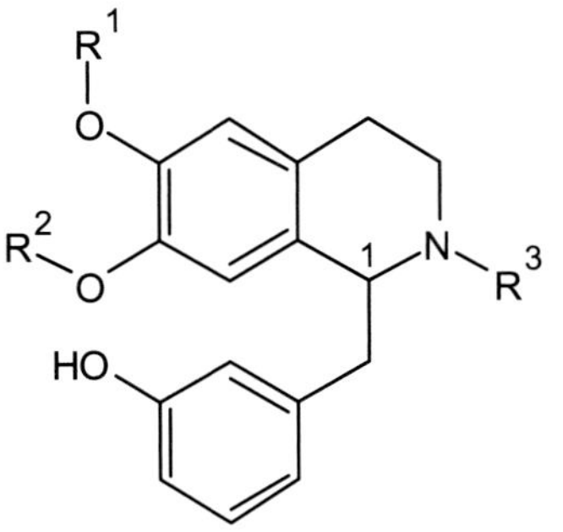

15 R^1=R^2=Me, R^3=H, 1R
16 R^1=Me, R^2= R^3=H 1S
17 R^1= R^3=Me, R^2=H 1S
18 R^1= R^2= R^3=H

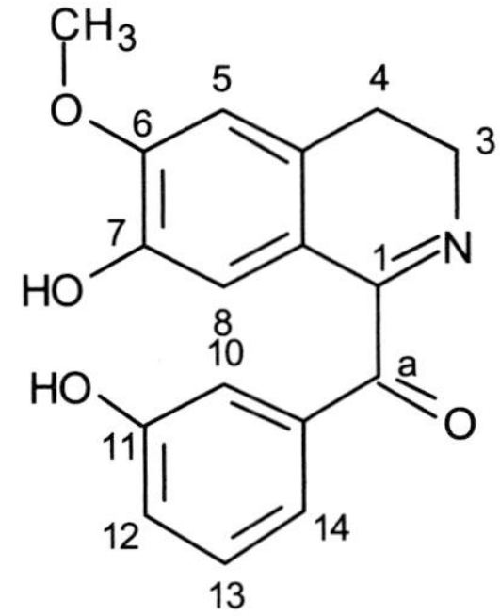

19

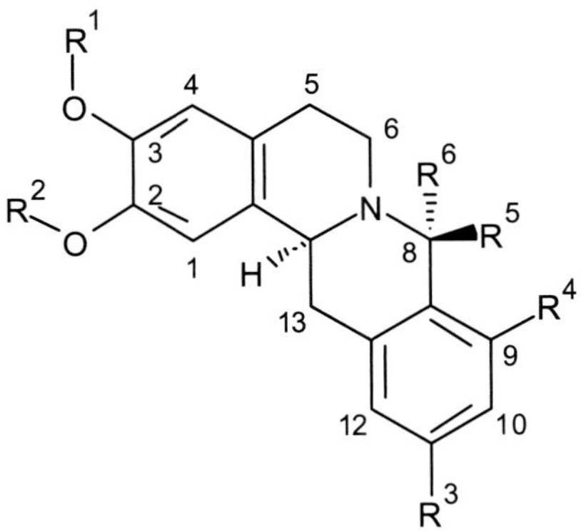

20 R^1=Me, R^2= R^3= R^5= R^6=H, R^4=OH
22 R^1=Me, R^2= R^4= R^5= R^6=H, R^3=OH
24 R^1= R^6=Me, R^2= R^4= R^5=H, R^3= OH
25 R^1= R^5=Me, R^2= R^6= R^4=H, R^3= OH
26 R^1= R^6=Me, R^2= R^5= R^3=H, R^4= OH

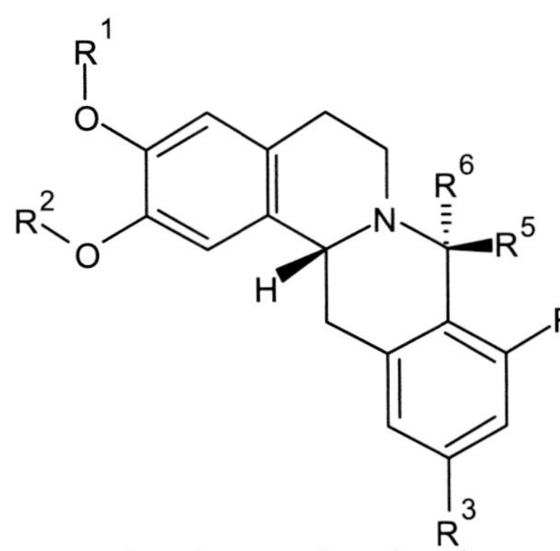

21 R^1= R^2=Me, R^3= R^5= R^6=H, R^4=OH
23 R^1= R^2=Me, R^6= R^5= R^4=H, R^3=OH

Figure 12.3: *Aniba* isoquinoline alkaloids.

In *Cryptocarya*, several isoquinoline alkaloids were already described. Curiously, the substances appear to be specific to each species, as: cryptopleurine from *Cryptocarya lævigata* (Hoffmann *et al.*, 1978); orientaline and laudanidine from *C. amygdalina* stem bark (Borthakur *et al.*, 1981); velucryptine (38) and ateroline, *C. velutinosa* leaves (Lebceuf *et al.*, 1989) and (+)-(1R, 1Ra)-1a-hydroxymagnocumarine from *C. konishii* (Lee *et al.*, 1993). *Cryptocarya chinensis* is one of the most studied lauraceae species because of its alkaloid content. (±)-Romneine (Lee and Chen, 1993); (-)-isocaryachine-

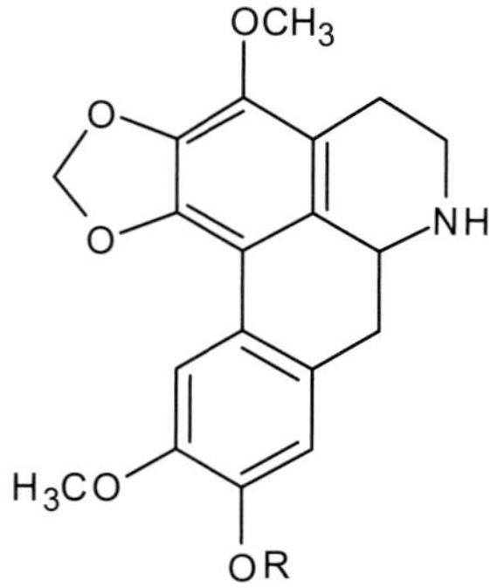

27 R=H
28 R=CH_3

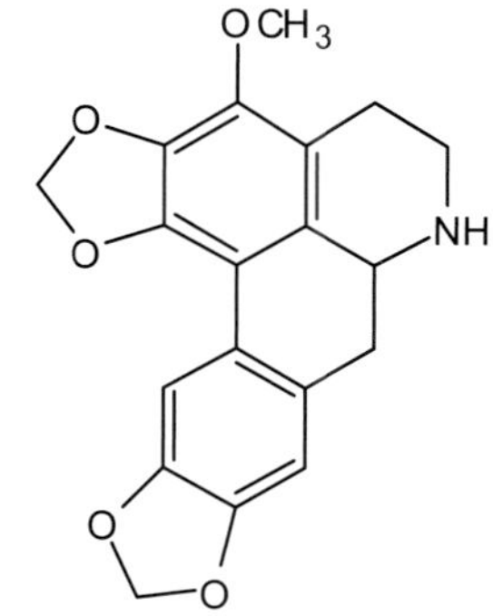

29

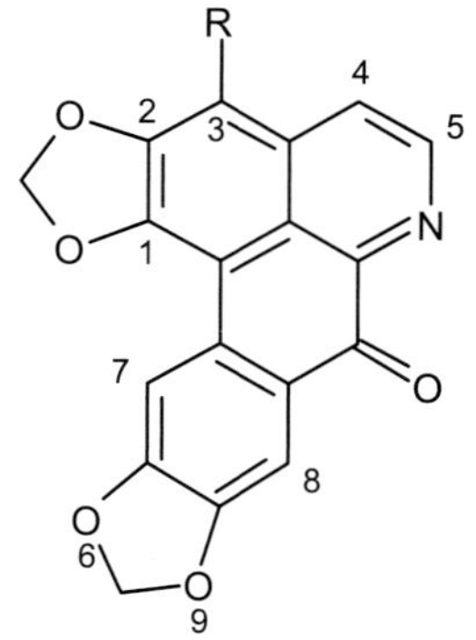

30 R=OCH_3
31 R=H

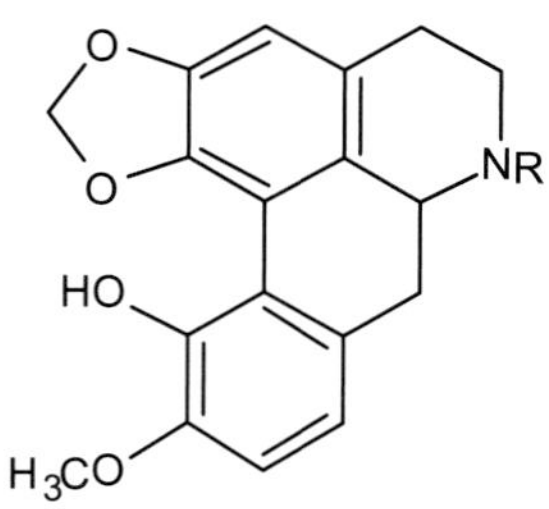

32 R=H
33 R=CH_3

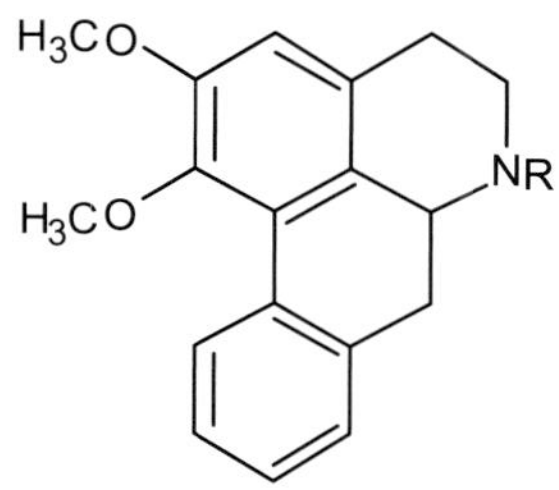

34 R=H
35 R=CH_3

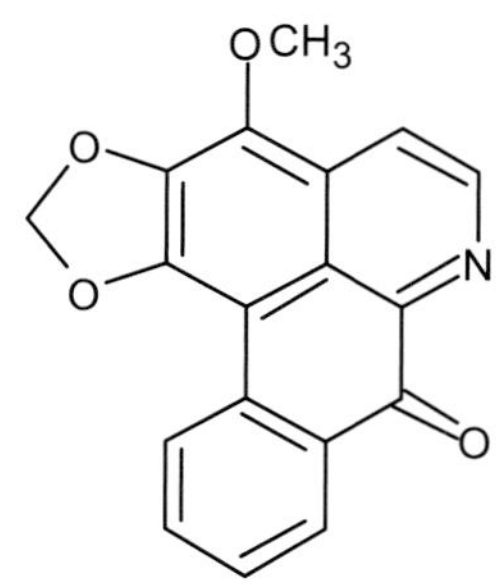

36

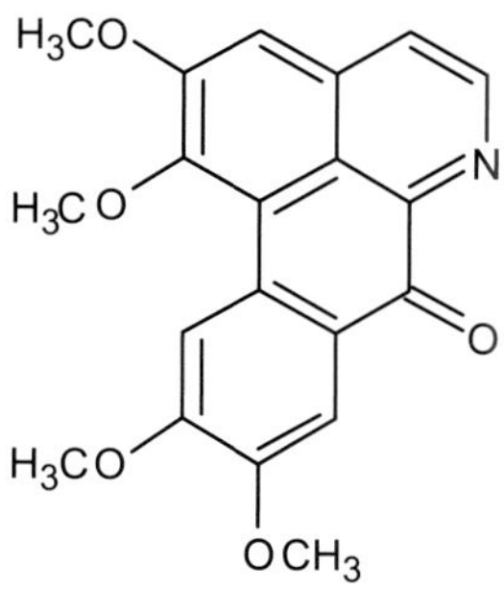

37

Figure 12.4: *Cassytha* isoquinolines alkaloids.

N-oxide (39), isoboldine-β-N-oxide (40), 1-hydroxycryprochine (41), (+)-isocaryachine (42), (+)-caryachine (43), (-)-caryachine (44), (-)-isocaryachine (45), (-)-munitagine (46), bisnorargeminine (47) (Lin *et al.*, 2001) were isolated from the leaves of this species. Wu and Lin (2001) isolated four pavine alkaloids from *C. chinensis* stem, (+)-

escholtzidine-N-oxide, (-)-12-hydroxycrychine, (-)-12-hydroxy-O-methylcaryachine and (-)-N-demethylcrychine and four proaporphine alkaloids: isocryprochine, prooxocryptochine, isoamuronine and (+)-8,9-dihydrostepharine. Substances isolated from the stem bark included (+)-cryprochine (Lee and Chen, 1993), (-)-isocaryachine-N-oxide B, (+)-caryachine-N-oxide, (-)-caryachine-N-oxide, 6,7-methylenedioxy-N-methylisoquinoline (48), (-)-neocaryachine, (+)-caryachine (43), (+)-cinnamolaurine, (-)-caryachine (44), (-)-mutagenine, (-)-isocaryachine (45), 1-hydroxycryprochine, 4,6,7-dimethyloxyisoquinoline-1-ylmethylfenol, (-)-2-O-norargemonine, (-)-N,N-dimethylcaryachine and (-)-eschscholtzidina (Lin *et al.*, 2002), besides three quaternary pavine alkaloids as salts N-metho-caryachine, neocaryachine and crychine from a *C. chinensis* callus culture (Chang *et al.*, 1998). Figure 12.5 shows some of these structures.

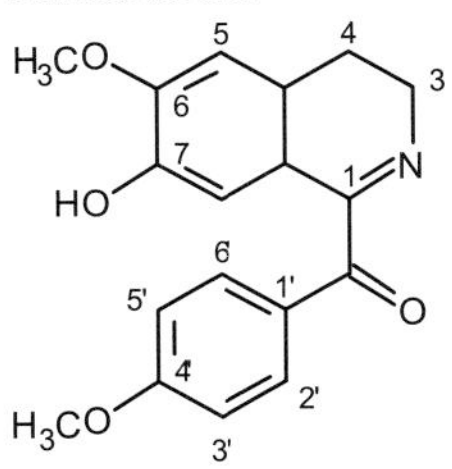

38

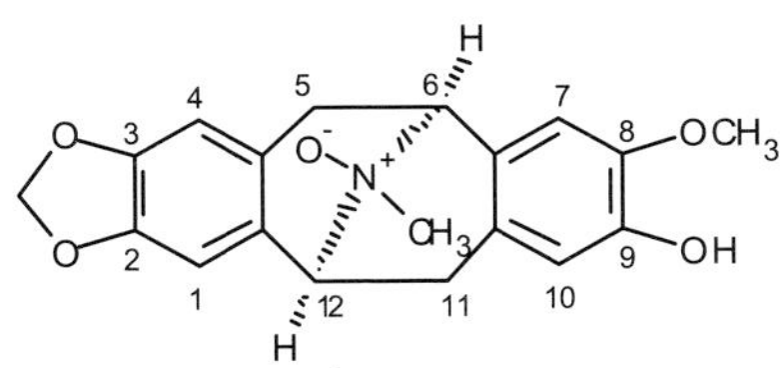

39

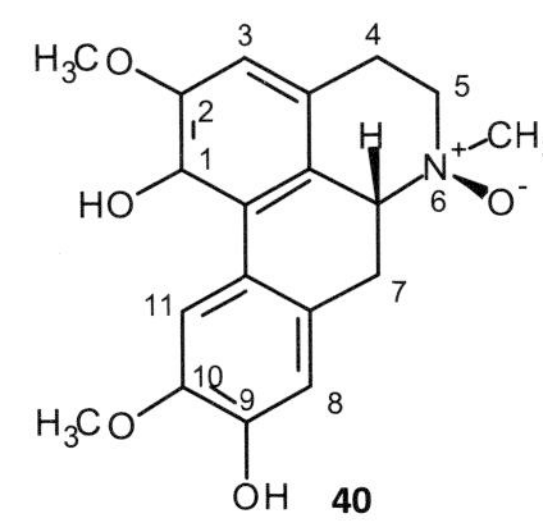

40

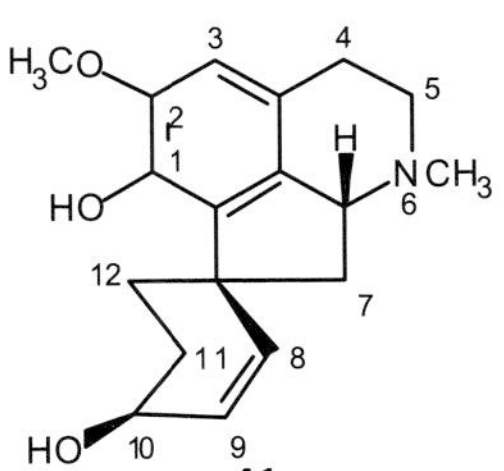

41

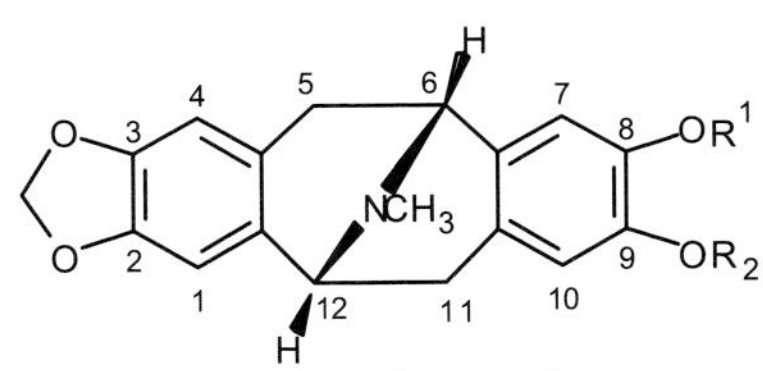

42 R^1=CH_3, R^2=H
43 R^1=H, R^2=CH_3

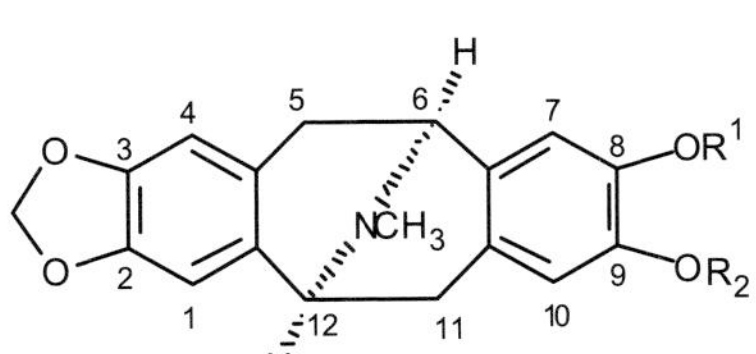

44 R^1=H, R^2=CH_3
45 R^1=CH_3, R^2=H

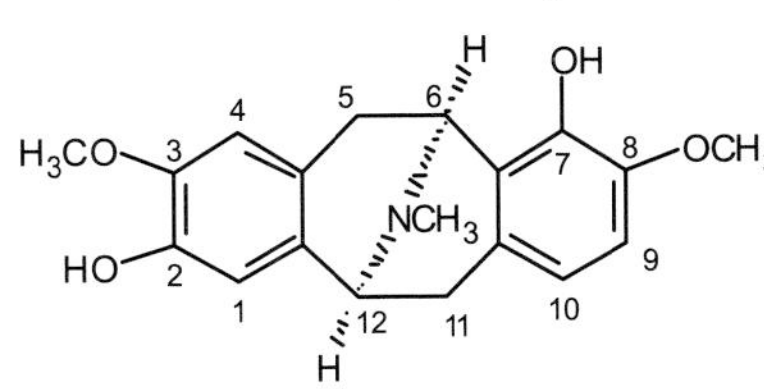

46

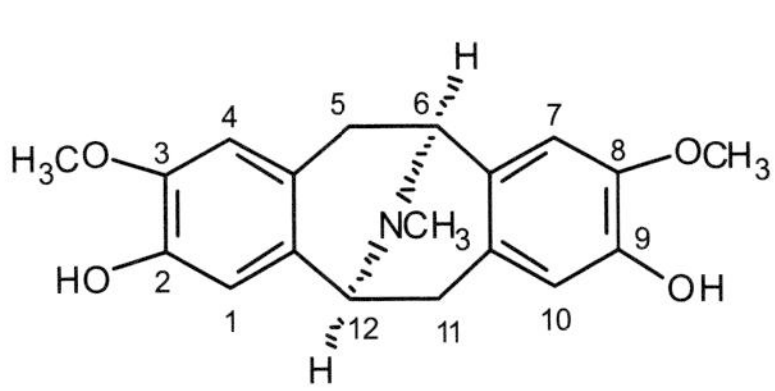

47

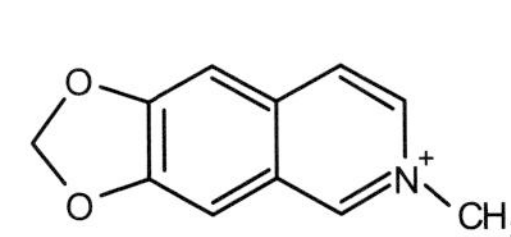

48

Figure 12.5: *Cryptocarya* isoquinoline alkaloids.

In the *Lindera* genus, Kiang and Sim (1967) isolated lindcarpine (50) and N-methyllindcarpine (51) from the *Lindera pipericarpa* root. Zhang *et al.* (2002) in a study of the *Lindera chunii* root, obtained ten aporphine alkaloids: hernandine (52), hernangerine (53), N-methylhernangerine (54), ocokriptine (N-methylhernandine) (55), hernandonine (56), 7-oxohernangerine (57), lindechunine A (58), lindechunine B, and 7-oxohernagine (59). More recently, Zhao *et al.* (2005) isolated norisocorydine from *Lindera angustifolia* and observed an antinociceptive and high free radical scavenging activity (SC_{50} de 14.1 μg/mL). Figure 12.6 shows some of these substances.

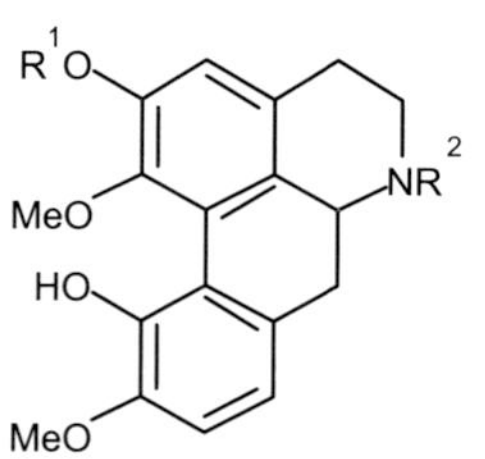

50 $R^1 = R^2 = H$

51 $R^1 = H, R^2 = Me$

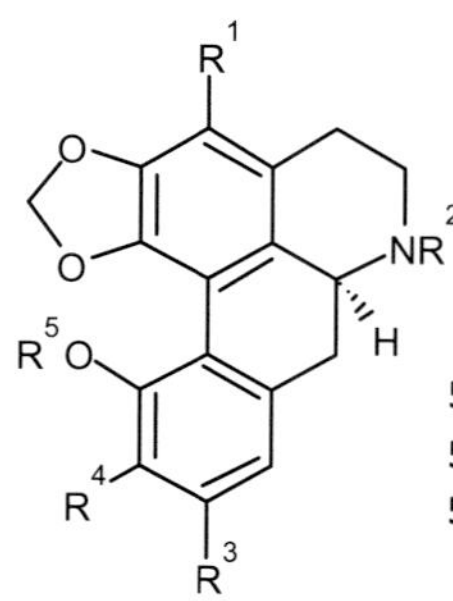

52 $R^1 = OCH_3, R^2 = R^3 = H, R^4 = OH, R^5 = CH_3$

53 $R^1 = R^2 = R^3 = H, R^4 = OH, R^5 = CH_3$

54 $R^1 = R^3 = H, R^2 = R^5 = CH_3, R^4 = OH,$

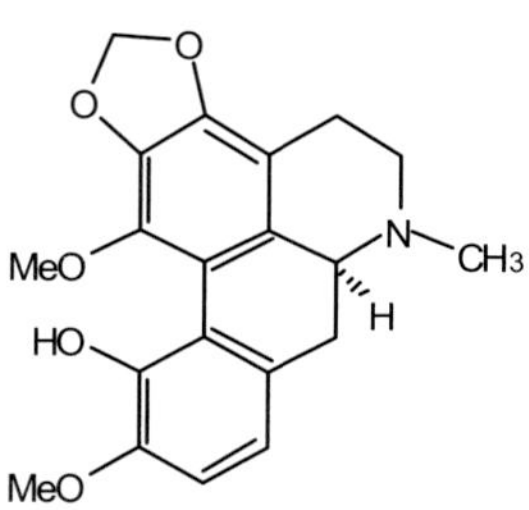

55

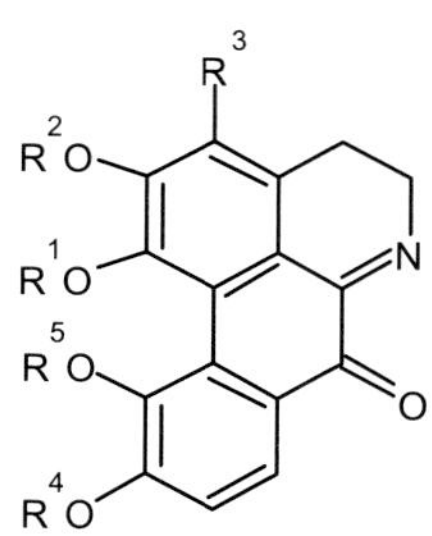

56 $R^1 + R^2 = R^4 + R^5 = CH_2, R^3 = H$

57 $R^1 + R^2 = CH_2, R^3 = R^4 = H, R^5 = CH_3$

58 $R^1 + R^2 = CH_2, R^3 = OCH_3, R^4 = H, R^5 = CH_3$

59 $R^1 = R^2 = R^5 = CH_3\ R^3 = R^4 = H$

Figure 12.6: *Lindera* isoquinoline alkaloids.

Lee *et al.* (1993) isolated from *Litsea cubeba* branches, the quaternary alkaloids from which included (-)-oblongine, (-)-8-O-methyloblogine, xantoplanine and (-)-magnocurarine. Borthakur and Rastogi (1979) isolated laetanine (60) from the *Litsea læta* barks, as well as laetine (61), N,O-dimethylharnovine (62) and glaucine (63) (Rastogi and Bortharkur, 1980). In the same study the authors obtained nordicentrine (64) and dicentrinone (65), both extracted from *Litsea salicifolia* leaves. In a review, Barbosa-Filho *et al.* (2006), list several alkaloids, specifically glaucine, with anti-inflammatory activity. Some of these structures can be observed at the Figure 12.7.

In the genus *Neolitsea*, benzilisoquinoline alkaloids were observed in the barks of *N. acuminatissia* (neolitacumonine, (-)-norushisuinina, N-mehtylactinodaphnine, (+)-cassitine, (-)-talicsimidine, (+)-O-methylflavinatine, (-)-anonaine and oxogalucine) (Chang *et al.*, 2002) and N-oxides of pallidine, reticuline (66 and 67), boldine, juziphine (68), N-methyllaurotetanine, (+)-corytuberine (69) and norisocorydine (70) were isolated from *N. sericea* leaves (Lee *et al.*, 2007). Figure 12.8 shows several of these substances.

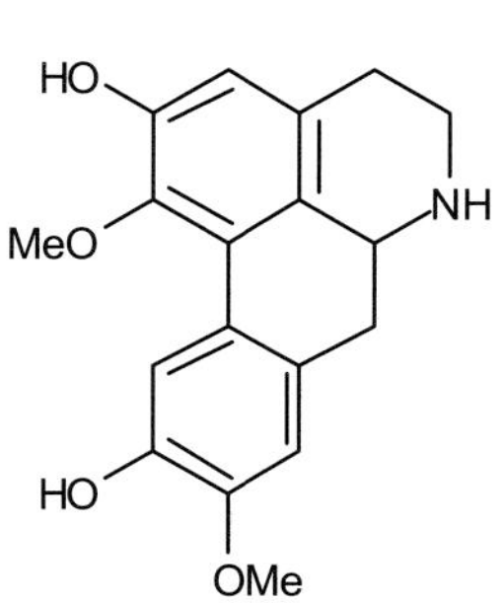

60

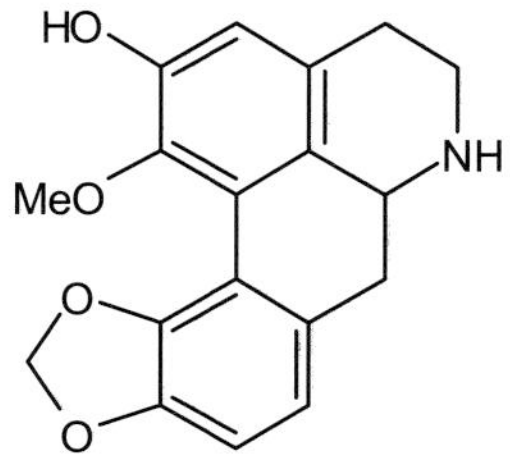

61

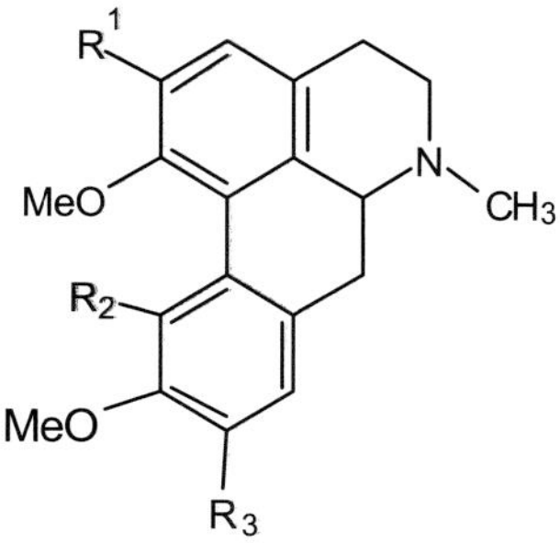

62 $R^1 = OH, R^2 = OMe, R^3 = H$
63 $R^1 = OMe, R^2 = H, R^3 = OMe$

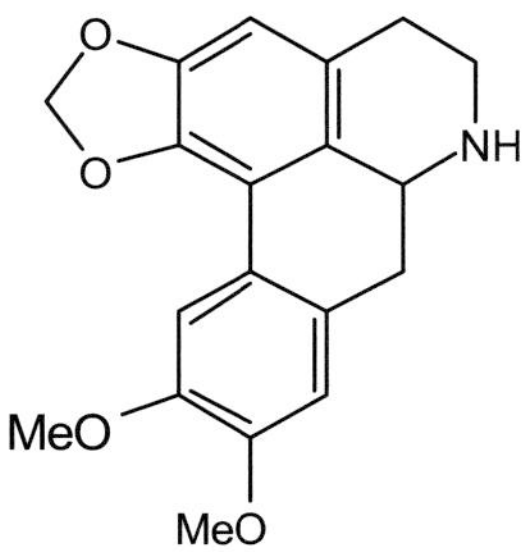

64

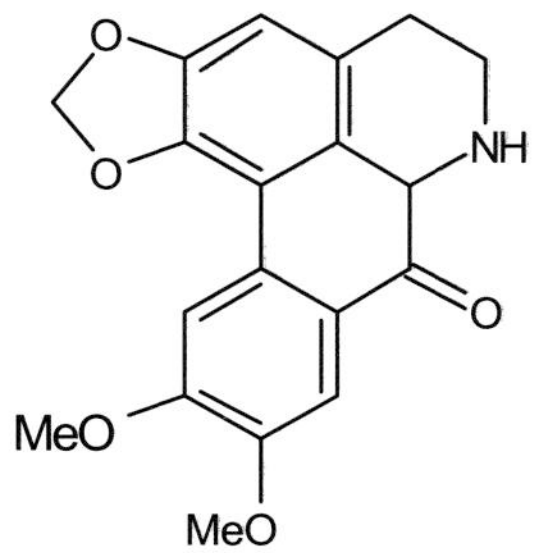

65

Figure 12.7: *Litsea* isoquinoline alkaloids.

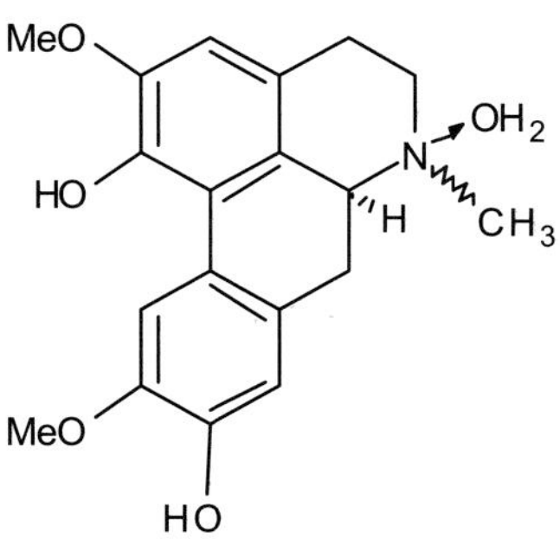

66 R = N_a-oxide
67 R = $N_ß$-oxide

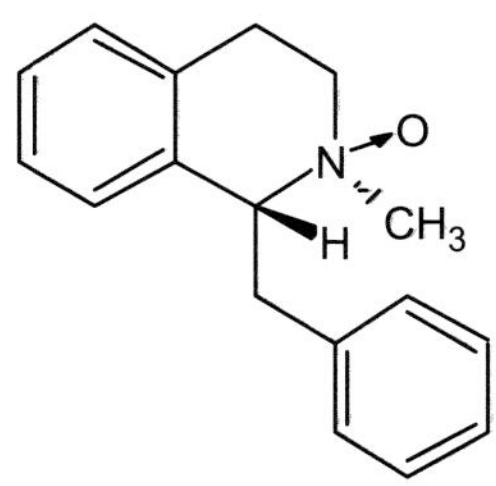

68

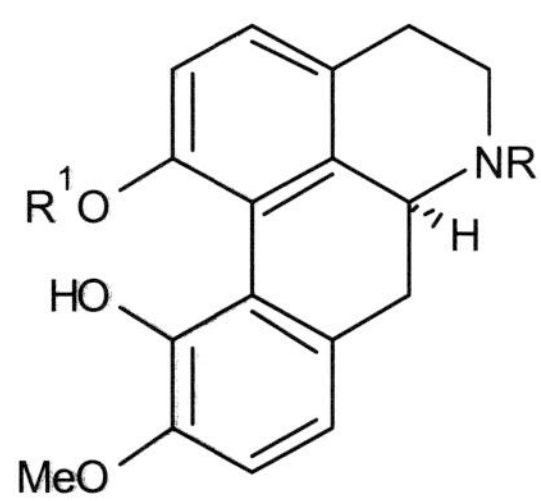

69 $R = Me, R^1 = H$
70 $R = H, R^1 = Me$

Figure 12.8: *Neolitsea* isoquinoline alkaloids.

In the genus *Ocotea* many alkaloids were already isolated, most notably aporphine. In *Ocotea vellosiana* nordicentrine, ocoteine, O-methyl-cassifoline, leucoxene, and ocotominarine were isolated from the branches; ocopodine and ocominarine in leaves; and glaucine and corydine in fruits (Garcez *et al.*, 1995). Da Silva and coworkers (2002) isolated coclaurine (71) from *Ocotea duckei* branches and stems.

Zanin and Lordello (2007), in a review of *Ocotea* alkaloids, described the occurrence of 54 aporphinoid in 17 species, being 39 aporphine, four oxoaporphine, five 6a,7dehydroaporphine, one didehydroaporphine, one C-3-aporphine, two phenanthrene, and one proaporphine. Among these structures are caaverine, from *O. glaziovii*; nantenine and dehydronantenine, from *O. macrophylla*; and isodomesticine, didehydroocoteine, from *O. insularis*. Barrera and Suárez (2009) isolated from leaves of *O. macrophylla* dehydronantenine, (+)-nantenine (72), (+)-neolitsine, (+)-N-acetyl-nornantenine, (+)-cassitidine and didehydroocoteine. Pabon and Cuca (2010) isolated from the *O. macrophyla* stem four alkaloids identified as (S)-3-methoxynordomesticine (73), (S)-N-ethoxycarbonyl-3-methoxynordomesticine (74), (S)-N-formyl-3-methoxynordomesticine (75) and (S)-N-methoxycarbonyl-3-methoxynordomesticine (76). Figure 12.9 shows some *Ocotea* isoquinoline alkaloids.

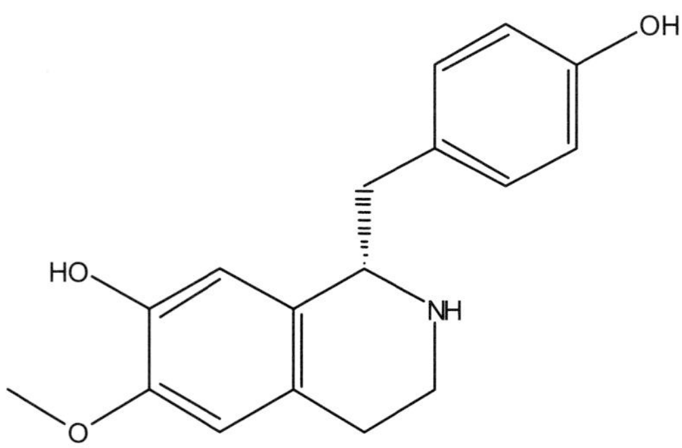

71

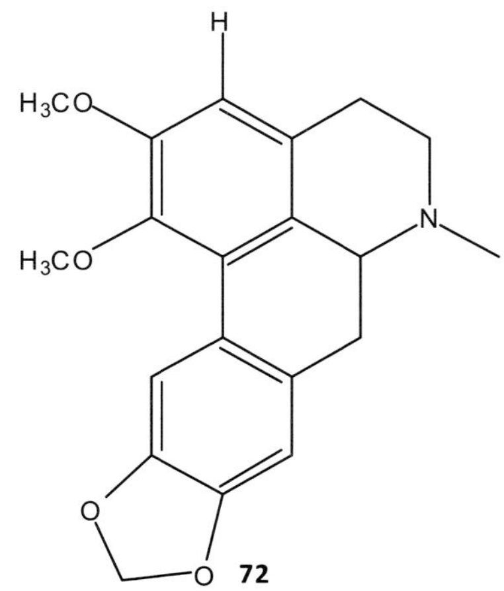

72

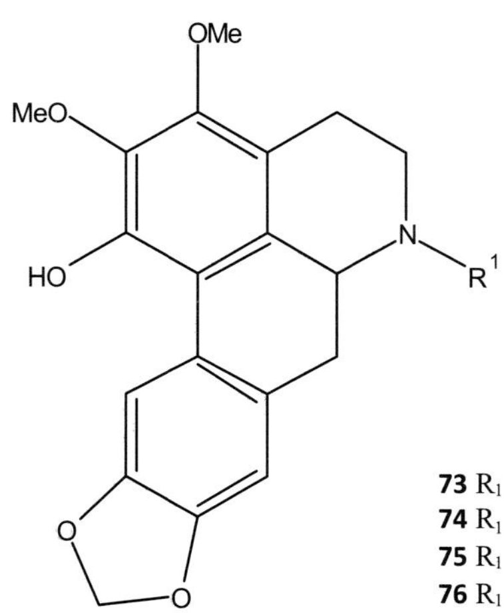

73 $R_1 = H$
74 $R_1 = COOCH_2CH_3$
75 $R_1 = COH$
76 $R_1 = COOCH_3$

Figure 12.9: *Ocotea* isoquinoline alkaloids.

Among the isoquinoline alkaloids noticed in the genus *Phoebe*, some aporphine pentasubstituted were found in *Phoebe molicella* stem bark: norpurpureine (77), purpureine (78), preocoteine (79) and norpreocoteine (80) (Stermitz, 1983). In the *Phoebe pittieri* stem bark were isolated 1,2,3-trimetoxy-9,10-methylenedioxynorarporphine and 1,2,9-trimetoxy-10-hydroxynorarporphine (new for this species), beyond the norpurpureine (Castro *et al.*, 1985). For the species *Phoebe grandis*, lindecarpine were isolated in the stem bark and two proaporphine in the leaves. These included the A and B phoebegrandines (Mukhtar *et al.*, 1997). A few of the *Phoebe* aporphine alkaloids are presented in Figure 12.10.

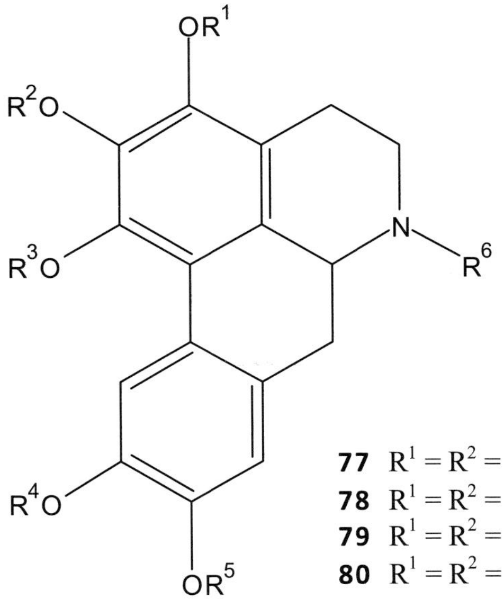

77 $R^1 = R^2 = R^3 = R^4 = R^5 = CH_3, R^6 = H$
78 $R^1 = R^2 = R^3 = R^4 = R^5 = R^6 = CH_3$
79 $R^1 = R^2 = R^4 = R^5 = R^6 = CH_3, R^3 = H$
80 $R^1 = R^2 = R^4 = R^5 = CH_3, R^3 = R^6 = H$

Figure 12.10: *Phoebe* isoquinoline alkaloids.

From *Sassafras albidum* root bark, norcinnamolaurine and cinnamolaurine were isolated (Chowdhury *et al.*, 1976). Le Quesne *et al.* (1980) obtained laurelliptine, an aporphine alkaloid, isolated from *Nectandra rigida* leaves and branches. Coy and Cuca (2008) isolated pleurotirine from *Pleurothyrium cinereum* leaves, which is an oxoaporphine alkaloid.

Indole Alkaloids

The indole alkaloids are benzopyrrole structures where the indole core (81) are formed by the fusion of the benzene ring and pyrrole ring at positions 2 and 3. When this fusion occurs at the 3 and 4 positions of the pyrrole ring there is the isoindole (82) core formation. The numbering of the atoms begins at the atom next to the junction in the pyrrole ring, proceeding the other atoms around the indole core (Figure 12.11) (Houlihan, 1972).

Klausmeyer *et al.* (2004), in a study of *Aniba panurensis*, isolated the quaternary alkaloid 6,8-didec-(1*Z*)-enyl-5,7-dimethyl-2,3-dihydro-1*H*-indolizidinium (83) as

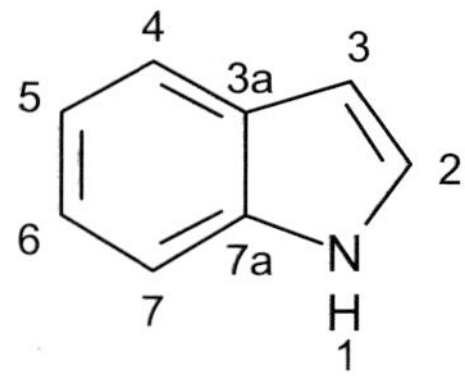

81

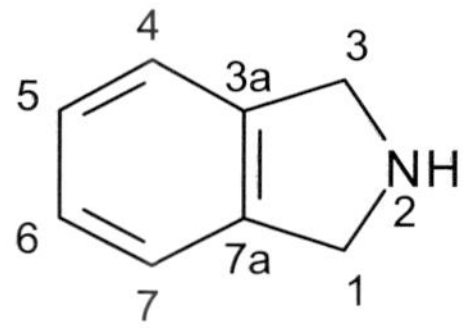

82

Figure 12.11: Indole and isoindole cores.

trifluoroacetic acid salt. Aguiar *et al.* (1980) isolated from *Aniba santalodora* trunk cecilin (84), a β-carboline alkaloid. Garcez *et al.* (2005) isolated from *Ocotea minarum* fruits a new indole alkaloid, the triptofol-5-O-β-D-glucopyranoside (Figure 12.12).

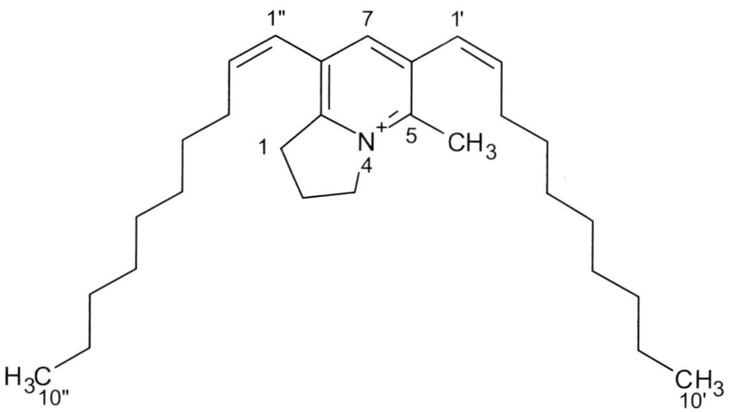

83

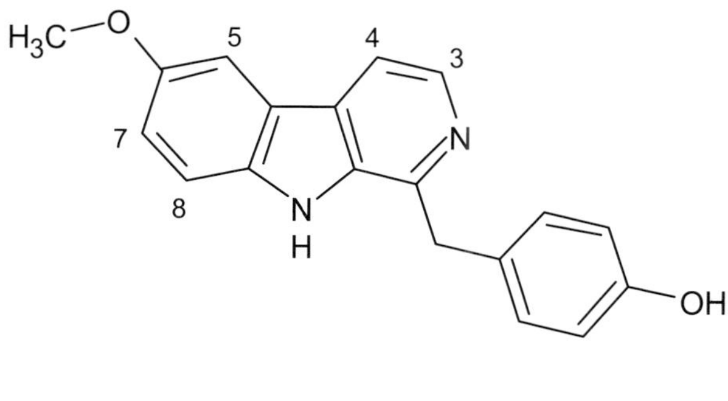

84

Figure 12.12: Lauraceae indole alkaloids.

Pyridine Alkaloids

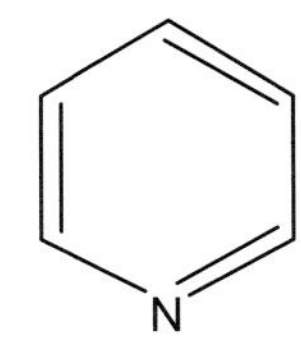

85

Figure 12.13: Pyridine core.

The pyridine alkaloids present a pyridine ring (85) which is formed from nicotinic acid (Dewick, 2002) (Figure 12.13).

They are also less frequently found in the Lauraceae family, as well as in indole alkaloids. There has been reported in *Aniba rosaeodora* the presence of two tertiary structures, anibine (86) (Mors *et al.*, 1957) and duckeine (87) (Correa and Gottlieb, 1975). Both of these were obtained from the stem together with a pyridine quaternary alkaloid, anibamine (88) (Jayasuriya *et al.*, 2004). The anibine is also reported in *Aniba coto* (Mors and Gottlieb, 1959) and *Aniba fragrans* was also obtained from the stems of the species. Gonçalves *et al.* (1958) reported the analeptic activity of this alkaloid (Figure 12.14).

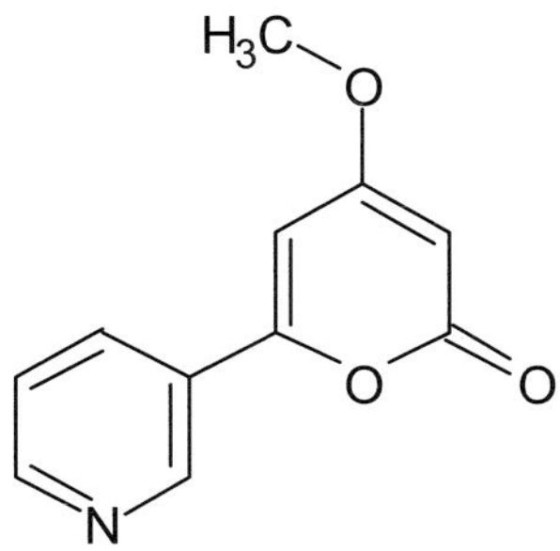

86

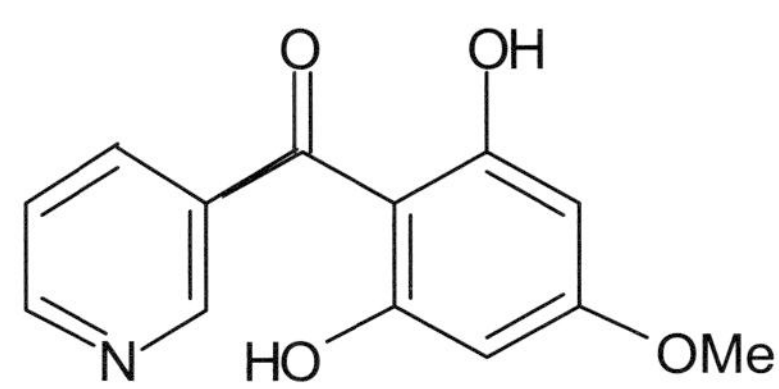

87

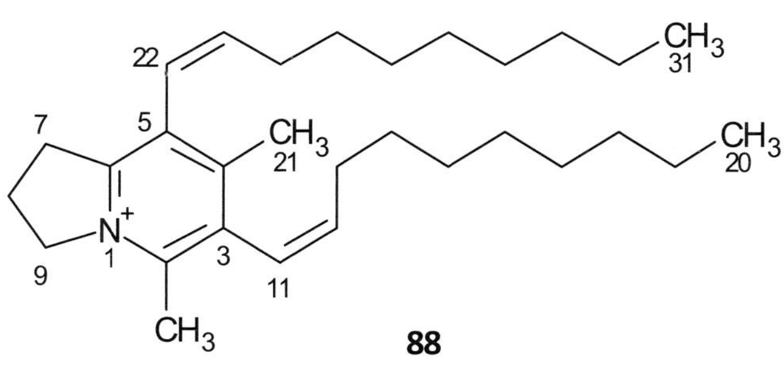

88

Figure 12.14: Lauraceae pyridine alkaloids.

Other Alkaloid Classes

Besides the isoquinoline, indole and pyridine alkaloids, the Lauraceae family presents other alkaloids classes. Lebeceuf *et al.* (1989) isolated the dibenzopyrrolidine alkaloids cryptowoline (89), O-methyl-cryptowoline (90) cryptowolinol (91) and cryptowolidine, from the *Cryptocarya phyllostemon* stem bark; crystautoline and cryptowolinol, from the stem bark; and cryptowolinol from *Cryptocarya oubatchensis* leaves.

Adrianaivoravelona and others (1999), in a study of *Ravensara anisata*, isolated the alkaloid *N*-(*p*-coumaroil)-tryptamine derived of tryptamine from a stem bark extract. Mukhtar and coworkers (2004), in a study of *Dehaasia longipedicellata* leaves, isolated five morphinandienone alkaloids, including the (-)-pallidime, (+)-milonine,

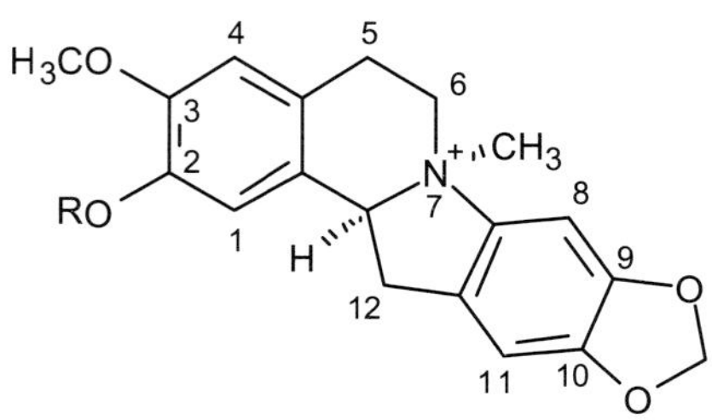

89 R=H
90 R=Me

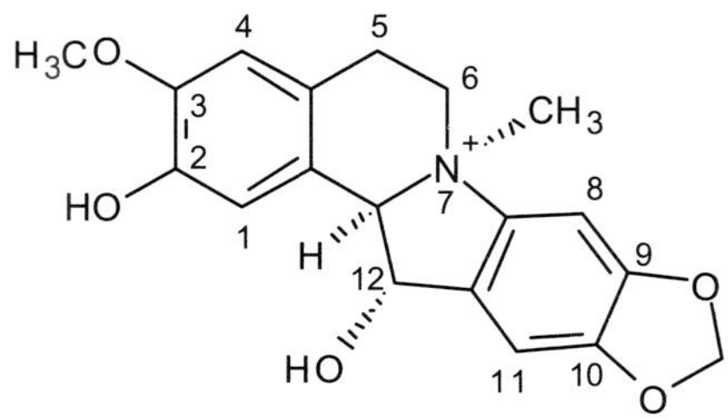

91

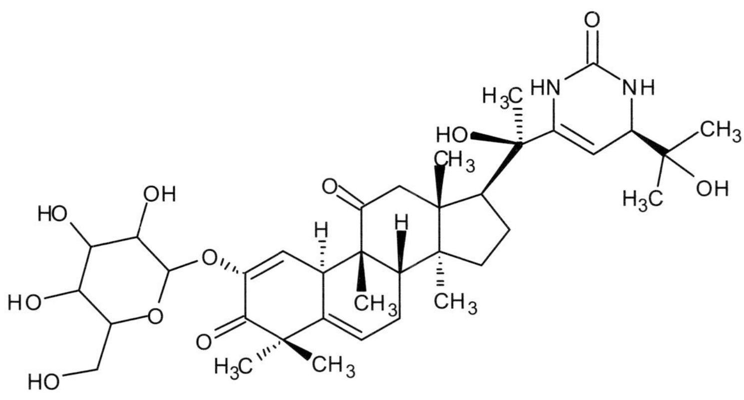

92

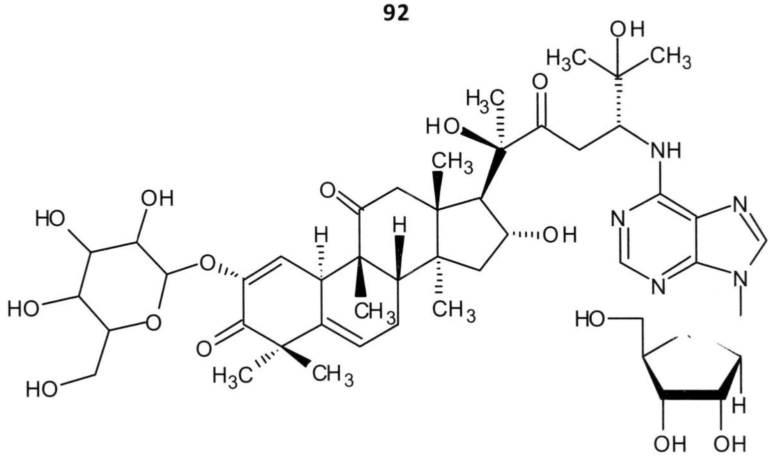

93

Figure 12.15: Lauraceae others classes alkaloids.

(-)8,4-dehydrosalutaridine, (-)-sinoacutine and (+) -pallidinine, a new compound in the species. From the study of *Machillus yaoshansis* stem bark, two triterpene glycoside alkaloids were isolated, called machilaminoside A (92) and machilaminoside B (93), as novel substances in this species (Liu *et al.*, 2007). Figure 12.15 shows some alkaloids of other classes described in Lauraceae.

Final Considerations

According to the data presented in this chapter, we can observe that the Lauraceae family presents great variety of alkaloids with aporphine, isoquinoline, benzyltetrahydroisoquinoline and pavine skeletons, together with rarely observed pyridine and indole. Some of these substances present a restricted distribution to certain genera or even species, showing the possibility of using them as chemical markers. They may also play an important role in chemotaxonomy and could show several interesting pharmacological properties, although most of them have never been evaluated in relation to biological activities.

References

Aguiar, L.M.G., Braz-Filho, R., Gottlieb, O.R., Maia, J.G.S., Pinho, S.L.V., and Sousa, J.R. (1980). Cecilin, a 1-benzyl-β-carboline from *Aniba santalodora*. *Phytochemistry*, **19**: 1859-1860.

Andrianaivoravelona, J.O., Terreaux, C., Sahpaz, S., Rasolondramanitra, J., and Hostettmann, K. (1999). A phenolic glycoside and *N*-(*p*-coumaroyl)-tryptamine from *Ravensara anisata*. *Phytochemistry*, **52**: 1145-1148.

Apers, S., Vlietinck, A., and Pieters, L. (2003). Lignans and neolignans as lead compounds. *Phytochemistry Reviews*, **2**: 201–217.

Babcock, P.A., and Segelman, A.B. (1974). Alkaloids of *Lindera benzoin* (Lauraceae). I. Isolation and identification of laurotetanine. *Journal of Pharmaceutical Sciences*, **63**: 1495-1496.

Barbosa-Filho, J.M., Vargas, M.R.W., Silva, I.G., Franca, I.S., Morais, L.C.S.L., Da Cunha, E.V.L., Da Silva, M.S., Souza, M.F.V., Chaves, M.C.O., Almeida, R.N., and Agra, M.F. (1999). *Ocotea duckei*: exceptional source of yangambin and other furofuran lignans. *Anais da Academia Brasileira de Ciências*, **71**: 231-238.

Barbosa-Filho, J.M., Piuvezam, M.R., Moura, M.D., Silva, M.S., Lima, K.V.B., da-Cunha, E.V.L., Fechine, I.M. and Takemura, O.S. (2006). Anti-inflammatory activity of alkaloids: A twenty-century review. *Revista Brasileira de Farmacognosia*, **16**: 109-139.

Barrera, E.D.C., and Suárez, L.E.C. (2009). Aporphine alkaloids from leaves of *Ocotea macrophylla* (Kunth) (lauraceae) from Colombia. *Biochemical Systematics and Ecology*, **37**: 522-524.

Bick, I.R.C., Preston, N.W., and Potier, P. (1972). Alkaloids of *Cryptocarya odorata* (Lauraceae). *Bulletin de la Societe Chimique de France*, **12**: 4596-4597.

Borthakur, N., and Rastogi, R.C. (1979). Laetanine, a new aporphine alkaloid from *Litsea laeta*. *Phytochemistry*, **18**: 910-911.

Borthakur, N., Mahanta, P.K., and Rastogi, R.C. (1981). Alkaloids and oleofinic acids from *Cryptocarya amygdalina*. *Phytochemistry*, **20**: 501-504.

Bravo, J.A., Sauvain, M., Balderrama, L., Moretti,C., Richomme, P., and Bruneton, J. (1996). Alcaloides de la *Aniba muca*. *Revista Boliviana de Química*, **13**: 19-22.

Castro, O.C., López, J.V., and Vergara, A.G. (1985). Aporphine alkaloids from *Phoebe pittieri*. *Phytochemistry*, **24**: 203-204.

Cava, M.P., Rao, K.V., Douglas, b., and Weisbach, J.A. (1968). The alkaloids of Cassytha Americana (C. filiformis L.). *The Journal of Organic Chemistry*, **33**: 2443-2446.

Chang, F.R., Hsieh, T.J., Huang, T.L., Chen, C.Y., Kuo, R.Y., Chang, Y.C., Chiu, H.F., and Wu, Y.C. (2002). Cytotoxic constituents of the stem bark of *Neolitsea acuminatissima*. *Journal of Natural Products*, **65**: 255-258.

Chang, W.T., Lee, S.S., Chueh, F.S., and Liu, K.C.S. (1998). Formation of pavine alkaloids by callus culture of *Cryptocarya Chinensis*. *Phytochemistry*, **48**: 119-124.

Chou, G.-X., Norio, N., Ma, C.-M., Wang, Z.-T. and Masao, H. (2005). Isoquinoline alkaloids from *Lindera aggregate*. *Zhongguo Tiamran Yaowu*, **3**: 272-275.

Chowdhury, B.K., Sethi, M.L., Lloyd, H.A., and Kapadia, G.J. (1976). Aporphine and tetrahydrobenzylisoquinoline alkaloids in *Sassafras albidum*. *Phytochemistry*, **15**: 1803-1804.

Corrêa, D.B., and Gottlieb, O.R. (1975). Duckein, an alkaloid from *Aniba duckei*. *Phytochemistry*, **14**: 271-272.

Coy, E.D., and Cuca, L.E. (2008). Nuevo alcaloide oxoaporfínico y otros constituyentes químicos aislados de *Pleurothyrium cinereum* (Lauraceae). *Revista Colombiana de Química*, **37**: 127-134.

Da Silva, I.G., Barbosa-Filho, J.M., da Silva, M.S., de Lacerda, C.D.G., and da Cunha, E.V.L. (2002). Coclaurine from *Ocotea duckei*. *Biochemical Systematics and Ecology*, **30**: 881-883.

Dewick, P.M. (2002). Medicinal natural products: a biosynthetic approach. John Wiley and Sons Ltd, Chichester.

Dias, K.L.G., Dias, C.S., Barbosa-Filho, J.M., Almeida, R.N., Correia, N.A. and Medeiros, I.A. (2004). Cardiovascular effects induced by reticuline in normotensive rats. *Planta Medica*, **70**: 328-333.

Din, L.B., Hadi, A.H.A., and Latiff, A. (1994). Isolation of dicentrine from *Actinodaphne sesquipedalis* (Lauraceae). *ACGC Chemical Research Communications*, : 5-6.

Garcez, W.S., Garcez F.R., Silva L.M.G.E., and Shimabukuro, A.A. (2005). Indole Alkaloid and other Constituents from *Ocotea minarum*. *Journal of the Brazilian Chemical Society*, **16**: 1382-1386.

Garcez, W.S., Yoshida, M., and Gottlieb, O.R. (1995). Benzylisoquinoline alkaloids and flavonols from *Ocotea vellosiana*. *Phytochemistry*, **39**: 815-816.

Gonçalves, N.B., Correa Filho, J.C., and Gottlieb, O.R. (1958). Analeptic Action of Anibine. *Nature*, **182**: 938-939.

Gottlieb, O.R. (1972). Chemosystematics of the Lauraceae. *Phytochemistry*, **11**: 1537-1570.

Henriques, A.T., Kerber, V.A., and Moreno, P.R.H. (1999). Alcalóides: Generalidades e aspectos básicos. In: Farmacognosia: da planta ao medicamento. Ed. By Simões, C.M.O. Ed. Universidade/UFRGS/Ed. da UFSC, Brasil, pp. 641-738.

Hoet, S., Stévigny, C., Block, S., Opperdoes, F., Colson, P., Baldeyrou, B., Lansiaux, A., Bailly, C. and Quentin-Leclercq, J. (2004). Alkaloids from *Cassytha filiformis* and related aporphines: Antitrypanosomal activity, cytotoxicity, and interaction with DNA and topoisomerases. *Planta Medica*, **70**: 407-413.

Hoffmann, J.J., Luzbetak, D.J., Torrance, S.J., and Cole, J.R. (1978). Cryptopleurine, cytotoxic agent from *Boehmeria caudata* (Urticaceae) and *Cryptocarya laevigata* (Lauraceae). *Phytochemistry*, **17**: 1448.

Houlihan, W.J. (1972). Indoles. Part One. *In:* The chemistry of heterocycle compounds: a series of monographs, Ed. By Weissberger, A., and Edward C. Taylor, Wiley-Interscience, USA, pp.1-587.

Jayasuriya,H., Herath, K.B., Ondeyka, J.G., Polishook, J.D., Bills, G.F., Dombrowski, A.W., Springer, M.S., Siciliano, S., Malkowitz, L., Sanchez, M., Guan, Z., Tiwari, S., Stevenson, D.W., Borris, R.P., and Singh, S.B. (2004). Isolation and structure of antagonists of chemokine receptor (CCR5). *Journal of Natural Products*, **67**: 1036-1038.

Johns, S. R.; Lamberton, John A.; Sioumis, A. A. (1969). Alkaloids of *Actinodaphne nitida* (Lauraceae). *Australian Journal of Chemistry*, **22**: 2257.

Johns, S.R., Lamberton, J.A., and Sioumis, A. A. (1966). *Cassytha* alkaloids. II. Alkaloids of *Cassytha pubescens*. *Australian Journal of Chemistry*, **19**: 2331-2338.

Kiang, A.K., and Sim, K.Y. (1967). Lindcarpine, an alkaloid from *Lindera pipericarpa* Boerl. (Lauraceae). *Journal of Chemical Society*, 282-283.

Klausmeyer, P., Chmurny, G.N., McCloud, T.G., Tucker, K.D., and Shoemaker, R.H. (2004). A novel antimicrobial indolizidinium alkaloid from *Aniba panurensis*. *Journal of Natural Products*, **67**: 1732-1735.

Lajis, N.H., Sharif, A.M., Kiew, R., Khan, M.N., and Samadi, Z. (1992). The alkaloids of *Lindera pipericarpa* Boerl (Lauraceae). *Pertanika*, **15**: 175-177.

Lamberton, J. A., and Vashist, V. N. (1972). Alkaloids of *Litsea leefeana* and *Cryptocarya foveolate* (Lauraceae). *Australian Journal of Chemistry*, **25**: 2737-2738.

Le Quesne, P.W., Larrahondo, J.E., and Raffauf, R.F. (1980). Antitumor plants. X. constituents of *Nectandra rigida*. *Journal of Natural Products*, **43**: 353-359.

Lebceuf, M., Cavé, A., Ranaivo, A., and Moskowitz, H. (1989). Cryptowolinol et cryptowolidine, nouveaux alcaloïdes de type dibenzopyrrocoline. *Canadian Journal of Chemistry*, **67**: 947-952.

Lebceuf, M., Ranaivo, A., Cavé, A., and Moskowitz, H. (1989). La velucryptine, nouvel alcaloïde isoquinoléique isolé de *Cryptocarya velutinosa*. *Journal of Natural Products*, **52**: 516-521.

Leboeuf, M., Cave, A., Provost, J., and Forgacs, P. (1979). Alkaloids from *Litsea laurifolia* (Jacq.) Cordemoy, Lauraceae. *Plantes Medicinales and Phytotherapie*, **13**: 262-267.

Lee, S.S., and Chen, C.H. (1993). Additional alkaloids from *Cryptocarya chinensis*. *Journal of Natural Products*, **56**: 227-232.

Lee, S.S., Lai, Y.C., Chen, C.K., Tseng, L.H., and Wang, C.Y. (2007). Characterization of isoquinolinealkaloids from *Neolitsea sericea* var. *aurata* by HPLC-SPE-NMR. *Journal of Natural Products*, **70**: 637-642.

Lee, S.S., Lin, Y.J., Chen, C.k., Liu, K.C.S., and Chen, C.H. (1993). Quaternary alkaloids from *Litsea cubeba* and *Cryptocarya konishii*. *Journal of Natural Products*, **56**: 1971-1976.

Lin, F.W., Wu, P.L., and WuT.S. (2001). Alkaloids from the leaves of *Cryptocarya chinensis* Hemsl. *Chemical and Pharmaceutical Bulletin*, **49**: 1292-1294.

Lin, F.W., Wang, J.J., and Wu, T.S. (2002). New pavine N-oxide alkaloids from the stem bark of *Cryptocarya chinensis* Hemsl. *Chemical and Pharmaceutical Bulletin*, **50**: 157-159.

Liu, M.T., Lin, S., Wang, Y.H., He, W.Y., Li, S., Wang, S.J., Yang, Y.C., and Shi, J.G. (2007). Two Novel Glycosidic Triterpene Alkaloids from the Stem Barks of *Machilus yaoshansis*. *Organic Letters*, **9**: 129-132.

Lu, S.T., and Lin, F.M. (1967). Alkaloids of Formosan lauraceous plants. XI. Alkaloids of *Litsea cubeba*. 2. *Yakugaku Zasshi*, **87**: 878-879.

Lu, S.T., and Su, T.L. (1973). Alkaloids of Formosan Lauraceous plants. XVII. Alkaloids of *Phoebe formosana*. *Journal of the Chinese Chemical Society*, **20**: 87-93.

Lu, S.T., and Wang, E.C. (1977). Studies on the alkaloids of Formosan Lauraceous plants. XXIII. Alkaloids of *Dehassia triandra* Merr. (1). Isolation of isocorydine and obaberine. *Taiwan Yaoxue Zazhi*, **29**: 49-53.

Marques, C.A. (2001). Importância econômica da família Lauraceae Lindl., *Floresta e Ambiente*, **8**: 195 – 206.

Morais, L.C.S.L., Barbosa-Filho, J.M. and Almeida, R.N. (1998). Central depressant effects of reticuline extracted from *Ocotea duckei* in rats and mice. *Journal of Ethnopharmacology*, **62**: 57-61.Mors, W.B., and Gottlieb, O.R. (1959). Anibine, the alkaloid of Coto bark. *Anais da Associação Brasileira de Química*, **18**: 185-187.

Mors, W.B., Magalhães, M.T., and Gottlieb, O.R. (1960). The chemistry of the genus Aniba. X. *Aniba fragrans* Ducke, a valid species. *Anais de Associação Brasileira de Química*, **19**: 193-197.

Mors, W.B.,Gottlieb, O. R., and Djerassi, C. (1957). The Chemistry of rosewood. Isolation and Structure of Anibine and 4-Methoxyparacotoin. *Journal of American Chemical Society*, **79**: 4507-4511.

Mukhtar, M.R., Martin, M.T., Domansky, M., Pais, M., Hadis, H., and Awang, K. (1997). Phoebegrandines A and B, proaporphine- tryptamine dimmers, from *Phoebe grandis*. *Phytochemistry*, **45**: 1543-1546.

Mukhtar, M.R., Hadi, A.H.A., Litaudon, M., and Awang, K. (2004). Morphinandienone alkaloids from *Dehaasia longipedicellata*. *Fitoterapia*, **75**: 792-794.

Mukhtar, M.R., Hadi, A.H.A., Rondeau, D., Richomme, P., Litaudon, M., Mustafa, M.R., and Awang, K. (2008). New proaporphines from the bark of *Phoebe scortechinii*. *Natural Product Research, Part A: Structure and Synthesis*, **22**: 921-926.

Nakasato, T., Asada, S., and Koezuka, Y. (1966). Alkaloids of Lauraceae plants. V. Alkaloids isolated from the trunk bark of *Neolitsea sericea*. *Yakugaku Zasshi*, **86**: 129-134.

Nguyen, V.H., and Nguyen, V.T. (2004). Aporphine alkaloids from *Phoebe chinensis* (Lauraceae) growing in Vietnam. *Tap Chi Hoa Hoc*, **42**: 205-209.

Oger, J.M., Duval, O., Richomme, P., Bruneton, J., Guinaudeau, H., and Fournet, A. (1992). (R)-(+)-noranicanine a new type of trioxygenated benzylisoquinoline isolation and synthesis. *Heterocycles*, **34**: 17-20.

Oger, J.M., Fardeau, A., Richomme, P., Guinaudeau, H., and Fournet, A. (1993). Nouveaux alcaloïdes isoquinoléiques isolés d'une Lauraceae bolivienne: *Aniba canelilla* H.B.K. *Canadian Journal of Chemistry*, **71**: 1128-1135.

Pabon, L.C., and Cuca, L.E. (2010). Aporphine alkaloids from *Ocotea macrophylla* (Lauraceae). *Quimica Nova*, **33**: 875-879.

Pech, B., and Bruneton, J. (1982). Alkaloids of *Laurus nobilis*. *Journal of Natural Products*, **45**: 560-563.

Rachmatiah, T., Mukhtar, M.R., Nafiah, M.A., Hanafi, M., Kosela, S., Morita, H., Litaudon, M., Awang, K., Omar, H., Hadi, A.H.A. (2009). (+)-N-(2-hydroxypropyl)lindcarpine: a new cytotoxic aporphine isolated from *Actinodaphne pruinosa* Nees. *Molecules*, **14**: 2850-2856.

Rastogi, R.C., and Borthakur, N. (1980). Alkaloids of *Litsea laeta* and *L. salicifolia*. *Phytochemistry*, **19**: 998-999.

Santos Filho, D., and Gilbert, B. (1975). The alkaloids of *Nectandra megapotamica*. *Phytochemistry*, **14**: 821-822.

Souza, V.C., and Lorenzi, H. (2005). Botânica sistemática: guia ilustrado para identificação das famílias de Angiospermas da flora brasileira, baseado em APG II. Instituto Plantarum, Nova Odessa.

Stermitz, F.R. (1983). Pentasubstituted aporphine alkaloids from *Phoebe molicella*. *Journal of Natural Products*, **46**: 913-916.

Stévigny, C., Block, S., De Pauw-Gillet, M.C., Hoffmann, E., Llabrés, G., Adjakidjé, V., and Quetin-Leclercq, J. (2002). Cytotoxic aporphine alkaloids from *Cassytha filiformis*. *Planta Medica*, **68**: 1042-1044.

Tsai, T.H., Wang, G.J., and Lin, L.C. (2008). Vasorelaxing alkaloids and flavonoids from *Cassytha filiformis*. *Journal of Natural Products*, **71**: 289-291.

Uprety, H., Bhakuni, D.S., and Dhar, M.M. (1972). Aporphine alkaloids of *Litsea sebifera*, *L. wightiana* and *Actinodaphne obovata*. *Phytochemistry*, **11**: 3057-3059.

Vecchietti, V., Casagrande, C., and Ferrari, G. (1974). Alkaloids of *Ocotea brachybotra*. *Farmaco, Edizione Scientifica*, **32**: 767-779.

Wu, T.S., and Lin, F.W. (2001). Alkaloids of the wood of *Cryptocarya chinensis*. *Journal of Natural Products*, **64**: 1404-1407.

Wu, Y.C., Chao, Y.C., Chang, F.R., and Chen, Y.Y. (1997). Alkaloids from *Cassytha filiformis*. *Phytochemistry*, **46**: 181-184.

Zanin, S.M.W., and Lordello, A.L.L. (2007). Alcalóides aporfinóides do gênero *Ocotea* (Lauraceae), *Quimica Nova*, **30**: 92-98.

Zhang, C., Nakamura, N., Tewtrakul, S., Hattori, M., Sun, Q., Wang, Z., and Fujiwara, T. (2002). Sesquiterpenes and alkaloids from *Lindera chunii* and their inhibitory activities aginst HIV-1 integrase. *Chemical and Pharmaceutical Bulletin*, **50**: 1195-1200.

Zhao, Q.Z., Zhao, Y.M., and Wang, K.J. (2005). Alkaloids from the root of *Lindera angustifolia*. *Yao Xue Xue Bao*, **40**: 931-934.

Bioactive Phytochemicals: Perspectives for Modern Medicine Vol. 1 (2012) *Pages* **437–455**
Editor: **V.K. Gupta**
Published by: **DAYA PUBLISHING HOUSE, NEW DELHI**

13

Phytochemical and Pharmacological Profile of *Lepidium sativum* Linn.

Alok Shukla[1], C.S. Singh[1] and Papiya Bigoniya[1*]

ABSTRACT

The demand of the herbs over the last decades is increasing gradually with both medicinal and economic implications. Widespread use of herbs throughout the globe has raised the attention of scientist towards standardization of herbal for its quality, safety and efficacy parameters. So, accurate scientific study has become a prerequisite for acceptance of herbal health claims. Lepidium sativum Linn. (Cruciferae) commonly known as Asaliyo, is an erect, glabrous annual herb cultivated as a salad plant throughout India, Europe and United States. Its therapeutic importance has been recognized in different system of traditional (Ayurveda, Unani, Sidha and Homeopathy) and modern medicine for the treatment of different diseases and ailments. The plant possesses the multitude of chemical compounds like flavonoids, coumarins, sulphur glycosides (glucosinolates), triterpines, sterols and alkaloids (lepidine). These compounds are responsible for exerting the medicinal properties such as bronchodilatory, chemoprotective, hypoglycemic, cardiovascular, diuretic and hepatoprotective. It has been reported to have antioxident, antihypertensive, abortifacient, insecticidal, skeletal muscle stimulant as well as oral contraceptive properties. This review is a compilation of botanical, phytochemical, nutritional, ethnopharmacological and pharmacological arrays of commonly and abundantly used plant Lepidium sativum for medicinal and food purposes.

Keywords: Brassicaceae, Hypoglycaemic, *Lepidium sativum*, Lepidine, Sulphur glycosides.

1 Radharaman College of Pharmacy, Fatehpur Dobra, Ratibad, Bhopal – 462 002, M.P. India.

* *Corresponding author*: E-mail: p_bigoniya2@hotmail.com

Introduction

Nature always stands as a golden mark to exemplify the outstanding phenomena of symbiosis. In the western world, as the people are becoming aware of the potency and side effect of synthetic drugs, there is an increasing interest in the natural product remedies with a basic approach towards the nature. Natural products from plant, animal and minerals have been the basis of the treatment of human disease. In developing countries about 80 per cent of population still depends on traditional medicine. Alternative medicine is the need of the time. Herbal medicines are currently in demand and their popularity is increasing day by day (Kirtikar and Basu, 2006).

Lepidium sativum Linn (Cruciferae) commonly known as Asaliyo, is an erect, glabrous annual herb cultivated as a salad plant throughout India, Europe and United States. It is an important medicinal plant since the Vedic era (Anonymous, 1962). The genus *Lepidium* comprises several species growing in most temperate warm climate. Some species of *Lepidium* are used as salad and the pods are sometimes used as food. Several plants of this family are used as antidiabetic (Edddouks *et al.*, 2005), antifungal, anticancer, antirheumatic. The leaves are antiscorbutic, diuretic and stimulant (Uphof, 1959; Chopra *et al.*, 1986). Seeds are bitter, thermogenic, depurative, galactagogue, emmenagogue, tonic, aphrodisiac, ophthalmic and diuretic. It is useful in leprosy, skin diseases, dysentery, diarrhoea, dyspepsia, eye diseases, leucorrhoea, scurvy, asthma, cough and cold, seminal weakness and also used as aperient, tonic, demulcent, carminative and ruvegacient (Khory, 1999). The polutice of seed is applied for hurt and sprains and for bronchial ashthama (Annonymous, 1962). The plant also shows teratogenic effect (Nath *et al.*, 1992) and antiovulatory properties (Sharief *et al.*, 2004). The root is used in the treatment of secondary syphilis and tenesmus. Preliminery phytochemical study of *L. sativum* showed that it contains flavonoids, coumarins, sulphur glycosides, triterpeines, sterols and alkaloids (Afaf *et al.*, 2008). Four glucosinolates isolated from *L. sativum* are glucotropaelin, gluconapin, gluconasturtin and glucobrassicanapin. Isolation of 4-methoxy glucobrassin was reported from the seeds of the plant (Radwan *et al.*, 2007). *Lepidium sativum* used in folk medicine for antidiabetic and antibacterial property due to the presence of benzyl isothiacyanates (Mennicke *et al.*, 1988).

Family Brassicaceae

Brassicaceae or Cruciferae, also known as the Crucifers. The name Brassicaceae is derived from the genus Brassica. Cruciferae is an older name, it means "cross-bearing" because the four petals of their flowers are reminiscent of a cross. According to ICBN Art. 18.5 (Vienna Code) both Cruciferae and Brassicaceae are regarded as validly published, and are thus accepted as names for the family. The family is included in Brassicales according to the APG system. Older systems (*e.g.*, Arthur Cronquist's) placed them into the Capparales, a now defunct order which had a similar definition. A close relationship has long been acknowledged between Brassicaceae and the Caper family, because members of both groups produce glucosinolate (mustard oil) compounds. Recent research suggests that Capparaceae as traditionally circumscribed are paraphyletic with respect to Brassicaceae, with Cleome and several related genera being more closely related to Brassicaceae than to other Capparaceae. The APG II system therefore has merged the two families under the name Brassicaceae (Cherepnov *et al.,* 1995). Brassicaceae is one of the largest plant families consisting of about 330 genera and about 3,700 species. The largest genera are Draba (365 species), Cardamine (200 species, but its definition is controversial), Erysimum (225 species), Lepidium (230 species) and Alyssum (195 specieps), (Klaus *et al.,* 2009; Grossgeim, 1950).

Herbs are annual, biennial or perennial, sometimes sub shrubs or shrubs, with a pungent, watery juice. Trichomes are glandular, unicellular, simple, stalked or sessile, two to many forked, stellate, dendritic, or malpighiaceous rarely peltate and scale like. Glandular trichomes are multicellular with uniseriate or multiseriate stalk. Stems are erect, ascending or prostrate, sometimes absent. Leaves are simple, entire or variously pinnately dissected rarely trifoliolate or pinnately, palmately, or bipinnately. In basal leaf rosette may present or absent. Cauline leaves are almost alternate rarely opposite or whorled, petiolate or sessile and sometimes absent.

Inflorescence bracteate or ebracteate racemes, corymbs, or panicles, sometimes flowers are solitary on long pedicels originating from axils of rosette leaves. Flowers are hypogynous, mostly actinomorphic. Sepals are 4 (in 2 decussate pairs), free or rarely united, not saccate or lateral (inner) pair saccate. Petals are 4 alternate with sepals, arranged in the form of a cross rarely rudimentary or absent. Stamens are 6, in 2 whorls, tetradynamous rarely equal or in 3 pairs of unequal length, sometimes stamens are 2 or 4, very rarely 8-24.

Fruit are typically a 2-valved capsule, generally termed silique (siliqua) when length 3 times or more than width, or silicle (silicula) when length less than 3 times of width, dehiscent or indehiscent. Sometimes the fruits are schizocarpic, nutlet like, lomentaceous, or samaroid, segmented or terete, angled, or flattened parallel to septum or at a right angle to septum (angustiseptate), replum (persistent placenta) rounded, rarely flattened or winged; septum complete, perforated, reduced to a rim, or lacking; style 1, distinct, obsolete, or absent; stigma capitate or conical, entire or 2-lobed, sometimes lobes decurrent and free or connate. Seeds without endosperm are uniseriately or biseriately arranged in each locule, Wetted seeds are mucilaginous, cotyledons incumbent (embryo notorrhizal, radicle lying along back of 1 cotyledon), accumbent (embryo pleurorrhizal: radicle applied to margins of both cotyledons), or conduplicate (embryo orthoplocal: cotyledons folded longitudinally around radicle), rarely spirally coiled (embryo spirolobal). Germination of seeds is epigeal (Dorofeev, 1998; Dorofeev, 2002).

Genus Lepidium

Herbs are annual, biennial or perennial, sometimes subshrubs, rarely shrubs or climbers. Trichomes are absent or simple. Stems are erect or ascending, sometimes creeping, simple or branched basally and/or apically. Basal leaves are rosulate or simple, entire or pinnately dissected. Cauline leaves are petiolate or sessile, base cuneate, attenuate, auriculate, sagittate, or amplexicaul, margin entire, dentate, or dissected. Racemes are ebracteate, corymbose or elongated. Fruiting pedicels are terete, flattened or winged, erect or divaricate. Sepals are ovate or oblong, rarely orbicular, base of lateral pair are not saccate. Petals are white, yellow or pink, erect or spreading, sometimes rudimentary or absent. Stamens are 2 and median, sometimes 6 and tetradynamous or sub equal in length, rarely 4 and all median or 2 median and 2 laterals. Anthers are ovate or oblong. Fruits are dehiscent silicles, oblong, ovate, obovate, cordate, obcordate, elliptic or orbicular, strongly angustiseptate (Kirtikar and Basu, 2004; Harkevitch, 1988). Five species commonly occur in India of which*L. sativum* is widely cultivated. In India *L. draba, L. latifolium, L. sativum, L. iberis, L. perfoliatum* and *L. ruderale* are also found (Anonymous, 1962).

Unambiguous Synonyms

Lepidium sativum L., *Nasturtium sativum*

Vernacular Name

Language	*Name*
English:	Garden cress, Garden pepperwort, Gardencress pepperweed
Hindi:	Aselio, Halim
Sanskrit:	Chandrika, Raktabija
Punjabi:	Halon, Tezak
Marathi:	Alhiv, Aliv
Bengali:	Halim-Shak
Gujarati:	Asaliya
Assamese:	Halim-Shak
Oriya:	Hidamba Saga
Tamil:	Ali
Kannada:	Allibija, Kurthike
Urdu:	Halim
Arabic:	Rashad, Thuffa, Hurf

Taxonomical Classification

Domain:	*Eukaryota*
Kingdom:	*Plantae*
Subkingdom:	*Viridaeplantae*
Phylum:	*Tracheophyta*
Subphylum:	*Euphyllophytina*
Infraphylum:	*Radiatopses*
Class:	*Magnoliopsida*
Subclass:	*Dilleniidae*
Superorder:	*Violanae*
Order:	*Capparales*

Suborder:	*Capparineae*
Family:	*Brassicaceae*
Genus:	*Lepidium*
Specific epithet:	*sativum*
Botanical name:	*Lepidium sativum*

Botanical Description

Common cress (*L. sativum*), with regard to the anatomy of the leaf, stem and root, has been divided into three botanical varieties: *vulgare*, *crispum* and *latifolium*. The latter is the most mesomorphic, *crispum* the most xeromorphic and *vulgare* intermediate. Cress is an annual, erect herbaceous, allogamous plant with self-compatible and self-incompatible forms and with various degrees of tolerance to prolonged autogamy, growing up to 50 cm. There are diploid forms, $2n = 2\times=16$, and tetraploid forms, $2n=4\times=32$. The basal leaves have long petioles and are lyrate-pinnatipartite; the caulinar leaves are laciniate-pinnate while the upper leaves are entire (Figure 13.1). Upper leaves are linear, full and acute. Bottom leaves are irregularly pinnatisect or bipinnatisect and ovate. The inflorescences are in dense racemes, a degree of variability is noted in the character of the basal leaves which are cleft or split to a greater or lesser degree, a character which is controlled by a single incompletely dominant gene. The stem is solitary, upright, paniculate, with straight branches.

The flowers are strongly elongated, loose, usually with an absolutely bare rachis with white or slightly pink petals, measuring 2 mm. Pedicels are cylindrical, bare, one half to three quarters the length of a silicle. Silicles are elliptical, elate from the upper half, glabrous orbicular-oval, emarginate, winged from the middle or lowermost third to the top, 5-6 mm in length and 4 mm in width. The pods are obovate or broadly ellipticrotundate, emarginated (occasionally with 3 valves), slightly but thickly winged above (Kirtikar and Basu, 2004). The seeds are reddish in colour, oblong, somewhat angular and curved slightly on one side, surface rugous (Figure 13.2). Near the point of attachment there is a white scar, from which a small channel extends to 1/3 the length of the seeds. Seeds are odorless and taste is pungent and mucilaginous. (Kory, 1999). Cress flowers in the wild state between March and June. Blossoms in April/May and bears fruit in June/August.

Geographical Distribution

The genus *Lepidium* is distributed throughout almost all temperate and subtropical regions of the world. The general distribution area includes Egypt, Ethiopia, Afghanistan, Iran, Israel, Jordan, Lebanon, Syria, Turkey, Mesopotamia, Palestine and India (Punjab and the Western Himalayas). The species also occurs in the Southern and Middle European part up to the Upper Dnieper and Upper Volga areas, Crimea and Caucasus (Tsvelev, 2000).

Traditional Uses

All parts of the herb are used medicinally. The herb is commonly used in many parts for the treatment of asthma, cough with expectoration, bleeding piles and

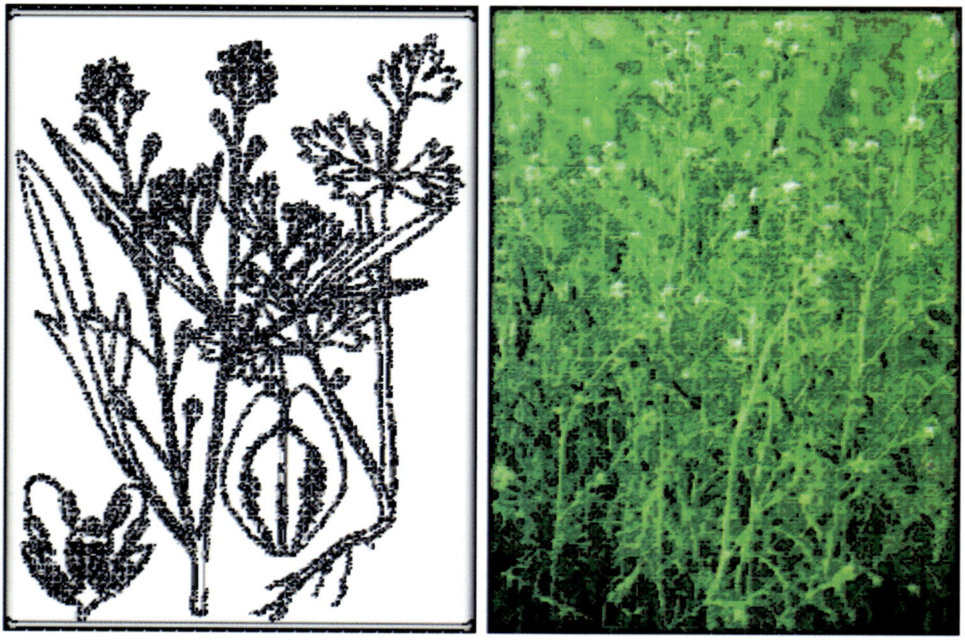

Figure 13.1: Photograph of *L. sativum* plant.

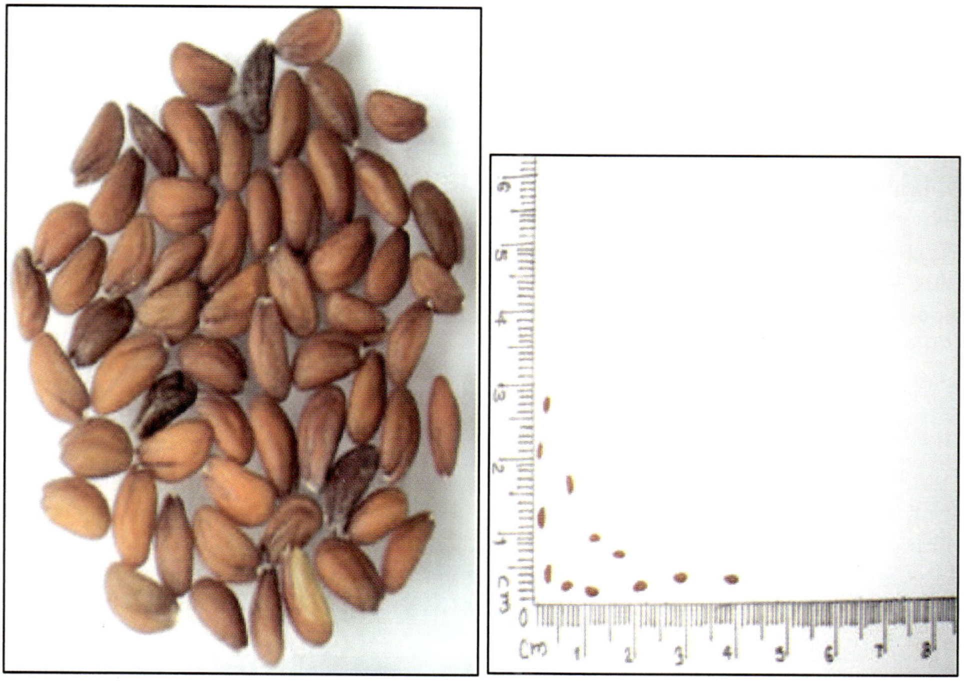

Figure 13.2: Photograph of *L. sativum* seeds.

scroulous diseases. The leaves are stimulant and diuretic, made into a salad and they are commonly eaten with great benefit by those suffering from scorbutic diseases. The seeds have tonic, alternative, aphrodisiac, stimulant and aperients properties. They are effective in hiccough, dysentery, diarrhea and skin diseases caused by impurity of blood. They are also recommended in enlargement of spleen and as galactogogue. They are given either as decoction, one in twenty or as a cold infusion, one in ten. Coarsely powdered seeds mixed with sugar are equally effective for the treatment of indigestion, dysentery and diarrhea. Seeds boiled with milk are given as an abortifacient. A poultice of the bruised seeds made with lime juice is applied for relief of internal inflammation and rheumatic pain. The roots are used in secondary syphilis tenesmus (Annonymous, 1962).

Phytochemistry

Analysis of leaves have the following compositions: water 82.3 per cent, protein 5.8 per cent, fat 1.0 per cent, carbohydrate 8.7 per cent, mineral matter 2.2 per cent, calcium 0.36 per cent and phosphorus 0.11 per cent. Trace elements are iron (28.6 mg/100g), nickel (40 μg/kg), cobalt (12 μg/kg) and iodine (110 μg/kg). Vitamins present are vitamin A 2970 i.u., thiamine 0.11 mg/100g, riboflavin 0.17 mg/100g, niacin 1.0 mg/100g and ascorbic acid 87 mg/100 g. Cooked leaves contain: vitamin A 3300 i.u., thiamine 70 μg/100g, riboflavin 0.15 mg/100g, niacin 0.8 mg/100g and ascorbic acid 39mg/100g.

On steam distillation the plant yields 0.115 per cent of a colorless volatile oil with a pungent odour, containing variable proportions of benzyl isothiocynate and benzyl cyanide. Analysis of cress seeds reveals the following values: moisture 5.69 per cent, protein 23.5 per cent, fat 15.91 per cent, ash 5.7 per cent, phosphorous 1.65 per cent, calcium 0.31 per cent and sulphur 0.9 per cent.

The seeds contain an alkaloid (0.19 per cent), glcotropaeolin, sinapin, sinapic acid, mucilaginous matter (5 per cent) and uric acid (Figure 13.3). The seeds yield up to 25.5 per cent of a yellowish brown semi drying oil with a peculiar disagreeable odour. The oil has the following characteristics sp.gr $^{33°}$ 0.909, n$^{31°}$ 1.4695, acid value 0.96, saponification value 185.0, iodine value 131.4 and unsaponification matter 1.8 per cent. The percentage of saturated and unsaturated acids in the oil is as follows: palmitic 1.27 per cent, stearic 6.01 per cent, arachidic 1.54 per cent, behenic 1.73 per cent, lignoceric 0.2 per cent, oleic 61.25 per cent and linolenic 28.0 per cent. The unsaponifiable matter contains β-sitosterol and α-tocopherol (1830 μg/g oil). The seed mucilage consists of a mixture of cellulose (18.3 per cent) and uronic acid containing polysaccharide (Anonymous, 1962).

Alexander *et al.* (1976) reported the presence of eleven components in volatile part of garden cress. In which eight were identified, all are glucosinolate degradation products (isothiocyanates and nitriles). Benzyl derivatives from glucotropaeolin were the most abundant but thiocynates were absent (Figure 11.3).

A new alkaloid lepidine was isolated from the seeds along with sinapic acid ethyl ester, it was characterized as N, N′- dibenzylthiourea and N, N′- dibenzylurea. 5,4′- dihydroxy- 7,8,3′,5′- tetramethoxyflavone. Two new isomeric flavones 5,3′-

dihydroxy- 7,8,4′- tetramethoxyflavanone and 5,3′- dihydroxy-6,7,4′-trimethoxyflavanone were also isolated and their structure determination and confirmation done by synthesis (Rastogi *et al.*, 1998). The seeds of *L. sativum* afforded five new dimeric imidazole alkaloids lepidine B, C, D, E and F in addition to the known imidazole alkaloids. Lepidine and two new monomeric imidazole alkaloids semilepidinoside A and B were identified and their structures were elucidated on the basis of spectroscopic evidence (Maier *et al.*, 1998).

The seeds of *L. sativum* were found to contain allyl, 2- phenethyl and benzyl glucosinolates. The effect of temperature, pH of the extraction medium and the length of time allowed for autolysis were assessed on the benzyl glucosinolate degradation

Figure 13.3: Isolated compounds of *Lepidium sativum.*

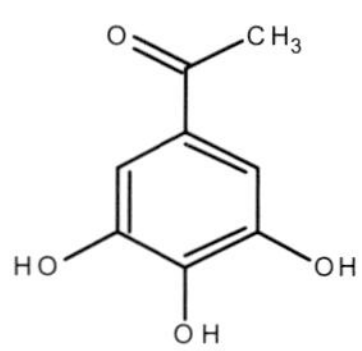

Gallic acid

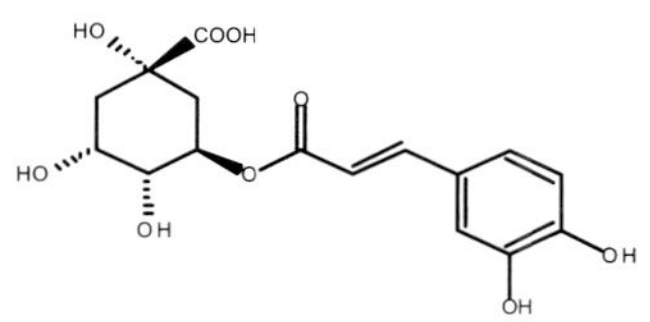

Chlorogenic acid

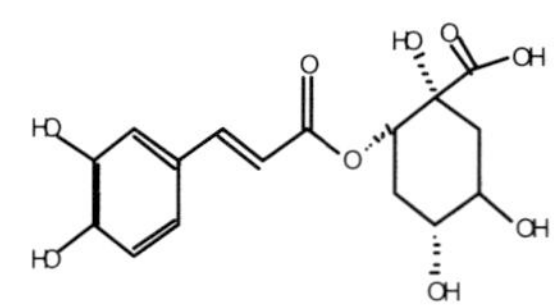

Neochlorogenic acid

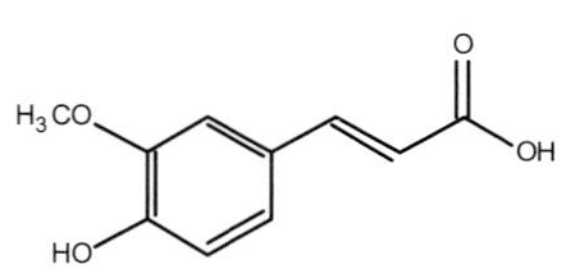

Ferulic acid

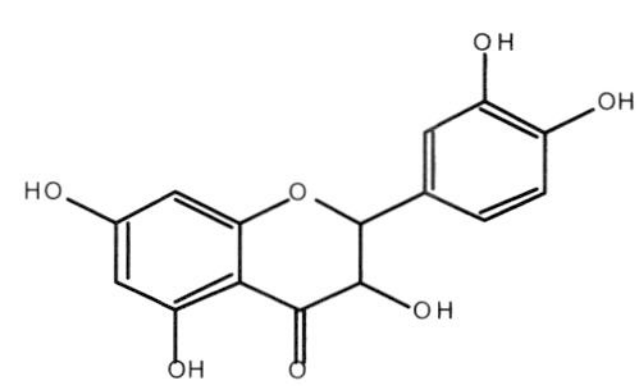

Dihydroquerceti n

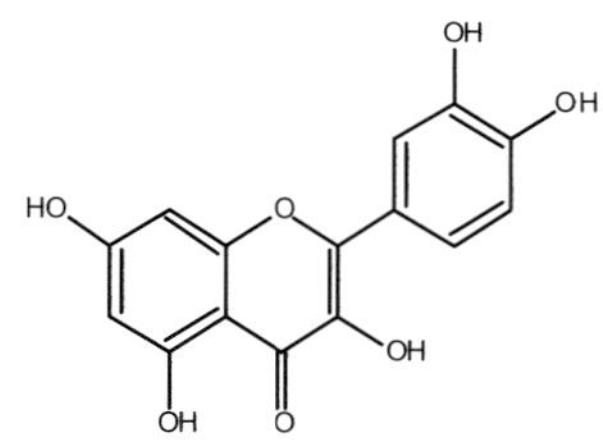

Quercetin

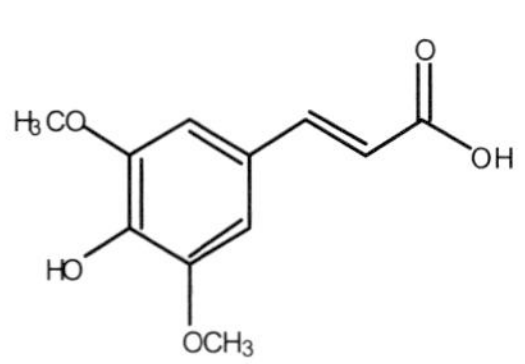

Sinapic acid

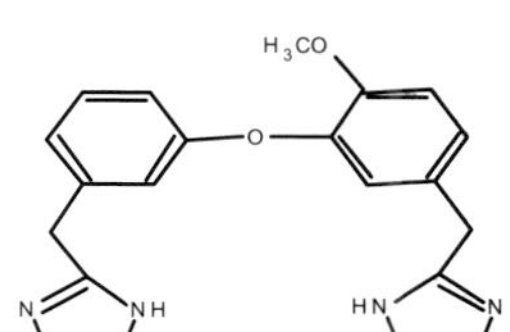

Lepidine

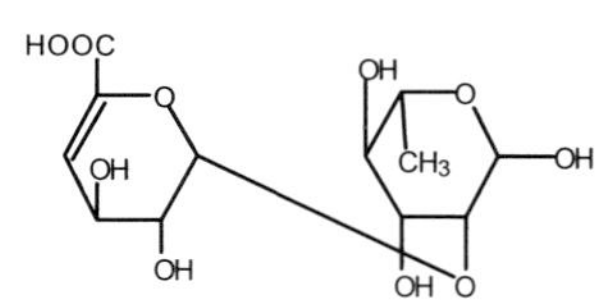

Lepidimoide

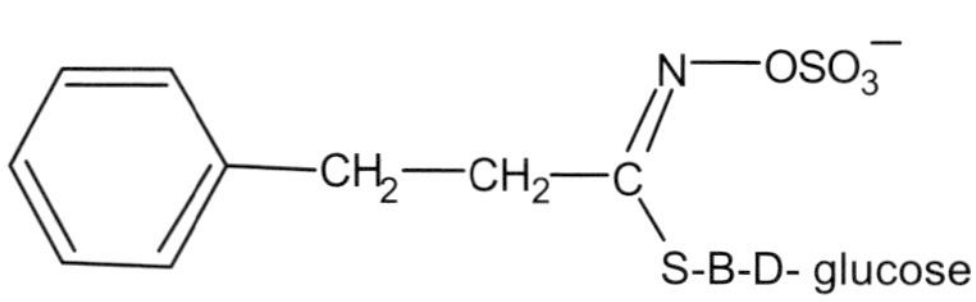

2-phenyl ethyl glucosinolate (Gluconasturiin)

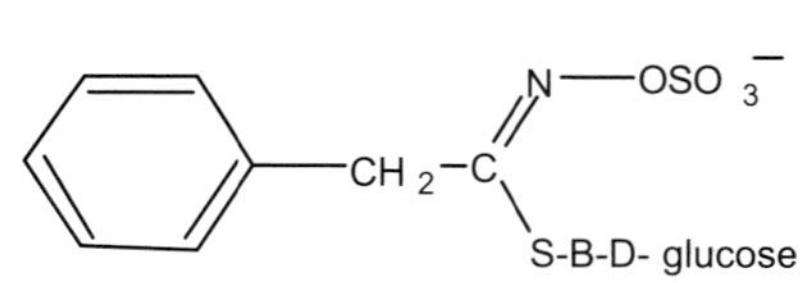

Glucotropaeolin

Contd...

Figure 13.3–*Contd...*

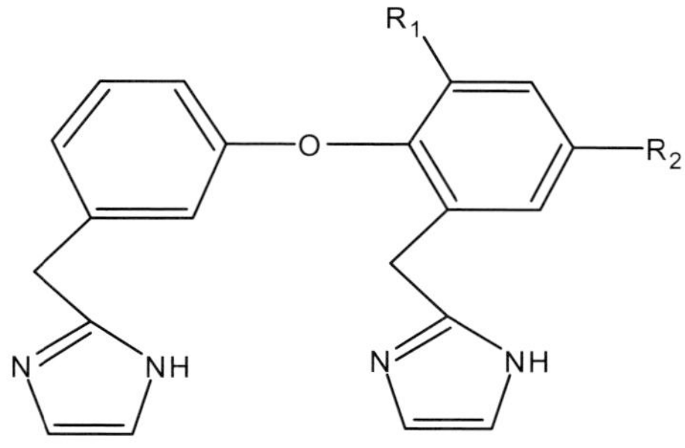

	R_1	R_2
Lepidine A	OCH_3	H
Lepidine B	OH	H
Lepidine C	H	OCH_3
Lepidine D	H	OH

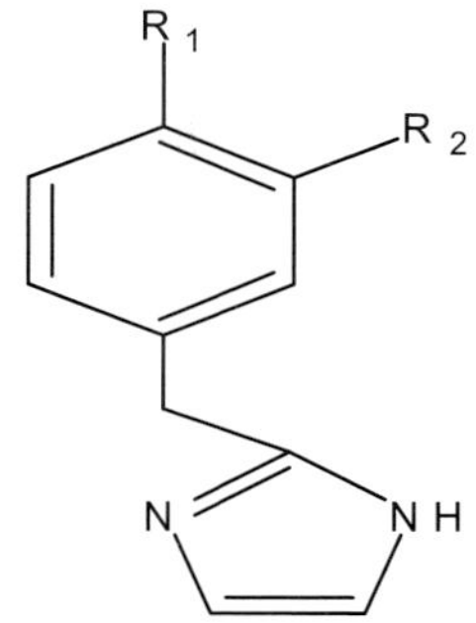

	R_1	R_2
Semilepidine	OH	H
Semilepidine	OH	OCH_3

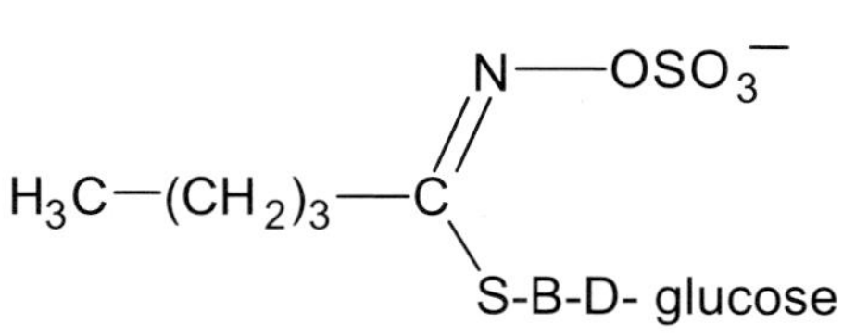

Glucobenzosisbbrin

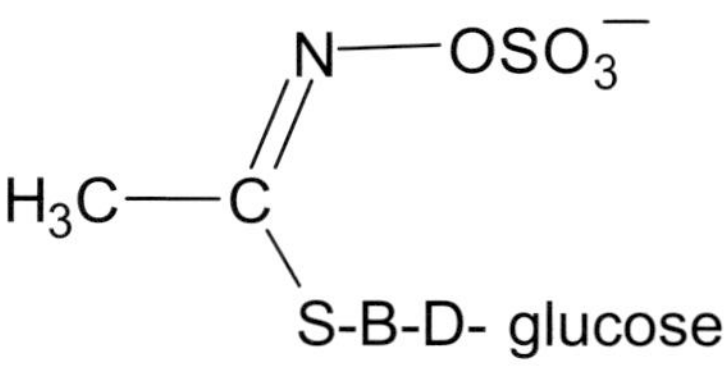

Methyl glucosinolate (Glucocapprin)

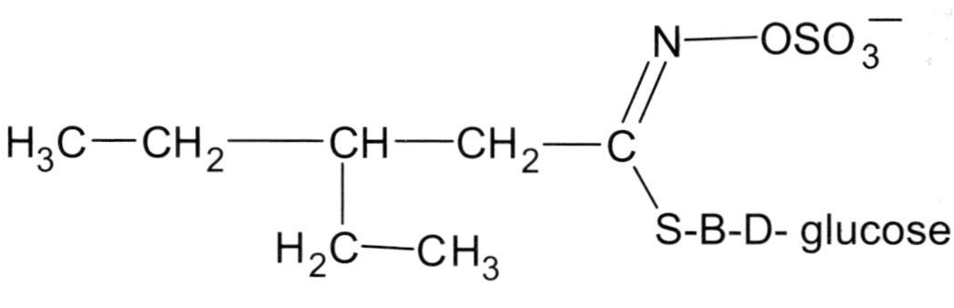

2- ethyl butyl glucosinolate

products in seed extracts. Benzyl thiocynate was not produced at higher temperatures but at ambient and lower temperatures it exceeded isothiocyanate. Five new possible benzyl glucosinolate degradation products were detected and evidence supports that benzaldehyde and benzyl alcohol could be secondary products formed thermally from isothiocyanate and thiocynate respectively. Benzyl mercaptan and benzyl methyl sulphide also appeared to be produced thermally (Gil *et al.*, 1980).

A lectin was isolated from extract of seeds of *L. sativum* by affinity chromatography on human immunoglobulin-Sepharose. As reported by Ziska *et al.* (1982) the lectin reacts with human erythrocytes without specificity for the A, B and O blood group constituents.

A new allelopathic substance that promoted the shoot growth of different plant species but inhibited the root growth was isolated as an amorphous powder from mucilage of germinated cress (*Lepidium sativum* L.) seeds. This substance was identified as sodium 2-O-rhamnopyranosyl-4-deoxy-threo-hex-4-enopyranosiduronate (Hasegawa *et al.*, 1992).

Radwan *et al.* (2007) investigated biological activity of *L. sativum* grown in Egypt. The study of the glucosinolate contents of *L. sativum* seeds revealed the isolation and identification of glucotropaeolin and 2-phenyl ethyl glucosinolate while the study of the glucosinolates contents of fresh herb revealed the presence of 2-ethyl butyl glucosinolates, methyl glucosinolate, butyl glucosinolate and glucotropaeolin. The identification of the isolated glucosinolates was substantiated through different chemical and spectroscopic determinations.

Orlovskaya *et al.* (2007) reported the carbohydrate and phenolic compounds from seeds of *L. sativum*. The water soluble polysaccharides (5.44 per cent), pectinic substances (2.74 per cent) and hemicelluloses (4.58 per cent) were determined by chromatographic technique. The qualitative composition of the phenolic compounds from *L. sativum* seed extract (70 per cent ethanol) was studied by HPLC. The mobile phase $CH_3OH:H_2O:H_3PO_4$ (400:600:5) was eluted at a flow rate of 0.5 ml/min in room temperature for 120 min at 254 nm. A total of 12 compounds were isolated from seeds. Gallic acid (9.44 per cent), chlorogenic acid (14.77 per cent), ferulic acid (5.63 per cent), neochlorogenic acid (2.22 per cent), luteolin-7-glucoside (14.67 per cent), dihydroquercetin (4.37 per cent) and quercetin (3.15 per cent) were identified. The contents of total phenolic compounds calculated as chlorogenic acid in *L. sativum* seeds were 0.85 per cent.

A qualitative and quantitative analysis method was established by Nayak *et al.* (2009) to improve quality assessment standards for *L. sativum* seeds. The sinapic acid was identified by comparing with standards and quantified simultaneously by high performance thin layer chromatography (HPTLC). HPTLC of *L. sativum* methanolic extract was performed on Silica gel $60F_{254}$ [20 cm ×10 cm] plates with butanol:acetic acid:water (4:1:5) as mobile phase. Quantitative evaluation of the plate was performed in the absorbance- reflectance mode at 326nm. The sinapic acid was separated on thin layer of silica gel and determined by HPTLC- photo densiometry. They concluded that this method can be used for identification and quantitative determination of sinapic acid in *L. sativum*.

Pharmacology (Table 13.1)

Cardiovascular and Respiratory Effect

Vohra *et al.* (1977) reported marked rise in blood pressure (40-80 mmHg, 5-15 min) of anesthetized cats with ethanolic extract of seeds of *L. sativum* (10-20 mg/kg, i.v.). The hypertensive effect was associated with slight respiratory stimulation but this effect was transient duration (0.5-1 min). It was further observed that the activity gradually decreased if the emulsion was stored even under refrigeration. The extract did not potentiate or depress the pressor responses of adrenaline (2 μg/kg, i.v.) and carotid occlusion (45 seconds). The hypertensive effect of the extract was completely blocked by pre- treatment of the animals with 5 mg/kg, i. v., priscoline. ECG record of anesthetized cats exhibited rhythm disturbances, inversion of T- wave and QRS-complex. The cardio stimulant action was also observed on isolated rabbit auricled (0.5-1.0 mg/ml). It was noted that the effect progressively diminished on repeated additions of the axtracts. However, if the interval between the two is more than 30 min, tachyphlaxis was not observed. On isolated perfused frog heart preparation, the extract (2-20 mg spot doses) caused cardiac arrest in diastole for 30 sec; the rate and force returned to normal after this period.

Table 13.1: Biological activity of *L. sativum.*

Part Used	*Extract*	*Activity*	*Reference*
Seeds	Aqueous extract	Tachyphylaxis	Vohora *et al.*, 1977
Seeds	Aqueous extract	Abortifacient activity	Nath *et al.*, 1992
Seeds	Ethanolic extract	Analgesic, antipyretic and anti-inflammatory activity	Al-Yaha *et al.*, 1994
Arial part	Juice	Chemoprotective activity	Kassie *et al.*, 2002
Seeds	Seeds powder	Oral contraceptive activity	Sharief *et al.*, 2004
Seeds	Aqueous extract	Hypoglycaemic activity	Eddouks *et al.*, 2005
Seeds	Aqueous extract	Antihypertensive and diuretic activity	Maghrani *et al.*, 2005; Patel *et al.*, 2009
Seeds	Ethanolic extract	Insecticidal activity	Radwan *et al.*, 2007
Seeds	Seeds powder	Fracture healing activity	Juma, 2007
Seeds	Methanolic extract	Hepatoprotective activity	Afaf *et al.*, 2008
Seeds	Ethanolic extract	Bronchodilatory activity	Mali *et al.*, 2008
Seeds	Powder	Antiasthamatic activity	Archana *et al.*, 2006
Seeds	Aqueous extract	Nephroprotective activity	Shinde *et al.*, 2010
Seeds	Methanolic extract	Antibacterial activity	Gupta *et al.*, 2010

Smooth and Skeletal Muscles

The ethanolic extract (1-5 mg/ml) elicited no significant response on smooth muscles (rat ileum and rat uterus). The ethanolic extract (2-5 mg/ml) showed contractile action on frog rectus abdominis muscle, in a matching assay with equipotent concentrations (per ml of bathing solution) of acetylcholine.

General Behavioral/Toxic Effects

Vohra *et al.* (1977) studied the general behavior and toxic effects of *L. sativum* seed extract in mice. The extract was given in doses of 100, 200, 500, 750 and 1000 mg/kg, i.p. The injected mice were observed continuously for 1 hr and intermittently for further 3 hrs. None of the mice showed any gross behavioral effects and there was no mortality upto a 48 hrs period of observation signifying its non-toxic effect.

A perusal of the results of those experiments shows cardiac and skeletal muscle stimulant actions in the ethanolic extract of the seeds of *L. sativum*. Evidence suggests the presence of a cardio-active substance in the extract. The substance appeared to be unstable in solution, showed tachyphylaxis and probably exerts its actions through adrenergic mechanism.

Abortifacient Activity

The aqueous extracts of *L. sativum* seeds were orally administered to rats in 125, 175, 250, 270 and 350 mg/kg dose. Total number of fetuses total number of live fetuses, total number of dead fetuses/total number of early/late resorptions, body weight (gm) of each foetus and body length crown to rump (cm) of each foetus were noted. The abortifacient activity of *L. sativum* seed extract was found below 50 per cent as reported by Nath *et al.* (1992).

Analgesic and Anti-inflammatory Activity

Al-Yaha *et al.* (1994) studied anti-inflammatory, antipyretic and analgesic activity of ethanolic extract of *L. sativum* seeds. The extract significantly inhibited carrageenan-induced paw edema and reduced the yeast-induced hyperpyrexia. It also prolonged the reaction time of mice on the hot plate. The extract exacerbated indomethacin-induced gastric mucosal damage. The coagulation studies showed a significant increase in fibrinogen level and an insignificant decrease in prothrombin time, conforming its coagulating property. The toxicity test showed that the administration of extract in single dose of 0.5 to 3.0 gm/kg did not produce any adverse effects or mortality in mice, whereas the animals treated with extract (100 mg/kg/day) for a period of 3 months in drinking water showed no symptom of toxicity. The seeds of *L. sativum* possess significant anti-inflammatory, antipyretic, analgesic and coagulant activities, and are free from serious side or toxic effects.

Chemoprotective Effects

The chemoprotective effects of *L. sativum* juices towards benzo(a)pyrene B(a)P-induced DNA damage using the single cell gel electrophoresis (SCGE)/Hep G2 test system was reported by Kassie *et al.* (2003). Contrary to the results with the juices, unexpected synergistic effects were observed with benzyl isothiocyanate (BITC, 0.6 μM), a breakdown product of glucotropaeolin contained abundantly in garden cress. Although these concentrations of benzyl isothiocyanate did not cause DNA damage per se, at higher concentrations (> or = 2.5 μM), the compound caused a pronounced dose-dependent DNA damage by itself. With phenethyl isothiocyanate (PEITC), the breakdown product of gluconasturtin contained in water cress, no synergistic effects with B(a)P were seen; however, significant induction of DNA damage was observed when the cells were exposed to the pure compound at concentrations > or = 5 μM. In experiments with (+/-)-anti-benzo(a)pyrene-7,8-dihydrodiol-9,10-epoxide (BPDE, 5.0 μM), the ultimate genotoxic metabolite of B(a)P, and the juices, only moderate protective effects were seen indicating that detoxification of BPDE is not the main mechanism behind the protective effect of the juices against B(a)P-induced DNA damage.

The chemoprotective effect of *L. sativum* and its constituents, glucotropaeolin and benzylisothiocyanate, a breakdown product of glucotropaeolin was investigated towards 2-amino-3-methyl-imidazo [4,5-f] quinoline (IQ)-induced genotoxic effects and colonic preneoplastic lesions. Pretreatment of F344 rats with either fresh*L. sativum* juice (0.8 ml), glucotropaeolin (150 mg/kg) or benzylisothiocyanate (70 mg/kg) for three consecutive days caused a significant reduction in IQ (90 mg/kg, 0.2 ml corn oil/animal)-induced DNA damage in colon and liver cells in the range of 75-92 per cent. Chemical analysis of *L. sativum* juice showed that benzylisothiocyanate does not account for the effects of the juice as its concentration in the juice was found to be 1000-fold lower than the dose required to cause a chemoprotective effect. Parallel to the chemoprotection experiments, the modulation of the activities of cytochrome P4501A2, glutathione-S-transferase (GST) and UDP glucuronosyltransferase (UDPGT) by *L. sativum* juice, glucotropaeolin and benzylisothiocyanate was studied. *L. sativum* juice caused a significant increase in the activity of hepatic UDPGT-2. In the Aberrant erypt foci assay, IQ was administered by gavages on 10 alternating days in corn oil (100 mg/kg). Five days before and during IQ treatment, subgroups received drinking water which contained 5 per cent cress juice. The total number of IQ-induced aberrant crypts and ACF as well as ACF with crypt multiplicity of > or =4 were reduced significantly in the IQ plus *L. sativum* juice group (Kassie *et al.*, 2002).

Oral Contraceptive

L. sativum seeds possess oral contraceptive activity as reported by Sharief *et al.* (2004). In the study, thirty two female mice were divided randomly into two groups. Sixteen mice of one group were fed for one week on a standard diet containing *L. sativum* seeds. Throughout the experiment, each four female mice were transferred and caged with two males for seventeen hours. Then, female mice were isolated in the cages alone for experimental feeding. The other group of sixteen female mice was fed on standard diet only and left with a male mice as a control. The rate of contraception was (100 per cent) in female mice in the treated group. In which, each mice received one gm/day of oral dose *Lepidium sativum* seeds. The pregnancy rate for the control group was 100 per cent. However interruption of oral dose for the same female mice was recovered with the ability for 80 per cent pregnancy.

Hypoglycaemic Effect

The hypoglycaemic effect of *L. sativum* seeds aqueous extract was investigated by Eddouks *et al.* (2005) in normal and streptozotocin-induced (STZ) diabetic rats. After acute (single dose) or chronic (15 daily repeated administration) oral treatments, the aqueous extract (20 mg/kg) produced a significant decrease on blood glucose levels in STZ diabetic rats. The blood glucose levels were normalised 2 weeks after daily repeated oral administration of aqueous extract (20 mg/kg). Significant reduction on blood glucose levels were noticed in normal rats after both acute and chronic treatment. In addition no changes were observed in basal plasma insulin concentrations after treatment either in normal or STZ diabetic rats indicating that the underlying mechanism of this pharmacological activity seems to be independent of insulin secretion. Aqueous extract exhibits a potent hypoglycaemic activity in rats without affecting basal plasma insulin concentrations.

Antihypertensive and Diuretic Effects

Maghrani *et al.* (2005) studied antihypertensive and diuretic effects of the aqueous extract in normotensive and spontaneously hypertensive rats. Daily oral administration of the aqueous *L. sativum* extract (20 mg/kg for 3 weeks) exhibited a significant decrease in blood pressure in spontaneously hypertensive rats while in normotensive rats, no significant change was noted during the period of treatment. The systolic blood pressure was decreased significantly from the 7th day to the end of treatment in spontaneously hypertensive rats. The aqueous*L. sativum* extract enhanced significantly the water excretion in normotensive rats but no statistically significant change was observed in spontaneously hypertensive rats. Furthermore, oral administration of aqueous *L. sativum* extract at a dose of 20 mg/kg produced a significant increase of urinary excretion of sodium, potassium and chlorides in normotensive rats. In spontaneously hypertensive rats, the aqueous extract administration induced a significant increase of urinary elimination of sodium, potassium and chlorides. Glomerular filtration rate showed a significant increase after oral administration of *L. sativum* in normal rats while in spontaneously hypertensive rats, no significant change was noted during the period of treatment. No significant changes were noted on heart rate after *L. sativum* treatment in spontaneously hypertensive rats as well as in normotensive rats.

Patel *et al.* (2009) investigated diuretic activity of aqueous and methanol extracts of *L. sativum* on rats. Aqueous and methanol extract of *L. sativum* seeds were administered to experimental rats orally at doses of 50 and 100 mg/kg. Hydrochlorothiazide (10 mg/kg) was used as positive control in study. Urine volume was significantly increased by the two doses of aqueous and methanol extracts in comparison to control group. While the excretion of sodium was also increased by both extracts, potassium excretion was only increased by the aqueous extract at dose of 100 mg/kg. There was no significant change in the conductivity and pH of urine after administration of the *L. sativum* extracts. Aqueous and methanol extract of *L. sativum* have notable diuretic effect which appeared to be comparable to that produced by the reference diuretic hydrochlorothiazide.

Insecticidal Activity

Radwn *et al.* (2007) reported the insecticidal activity of alcoholic seed extract (2 per cent), alcoholic herb extract (2 per cent), total glucosinolates (1 per cent), butanol fraction (2 per cent), glucotropaeoline (0.5 per cent), petroleum ether seed extract (2 per cent) and petroleum ether herb extract (2 per cent) carried on the white fly (*Bemisia tabaci*). Glucotropaeolin reduces the fecundity to 3.92 eggs in comparision to 159.8 eggs/female for the control with 92.5 per cent mortality. The majority of eggs failed to hatch and the percentage dropped to 13.2 per cent when glucotropaeolin was used.

Hepatoprotective Activity

Afaf *et al.* (2008) investigated the hepatoprotective effect of *Lepidium sativum* seeds against CCl_4 induced hepatic damage in rats. The methanolic seed extract at 200 mg/kg and 400 mg/kg dose reduced serum AST, ALT, ALP and bilirubin concentration. Toxicity evaluation of similar doses of the plant revealed no alteration in the parameters of serum AST, ALT, ALP and bilirubin.

Radwan *et al.* (2007) reported hepatoprotective activity of petroleum ether and 80 per cent alcoholic extract of *L. sativum* using hepatocyte monolayer culture from rat. Both the petroleum ether and 80 per cent ethanolic extracts showed hepatoprotective effect on the hepatocyte against CCl_4 cytotoxicity at the concentration of 50 µg/ml where, the LC_{50} were 150 µg/ml and 200 µg/ml respectively.

Fracture Healing

Juma, (2007) revealed the effect of *L. sativum* seeds on Fracture- induced healing in Rabbits. The study was carried out by inducing fractures in the midshaft of the left femur of 6 adult New Zealand White rabbits. X-rays of the induced fractures were taken at 6 and 12 weeks postoperatively to assess the healing of the fractures and documenting the healing by direct measurements of callus formation in millimeters at the longitudinal medial and longitudinal lateral and circumferential areas. The *L. sativum* showed a statistically significant increase in fractures healing.

Bronchodilatory Effect

Mali *et al.* (2008) studied the bronchodilatory effect of *L. sativum* against allergen induced bronchospasm in guinea pigs. The ethanolic extract of *L. sativum* seeds and its various fractions were tested for their bronchodilatory effect against histamine and acetylcholine induced acute bronchospasm in guinea pigs. The ethanolic extract and its all the fractions *viz.*, ethyl acetate, n-butanol and methanol exhibited significant protection against bronchospasm. The n-butanol fraction also exhibited significant protection which was comparable with that of ketotifen (1 mg/kg) and atropine sulphate (2 mg/kg).

Archana *et al.* (2006) investigated the efficacy and safety of *L. sativum* in patients of bronchial asthma. Seed powder was given at a dose of 1 gm thrice a day orally to 30 patients of either sex in the range of 15-80 years with mild to moderate bronchial asthma without any concurrent medication. The respiratory functions like Forced Vital Capacity (FVC), Forced Expiratory Volume in 1 sec, The average expired flow over the middle half of the FVC manoveure (FEF25-75 per cent) and Maximum voluntary ventilation were assessed using a spirometer prior to and after 4 weeks of treatment. Efficacy of the drug in improving clinical symptoms and severity of asthmatic attacks was evaluated by inter-viewing the patient and by physical and hematological examination at the end of the treatment. 4 weeks treatment with the drug showed statistically significant improvement in various parameters of pulmonary functions in asthmatic subjects. Also significant improvement was observed in clinical symptoms and severity of asthmatic attacks. None of the patient showed any adverse effect with *L. sativum*.

Antibacterial Activity

The methanolic extract of *L. sativum* seeds showed antibacterial activity against the pathogens *Escherichia coli*, *Salmonella typhi*, *Pseudomonas aeruginosa*, *Staphylococcus aureus*, *Bacillus cereus* and *Micrococcus luteus*. The minimum inhibitory concentrations (MIC) and minimum bactericidal concentration (MBC) were determined by tube dilution method and subculturing method respectively. The MIC values of the methanolic extract ranged from 1.56 mg/ml to 25.0 mg/ml whereas the MBC values ranged from 6.25 mg/ml to 25.0 mg/ml as reported by Gupta *et al.* (2010).

Nephroprotective Activity

Shinde *et al.* (2010) reported the protective effect of *L. sativum* aueous extract against doxorubicin-induced nephrotoxicity in rats. The levels of tissues malondialdehyde (MDA), the activities of superoxide dismutase (SOD), catalase (CAT), reduced glutathione (GSH) and serum creatinine and blood urea nitrogen were measured. Significantly elevated serum urea and creatinine levels in the doxorubicin alone treated group were reduced in the *L. sativum* (200 and 400 mg/kg, p.o) treated groups. The activities of SOD, CAT and level of GSH were elevated and level of malondialdehyde were declined significantly in the *L. sativum* (200 and 400 mg/kg) treated groups. Histopathological examination showed that *L. sativum* markedly ameliorated doxorubicin -induced renal tubular necrosis.

Discussion and Conclusion

In the present review we have made an attempt to congregate the taxonomical, botanical and ethnopharmacological information on *L. sativum*, a medicinal herb used in the Ayurveda. Literature survey reveals the presence of flavonoids, coumarins, sulphur glycosides, triterpenes, sterols and various imidazole alkaloids. The leaves of the plant are rich in minerals and vitamins. The plant belongs to family Brassicaceae since it contains benzyl isothiocynate and benzyl cyanide which is responsible for its characteristic odour. The major secondary compounds of this plant are glucosinolates. The alkaloids of *L. sativum* are member of the rare imidazole alkaloids that is known as lepidine. Carbohydrates present in the plant are polysaccharides, pectin substances and hemicelluloses. The plant also contains phenolic compounds. Several phytoconstituents in the plant have shown promising cardiovascular, respiratory, abortifacient, analgesic, anti-inflammatory, chemoprotective, oral contraceptive, hypoglycaemic, antihypertensive, diuretic, insecticidal, hepatoprotective, fracture healing, bronchodilatory and antibacterial activity.

The alcoholic extract of seed increases 40-80 mmHg of blood pressure. It possess cardiostimulant action on rabbit. Cardiac disease claims several million deaths every year on a global basis which is mainly due to change in life style of human being. In spite of the fact that clinically used cardiovascular drug, digitoxin is originally derived from plants, further search for isolation and identification of new cardioactive drugs from natural sources are extremely limited. Ethnopharmacological approach in the search for new cardiovascular compounds from plants appears to be helpful compared to the random screening approach. However a promising phytopharmacological basis is needed to use phytoactive constituent as templates for designing new derivatives with improved cardioactive properties.

According to World Health Organization (WHO, 2009) at least 171 million people worldwide have diabetes. Around 3.2 million deaths every year are attributable to complications of diabetes; six deaths every minute. If not checked, an estimated 360 million people worldwide are expected to get diabetes by 2030, with the largest increase occurring in the developing countries. The *L. sativum* is widely used in diabetes as evidenced by the study of Eddouks, (2005) that aqueous extract exhibits a potent hypoglycaemic activity in rats without affecting basal plasma insulin concentrations. The mode of action, pharmacokinetic and pharmacodynamic of drug is not explored. The further detailed study on the seed may lead to a safe drug for controlling diabetes.

The *L. sativum* has a wide use in treating different ailments from ancient times. Very little pharmacological work has been done on medicinal application of the isolated compounds so imperative that more pharmacological and clinical studies should be conducted to investigate unexploited potential of this plant. Exploration of chemical constituents and further pharmacological evaluation will give us basis for its therapeutic use in asthma, diabetes and liver complications. Very less information is available regarding the chemicals constituents like flavonoids and alkaloids of this plant due to lack of phyto-pharmacological studies. Depending on the primary information available further studies can be carried out like phyto-pharmacological standardization of extracts, isolation and identification of active constituents, pharmacological studies on isolated compounds and toxicity study. These studies may be followed by development of active molecules and clinical trial as a tool for modern drug development and serve the purpose of Ayurvedic formulation development.

Acknowledgements

The authors are thankful to Director NISCAIR, New Delhi for providing library facility to carry out the literature survey.

References

Afaf, I., Nuha, H.S., and Mohammed, A.H. (2008). Hepatoprotective effect of *Lepidium sativum* against carbon tetrachloride induced damage in rats. *Research Journal of Animal and Veterinary Sciences*, **3**: 20-23.

Alexander, J.M., and Islam, R. (1976). Volatile components of garden cress. *Journal of the Science of Food and Agriculture*, **27**: 909-912.

Al-Yaha, M.A., Mossa, J.S., Ageel, A.M., and Rafatullah, S. (1994). Pharmacological and safety studies on *Lepidium sativum* L. seeds. *Phytomedicine*, **1**: 155-159.

Anonymous. (1962). The wealth of India, (Raw Material), Vol. VI. New Delhi, India: CSIR Publication, pp 71-73.

Archana, P.N., and Mehta, A.A. (2006). A study on clinical efficacy of *Lepidium sativum* seeds in treatment of bronchial asthma. *Iranian Journal of Pharmacology and Therapeutics*. **5(1)**: 55-59.

Cherepanov, S.K. (1995). Plantae Vasculares Rossicae et Civitatum Collimitanearum (in limicis USSR olim). St. Petersburg: Mir I Semia, pp. 990.

Chopra, R.N., Nayar, S.L., and Chopra, I.C. (1956). Glossary of Indian Medicinal Plants (Including the Supplement). New Delhi, India: CSIR Publication, pp 227-228.

Dorofeev, V.I. (1998). Family Cruciferae (Brassicaceae) middle Zone of the European part of the Russian Federation. *Turchaninowia, Barnaul*, **1(3)**: 94.

Dorofeev, V.I. (2002). Cruciferae (Brassicaceae) of European Russia. *Turchaninowia, Barnaul*, **5(3)**: 115.

Eddouks, M., Maghrani, M., Zeggwagh, N.A., and Michel, J.B. (2005). Study of hypoglycaemic activity of *Lepidium sativum* L. aqueous extract in normal and diabetic rat. *Journal of Ethnopharmacology*, **97**: 391-395.

Mali, G.R., Mahajan, G.S., and Mehta, A.A. (2008). Studies on bronchodilatory effect of *Lepidium sativum* against allergen induced bronchospasm in guinea pigs. *Pharmacognosy Magzine*, **4**: 189-192.

Gill, V., and Macleod, A.J. (1980). Studies on glucosinolate degradation in *Lepidium sativum* seed extract. *Phytochemistry*, **19**: 1369-1374.

Grossgeim, A.A. (1950). Flora of the Caucasus. Vol. IV. Moscow-Leningrad, pp 117.

Gupta, P.C., Devki, P., Joshi, P., and Lohar, D.R. (2010). Evaluation of antibacterial activity of *Lepidium sativum* Linn. seeds against food-borne pathogens. *International Journal of Chemical and Analytical Science*, **1(4)**: 74-75.

Harkevitch, S.S. (1988). Vascular Plants of the Soviet Far East. Vol. III. Leningrad: Nauka, pp 42.

Hasegawa, K., Mizutani, J., Kosemura, S., and Yamamura, S. (1992). Isolation and identification of lepidimoide, a new allelopathic substance from mucilage of germinated cress seeds. *Plant Physiology*, **100(2)**: 1059-1061.

Juma, A.H. (2007). The effects of *Lepidium sativum* seeds on fracture induced healing in rabbits. *Medscape General Medicine*, **9(2)**: 23 available online http: //www.ncbi.nlm.nih.gov/pmc/articles/PMC1994840/< accessed on 22 June 2010.

Kassie, F., Laky, B., Gminski, R., Mersch-Sundermann, V., Scharf, G., Lhoste, E., and Kansmuller, S. (2003). Effects of garden and water cress juices and their constituents, benzyl and phenethyl isothiocyanates, towards benzo(a)pyrene-induced DNA damage: a model study with the single cell gel electrophoresis/ Hep G2 assay. *Chemico- Biological Interactions*, **142(3)**: 285-96.

Kassie, F., Rabot, S., Uhl, M., Huber, W., Qin, H.M., Helma, C., Schulte-Hermann, R., and Knasmuller, S. (2002).Chemoprotective effects of garden cress (*Lepidium sativum*) and its constituents towards 2-amino-3-methyl-imidazo[4,5-f]quinoline (IQ)-induced genotoxic effects and colonic preneoplastic lesions. *Carcinogenesis*, **23(7)**: 1155-61.

Khory, R. (1999). Materia Medica of India and Their Therapeutics, Delhi, India: Komal Prakashan, pp 63-64.

Kirtikar, K.R., and Basu, B.D. (2006). Indian Medicinal Plants, Vol. I. Allahabad, India: Popular Prakashan, pp 174-175.

Klaus, M., Alexander, P., Andreas, M., and Gunter, T. (2009). Lepidium as a model system for studying the evolution of fruit development in Brassicaceae. *Journal of Experimental Botany*, **60(5)**: 1503-1513; available online http: //jxb.oxfordjournals.org/cgi/content/full/60/5/1503.

Maghrani, M., Zeggwagh, N.A., Michel, J.B., and Eddouks, M.J. (2005). Antihypertensive effect of *Lepidium sativum* L. in spontaneously hypertensive rats. *Journal of Ethnopharmacology*, **22**: 193-197.

Maier, U.H., Gundlach, H., and Zenk, M.H. (1998). Seven imidazole alkaloids from *Lepidium sativum. Phytochemistry*, **49(6)**: 1791-1795.

Mennicke, W.H., Goerler, K., Krumbiegel, G., and Rittman, N. (1988). Studies on the metabolism and excretion of benzyl isothiocyanate in man. *Xenobiotica*, **18**: 441-447.

Nath, D., Sethi, N., Singh, R.K., and Jain, A.K. (1992). Commonly used Indian abortifacient plants with special reference to their teratologic effects in rats. *Journal of Ethnopharmacology*, **36**: 147-154.

Nayak, P.S., Upadhyaya, S.D., and Upadhyaya, A.A. (2009). HPTLC densiometry of sinapic acid in chandrasur (*Lepidium sativum*). *Journal of Scientific Research*, **1(1)**: 121-127.

Orlovskaya, T.V., and Chelombit'ko, V.A. (2007). Phenolic compounds from *Lepidium sativum. Chemistry of Natural Compounds*, **43(3)**: 306, 307, 323.

Patel, U., Kulkarni, M., Undale, V., and Bhosale, A. (2009). Evaluation of diuretic activity of aqueous and methanol extracts of *Lepidium sativum* garden cress (Cruciferae) in rats. *Tropical Journal of Pharmaceutical Research*, **8(3)**: 215-219.

Radwan, H.M., El-Missiry, M.M., Al-Said, W.M., Ismail, A.S., Abdel, S.K.A., and Seif-El, N. (2007). Investigation of the glucosinolates of *Lepidium sativum* growing in Egypt and their biological activity. *Research Journal of Medical Science*, **2(2)**: 127-132.

Rastogi, R.P., and Mehrotra, B.N. (1995). Compendium of Indian Medicinal Plant, Vol. IV, Lucknow, India: Central Drug Research Intitute, pp 429.

Sharief, M., and Zainab, H. (2004). Garden cress (*Lepidium sativum*) seeds as oral contraceptive plant in mice. *Saudi Medical Journal*, **25(7)**: 965-966.

Shinde, N., Jagtap, A., Undale, V., Kakade, S., Kotwal, S., and Patil, R. (2010). Protective effect of *Lepidium sativum* against doxorubicin-induced nephrotoxicity in rats. *Research Journal of Pharmaceutical, Biological and Chemical Sciences*, **1(3)**: 42.

Tsvelev, N.N. (2000). Vascular Plants of Russia and the Contiguous States (Determinant) (Leningrad, Pskov and Novgorod district). St. Petersburg: Publishing House of SPHFA, pp 781.

Uphof. J. C. (1959). The Dictionary of Economic Plants. Weinheim.

Vohra, S.B., and Khan, M.S.Y. (1977). Pharmacological studies on *Lepidium sativum* Linn.*Indian Journal of Physiology and Pharmacology*, **21(2)**: 118-120.

World Health Organization. (2009). Global strategy on diet, physical activity and health: Diabetes. Available online: http: //www.who.int/dietphysicalactivity/publications/facts/diabetes/en/. Accessed on: 22nd May 2009.

Ziska, P., Kindt, A., and Franz, H. (1982). Isolation and characterization of a lectin from garden cress, *Acta Histochem*, **71(1)**: 29-33.

Bioactive Phytochemicals: Perspectives for Modern Medicine Vol. 1 (2012) *Pages* **457–475**
Editor: **V.K. Gupta**
Published by: **DAYA PUBLISHING HOUSE, NEW DELHI**

14

Chemistry and Pharmacology of Selected Asian and American Medicinal Species of *Justicia*

Juan Carlos Gomez-Verjan[1*], Ricardo Reyes-Chilpa[2] and María Isabel Aguilar[3]

ABSTRACT

Justicia is one of the biggest and complex genus among the Acanthaceae family, constituted by around 600 and 700 species in the world, two hundred of these grow in America. In Latin America, three species are the most widely used for medicinal purposes: Justicia spicigera, Justicia secunda and Justicia pectoralis; however there are very few studies related to their chemical composition and pharmacological properties. On the other side, Asian species like Justicia procumbrens or Justicia adhatoda have been deeply studied showing interesting properties as antiviral, cytotoxic and broncodilatory activities attributed mainly to alkaloids, lignans and flavonoids. In this chapter we review the studies of the species most widely used in Asia and Latin America are reviewed and their chemistry and biological properties (antimicrobial, antiinflamatory, antioxidant among others) are compared.

Keywords: *Justicia* sp., *Adhatoda vasica*, Lignans, Antiviral, Cytotoxic.

1 Posgrado en Ciencias Biológicas, Facultad de Ciencias,

2 Instituto de Química,

3 Facultad de Química. Universidad Nacional Autónoma de México. Av. Universidad 3000. Ciudad Universitaria, D.F., CP04510.

* *Corresponding author*: E-mail: poison132@hotmail.com; Tele: (52) 55 56225290.

Abreviations

Justicia sp.: *J.* sp.; *Adhatoda vasica*: *A. vasica*; *Mycobacterium tuberculosis*: *M. tuberculosis*; *Pseudomonas aeruginosa*: *P. aeruginosa*; HPLC: High Performance Liquid Chromatography; GC/MS: Gas Chromatography/Mass Spectrometry; MIC: Minimal inhibitory concentration; CNS: Central Nervous System, MTT: Yellow tetrazolium salt.

Symbols and Units

% Inhibition, µg/ml, Gallic Acid Equivalents/100 grams of plant, Catechin Equivalents/100g.

Introduction

The genus *Justicia* is one of the largest and most complex among the Acanthaceae family. It comprises about 600-700 perennifolius species, mostly weeds and bushes widely used as ornament (Graham, 1988), most of them are tropical and subtropical species. Nearly 300 species are found in the American continent and about 400 in Asia (Ezcurra, 1999b). In Mexico, there are about 75 species (Daniel, 1993), 85 in Colombia (Leonard, 1951), 27 in Ecuador (Joergensen and LeonYanez, 1999), 50 in Peru (Brako and Zarucchi, 1993) and 28 in Argentina (Ezcurra, 1993a). These species are ecologicaly important; they are abundantly distributed in wet forests, but can also be found in semiarid environments (Ezcurra, 1999b). Many of these species are ethnopharmacological significant, since ethnic groups and peasants use them as medicines.

History and Taxonomy of the Genus

The *Justicia* genus was proposed by Linne in 1753. A century later, in his treatise on the global Acanthaceae, Nees (1847) delimited the genus from more than 600 species which had been described under the name of *Justicia* to only 12 species in Asia and Africa. On the other hand, he created several new genus related to *Justicia* to locate a great number of species recently described in the New World. Later, Bentham (1876) and Lindau (1893) broadened Nee's concept of *Justicia* and reduced many genus to synonyms. Currently, as proposed by Graham in 1988, most authors consider *Justicia* in its broadest sense, which includes 600-700 species (Graham, 1988; McDade *et al.*, 2000). A preliminary molecular analysis performed by McDade and Daniel (2000) indicates that *Justicia s.* lat. conforms a separate lineage within the tribe Justicieae and the great morphological diversification and the high rate of speciation has experimented very little change concomitantly at the molecular level in the loci analyzed so far. Following the concept of Graham (1988) the genus *Justicia* includes species characterized by bilabiate corollas with stylar groove on the rear inner, presence of 2 exerts stamens under the posterior lip with 2 teaks (rarely 1), an absence of staminoides, pollen subprolade to perprolade 2- or 3(4)-porate or colporate and capsules 4-seminades.

Asian Species of Justicia

Justicia adhatoda or Adhatoda vasica

Several species of *Justicia*, mainly Asian have been widely investigated pharmacological and chemically. *Adhatoda vasica* also called *Justicia adhatoda* (Claeson *et al.*, 2000), is the most important and promising species of this genus. It has been widely used in Southeast Asia particularly in India in Unani and Ayurdevic medicine since almost 2000 years (Atal, 1980). It is known as the Malabar tree in the Traditional Hindu Medicine (Claeson *et al.*, 2000), and as Vasaka in Sanskrit (WHO,1990). Due to its properties, it is included in the "Manual of Traditional Medicine in Primary Health Care", published by the World Health Organization, where it is recommended for the treatment of cough, asthma, phlegm, bleeding hemorrhoids, both for adults and youngsters (WHO, 1990).

As for this species, vasicine, a quinazoline alkaloid (Figure 14.1) has been isolated from the flowers, leaves and roots (Dymock *et al.*, 1890). The leaves and roots contain also alkaloids such as vasicinone, vasicinol, adhatodine, adhatodinine, adhavasinone, anisotine and peganine (Huq *et al.*, 1967; Willaman *et al.*, 1970; Bhat*et al.*, 1978; Atal, 1989; Chowdhury and Bhattacharyya, 1987). The flowers contain some important flavonoids such as astragaline, kaempferol and quercetin, as well as the triterpenoid α-amyrin (Huq *et al.*, 1967).

The numerous pharmacological studies of this species show the relaxing activity on tracheal vascular smooth muscle of guinea pig induced by the essential oil of the aerial parts (D´Cruz *et al.*, 1979), the hypoglycemic activity in mice and rabbits induced by the ethanolic extract of aerial parts (Modak *et al.*, 1966; Dhar *et al.*, 1968) and antiallergic and antiasthamatic activities of methanol extract of the whole (Muller *et al.*, 1993). Infusion of the aerial parts has shown activity in isolated microflora from patients with gingivitis (Patel *et al.*, 1984). However, Naovi *et al.* (1991) did not observe any antimicrobial activity on gram (+) and gram (-) bacteria, yeasts or filamentous fungi. The ethanol extract of roots showed antihelmintic activity, proving that not only the aerial parts are responsible for many of its biological properties (Jabbar *et al.*, 2003). Also, aqueous and methanol extracts of aerial parts showed activity against *Mycobacterium tuberculosis* (Chopra, 1955; Kamilia *et al.*, 2003). Other studies showed a significant protective effect on radiation-induced damaged chromosomes (Kumar, 2007).

One of the most promising compounds studied in this species is the alkaloid vasicine (Figure 14.1). This compound showed a significant bronchodilator activity both *in vivo* and *in vitro* (Atal, 1980). From this compound bromhexine, and its main metabolic product in man, ambroxol (Figure 14.1) were obtained by semisynthesis, the latter showing a significant mucolytic activity; currently both compounds are highly used in various pharmaceutical preparations (Grange *et al.*, 1996). Vasicine has also shown to stimulate rhythmic contractions in human myomether demonstrating an effect which is comparable to that of oxytocin (Atal, 1980). Pharmacokinetic and pharmacodynamic studies on vasicine have demonstrated its half life of 5-7 minutes if applied intravenously and 1.5-2 hours intramuscularly, it is metabolized in the liver to vasicinone and other metabolites, and excreted mainly in

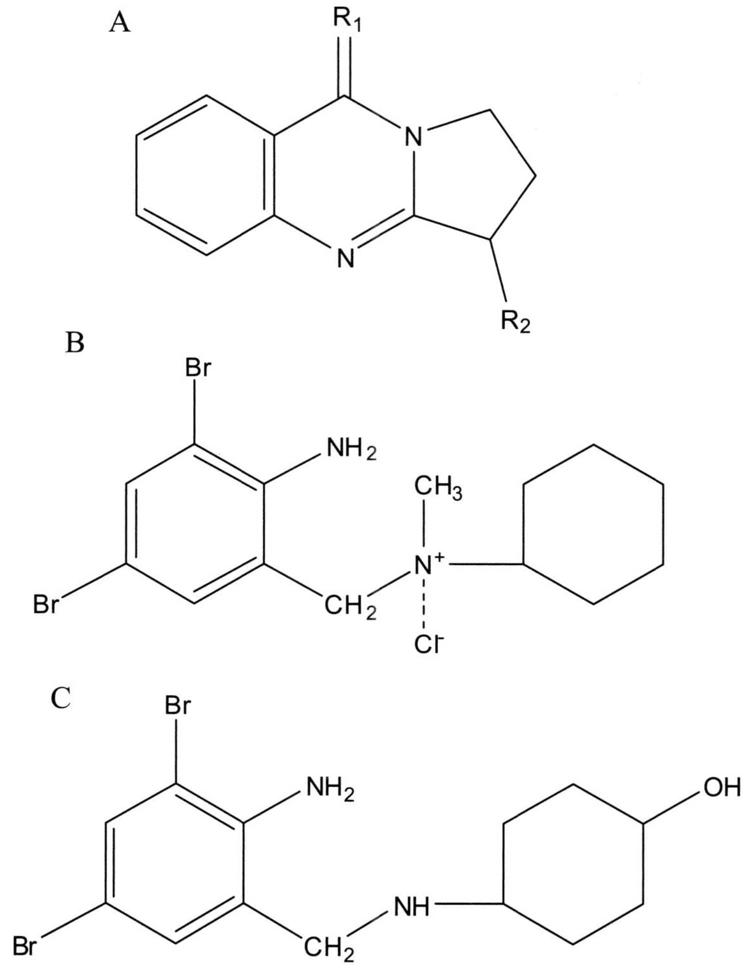

Figure 14.1: Chemical structures of the main alkaloids isolated from *A. vasica*. (A) Vasicine (R_1=H2, R_2=OH) and Vasicinone (R_1=O, R_2=OH) and semisynthetic derivatives such as alkaloids; (B) Bromhexine and (C) Ambroxol.

the urine (Atal, 1980). Many toxicological studies have been carried out with different protocols and preparations, and either extracts or pure vasicine have not shown any evidence of risks (Claeson, 2000). In addition, in three clinical studies with preparations containing *A. vasica* with 130 patients, no adverse toxic effects were detected, showing it is safe to use (Shete, 1993; Iyengar *et al.*, 1994; Thom and Wollan, 1997).

Other Asian Species

Justicia procumbrens is one of the most studied species to date, it is found mainly in Southeast Asia and China where it is used as an antipyretic, to treat pain, respiratory tract infections and against different types of cancer (Day *et al.*, 2002). Compounds isolated from this species are neojusticine-A, neojusticine-B, and taiwanine E as well as juticidines-A, B, C and D (Ohta *et al.*, 1970). It has been demonstrated that neojusticine-A can induce platelet aggregation (Chen *et al.*, 1996), while neojusticine-B shows antiarrhythmic activity in rats (Lin and Zhong, 1982). One of the most promising areas of research in these species is as an antiviral, since the lignans justicidine- A, B, C and D; justicidinosides A, B and C, and the dyphiline apioside isolated from aerial parts of *J. procumbrens* (Figure 14.2) have demonstrated significant activity against the vesicular stomatitis virus. Also, in this study an important cytotoxic activity in rabbit lung cells was found (Asano, 1996). The flavonoids peonidine 3-glucoside and dyphiline were also isolated (Fukamiya *et al.*, 1986) and showed potent activity against this virus (Asano *et al.*, 1996). Day *et al.* (2002) found important cytotoxic activity and increase in the production of nitric oxide and tumor necrosis factor-*a* in mouse cells by justicidian-C, E, D, and A, procumbrenoside, tuberculatine, diphyline and secoisolariciresinol isolated from aerial parts of *Justicia procumbrens*.

Justicia hyssopifolia endemic to the Canary Islands, is an African species which contains two lignans called J1 and J2, as well as an abundant arilnaftalen lignan named ellenoside (Figure 14.2) shown to be a central nervous system depressant (Navarro *et al.*, 2004a) and to be able to inhibit intestinal motility *in vitro* (Navarro *et al.*, 2006b). *Justicia prostate* grows mainly in India; it contains arylnaftalid lignans, like protalidine-A, B and C, as well as, retoquinesine, found in the aerial parts, which have demonstrated an antidepressant activity in albino mice (Ghosal *et al.*, 1979a). Also, both aqueous and alcoholic extracts from this species have demonstrated an anti-inflammatory activity in acute and subacute inflammation models (Sammugapriya *et al.*, 2005). *Justicia simplex* a species native of India has also been widely investigated. The less polar extracts of aerial parts have shown an hepatoprotective activity (Singh *et al.*, 2007) and furofuran lignans have been isolated, including simpletoxine, sesamoline, sesamine, asarinine, as well as β-sitosterol (Ghosal *et al.*, 1979a), 3-arylnaftalide lignans, justicines C and E (Sastry *et al.*, 1979). Ghosal *et al.* (1980b) isolated other furofuran lignans such as justisoline and simplexoside, and a triterpenic saponine called justicisaponin which showed an strong activity as anti-fertility agent in female rats. In contrast, the aqueous extract of aerial parts from *J. insulinarias* increased fertility in female rats (Telefo *et al.*, 1998). Other Indian species, like *J. gendarussa*, contain β-sitosterol and aromatic amines (Chakravarty *et al.*, 1982); the ethanol extract of aerial parts of this species showed an important anthiarthritic effect in two different physiological models (Paval, 2009). Other Asian species that also exhibit an interesting biological activity are: *J. ciliata* which contains a huge amount of lignans with a potent cytotoxic *in vitro* activity against various tumor lines (Day *et al.*, 1999), the infusion of *J. extensa* presented high toxicity against *Tilapia nilotica* (Ibrahim *et al.*, 2000) in an assay proposed to asses toxicity such as the *Artemia salina* model.

It is noteworthy that many Asian species of *Justicia* contain lignans, such as *J. tranquebariensis* in which aryltetraline, (+)=laricireasinol, and (+)-medioresinol have been found (Raju *et al.*, 1989). *Justicia glauca* contains furanoid lignans such as justiciresinol (Subbaraju *et al.*, 1991) and jusglacucinol (Rajendrian and Subramanian, 1991). In addition, *J. flava* contains the lignans justicinol, helioxanthine and (+)-

Figure 14.2: Structures of some of the main chemical compounds isolated from the main *Justicia* species of the world that posses important antiviral and cytotoxic activities.

(A) R = OCH_3-Justicidine A, R = H-justicidine B, R = OH-diphyline; (B) justicidine C; (C) justicidine D; (D) justicinioside A; (E) R= OCH_3-justicionioside B, R= H-justicionioside C. (F) Ellenoside R= glucoside.

A

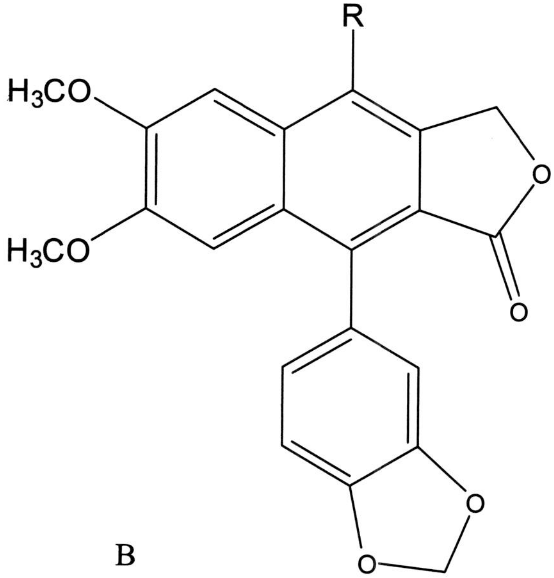

B

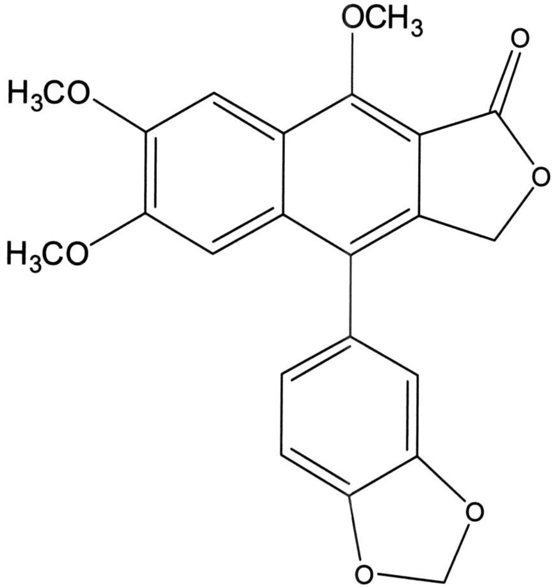

Contd...

Figure 14.2–*Contd...*

C

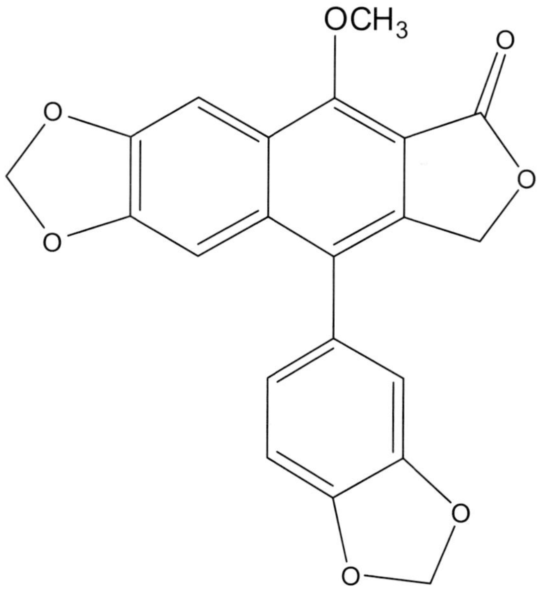

D

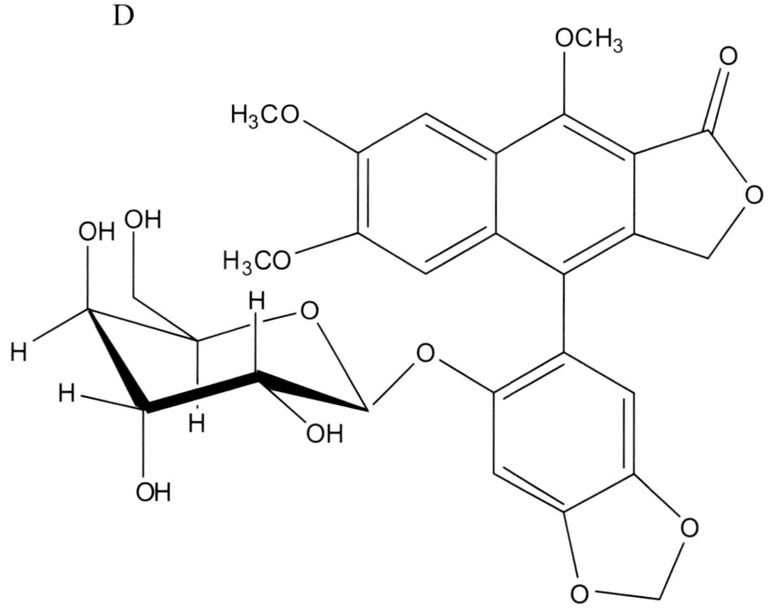

Contd...

Very little is known about the metabolic contents of *J. spicigera*. However, Euler and Alam (1982) isolated the flavonoid kampferitrine and Dominguez *et al.* (1990) isolated *O*-sitosteryl-3β-glucoside, allantoin and cryptoxanthin (Table 14.1). In the

Figure 14.2–*Contd...*

Table 14.1: Chemical compounds isolated from of the species of *Justicia* genus in America

J. spicigera	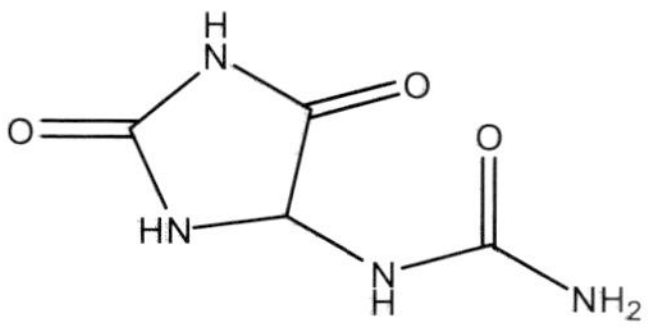	Alantoine	Domínguez *et al.*, 1990
	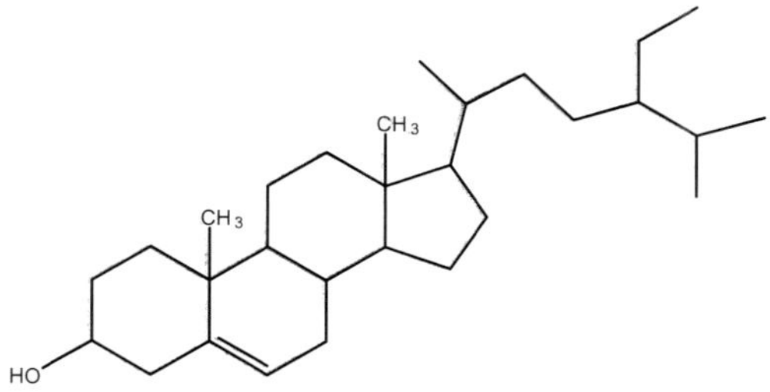	β-sitosterol	Domínguez *et al.*, 1990
	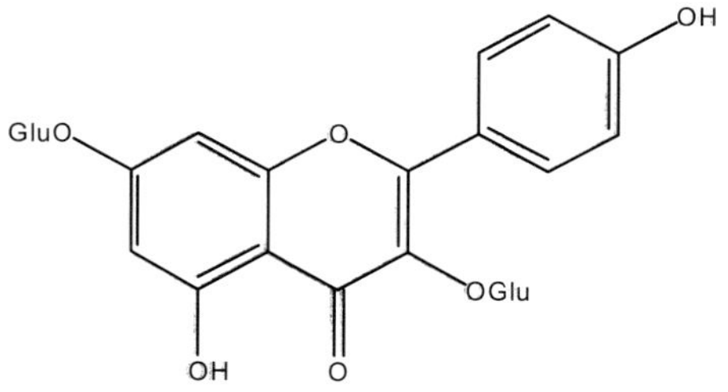	Kampferitrine	Alam *et al.*, 1982
J. pectoralis	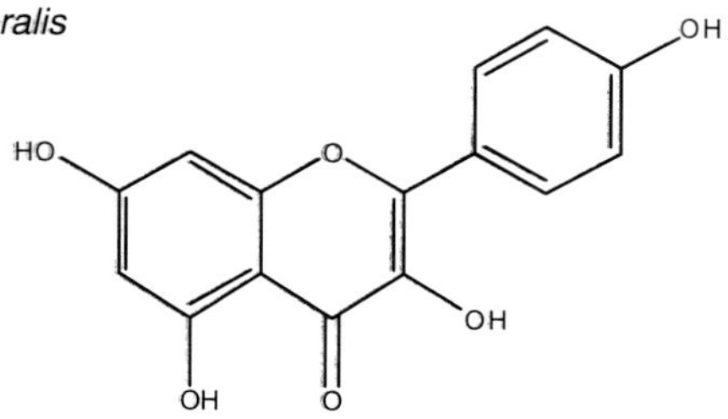	Kaempferol	Olveira *et al.*, 2000
	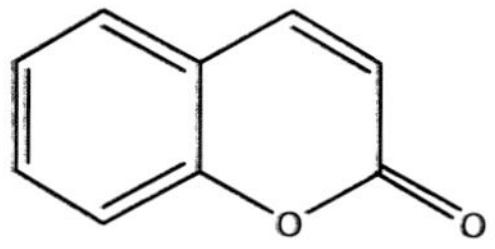	1,2-benzopirone	de Vries *et al.*, 1988 Olveira *et al.*, 2000
	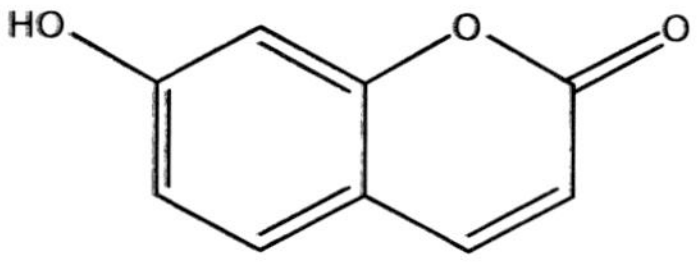	Umbeliferone	de Vries *et al.*, 1988 Olveira *et al.*, 2000

Contd...

Table 14.1–*Contd...*

	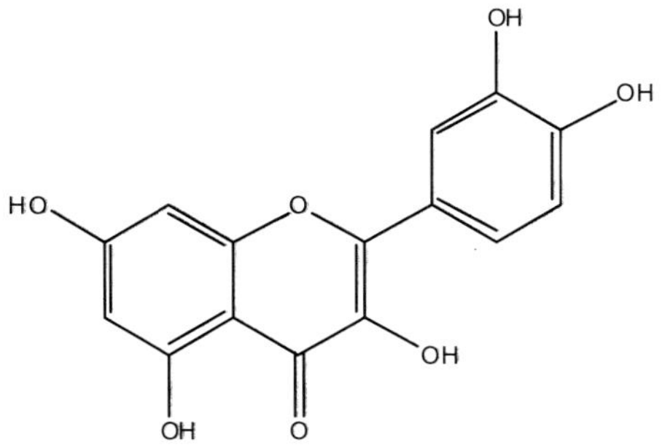	Quercetine	Olveira *et al.*, 2000
	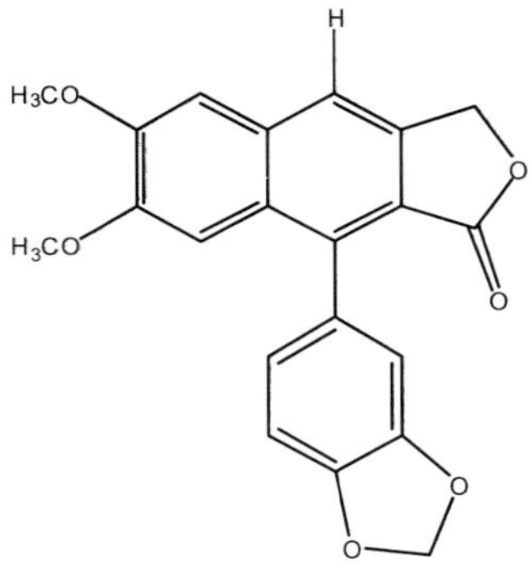	Justicidiane B	Joseph *et al.*, 1988
J. secunda	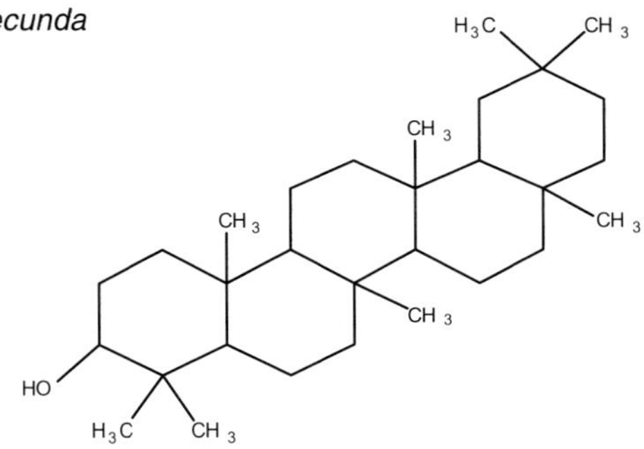	Taraxerol	Herrera-Mata *et al.*, 2001
	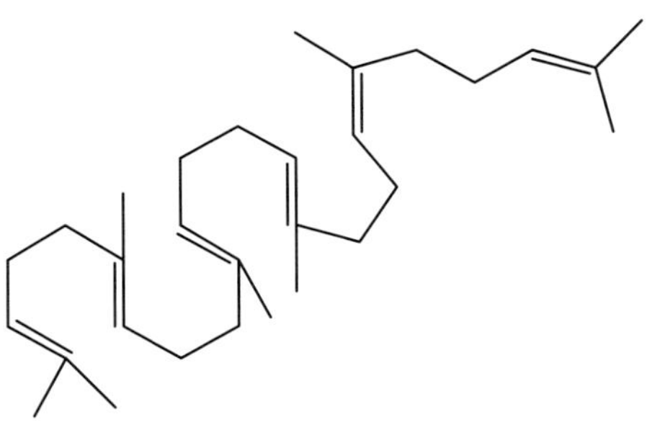	Escualene	Herrera-Mata *et al.*, 2001

most comprehensive study done to date, Sepulveda-Jimenez*et al.* (2009) found a total content of polyphenols in methanol and water extracts of 1.33 to 5.01 g of GAE/100g of plants, which include flavonoids that represented 0.18 and 1.30 g of CE/100g of the plant; it is noteworthy that leaves and stems were the organs with the highest amounts of flavonoids. Since, a large amount of polyphenols have been detected in this species, a study was conducted to analyze antioxidant activity. The methanol extract of the leaves showed an IC_{50}=48.9 µg/mL scavengers of reactive oxygen species (Sepulveda-Jimenz *et al.*, 2009).

Justicia pectoralis

Justicia pectoralis is a native species of the American tropics, it is found in the mainland of Central and South America. In Cuba it is known as "Tilo or Tila", and in Brazil as "Chamba", where it is most common ethnomedical use is as a sedative, but has also been used as an expectorant ("pectoral"). Lino *et al.* (1997) demonstrated that coumarin and umbeliferone in*J. pectoralis* are responsible for the antiinflammatory and analgesic properties popularly attributed to this species in the Caribbean Islands and Central America. Genotoxicity assessment through the Ames test for detecting gene mutation and micronucleus in the mouse bone marrow, demonstrated its safety and its potential as a raw material to prepare a phytomedicine. It is important to note that this species is specially important in Brazil, as Martins and colleagues report that is widely used in several densely populated communities of Rio de Janeiro as an antipyretic and analgesic (Martins, 2005).

In Trinidad and Tobago this plant is used to treat prostate problems, for the treatment of respiratory tract infections and to relieve cough. Recently it has been found that alcoholic extracts exhibit a bronchodilator activity in guinea pigs (Mills *et al.*, 1986). On the other hand, the alcoholic extracts of this plant have shown an insecticide activity against the mosquito larvae of*Aedes aegypti* Linn. vector of Dengue disease. It is important to note that*J. pectoralis* is a component of some hallucinogenic preparations of several ethnia of South America, but there are only two ethnobotanical studies on this aspect (MacRae *et al.*, 1984; de Smet *et al.*, 1985), however, in none of these studies the active principles responsible of such activities were isolated.

Justicia pectoralis is the chemically most studied American species (Table 14.1). In an analysis by GC/MS the coumarins, dihydrocoumarine and umbelliferone were found (Olveira *et al.*, 2000). It has also been isolated the lignan justicidiane-B (which later was demonstrated to posses cytotoxic activity), and a glycosylflavone (Joseph *et al.*, 1988). Lino*et al.* (1997) analyzed the effect of hydroalcoholic extract of aerial parts as well as their constituents (coumarin and umbelliferone) in the model of rat paw oedema induced by carrageenan. It was demonstrated that both the hydroalcoholic extract and these compounds have antiinflammatory and antinociceptive effects, probably by acting on the nitric oxide system.

On the other hand, in one of the most comprehensive phytochemical studies of this species, the analysis of the methanol extract of leaves (which traditionally is the most used part) was found to contain coumarins, 1,2-benzopyrene and umbelliferone as well as the flavonoids quercetin, kaempferol and stigmasterol (Table 14.1), suggesting that the activity attributed to this plant is due to these compounds (Olveira *et al.*, 2000). Recently, Rodiguez-Chanfrau *et al.* (2008) developed an HPLC method as a possible quality test to quantify coumarins for dry extracts of *J. pectoralis*. The same authors also obtained raw material from a 30 per cent hydroalcoholic extract of pharmaceutical quality of the aerial parts prepared by a spray-drying methodology (Rodiguez-Chanfrau *et al.*, 2008). The previously reviewed studies highlight the importance of coumarins as the probably most important active principles of *J. pectoralis* (Lino *et al.*, 1997). Those coumarins have been isolated from other species, and have shown anticancer activity, anti-oedema and capability to modulate inflammation, however, these activities have not been evaluated up to date in *J. pectoralis*, as neither has the potential hepatotoxicity been documented for other coumarins (Yarnell and Abascal, 2009).

Justicia secunda

Justicia secunda is widely distributed in Central America and northern South America and it is used in traditional medicine to treat kidney stones. In Venezuela it is used as antipyretic and is known as "sanguinaria" (Herrera-Mata *et al.*, 2002). In Colombia it is also used for glycemic disorders and to treat different infectious pathologies (Rojas, 2006). In Trinidad and Tobago is used to treat pain during menstruation and nonspecific dermal infections (Lans, 2007b); it also has an ethno-veterinary application for the treatment of injuries, snake bites and dysentery problems of hunting dogs (Lans *et al.*, 2001a).

Toxicological studies performed with aerial parts of this plant on *Artemia franciscana* showed activity for aqueous (CL_{50}= <200µg/mL) and dichlorometane extracts (CL_{50}=42.23µg/mL), while methanol extract was inactive (CL_{50}>1000mg/mL) (Cantilla *et al.*, 2007). Activity over *Artemia salina* was also found in aqueous extracts (CL_{50}=37.93µg/mL) (Herrera-Mata *et al.*, 2002). Antimicrobial activity was tested with the methanol extracts of aerial parts and showed activity against *E. coli* and *C. albicans* (MIC of 0.6 µg/mL for both) (Herrera-Mata *et al.*, 2002). On the other hand in a bioprospecting screening with 11 plants from Panama, cytotoxicity of *J. secunda* dichloromethane and methanol extracts of leaf, steam and roots were tested against 3 cancer cell lines MCF-7 (breast cancer), H460 (lung carcinoma) and SF-268 (CNS carcinoma). The most relevant activity was found in the dichloromethane extract of root with IC_{50}= 47 µg/mL against MCF-7 cell line, 40 µg/mL for H460, and 42 µg/mL for SF-268 (Calderon *et al.*, 2003), although cytotoxic properties were not attributed to any metabolite or metabolites in specific.

Red and blue pigments have been obtained from the aqueous and alcoholic extracts from aerial parts of *J. secunda*, which are used in some pharmaceutical and aesthetic products. Within the few compounds isolated from this plant, it has been reported that 4,6-diphenyl-2-pyrimidinilamine, carboxylic and eicosanoid acids, and as component of active fractions against *A. franciscana*, taraxerol, squalene, as well as 11-hexadecanoic acid (Table 14.1) (Herrera-Mata *et al.*, 2002) were found.

Justicia reptans

There is only one study of this species endemic of Guatemala (Alcami *et al.*, 2008). Based on the phylogenetic relationship of this species compared with other

Asian species reported with an important activity against VSV (Asano *et al.*, 1996). This study was completed in two models, the MTT and the recombinant virus assays. The ethanol extract of aerial parts, as well as its fractions were tested; the most outstanding effect was found for the ethanolic extract with IC_{50} of 34.6 µg/mL in the MTT assay and IC_{50} of 41.3 µg/mL in the recombinant virus assay. Such properties were attributed to the flavonoids contained in this species; however such flavonoids were not isolated in this study (Alcami, 2008).

Conclusion

It is important to highlight that the Asian species of this genus have been widely studied, obtaining very interesting results about their pharmacological and chemical properties, showing their high contents mainly in lignans and alkaloids some of which are widely used in pharmaceutical formulations. Asian species have been notoriously relevant against virus and cytotoxicity in contrast, with the exception of *J. pectoralis*. There are few studies about the pharmacological effectiveness of the American species, however *Justicia* species are widely cited in Traditional Medicine of several countries in Latin America. To date, American species of *Justicia* have been found to contain some flavonoids and coumarins so it could be important to analyze their content of alkaloids and lignans like in the Asian species. Also in the biological activities of all the American species it could be important to analyze the antiparasitic, antiinflammatory activities as well as the toxicity of all this species more specifically.

It is important to emphasize that there are efforts of *J. pectoralis* to develope a serious phytomedicament, although there are not important investigations on the toxicology of this species.

Acknowledgments

The first author is grateful to CONACyT for awarding a M.Sc. Scholarship (262193) and also to UNAM for the economical support PAPIIT IN223411 and PAPIIT IN203810.

References

Alam M. and Euler K.L. (1982). Isolation of Kaempferitrin from *Justicia spicigera*. *Journal of Natural Products*, **2**: 15-19.

Alcami J., Caceres A.S., Garcia P.A., Escarcena R., Gaitan I., Cruz S.M., Palomino-Sanchez S.S., Bermejo M., Bedoya L.M. (2008). Guatemalan plants extracts as virucides against HIV-1 infection. *Phytomedicine*, **15**: 520-524.

Asano J, Chiba K, Tada M, Yoshii T (1996). Antiviral activity of lignans and their glycosides from *Justicia procumbens* L. *Phytochemistry*, **42**: 713–717.

Atal, C.K. (1980). Chemistry and Pharmacology of Vasicine. A New Oxytocic and Abortifacient. Regional Research Laboratory, Jammu-Tawi. **16**: 34-36.

Bentham, G. (1876). Acanthaceae. In G. Bentham and J. D. Hooker, Genera Plantarum. **2(2)**: 1060-1122.

Bhat V.S., Nasavatl D.D., Mardikar B.R. (1978). *Adhatoda vasica*–an Ayurvedic medicinal plant. *Indian Drugs*, **15**: 62–66.

Caceres A. Giron L.M., Alvarado S.R., Torres M.F. (1987). Screening of antimicrobial activity of plants popularly used in Guatemala for the treatment of dermatomucosal Diseases. *Journal of Ethnopharmacology*, **20**: 228-237.

Càceres-Cortes M.E., Moreno-Alvarado M., Ramírez-Nieves M.E. (2001). Transfection of the TF-1 cell line with the human proto-oncogene bcl-2 favors short term cell survival and does not change phenotype. *Revista de Investigación Clínica*, **52**: 645-653.

Calderón A.I., Terreaux C., Gupta M.P., Hostettmann K. (2003). *In vitro* cytotoxicity of 11 Panamanian plants. *Fitoterapia*, **74**: 378–383.

Cantillo J., Güete J., Baldiris R., Jaramillo B., Olivero J. (2007). Evaluación de la toxicidad aguda (CL_{50}) Frente a*Artemia franciscana* y la actividad hemolítica de los extractos acuosos, en diclorometano y metanólico parcial de *Justicia secunda* (Vahl.). *Sciencia et Technica* III : 3.

Chakravarty AK, Dastidar PPG, Pakrashi SS (1982). Studies on Indian medicinal plants. Part 67. Simple aromatic amines from *Justicia gendarrusa*. Carbon-13 NMR spectra of the bases and their analogs. *Tetrahedron*, **38**: 1797–1802.

Chen, C.C. Wen-C. H., Ko F.N., Yu-Lin H., Jun-Chih O., and Che-Ming T. (1996). Antiplatelet Arylnaphthalide Lignans from *Justicia procumbens*. J. Nat. Prod., **59** (12): 1149–1150.

Chopra R.N. (1955). A Review of Work on Indian Medicinal Plants. Indian Council of Medical Research, New Delhi, p. 23.

Chowdhury B.K., Bhattacharyya P. (1987). Adhavasinone: a new quinazolone alkaloid from *Adhatoda vasica* Nees. *Chemical Industry* (*London*), **1**: 35–36.

Claeson U. P, Malmfors T., Wikman G., Bruhn J. G. (2000). *Adhatoda vasica*: a critical review of ethnopharmacological and toxicological data. *Journal of Ethnopharmacology*, **72**: 1–20.

D'Cruz, J.L., Nimbkar, A.Y., Kokate, C.K. (1979). Evaluation of essential oil from leaves of *Adhatoda vasica* as an airway smooth muscle relaxant. *Indian Journal of Pharmaceutical Sciences*, **41**: 247.

Daniel, T. F. (1993a). New and reconsidered Mexican Acanthaceae III, Justicia. *Contr. Univ. Michigan Herb.*, **17**: 133-137.

Day S.H., Chen-Lin Y., Mei-Lin T., Tsa L.T., Horng-Huey K. Mei-Ing C., Chang Lee J., y Chun-Nan L. (2002). Potent citotoxic lignans from *Justicia procumbens* and their effects on Nitric Oxide and Tumor Necrosis Factor-α Production in Mouse Macrophages. *J. Nat. Prod.*, **65**: 379-381.

de Smet PA (1985): A multidisciplinary overview of intoxicanting snuff rituals in the western hemisphere. *J Ethnopharmacol.*, **13**: 3–49.

Dhar, M.L., Dhar, M.M., Dhawan, B.N., Mehrotra, B.N., Ray, C. (1968). Screening of Indian plants for biological activity: part I. *Indian Journal of Experimental Biology*, **6**: 232–247.

Domínguez X.A., Achenbach H., González C., Amare F.D. (1990). Estudio químico del muitle (*Justicia spicigera*). *Rev. Latinoamericana de Química*, 21: 142-143.

Dymock, W., Waeden, C.J.H., Hooper, D. (1890). Pharmacographia Indica, A History of the Principal Drugs of Vegetable Origin. Paul, Trech, Trubner and Co. Ltd, London, pp. 50–54.

Ezcurra C. (1993a). Acanthaceae. In A. L. Cabrera (editor), Flora (le la Provincia de Jujuy 9: 278-359. Colee 3i. 1NTA, Buenos Aires

Ezcurra C. (1999b). Acanthaceae. In F. O. Zuloaga and O. Mo- rrone (etlitors), Catalogo de las Plantas Vaseulares de la Republica Argentina. *Monogr. Syst. Bot. Missouri Bot. Gard.*, **74**: 1-14.

Fukamiya N, Lee KH (1986): Antitumor agents, 81. Justicidin-A and diphyllin, two cytotoxic principles from *Justicia procumbens*. *J Nat Prod.*, **49**: 348–350.

Garcia, S.K. y Dimayuga, R.E. (1991). Antimicrobial screening of medicinal plants from Baja California Sur, México. *Journal of Ethnopharmacology*, **31**: 181-192

Ghosal S, Banerjee S, Frahm AW (1979a): Chemicalconstituents of *Justicia*. III. Prostalidins A, B, C and retrochinensis: a new antidepressant; 4-aryl-2,3-naphtalide lignans from *Justicia prostrata*. *Chem Ind.*, **23**: 854–855.

Ghosal S, Banerjee S, Jaiswal DK (1980b). Chemical constituentsof *Justicia*. Part 2. New furofurano lignans from *Justicia simplex*. *Phytochemistry* **19**: 332–334.

Graham, V. (1988). Delimitation and infra-generic classification of *Justicia* (*Acanthaceae*). *Kew Bulletin*, **43**: 551-624.

Grange J. M., Noel J.C. Snell. (1996). Activity of bromhexine and ambroxol, semi-synthetic derivatives of vasicine from the Indian shrub *Adhatoda vasica*, against *Mycobacterium tuberculosis in vitro*. *Journal of Ethnopharmacology*, **50**: 49-53.

Herrera-Mata H., Rosas-Romero A. and Crescente O. (2002). Biological Activity of "Sanguinaria" (*Justicia secunda*) Extracts. *Pharmaceutical Biology*, **40(3)**: 206–212

Huq M.E., Ikram M., Warsi S.A. (1967). Chemical composition of *Adhatoda vasica* Linn. II. *Pakistan Journal of Scientific and Industrial Research*, **10**: 224–225.

Ibrahim B, M'batchi B, Mounzeo H, Bourobou BHP, Posso P (2000). Effect of *Tephrosia vogelii* and *Justicia extensa* on *Tilapia nilotica in vivo*. *J. Ethnopharmacol.*, **69**: 99–104.

Iyengar M.A., Jambaiah K.M., Kamath M.S., Rao G.O. (1994). Studies on an antiasthma Kada: a proprietary herbal combination, Part I. Clinical study. *Indian Drugs*, **31**: 183–186.

Jabbar A., Lateef M., Iqbal Z., Khan M. N., Akhtar M. S. (2003). Anthelmintic activity of *Adhatoda vasica* roots. *International Journal of Agriculture and Biology*, **5**: 86-90

Jorgensen, P. M. and S. Leon-Yanez. (1999). Catalogo de las Plantas Vasculares del Ecuador. Monogr. *Syst. Bot. Mis- souri Bot. Gard*., **75**: 453-465.

Joseph H, Gleye J, Moulis C, Mensah LJ, Roussakis C, Gratas C (1988). Justicidin B, a cytotoxic principle from *Justicia pectoralis*. *J Nat Prod.*, **51**: 599–600.

Sanmugapriya, E., Shanmugasudraram, P., Venkataraman, S. (2005). Anti-inflammatory activity of *Justicia próstata* gamble in acute and sub-acute models of inflammation. *Inflammopharmacology*, **13**: 493-500

Sastry KV, Rao EV, Pelter A, Ward RS (1979). 4-Aryl-2,3-naphtalide lignans from *Justicia simplex*. *Indian J Chem Sect B*. (**17B**): 415–416.

Sepulveda-Jimenez G., Reyna-Aquino C., Bermudez-Torres K., Rodriguez-Monroy M. (2009). Antioxidant activity and content of phenolic compounds and flavonoids from *Justicia spicigera*. *Journal of Biological Sciences*, **1**: 1-4

Shete, A.B. (1993). Femiforte, indigenous herbomineral formulation in the management of non-specific leucorrhoea. *Doctor's News*, **5**: 13–14.

Singh K., Jasemine S., Srivastava R.S. (2007). Hepatoprotective Effect of Crude Extract and Isolated Lignans of justicia simplex Against CCl_4-Induced hepatotoxicity. *Pharmaceutical Biology*, **45(4)**: 247-277

Subbaraju, G.V., Kumar, K.K., Raju, B.L., Pillai, K.R., Reddy, M.C.(1991). Justiciresinol, a new furanoid lignan from *Justicia glauca*. *J Nat Prod.*, **54**: 1639–1641.

Telefo, P.B., Moundipa, P.F., Tchana, A.N., Tchouanguep, D.C.,Mbiapo, F.T. (1998). Effects of an aqueous extract of *Aloe buettneri, Justicia insularis, Hibiscus macranthus, Dicliptera verticillata* on some physiological and biochemical parameters of reproduction in immature female rats. *J Ethnopharmacol.*, **63**: 193–200.

Thom E., Wollan T. (1997). A controlled clinical study of Kanjang mixture in the treatment of uncomplicated upper respiratory tract infections. *Phytotherapy Research*, 11: 207–210.

Willaman, J.J., Li, H.L. (1970). Alkaloid-bearing plants and their contained alkaloids, 1957–1968. *Lloydia*, **33**S: 1-286.

World Health Organization (1990). The use of traditional medicine in primary health care. A Manual for Health Workers in South-East Asia, SEARO Regional Health Papers, No 19, New Delhi, pp. 1–2.

Yarnell E., Abascal K. (2009). Plants coumarins: Myths and realitie. *Alternative and Complementary Therapies*, **15 (1)**: 24-30.

Bioactive Phytochemicals: Perspectives for Modern Medicine Vol. 1 (2012) *Pages* **477–494**
Editor: **V.K. Gupta**
Published by: **DAYA PUBLISHING HOUSE, NEW DELHI**

15

Biological Activities of *Anoectochilus formosanus* Hayat and its Active Component

Xiao-Ming Du[1] and Yukihiro Shoyama[2*]

ABSTRACT

The extract of Anoectochilus formosanus showed significant activity in decreasing the levels of LDH, GOT and GPT, resulting prominent hepatoprotective activity against CCl_4 induced hepatotoxicity. In the test using aurothioglucose-induced obese mice, the extract of A. formosanus showed a significant antihyperliposis effect. The body and liver weights were significantly suppressed ameliorating TG levels in the liver and serum in the extract treated group. When the high TG volunteers were used, the administration of A. formosanus significantly decreased the levels of TC, VLDL and Apo E. The results suggest that A. formosanus may be useful for improvement of lipid-metabolism and the prevention of atherosclerosis. A. formosanus contains ten compounds including a major known component, kinsenoside. In an anti-hyperliposis assay using high-fat diet rats and in aurothioglucose-induced obese mouse, kinsenoside significantly reduced the weights of body and liver, and also decreased the triglyceride level in the liver compared to those of control rats.

Keywords: *Anoectochilus* species, Orchidaceae, Kinsenoside, Antihyperliposis, Hepatoprotective activity.

1 Central University for Nationalities, 27 Zhongguancun, South Avenue, Beijing 100081, China.

2 Faculty of Pharmaceutical Science, Nagasaki International University, 2825-7 Huis Ten Bosch, Sasebo, Nagasaki 859-3298, Japan.

* *Corresponding author* E-mail: shoyama@miu.ac.jp

Introduction

The *Anoectochilus* species (Orchidaceae) is perennial herbs which comprise more than 35 species that are widespread in the tropical regions, from India through the Himalayas and southeast Asia to Hawaii (Asahishinbun, 1997). Several species have been used in Chinese folk medicines (Jiangsu New Medical College, 1977). Among them, *A. formosanus* which is only found in Taiwan and Okinawa, has been used for hypertension, lung and liver diseases and underdeveloped children as a folk medicine (Kan, 1986). It becomes evident that the natural resources of *A. formosanus* are becoming exhausted, therefore the other *Anoectochilus* species such as *A. koshunensis* and a different genus, *Goodyera* species are commercialized as substitutes used for the same purpose in the recent market (Lin and Namba, 1981a,b). From such situation we started to investigate the micropropagation of this species by tissue culture techniques, and worked on its chemical components and pharmacological profiles (Du *et al.*, 1998; 2000a,b).

Since we isolated a great amount of kinsenoside without its methyl ester by silica gel column chromatography eluting with chloroform-ethanol solvent system, it is easily suggested that some artificial conversion occurred during the separation procedure. This result inspired us to investigate the existence and concentrations of kinsenoside and its analogues in *Anoectochilus* species. Purified kinsenoside had antihyperliposis and hepatoprotective activity.

This review demonstrated the clinical evidences using volunteers will be also discussed.

1. Micropropagation of A. formosanus and its Components

The ripened fruits of *A. formosanus* were sterilized, and seeds in fruits were cultured on 1/2 MS medium (Murashige and Skoog, 1962) supplemented with 1 mg/l 6-benzylaminopurine (BA) and 2 g/l peptone. After 30 days the seeds germinated and formed protocorms at 25°C. The seedlings, 6–8 cm in length, were transferred to 1/2 MS liquid medium to produce the multiple shoot complex. They were cultured in 1/2 MS liquid medium supplemented with 0.3 mg/l BA and 0.03 mg/l α-naphthaleneacetic acid (NAA) under shaking at 30 rpm. After 2 months they were transferred to 1/2 MS liquid medium without growth regulator and shaken for 4 more months. The regenerated plantlets were grown for 6–8 months as indicated in Figure 15.1. Since the wild and cultured *A. formosanus* had the completely same composition, the cultured plants were used for further investigations.

The regenerated plants at three different stages of culturing: (a) multiple shooting, (b) shoot elongation and (c) rooting were analyzed. The results suggested that the cultured segments, a, b and c and the original plant had the same pattern of composition, although the concentrations were somewhat different. Therefore, it is evident that micropropagation of this species using plant biotechnological technique will be available to enable maintenance of this important crude drug.

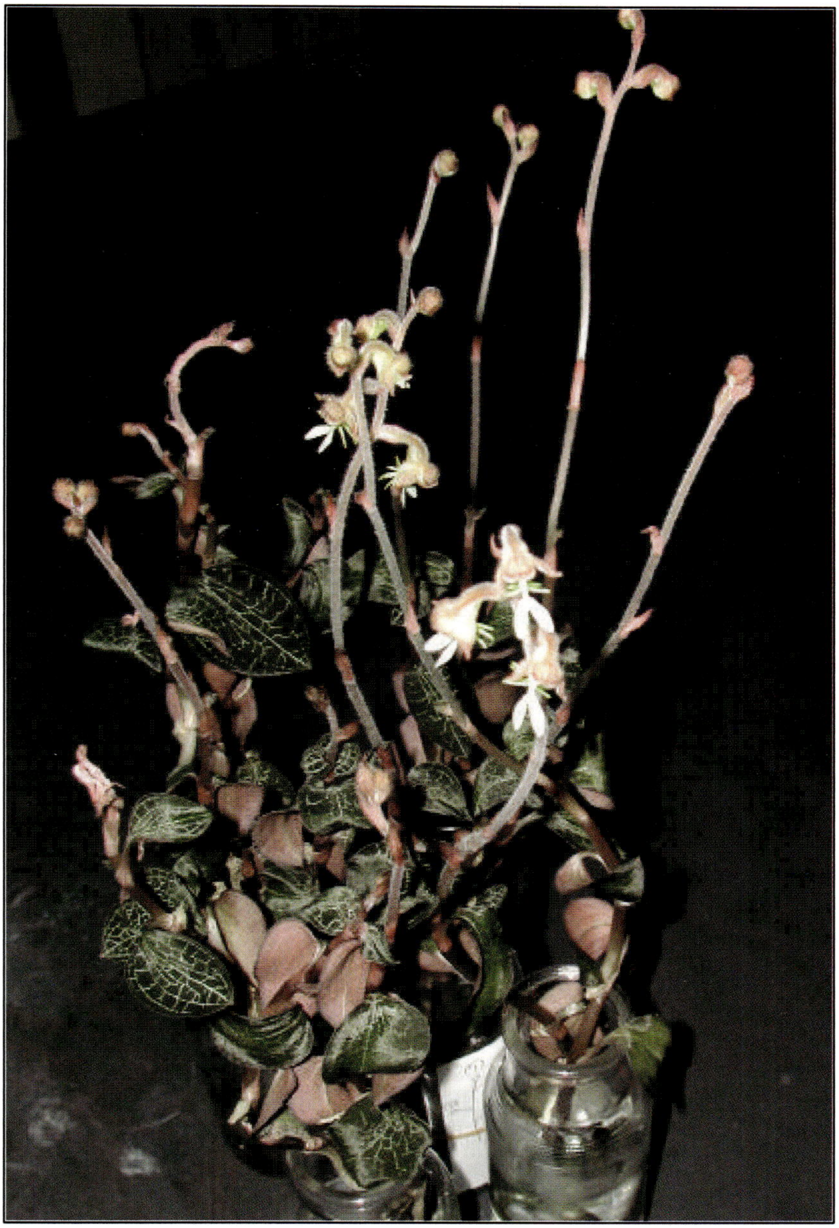

Figure 15.1: Flowering of cultured *Anoectochilus formosanus* Hayata.

2. Antihyperliposis Activity of Crude Extract of A. formosanus

The hyperlipidemia and obesity following customs of livelihood is a major health problem in many countries with the escalation of obesity-related disease. The prevalence is increasing even in developing countries. This condition is associated

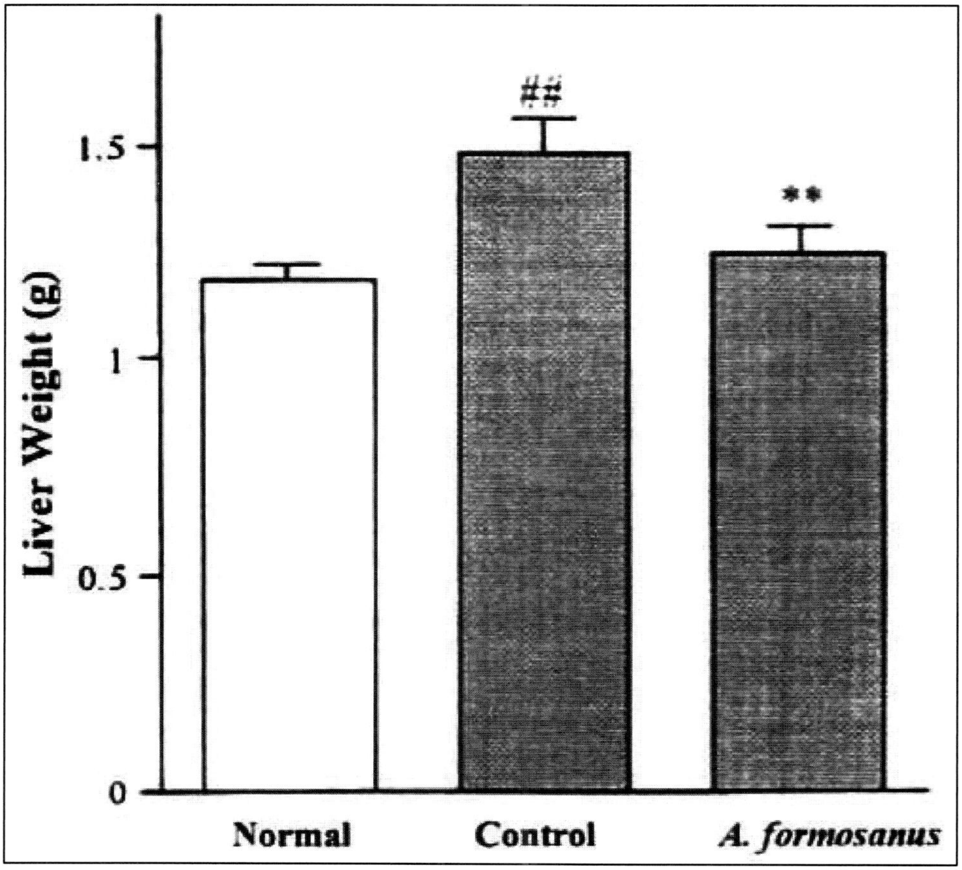

p < 0.01 significantly different from the normal group.
** p < 0.01 significantly different from the control group.

Figure 15.3: Effect of *Anoectochilus formosanus* crude extract on liver weight of mice.

for hyperliposis, especially for fatty liver. Moreover, the improvement of lipid-metabolism might be closely related to the hepatoprotective activity of *A. formosanus*.

Clinical Evidences

The higher levels of TC and TG in serum than 220 mg/dl and 150 mg/dl, respectively, were considered to be hyperlipidemia. Since the VLDL and LDL levels are depend on the increases of TC and TG, it is considered that the high-TC or TG levels may possibly induce high-lipoprotein. Cholesterol status became to be considered as an important factor since the correlation has been established between the serum cholesterol level and risk of coronary heart disease as well as the severity of atherosclerosis (Brecher *et al.*, 1965; Kannel *et al.*, 1971; Goldburt *et al.*, 1985; Stamler *et al.*, 1986). Moreover, the increases of VLDL and LDL levels were also observed in the disease of obesity, diabetes and nephrosis.

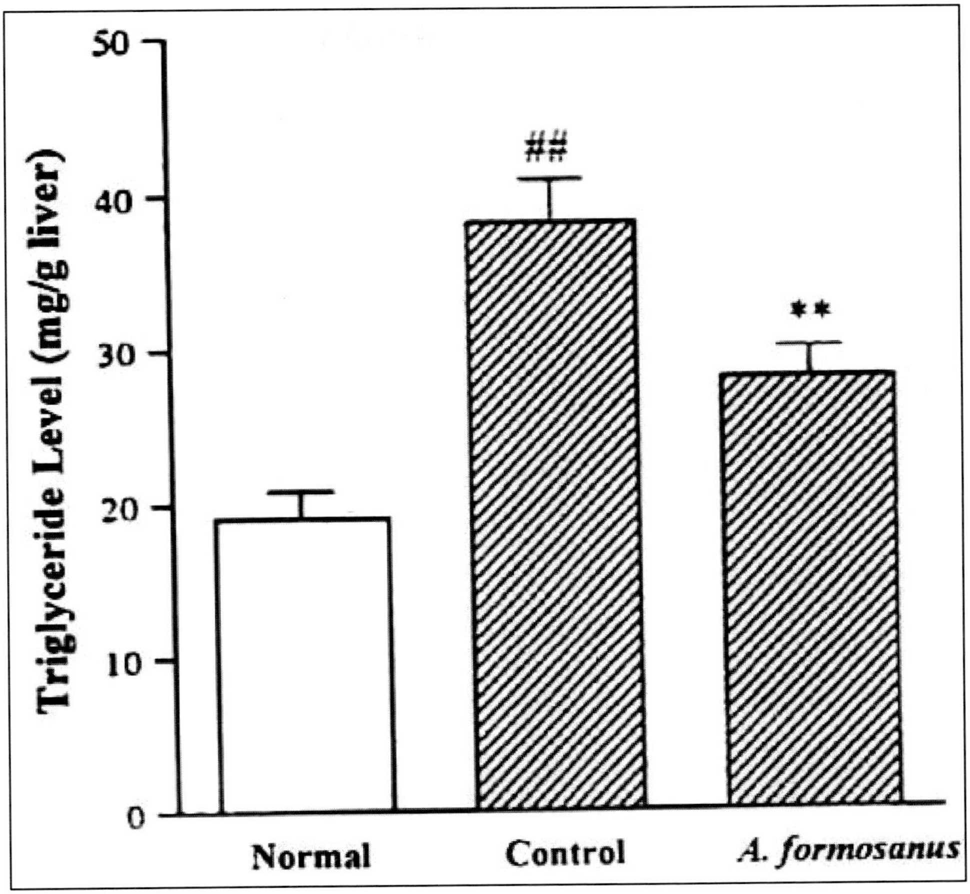

p < 0.01 significantly different from the normal group.
** p < 0.01 significantly different from the control group.

Figure 15.4: Effect of *Anoectochilus formosanus* crude extract on triglyceride level on the liver of mice.

There were no significant differences in all anthropometry and serum biochemical parameters during 6 months of the administration period in normal health subjects. On the other hand, the level of Apo E decreased significantly after 12-months-treatment and that of VLDL did remarkably (Table 15.2).

When the high TG volunteers were used, the administration of *A. formosanus* significantly decreased the levels of TC, VLDL and Apo E (Table 15.3). The results of the present study suggest that *A. formosanus* may be useful for improvement of lipid-metabolism and the prevention of atherosclerosis. On the other hand, Nomura *et al.* confirmed the close correlation between hyperlipidemia, fatty liver and obesity by the previous investigation of nosographic study (Nomura *et al.*, 1988).

The levels of AST and ALT were significantly lower after 6-months-treatment, these levels, however, return to the original values. In the present study, 11 volunteers

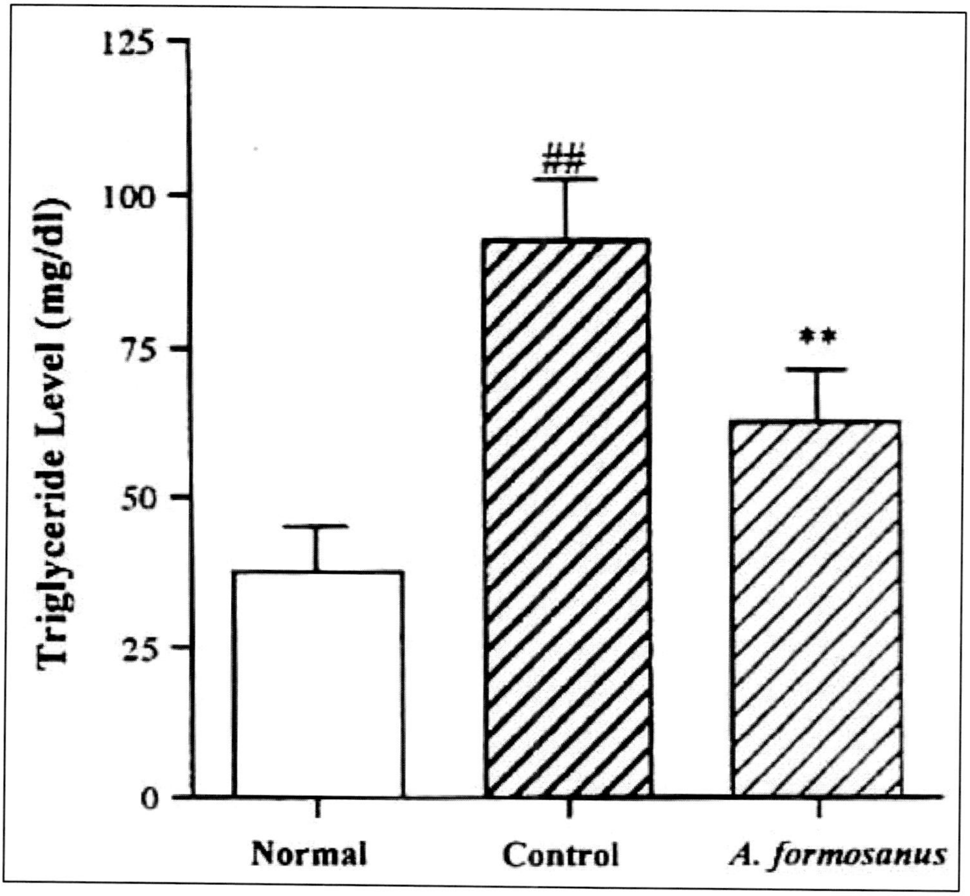

p < 0.01 significantly different from the normal group.
** p < 0.01 significantly different from the control group.

Figure 15.5: Effect of *Anoectochilus formosanus* crude extract on serum triglyceride level in mice.

were high-ALT, AST levels, and they also have higher levels of BMI, VLDL and LDL compared to those of the normal volunteers. The levels of VLDL and Apo E were significantly lower after 12-months-treatment, although no difference was observed after 6 months-treatment (Table 15.4). The level of TG was decreased gradually during 12 months.

After administration of *A. formosanus* for 6 months, the levels of AST and ALT were significantly reduced, and after 12 months of treatment, the levels of TC, VLDL and LDL were also significantly reduced when used high TG and TC volunteers (Table 15.5). From these results, it was believed that the improvement of lipid-metabolism effect of *A. formosanus* might be closely related to the improvement of liver function. Liver, the key organ of metabolism and excretion is continuously and variedly exposed to xenobiotics because of its strategic placement in the body. The effect of *A. formosanus* on liver function will be further investigated.

Table 15.2: Effect of *Anoectochilus formosanus* crude extract on the lipid metabolism in normal health subjects.

	36 Volunteers		*21 Volunteers*	
	0 Months	*6 Months*	*6 Months*	*12 Months*
BMI (kg/m²)	23.9±32	23.9±3.1	23.7±3.1	23.8±3.3
Percentage body fat (per cent)	28.1±4.6	29.4±4.1	28.5±4.4	28.2±3.9
TG (mg/dl)	90.1±30.7	95.7±41.4	93.9±27.0	80.7±25.9
TC (mg/dl)	177.9±31.4	183.7±33.0	189.3±25.3	178.3±28.8
HDL-C (mg/dl)	58.8±13.2	54.5±10.1	60.2±15.1	54.7±11.9
LDL (mg/dl)	100.1±26.2	109.3±26.9	106.3±21.9	107.4±26.9
VLDL (mg/dl)	124.9±56.4	129.6±61.8	129.9±53.5	85.8±36.5**
Apo A-T (mg/dl)	147.6±20.7	149.3±21.8	148.8±22.2	147.1±27.6
Apo B (mg/dl)	58.8±13.2	79.9±21.5	85.2±17.0	93.5±363
Apo E (mg/dl)	5.1±1.6	5.1±1.3	5.1±1.4	4.2±0.9*
AST (IU/l)	16.3±5.5	16.9±6.2	17.7±6.5	18.2±6.3
ALT (IU/l)	17.7±10.5	18.5±11.7	19.1±12.2	18.9±10.3
ALP (IU/l)	162.6±53.2	160.4±43.0	165.2±63.9	159.0±58.8
γ-OPT (IU/l)	30.8±34.2	31.8±37.6	27.5±19.5	31.5±34.0

Values are presented as mean±SD.

*$p < 0.05$. **$p < 0.01$.

Significantly different compared to values before treatment.

Table 15.3: Effect of *Anoectochilus formosanus* crude extract on the lipid metabolism in high triglyceride subjects.

	14 Volunteers		*7 Volunteers*	
	0 Months	*6 Months*	*6 Months*	*12 Months*
BMI (kg/nr)	25.6±4.2	25.5±4.4	25.4±1.8	25.3±2.3
Percentage body fat (per cent)	26.8±7.2	27.8±8.1	26.7±6.6	26.7±9.2
TG (mg/dl)	242.4±77.6	204.3±48.2	207.6±38.1	159.3±34.7
TC (mg/dl)	208.2±50.4	203.9±36.4	223.7±56.2	202.4±47.6*
HDL-C (mg/dl)	45.9±10.5	44.0±11.5	49.9±9.3	47.7±10.2
LDL (mg/dl)	115.6±46.0	119.0±33.2	132.2±48.8	122.9±45.3
VLDL (mg/dl)	323.2±87.3	321.7±82.7	329.0±77.7	165.0±37.4**
Apo A-I (mg/dl)	141.6±29.0	140.0±23.7	146.1±21.2	158.6±33.6
Apo B (mg/dl)	104.6±24.6	102.4±24.4	108.1±29.9	99.9±53.9
Apo B (mg/dl)	7.2±2.3	6.9±14	7.3±2.0	5.8±1.2*
AST (IU/l)	24.6±10.6	21.6±6.7	23.4±12.9	19.4±6.5
ALT (IU/l)	31.7±19.5	27.6±18.4	27.9±20.6	22.0±10.5
ALP (IU/l)	204.2±50.3	198.3±54.6	198.0±59.8	203.1±77.9
γ-GPT (IU/l)	62.1±65.2	52.9±43.1	56.1±74.1	55.4±61.2

Values are presented as mean±SD.

*$p < 0.05$. **$p < 0.01$.

Significantly different compared to values before treatment.

Table 15.4: Effect of *Anoectochilus formosanus* crude extract on the lipid metabolism in high cholesterol subjects.

	11 Volunteers		
	0 Months	*6 Months*	*12 Months*
BMI (kg/m³)	25.8±2.7	25.6±3.1	25.6±3.0
Percentage body fat (%)	25.6±5.3	26.6±5.8	25.4±5.0
TG (mg/dl)	227.0±54.7	166.6±46.6	143.7±503
TC (mg/dl)	248.5±24.2	239.9±18.5	235.8±25.7
HDL-C (mg/dl)	53.9±12.5	50.3±13.0	53.1±14.8
LDL (mg/dl)	156.3±36.5	155.2±24.8	160.3±33.8
VLDL (mg/dl)	289.9±126.3	282.0±132.6	150.0±53.4*
Apo A-I (mg/dl)	153.2±31.2	146.0±27.1	156.6±39.5
Apo B (mg/dl)	125.2±14.5	120.0±20.5	128.0±56.3
Apo E (mg/dl)	7.2±2.9	6.9±1.5	5.9±1.5*
AST (IU/l)	27.6±10.0	21.3±6.8*	24.9±9.5
ALT (IU/l)	35.3±19.6	27.3±14.4*	35.6±18.4
ALP (IU/l)	208.6±53.8	207.0±48.4	211.7±56.5
γ-GPT (IU/l)	84.9±71.0	71.5±61.8	78.4±89.3

Values are presented as mean±SD.

*$p < 0.05$. **$p < 0.01$.

Significantly different compared to values before treatment.

Table 15.5: Effect of *Anoectochilus formosanus* crude extract on the lipid metabolism in high triglyceride and cholesterol subjects.

	5 Volunteers		
	0 Months	*6 Months*	*12 Months*
BMI (kg/m³)	25.2±2.2	24.7±2.1	23.7±1.5
Percentage body fat (%)	25.0±5.0	25.4±5.5	22.6±5.9
TG (mg/dl)	209.0±46.7	186.8±43.9	160.8±42.1
TC (mg/dl)	265.4±23.5	238.2±27.0*	237.5±22.5*
HDL-C (mg/dl)	52.6±10.2	48.8±10.4	53.0±10.5
LDL (mg/dl)	171.0±22.7	152.0±25.7*	143.5±39.1*
VLDL (mg/dl)	323.8±103.2	363.0±118.4	1703±28.1**
Apo A-I (mg/dl)	154.2±20.9	145.8±24.9	171.3±39.8
Apo B (mg/dl)	130.2±13.4	118.6±23.9	107.5±74.6
Apo E (mg/dl)	7.6±2.2	7.6±1.5	6.4±1.1
AST (IU/l)	30.6±13.5	23.2±8.0*	22.3±7.3*
ALT (IU/l)	40.0±27.5	29.2±19.6*	23.0±14.2*
ALP (IU/l)	210.8±69.2	203.2±48.9	199.0±1.5
γ-GPT (IU/l)	96.2±93.7	71.6±573	70.8±81.8
Glucose (mg/dl)	100.8±13.4	101.4±21.2	89.7±7.5
HbA1C (per cent)	5.7±0.8	5.7±0.6	5.3±0.3

Values are presented as mean±SD.

*$p < 0.05$. **$p < 0.01$.

Significantly different compared to values before treatment.

In general *A. formosanus* has been used 4 to 40 g of fresh weight per day, although the present study only used a very lower dose for volunteers (450 mg/day). The acute toxicological effects of water extracts of *Anoectochilus* species including *A. formosanus* were administered in single dose of 5000 mg/kg p.o. No gross abnormalities were found in any organs of the treated animals at the necropsy, but the change of body weight of tested rats showed significant decrease in male and female rats at 7 and 14 days. It becomes evident that *Anoectochilus* species were non-or less toxic products.

Chemical Composition of Cultured A. koshunensis

The dried whole plants cultured were extracted with MeOH at room temperature, and the concentrate was suspended in H_2O and partitioned successively with $CHCl_3$ and *n*-BuOH. The residues obtained from the H_2O layer and the *n*-BuOH layer were separately subjected to normal-phase and reversed-phase silica gel column chromatography to give ten compounds. The structures of the known compounds were identified as glucose, sucrose, kinsenoside (**1**) (Ito *et al.*, 1994), 3-(*R*)-3-β-D-glucopyranosyloxy-4-hydroxybutanoic acid (**2**) (Du *et al.*, 1998; 2000a), 1-*O*-isopropyl-β-D-glucopyranoside (**4**) (Du *et al.*, 1998b), (*R*)-(+)-3,4-dihydroxybutanoic acid γ-lactone (**5**) (Ito *et al.*, 1994), 4-(β-D-glucopyranosyloxy)benzyl alcohol (**6**) (Pabst et al., 1992) (Taguchi *et al.*, 1981), (6*R*,9*S*)-9-hydroxy-megastigma-4,7-dien-3-one-9-*O*-β-D-glucopyranoside (**7**) (Pabst *et al.*, 1992), and corchoionoside C (**8**) (Pabst *et al.*, 1992), by comparing their spectral data with those previously reported.

The positive ion FAB mass spectrum of unknown components, **2** showed a $[M+H]^+$ peak at m/z 283 suggesting that it had the molecular formula $C_{10}H_{18}O_9$. The ^{13}C NMR spectrum indicated the existence of a free carboxylic acid group (δ179.6), an oxygenated carbon at δ66.0 and a hexose moiety at δ104.1 (see Experimental). The ^1H NMR spectrum showed some readily assignable signals, such as two methylene groups δ2.38 (1H, *dd*, *J*=14.8, 5.9 Hz), 2.46 (1H, *dd*, *J*=14.8, 7.3 Hz) and δ3.59 (1H, *dd*, *J*=12.5, 5.9 Hz), 3.64 (1H, *dd*, *J*=12.5, 4.3 Hz), and a methine signal 4.12 (*dddd*, *J*=7.3, 5.9, 5.9, 4.3 Hz). These data suggested the presence of 3,4-dihydroxy butylic acid in **2**. When **2** was exposed to mild acid conditions, compound **3** was obtained. From the above evidence, the structure of **2** was determined to be 3-*O*-β-D-glucopyranosyl-(3*R*)-4-dihydroxy butanoic acid. From these results the stereochemistry of the C-3 hydroxyl group of **2** was confirmed to be *R*. Figure 15.6 indicated the structures of components isolated from cultured *A. koshunensis*.

In order to confirm the exact structure of kinsenoside, X-ray diffraction analysis of the corresponding peracetate was investigated. The structure of kinsenoside (**1**), including the stereochemistry on the hydroxyl group at C-3 was identified unambiguously to be 3-*O*-β-D-glucopyranosyl-(3*R*)-4-dihydroxy butanolide, isolated from *A. koshunensis* and named as kinsenoside by Ito *et al.*, 1994, as indicated in Figure 15.7.

Antihyperliposis and Hepatoprotective Active Compound, Kinsenoside

The crude extracts of *in vitro* cultured *A. koshunensis* were purified guided by anti-hyperliposis assay using high-fat diet rats to isolate kinsenoside as an active component.

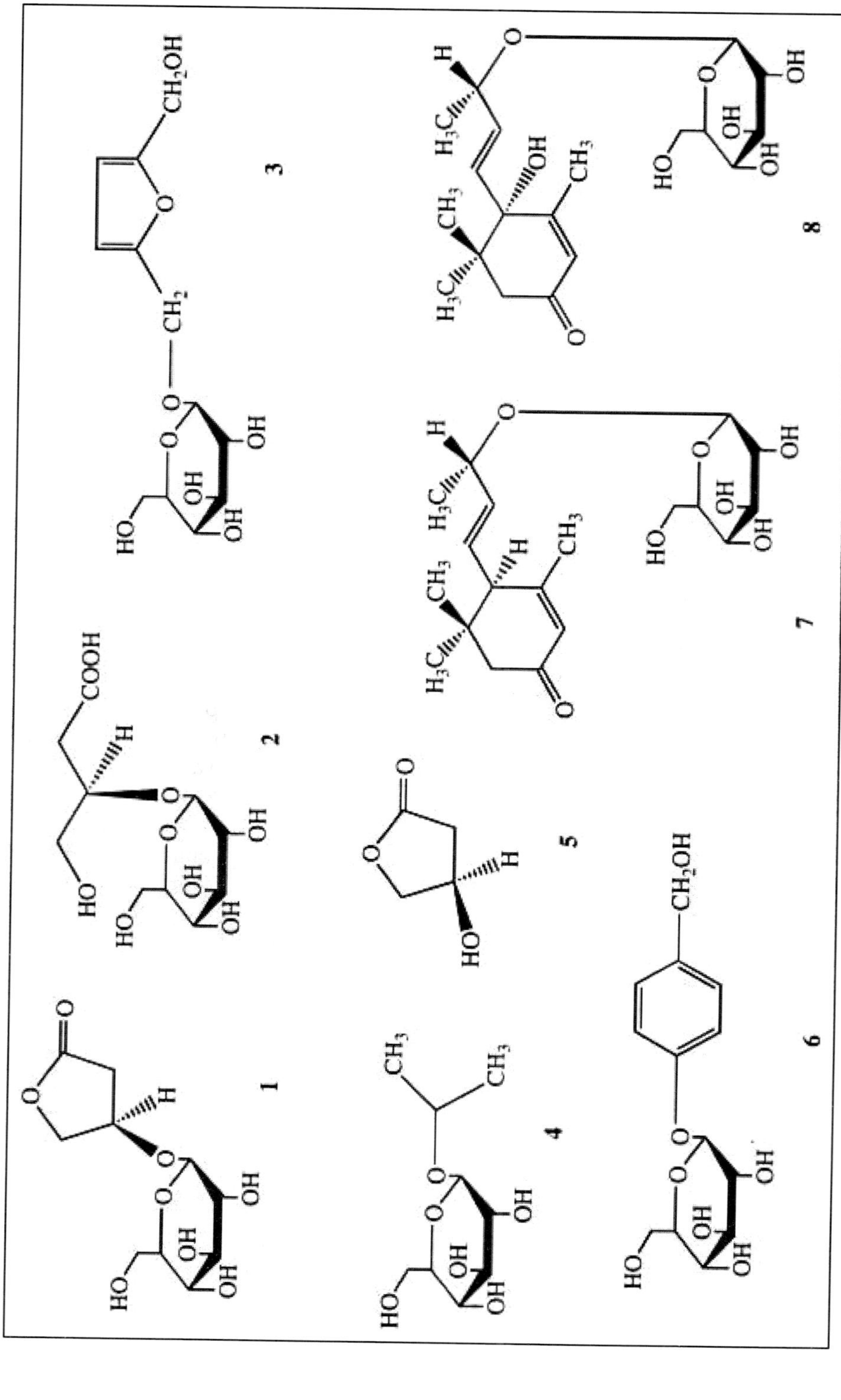

Figure 15.6: Structure of components isolated from *Anoectochilus formosanus*.

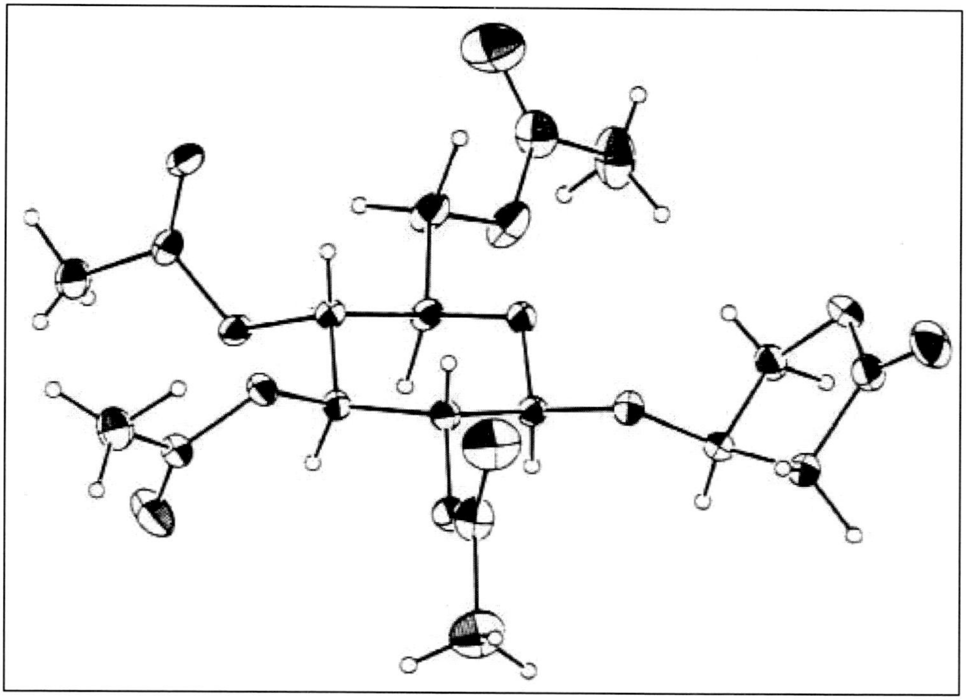

Figure 15.7: X-ray analysis of peracetyl-kinsenoside.

In an assay for anti-hyperliposis effect using high-fat diet rats, kinsenoside significantly ameliorated the TG level in liver. The liver and body weights were lower than those of control group. Table 15.6 shows the change in body weight and liver weight when 6-week-old male SD rats were fed HFD (to make hyperlipemia model rats) and the same diet plus oral administration of kinsenoside [(50 mg/kg (being equal to 300-400 mg dried whole plant of *A. formosanus*) and 100 mg/kg (being equal to 600-800 mg plant)] for 6 days, respectively. The body weight increase was seen in the normal group and control group, although no difference was observed between these two groups. However, weight was suppressed in kinsenoside administered groups. Especially, the 100 mg/kg kinsenoside administered group exhibited significantly lower weight than the control group.

The liver weight of the control group was significantly higher than that of the normal group. However, the liver weight of both the 50 mg/kg kinsenoside group and 100 mg/kg kinsenoside group was significantly lower than that of the control group.

Figure 15.8 shows the value of TG in liver of rats TG, a neutral lipid, is a risk factor implicated in obesity and other diseases. The TG level in liver of the control group was significantly higher than in the normal group. The levels in the 50 mg/kg kinsenoside group and the 100 mg/kg kinsenoside group were significantly lower than the control group. When compared to TG concentration per liver protein, the same result was obtained.

Table 15.6: Hepatoprotective activity of kinsenoside and compound 2 on the body and liver weight in rats.

Group	*Dose (p.o.) (mg/kg)*	*Body Weight (g)*	*Liver Weight (g)*
Normal	–	212.32±2.24	6.80±0.18
Control	–	213.19±4.23	8.81±0.33##
Kinsenoside	50	204.10±1.97	7.72±0.18**
Kinsenoside	100	202.18±2.39*	7.08±0.28**

##: $p < 0.01$ versus normal group; *$p < 0.05$; **$p < 0.01$ versus control group.

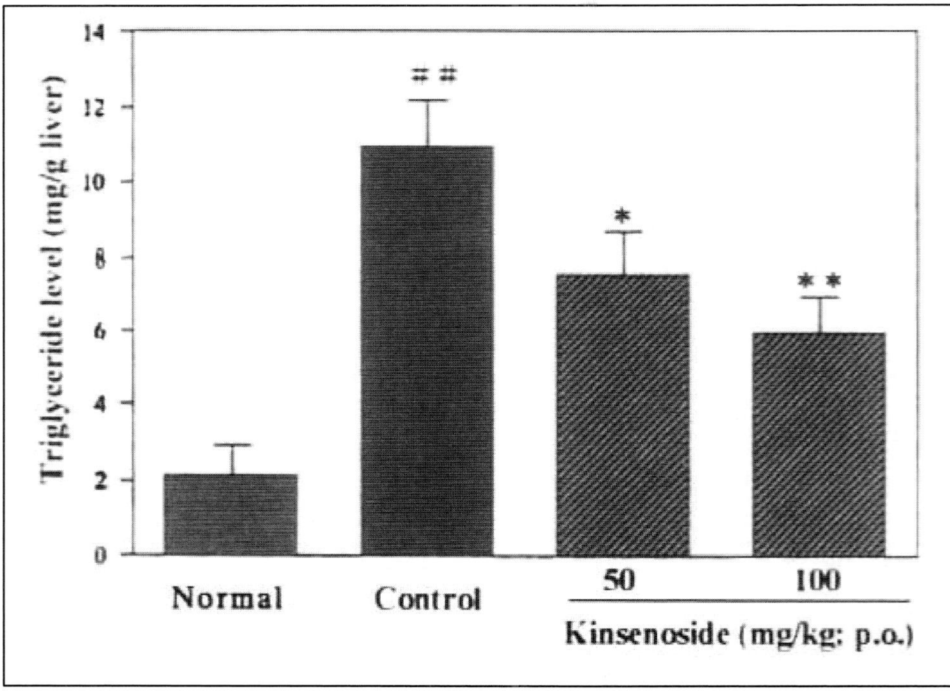

p < 0.01 significantly different from the normal group.
** p < 0.01 significantly different from the control group.
* p < 0.1significantly different from the control group.

Figure 15.8: Effect of kinsenoside on triglyceride level in liver of rats.

The effect of kinsenoside on antihyperliposis was also examined by using aurothioglucose-induced obese mouse (Pabst *et al.*, 1992; Brecher and Waxler, 1949). There was no significant difference in food consumption between normal and the control or kinsenoside treated groups. This is in agreement with the literature (Brobeck, 1946; Han and Liu, 1966). Diet amounts during the period were 3.93 g/d for the normal mouse, 4.18 g/d for the control mouse, 4.23 g/d and 4.09 g/d for kinsenoside treated mouse. Figure 15.9 shows the change in body weight for normal mice, and

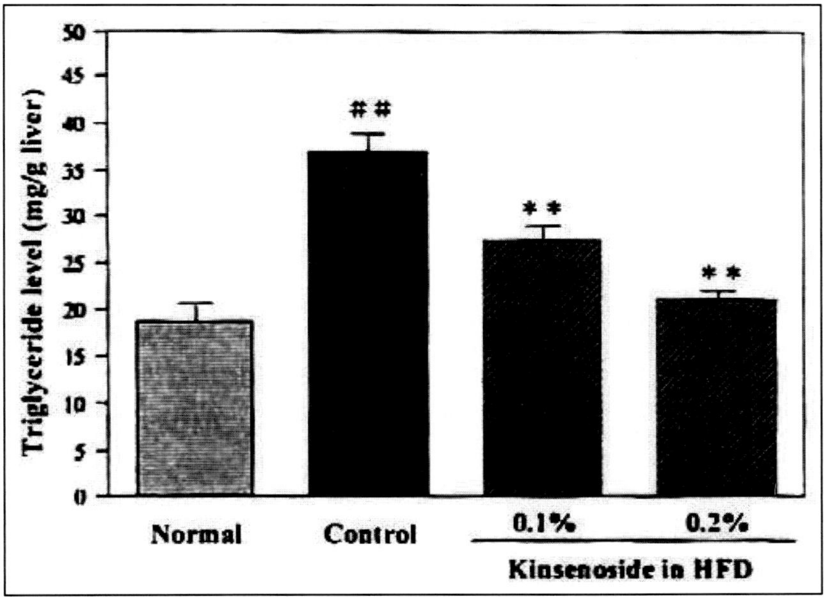

p <0.01 significantly different from the normal group.
** p < 0.01 significantly different from the control group.

Figure 15.9: Effect of kinsenoside on the triglyceride level in liver after aurothioglucose-induced obese mice for 6 weeks.

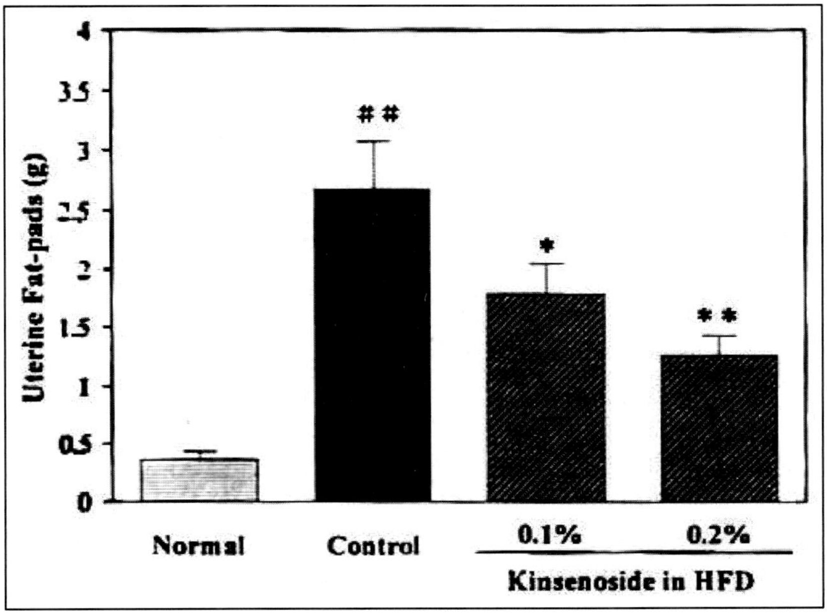

p < 0.01 significantly different from the normal group.
** p < 0.01 significantly different from the control group.
* p < 0.1 significantly different from the control group.

Figure 15.10: Effect of kinsenoside on uterine fat pads of aurothioglucose-induced obese mice after 6 weeks.

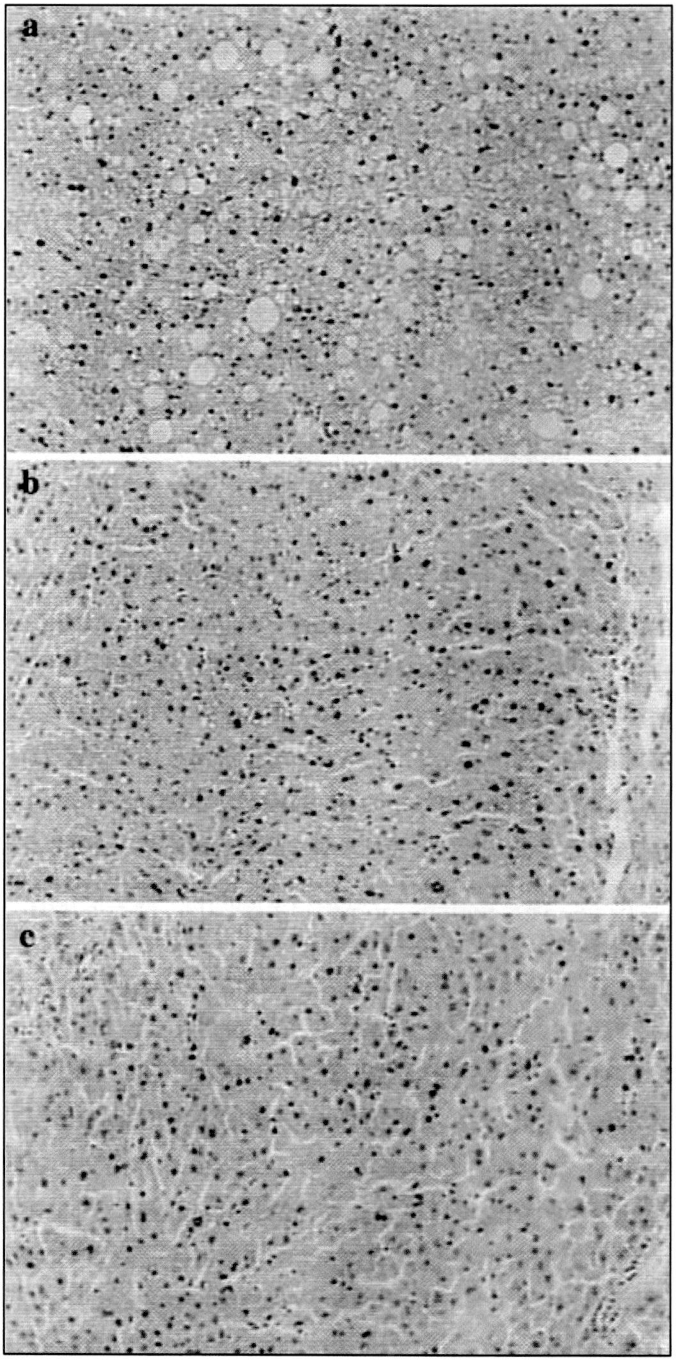

Figure 15.11: Photomicrographs of histopathological changes showing the effect of kinsenoside in the liver of aurothioglucose-induced obese mice after 6 weeks.

a: Control group **b**: 0.1% kinsenoside group **c**: 0.2% kinsenoside group.

when aurothioglucose-induced obese mice that were fed the HFD (as control) or the same diet containing 0.1 per cent or 0.2 per cent kinsenoside for 6 weeks, respectively. Rapid weight increase was observed in the control group, while it was suppressed in the kinsenoside treated groups. Especially, the 0.2 per cent kinsenoside administered group exhibited significantly lower weight than the control group. The weight increases of liver and uterine fat-pads were also observed in the control group, while in the kinsenoside treated groups, they were significantly decreased (Figure 15.10). The livers in the control group were considerably swollen, and the color and luster were those of fatty liver. These phenomena were not observed in the kinsenoside treated groups.

Figure 15.11 shows the typical histological views of the liver in the mice being fed the HFD and the diet with kinsenoside (0.1 per cent and 0.2 per cent, respectively) after 6 weeks. A great deal of accumulated fatty drops was observed in the control group, while it was significantly decreased in the kinsenoside administered groups. It is considered that the body weight increase was suppressed by the improvement of lipid-metabolism.

The findings of the present study indicate kinsenoside may be useful for the treatment for hyperliposis. In aurothioglucose-induced obese mouse, kinsenoside suppressed the body and liver weight increase, significantly ameliorated the triglyceride level in the liver, and also reduced the deposition of uterine fat-pads.

Acknowledgement

Clinical evidences were investigated by Prof. Jun Hayashi and co-workers in Kyushu University Hospital. We thank for their assistances.

References

Asahishinbun, *Asahi Encyclopedia the World of Plants*, Vol. 9. Asahishinbun Press, **1997**, pp. 243-244.

Brecher, G., Laquer, G.L., Cronkite, E.P., Edelman, P.M. and Schwartz, I.L. (1965). The brain lesion of Goldthioglucose obesity. *J Exp Med.*, **121**: 395-401.

Brecher, G. and Waxler, S.H. (1949). Obesity in albino mice due to single injections of gold thioglucose. *Pro Soc Exp Biol Med.*, **70:** 498-501.

Brobeck, J.R. (1946). Mechanism of the development of obesity in animals with hypothalamic lesions. *Physio. Rev.*, **26:** 541-559.

Clawson, G. A. (1989). Mechanisms of carbon tetrachloride hepatotoxicity. *Pathol. Immunopathol. Res.*, **8**: 104-112.

Du, X.M., Sun, N.Y., Chen, Y., Irino, N. and Shoyama, Y. (2000a). Hepatoprotective aliphatic glycosides from three *Goodyera* species. *Biol Pharm Bull.*, **23**: 731-734.

Du, X.-M., Sun, N.-Y. and Shoyama, Y. (2000b). Flavonoids from *Goodyera schlechtendaliana*. *Phytochemistry*, **53:** 997-1000.

Du, X.M., Yoshizawa, T. and Shoyama, Y. (1998). Butanoic acid glucoside composition of whole body and *in vitro* plantlets of *Anoectochilus formosanus*. *Phytochemistry*, **49**: 1925-1928.

Faroon, O., De Rosa, C.T. and Smith, L. (1994). Carbon tetrachloride: Health effects toxicokinetics, human exposure and environmental fate. *Toxic Indust Health*, **10:** 4-20.

Goldbourt, V., Holtzman, E. and Neufeld, N.N. (1985). Total and high density lipoprotein cholesterol in the serum and risk of mortality: evidence of a threshold effect. *Br Med J.*, **290**: 1239-1243.

Han, P.W. and Liu, A.C. (1966). Obesity and impaired growth of rats force fed 40 days after hypothalamic lesions *Am J Physiol.*, **211**: 229-231.

Ito, A., Yasumoto, K., Kasai, R. and Yamasaki, K. (1994). A Sterol with an unusual side chain from *Anoectochilus koshunensis. Phytochemistry*, **36:** 1465-1467.

Jiangsu New Medical College, *Dictionary of the Traditional Chinese Medicines*, Shanghai Scientific Technologic Publishing House, Shanghai, **1977**, pp. 1334-1335.

Kan, W. S. (1986). *Pharmaceutical botany*, National Research Institute of Chinese Medicine, Taipei, p. 647.

Kannel, W.B., Castelli, W., Gordon, T. and McNamara, P.M. (1971). T Serum cholesterol, lipoproteins, and the risk of coronary heart disease: the Framingham Study. *Ann Intern Med.*, **74**: 1-12.

Lin, C.C. and Namba, T. (1981a). Pharmacognostic studies on the crude drugs of Orchidacae from Taiwan 6. *Shoyakugaku Zasshi*, **35:** 262-271.

Lin, C.C. and Namba, T. (1981b). Pharmacognostic studies on the crude drugs of Orchidacae from Taiwan 7. *Shoyakugaku Zasshi*, **35**: 272-286.

Murashige, T. and Skoog, F. (1962). A revised medium for rapid growth and bioassay with tobacco tissue culture. *Physiol Plant.*, **15:** 473-497.

Nomura, H., Kashiwagi, S., Hayashi, J., Kajiyama, W., Tani, S. and Goto, M. (1988). Prevalence of fatty liver in a general population of Okinawa, Japan. *Jpn J Med.*, **27**: 142-–149.

Pabst, A., Barron, D., Sémon, E. and Schreier, P. (1992). Two diastereomeric 3-oxo-α-ionol β-D-glucosides from raspberry fruit. *Phytochemistry*, **31**: 1649-1652.

Raucy, J.L., Kraner, J.C. and Lasker, J. (1993). Bioactivation of halogenated hydrocarbons by cytochrome P450 2E1. *Crit Rev Toxicol.*, **23**: 1-20.

Stamler, J., Wenworth, D. and Neaton, J. (1986). Is relationship between serum cholesterol and risk of premature death from coronary disease continuous and graded? Findings in 356,222 primary screenees of the Multiple Risk Factor Intervention Trial (MRFIT). *JAMA*, **256**: 2823-2828.

Taguchi, H., Yoshioka, I., Yamasaki, K. and Kim, L. (1981). Studies on the constituents of *Gastrodia elata* Blume. *Chem Pharm Bul.*, **29**: 55-62.

Index

(+)-lariciresinol 4′-O-β-D-glucoside 287
(+)-lyoniresinol-3α-O-glucopyranoside 307
(+)-medioresinol 461
(+)-syringaresinol-O-β-D-glucoside 285
(+)-Tubocurarine 310
(-)-pinoresinol-4′-O-β-D-glucopyranoside 286
(-)-tubifolidine 308
(-)-Tubifoline 307
(7S, 8R)-balanophonin-4-O-β-D-glucopyranoside 285
@20R-Hydroxypregna-4,6-diene-3,12-dione 6
1-(3-pyridyl) ethanol 307
1-methyl-2-indoleacetate 308
1-nitro-2-phenylethane 262
10-gingerol 241
11-demethoxy-12-hydroxy-3-epi-myrtoidine 290
11-demethoxy-3-epi-myrtoidine 290
11-demethoxymyrtoidine 290
11-hexadecanoic acid 469
11b-HSD1 92
1,2-benzopirone 466
1,2-benzopyrene 468
1,2-epoxy-3-(p-nitrophenoxy)propane 121
12-Hydroxy-11-methoxy-N-acetylmon-C-fluorocurarimi 303
12-Hydroxy-11-methoxy-nor-C-fluorocurarine 303
12-Hydroxy-11-methoxydiaboline 303
12-Hydroxymalagashanine 299
12β-Hydroxypregna-4,6,16-triene-3,20-dione 7
13C NMR spectra 4
16-(S)-E-isositsirikine 303
16-Hydorxy-α-colubring 302
16β,17β-Epoxy-12β-hydroxypregna-4,6-diene-3,20-dione 6
17-O-methylakagerine 306
1,8-cineol 260
18-hydroxyisosungucine 312
19,20-Dihydroakuammicine 300
^{1}H-^{15}N gHMBC 385
2-(1,3-dithian-2-yl)-indole 307
2-cyano-3-ethyl-1-methyl-1,2,3,6-tetrahydropyridin 307

2-ethyl butyl glucosinolate 445
2-Hydroxy-3-methoxystrychnine 302
2-phenyl ethyl glucosinolate (Gluconasturiin) 444
20S,21-Dihydroxypregn-4-ene-3,12-dione 9
20S,21-Dihydroxypregna-4,6-diene-3,12-dione 9
21-Hydroxypregna-4,6-diene-3,12,20-trione 6
2,3-Di-O-methylmannopyranose 296
2,3,4,6-Tetra-O-methylgalactopyranose 296
2,3,6-Tri-O-methylmannopyranose 296
3-epi-myrtoidine 289
3-hydroxy-2-methyloctynoic acid 386
3-hydroxy-3-methyl-glutaryl-CoA (HMG-CoA) 92
3′-O-acetylloganic acid 301
3,4-dehydropalicoside 305
3,4-di-O-caffeoylquinic acid 288
3,4,5-trimethoxyphenol-1-O-β-D-apiofuranosyl-(1-6) 283
3,4,5,6-tetradehydrodolichantoside 296
3′,4′,5′,6′-tetradehydrolongicaudatine Y 305
3,4,5,6-tetradehydropalicoside 296
3,5-di-O-caffeoylquinic acid 288
3β-O-(4-O-Gentiobiosyl-D-dignosyl)-8,14-epoxy-5β14β-card-20(22)-enolide 30
3β-O-(4-O-gentiobiosyl-D-dignosyl)-8,14-epoxy- 5β,14β-card-16,20 30
3β-O-(D-Diginosyl)-14-hydroxy-5β,14β-card-16,20 (22)-dienolide 21
3β-O-(D-Diginosyl)-14,16β-dihydroxy-5β,14β-card-20 20
3β-O-(D-Diginosyl)-16β-acetoxy-14-hydroxy-5α,14β-card 16
3β-O-(D-Diginosyl)-8,14,16α,17-diepoxy-5β,14β-card 11
3β-O-(D-Digitalosyl)-14-hydroxy-5α,14β-card-20(22) 20
3β-O-(D-Digitalosyl)-8,14-epoxy-5β,14β-card-16,20 20
3β-O-(D-Glucosyl)-16b-acetoxy-14-hydroxy-5β,14β-card 20
3β-O-(D-Sarmentosyl)-14-hydroxy-5β,14β-card-20(22) 11
3β-O-(D-Sarmentosyl)-8,14-epoxy-5β,14β-card-16,20 11
3β-O-[β-D-glucopyranosyl-(1→4)-β-D-diginopyranosy 23
4′, 5′-trimethoxyflavone 88
4-Hydroxystrychnine 293
4-methoxy glucobrassin 438
4-O-(3,5-dimethoxy-4-hydroxybenzoyl) quinic acid 296
4′-O-acetylloganic acid 301
4″-O-β-D-glucopyranosyl-caffeoyl-calleryanin 283
5, 7-dihydroxy-3′ 88
5-fluorouracil (5-FU) 398
5″-O-trans-feruloyl-6′-O-β-D-apiofuranosylcall 282
5″-O-trans-feruloyl-6′-O-β-dapiofuranosylvanil 282
5′,6′- dehydroguiaflavine 292
5′,6′-dehydroguiachrysine 292
6-dehydrogingerdione 243
6-gingerol 241
6′-O-acetylloganic acid 301
6′-O-β-D-apiofuranosylcalleryanin 282
6-shogaol 244
7-O-acetylloganic acid 301
7-O-trans-caffeoylvanilloloside 282
7-oxohernangerine 424
7,12-dimethylbenz (a)anthracene 3,4-dihydrodiol 121

7β-hydroxypimara-8,15-dien-14-one 306
9-cis β-carotene 138
9-methoxy-Nb-methylgeissoschizol 291
9-methoxygeissoschizol 290
9α,4α-iminoethano-carbazole 298
α-glucosidases 91
α-humulene 261
α-phellandrene 260
α -pinene 260
α -terpinene 260
α -terpinolene 260
α -Tocopherol 136
β-caryophyllene 263
β-cells 81
β-hexosaminidase 229
β-phellandrene 260
β-sitosterol 461
δ-cadinene 261
γ-linolenic acid 143
γ-schisandrin 187
γ-terpinene 259
ß-lactamase 333
ß-lactum 333

A

Abortifacient 448
Abrus precatorius 353
Acacia catechu 353
Acalypha indica L. 228
Acanthus ilicifolius 406
Acetylmalagashanol 299
Achillea millefolium 353
Achyranthes aspera 353
Aconine 131
Acorus calamus 353
Actinidia rubricaulis 196
Actinodaphnine 414
Activating protein-1 216
Adenocalymma aliaceum 270
Adenocarcinomas 115, 118
Adenomas 115
Adhatoda vasica 218, 353, 457, 459
Adhatodine 459, 226
Adhatodinine 459
Adhavasinone 459
Adipocytes 90
Adipokine 130
Advanced glycation end-products (AGEs) 80
Aedes aegypti 468
Aegiceras corniculatum 406
Aegle marmelos 353
Aerobic 109
AFLD 128
Aframomum melegueta 353
Ag-Ab reaction 227
Agarose 398
AGE-immune complexes 81
Ageratum conyzoides 353
Akagerine 298
Akuammicine 300
Alangium salviifolium 353
Albizia lebbeck (L.) Benth. 226
Alchornea trewioides 195
Alginate 398
Alisma 146
Alkaline phosphatase 115
Alkaloids 131, 396, 413, 438
Allergic diseases 215
Allicin 141
Allium cepa L. 218, 353
Allium fistulosum 150
Allium sativum 270
Aloe vera 353
Alotamide A 386

Alpha-pinene 112
Alpha2µ-globulin 108
Alpinia speciosa 269
Alstonia scholaris 353
Alternative medicine 438
Amaranthus blitum 353
Ampelopsis megalophylla 182
Amydae carapax 203
Anabaena 383
Anaerobic 109
Analgesics 259, 448
Anaphylactic shock 226
Anaxagoras dolichocarpa 268
Anchusa strigosa 353
Andrographis paniculata 353
Andrographolide 137, 241
Aniba canelilla 256, 257, 262
Aniba coto 429
Aniba muca 420
Aniba panurensis 427
Aniba rosaeodora 256, 414
Aniba santalodora 428
Anisomeles malabarica 353
Anisotine 226, 459
Annona foetida 267
Anoectochili mxburghii 151
Anoectochilus formosanus 200, 477
A. koshunensis 478
Anthocyanidins 86
Anthocyanin 87
Anti-dinitrophenyl-immunoglobulin G 216
Anti-fatty liver disease 128
Anti-hepatofibrotic drugs 178
Antialgal 407
Antiallergic 459
Antiasthamatic 447, 459
Antibacterial 3, 407, 447
Antiblenorrágico 266
Anticancer 3, 382, 396, 438
Antidiabetic 407, 438
Antidiarrheal 266
Antidote 3
Antifungal 113, 334, 407, 438
Antihyperliposis 478, 490
Antihypertensive 447, 450
Antiinflammatory 3, 279, 407, 448, 468, 470
Antilarval 113
Antileprotic 3
Antillatoxin 386
Antimalarial 382
Antimicrobial 113, 382, 465
Antinociceptive 468
Antioxidant 396, 405
Antiparasitic 470
Antiprotozoal 382, 407
Antipyretic 469
Antirheumatic 259, 267, 438
Antiscorbutic 438
Antiviral 113, 407, 457
Aphrodisiac 438
Apigenin 88, 241
Apoptosis 117, 396
Aporphine 414
Aquilegia vulgaris 200
Arachidonic acid 144
Arbortristoside-A 242
Arrhythmia 3
Artemia franciscana 469
Artemia salina 269, 461, 469
Artemisia capillaries 151
Artemisia vulgaris 353
Arthritis 480

Arthrospira maxima 150
Asarinine 461
Ash bark 148
Asidospermine 316
Aspalathin 89
Aspalathus linearis 89
Aspergillus flavus 270
Asphodeline lutea 353
Asteracantha longifolia 353
Astragaline 459
Astrogalosides 189
Atherogenesis 81
Atherosclerosis 482
Atracurium 311
Aurothioglucose 480
Avena sativa 353
Avicennia alba 406
Avicennia marina 406
Axillarenic acid 228
Axillaroside 283
Ayurveda 227, 278

B

Baccharis glutinosa 354
Bacillus cereus 451
Bacillus subtilis 465
Backhousia citriodora 350
Baicalin 137, 189
Baliospermum montanum 228
Basophils 216
Bauhinia vahlii 354
Bemisia tabaci 450
Benziltetrahydroisoquinolines 414
Benzyl benzoate 264
Benzylisothiocyanate 449
Berberine 131, 179, 302
Beta1-elemene 192
Betaine 132, 181
Bidens bipinnata 182
Bilirubin 115
Bioactive pregnanes 1
Bioavailability 88
Biochanin A 92
Biodegradation 109
Biodiversity 218
Bioflavonoids 80
Biomphalaria glabrata 390
Bipolaris sorokiniana 265
Bisebromoamide 385
Bisnordihydrotoxiferine 295
Bixa orellana L. 256
Blue-green algae 382
Boerhavia diffusa L. 229
Boldine 416
Boswellia ameero 354
Boswellia elongata 354
Brassaiopsis palmata 354
Brassicaceae 437
Breviscapine 201
Bronchial asthma 218
Bronchodilatory 447, 451
Broth dilution method 349
Brucine 278, 293
Brucine N-oxide 301
Bruguiera cylindrica 406
Bruguiera gymnorrhiza 406
Bupleurum salicifolium 340
Burasaine 308
Buxus hildebrandtii 354

C

C-alkaloid A 309
C-alkaloid E 309
C-alkaloid F 309
C-alkaloid G 309
C-alkaloid H 309

C-alkaloid O 291
C-calebassine 310
C-curarine 309
C-dihydrotoxiferine 308
C-Jun N-terminal kinase (JNK) 84
C-mavacurine 300
C-profluorocurine 291
C-Toxiferine 308
CaCo-2 colon cancer cell line 407
Caffeic acids 335
Caffeoylcalleryanin 284
Calleryanin 284
Calluna vulgaris 354
Calophyllum inophyllum 354
Calothrix 383
Calotropis gigantea 354
Calyptranthes spruceana 269
Campesterol 464
Camphene 227
Cancer 396, 480
Candida albicans 266, 338
Cantleyoside 287
Capparis spinosa 354
Capsaicin 138
Capsosiphon fulvescens 401
Carcinogenic 114, 117
Cardenolide 3
Cardenolide monoglycoside 3
Cardenolide triglycoside 3
Cardenolides 1
Cardiospermum halicacabum 354
Cardiotonic properties 3
Cardiovascular 269
Cardiovascular disorder 480
Carica papaya 354
Carminative 269, 438
Carphalea obovata 354
Carrageenan 398, 465
Carvacrol 227
Carvone 113
Caryophyllene 227
Casca-preciosa 257
Cassia fistula 354
Cassia tora 354
Cassytha filiformis 420
Catafiline 420
Cataformine 420
Catha edulis 354
Celosia argentea 354
Centaurea appendicigera 354
Centaurium erythraea 354
Centella asiatica 354
Centrolobular hepatocytes 480
Ceriops decandra 406, 407
Chalcones 87
Champia feldmannii 398
Chelating metal ions 88
Chelerythrine 180
Chelidonium majus 354
Chemokine (C-C motif) ligand 11 216
Chemopreventive 114
Chemoprotective 447
Chemotherapeutic agent 332
Chicory Polysaccharide 142
Chiral molecule 108
Chlorofluorocarbons 113
Chlorogenic acid 444
Chloromycetin 333
Chlorotetracycline 333
Chondrococcus hornemanni 405
Chondroitin Sulfate 142
Chrysanthemum cinerariifolium 265
Cichorium intybus 355
Cineole 227

Cinnamaldehyde 262
Cinnamomum cassia 149
Cinnamomum iners 355
Cinnamomum zeylanicum 256
Cinnamon verum 262
Cirrhosis 128
Cis-3α-(O-Nitrophenyl) hexahydroindol-4-one 300
Cissampelos pareira 355
Cissus quandrangularis 355
Citrus acida 355
Citrus aurantifolia 355
Citrus aurantium 355
Citrus reticulata 112
Cladosiphon okamuranusa 399
Cladosporium cladosporioides 266
C. sphaerospermumas 266
Clausena excavata 355
Cleanser 269
Clematis cirrhosa 355
Cleome socotrana 355
Clerodendron serratum Spreng. 226
Clerodendrum indicum 355
Clerodendrum infortunatum 355
Clerodendrum serratum 355
Clidemia hirta 355
Clostridium botulinum 337
Cluster of differentiation 216
Cnidium monnieri 141
CNS depression 269
Coastal marine ecosystem 407
Coccoid 382
Coibamide A 385
Cola greenwayi 355
Colletotrichum gloeosporiodes 265
Colorectal cancer 114
Colpomenia sinuosa 397
Colubrine 293
Combretum apiculatum 355
Combretum woodii 336
Commelina communis 355
Commiphora myrrha 259
Commiphora parvifolia 355
COMPARE analysis 385
Complementary and alternative medicine 128
Conjugated linoleic acid 142
Cordyceps sinensis 155
Coronary heart disease 482
Corosolic acid 138
Cortex fraxini 148
Corydalis saxicola 180
Corydyceps polysaccharide 192
COSY 385
Coumarins 338, 438
COX-2 mRNA 136
Crataegus pinnatifida 146
Crescentia cujete 355
Crinipellis perniciosa 337
Crithmum maritimum 356
Croton cajucara 268
Croton hirtus 356
Croton palanostigma 268
Cryptocarya chinensis 421
Cryptocarya lævigata 421
Cryptocarya oubatchensis 429
Cryptocarya phyllostemon 429
Cryptolepine 315
Cryptowolidine 429
Cryptowoline 429
Cryptowolinol 429
Cucurbitacin 137, 188
Cudrania cochin chinensis 182
Curculigo orchioides Gaertn 226

Curculigoside A 226, 240
Curculigoside B 226
Curcuma longa L. 227
Curcumin 135, 184, 239
Curtisia dentata 356
Cuscuta reftexa 356
Cussonia spicata 356
Cyclea pehata 356
Cyclic adenosine monophosphate 216
Cyclin-dependent kinase inhibitor 1A (Cdkn1a) 89
Cymbopogon citratus 257
Cymodocea serrulata 408
Cyperus articulatus 257
Cyperus rotundus 356
Cyphostemma flaviflorum 356
Cyphostemma lanigerum 356
Cyphostemma natalitium 356
Cystadenocarcinoma 118
Cystostemon socotranus 356
Cytosolic ATP 84
Cytotoxic 383, 457, 469
Cytotoxic activity 3

D

d-galactose 399
d-limonene 108
d-mannose 399
d-xylose 399
Daidzein 239
Danshen 145
Danshensu 136
Datura stramonium 356
Daucus carota 356
Db/db mice 90
De novo 335
Deacetyldiaboline 289
Dean-stark procedure 112
Dehaasia longipedicellata 430
Dehydronantenine 426
Delphinium formosum 356
Demulcent 438
Depurative 438
Dermatitis 226
Desmos dumosus 356
Desoxycordifoline 297
Diabetes 79, 128, 482
Diabetes mellitus 80
Diabetic nephropathy 81
Diabetic neuropathy 81
Diabetic retinopathy 81
Diaboline 288
Diacylglycerol 84
Diallil sulfide 269
Diarrhoea 227
Dicentrine 414
Dictyota dichotoma 405
Didymocarpus crinita 356
Dietary ω-3 and ω-6 polyunsaturated fatty acids 143
Digitoxin 3
Diglycoside 3
Digoxin 3
Dihydroquercetin 444
Dihydrousambarensine 312
Dillapiole 266
Dillenia suffruticosa 357
Dioscorea membranacea 232
Dioscorealide A 242
Dioscorealide B 243
Dioscoreanone 243
Diosgenin 242
Diosmetin 88
Diosmin 89
Dipentene 108

Dipteryx odorata 257
Disk diffusion method 348
Disodium cromoglycate 216
Diterpenes 231
Diuretic 265, 269, 438
Docosahexaenoic acid 144
Dolastatins 383
Dolichantoside 297
Dombeya burgessiae 357
Dombeya cymosa 357
Dombeya rotundifolia 357
DPPH radical scavenging assay 406
Drug discovery 382
Drymaria diandra 339
Drynaria quercifolia 357
Dypterix odorata 268
Dysentery 227

E

Ecklonia cava 398
Eclipta alba 357
Eclipta prostrata 357
Eczema 216
Edwardsiella tarda 270
Eicosanoid acids 469
Eicosapentaenoic acid 143
Eicosapentaenoic acid ethyl ester 144
Eisenia bicyclis 398
Elaeocarpus tuberculatus 357
Elaeodendron transvaalense 357
Elephantopus scaber 357
Elephantorrhiza burkei 357
Eleusine indica 357
Ellagic acid 406
Embryotoxic 114
Emetine 311
Emilia sonchifolia 357
Emmenagogue 438
Emodin 135
Empetrum nigrum 357
Enhalus acoroides 407
Enicostema littorale 357
Enterobacter aerogenes 265, 270
Enterococcus faecalis 333
Enterococcus hirae 340
Environmental protection agency (EPA) 108
Epigallocatechin 89
Epigallocatechin-3-gallate 91, 134, 184
Epigallocatechin-3-O-gallate 243
Epilepsy 386
Epilobium angustifolium 357
Equisetum telmateia 357
Erigeron breviscapus 151
ERK signalling pathways 401
Eryngium creticum 357
Erythrophleum lasianthum 357
Escherichia coli 270, 451
Escualene 467
Essential oils 256, 338, 414
Eucommia ulmoides 93
Eugenol 227, 240, 262
Eugenol methyl ether 227
Eupatorium odoratum 357
Euphorbia antiquorum L. 228
Euphorbia hirta L. 227, 357
Euphorbia tirucalli L. 228
Euryops arabicus 358
Evening primrose 150
Evolvulus alsinodes L. 229
Excoecaria agallocha 406

F

Fagonia luntii 358
Fatty liver disease (FLD) 128
Fc epsilon RI 216

Febrifuge 267
Femiforte 226
Fenugreek 148
Fenugreek saponins 139
Ferulic acid 444
Festuclavine 314
Fetal bovine serum 216
Fibrosis 128
Ficus benghalensis 358
Ficus religiosa 358
Filipendula ulmaria 358
Flavones 86, 87
Flavonoids 79, 231, 336, 438, 459
Flavonols 86
Flavonone 86, 87
Flourocurarine 289
Fluorocurine 291
Folk medicine 267
Food and drug administration (FDA) 108
Forced vital capacity (FVC) 451
Formononetin 92
Forskolin 239
Fragrance 117
Fraxinus rhynchophylla 198
Fucoidan 398
Fucus evanescens 399
Fucus vesiculosus 399
Fusarium oxysporum 265

G

Galactagogue 438
Galactan 295
Galactomannan 295
Galaxaura marginata 397
Gallic acid 444
Ganoderma 201
GC/MS 458
Gelidiella acerosa 405
Gene expression 84
Genistein 89
Genotoxicity 404, 468
Geranium asphodeloides 358
Giardia duodenalis 465
Giardia lamblia 465
Gingivitis 459
Gingko biloba 133, 146, 195
Glomerulus 81
Glucobenzosisbbrin 445
Glucobrassicanapin 438
Glucocorticoids (GC) 91, 130
Gluconasturtin 438
Glucose 487
Glucose-6-phosphatase 91
Glucosinolates 335
Glucosuria 80
Glucotropaeolin 444, 449
GLUT2 132
GLUT4 90
Glutamine 140
Glycosides 232
Glycyrrhiza glabra 156
Glycyrrhiza uralensis 358
Glycyrrhizin 186
GOT 480
GPT 480
Gracilaria edulis 405
Green tea 133, 147
Guatteria juruensis 267
Guatteriopsis blepharophylla 267
Guiachrysine 291
Guiaflavine 292
Guianensine 290
Gunnera perpensa 358
Gymnadenia conopsea 232
Gymnantes lucida 358

Gymnema montanum 156
Gymnema sylvestre 156
Gynostemma pentaphyllum 150

H

H_1 receptor 216
H2BC 385
Haemostatics 259
Halodule pinifolia 407, 408
Halophila ovalis 408
Hantupeptin A 385
Harpephyllum caffrum 358
Hawthorn Leaf 133
Heart failure 386
Heartburn 114, 116
Hedyotis capitellata 358
Hedyotis congesta 358
HeLa cells 216
Hemidesmus indicus 358
Hemostatic 266
Henrietta lacks cells 216
Hepatic glutathione-S-transferase activity 121
Hepatocellular carcinogenesis 129
Hepatocellular carcinoma 128
Hepatoprotective 447
HepG2 cells 60
Heracleum platytaenium 358
Herbal drugs 334
Herbal medicines 438
Herbivores 407
Hernandine 424
Hernandonine 424
Hernangerine 424
Hesperidin 91, 92, 134
Heteromorpha trifoliata 358
Hevea brasiliensis 256
Hexosamine pathway 83, 85
Hibiscus sabdariffa 199
Hippophae rhamnoides 358
Hirudin 190
Histamine 227
Histamine H1 receptor (H1R) 216
HMBC 385
Holarrhena antidysenterica 358
Holotrichia diomphalia 203
Holstiine 293
Homeopathic medicine 128
Homeostasis 91
Honokiol 136
Hovenia acerba 148
HPLC 458
Hsian-tsao 201
HSQC-TOCSY 385
Human epidermal growth factor receptors 397
Hyaluronic acid 181
Hypercholesterolemia 80
Hyperglycaemia 80
Hyperlipidemia 482
Hyperliposis 482
Hypertriglyceridemia 80
Hypnea pannosa 405
Hypoglycaemic 437, 447, 449
Hypotensive 269
Hyptis crenata 268
Hyptis suaveolens 358

I

Icajine 294
IgE antibody 227
Immunomodulation 178, 396
In vitro 58, 82, 108, 181, 218, 335, 385, 420, 459, 461
In vivo 63, 181, 231, 351, 383, 459
Indole 413

Inflammation 216, 461, 480
Inflammatory cytokine 130
Inflammatory pathways 129
Insecticidal 447
Insecticide 113
Insulin-dependent diabetes mellitus (IDDM) 80
Insulin-like growth factor (IGF) 397
Interleukin-1 54
Interleukin-10 155
Interleukins 216
Intestinal parasitosis 227
Intrinsic pathways 398
Inula viscosa 358
Iridoid glycosides 335
Isoboldine 414
Isobrucine 302
Isobrucine-N-oxide 302
Isocorydine 414, 416
Isocryptolepine 315
Isoflavones 86, 87
Isoflavonoids 335
Isomers 117
Isoneocryptolepine 315
Isoquinoline 413
Isoretuline 292
Isostrychnine 302
Isostrychnine-N-oxide 302
Isostrychnopentamine 305
Isosungucine 312
Isotachioside 283

J

Jamaicamide A 386
Jatropha unicostata 358
Juglans regia 358
Juniperus lucayana 359
Justicia adhatoda 459
Justicia glauca 461
Justicia hyssopifolia 461
Justicia pectoralis 465
Justicia procumbrens 460
Justicia prostate 461
Justicia secunda 465, 469
Justicia simplex 461
Justicia spicigera 465
Justicidiane B 467
Justicisaponin 461

K

Kadsura coccinea 202
Kaempferia parviflora Wall. Ex. Baker. 228
Kaempferol 88, 241, 459
Kalanchoe farinacea 359
Kalanchoe pinnata 359
Kalkitoxin 386
Kappaphycus alvarezii 405
Kappaphycus striatum 403
Ketoacidosis 80
Kinsenoside 477, 487
Klebsiella pneumoniae 265, 270
Knema malayana 359
Kupffer cells 200
Kutkin 227, 240

L

L-arginine 141
l-limonene 108
Lagerstroemia speciosa 359
Laminaria angustata 398
Laminaria japonica 398
Laminaria religiosa 398
Lamium album 359
Lantana camara 359
Larrea tridentata 359
Lauraceae 413
Laurolitsine 414

Laurotetanine 414, 416
Laurus nobilis 261
LDH 480
LDL 484
Lectins 339
Leishmania donovani 388
Leishmania mexicana 388, 465
Lepidimoide 444
Lepidine 437, 444
Lepidium sativum 437
Leptin 155
Leptolyngbya sp. 385
Letospermum petersonii 350
Leucas aspera 359
Leucojum vernum 339
Leucoxene 425
Leukotrienes 216, 227
Licaria martiniana 264
Licaria puchury-major 257, 264
Lignans 457
Ligustrazine 141
Limonene 107, 269
Linalool 227, 262
Lindera angustifolia 424
Lindera chunii 424
Lindera pipericarpa 424
Lipogenesis 129
Lippia alba 257
Lippia nodiflora 359
Liquiritigenin 92
Liriodendrin 286
Liriodenine 414
Lisicamine 420
Lithium-2-(lithiomethyl)indole-1-carboxylate 308
Lithraea molleoides 359
Litsea coreana 182
Litsea læta 424
Litsea salicifolia 424
Liver fibrosis 178
Loganiaceae 278
Loganic acid 287
Loganin 287
Longicaudatine 313
Longicaudatine Y 305
Losartan 130
Lumnitzera racemosa 407
Luteolin 242
Lycium barbarum 148
Lycium barbarum Polysaccharides 142
Lycium europeum 359
Lycopene 138, 192
Lycopodium cernuum 359
Lygodium flexuosum 200
Lymphadenopathy 117
Lyngbya aestuarii 383
Lyngbya bouillonii 386
Lyngbya confervoides 383
Lyngbya majuscula 383
Lythrum salicaria 359

M

Machillus yaoshansis 431
Macrocarpamine 313
Macusine B 292
Magnolia officinalis 149
Malagashanine 299
Malagashanol 299
MALDI-TOFMS 278
Malignant tumors 397
Mallotus phillppensis 359
Malondialdehyde (MDA) 452
Malva moschata 359
Mangifera indica 359
Mangroves 405

Manzamine A 315
Mapania cuspidata 359
MAPK-PP1 pathways 90
Maranta arundinaceae 359
Marfey's analysis 388
Marine cyanobacteria 381
Marine natural compounds 396
Marsupin 92
Mass spectrometry (MS) 345
Mast cells 216
Mastigocoleus laminosus 383
Matopensine 303
Matricaria chamomilla 359
Matrine 179
Mavacurine 291
MDR reversal activity 3, 67
Medicinal plants 218, 331
Melastoma malabathricum 359
Melatonin 132, 191
Melicoccus bijugatus 360
Melinonine F 297
Memecylon excelsum 360
Mentha piperita 257
Mentha suaveolens 257
Mesangial cells 81
Messenger RNA 216
Metabolic disorder 80
Metabolic syndromes 128
Metastasis 397
Methyl benzoate 262
Methyl chavicol 227
Methyl glucosinolate (Glucocapprin) 445
MHC antigens 404
Micrococcus luteus 451
Micromeria nervosa 360
Millettia extensa 360
Mimosa pigra 360
Minfiensine 298
Minimal inhibitory concentration 458
Mitochondrial dysfunction 130
Mitochondrial pathway 118
Moandaensine 298
Modern medicine 278
MOLT-4 leukemia cell line 386
Momordica charantia 360
Monochordia vaginalis 360
Monostroma nitidum 398
Monoterpenes 117, 256, 261
Montanin 228, 241
Morin 88, 183
Moringa oleifera 360
Mortierella isabellina 155
Morus alba 204
MRNA 84
MRNA expression 216
MTT assay 55, 470
Multiplicity-edited HSQS 385
Murraya exotica 360
Murraya koenigii 360
Mutagenic 114
Mycobacterium tuberculosis 333, 458
Myrcetin 88
Myrcianthes cisplatensis 360
Myrtoidine 290

N

n-3 Polyunsaturated Gatty Acids 143
n-BuOH 487
N-desacetylisoretuline 303
N-desacetylretuline 303
N-desacetylspermostrychnine 303
N-formyl-asidospermidine 316
N-methyl-3-bromotyrosine 385
N-methylhernangerine 424

N-methylisocryptolepinium 315
N-methyllaurotetanine 414, 416
N-substituted D3-piperidein-2-ones 307
N1-methyl-δ-carboline 315
N_a-deacetyl-Na-methyl-SB 308
N_a-deacetyl-SB 308
NAFLD 128
Nantenine 426
Naringenin 88, 243
Naringenin-7-O-glucoside 89
Natural drugs 128, 178
Natural products 128, 382, 438
Nβ-methyl-21-β-hydroxy-mayumbine 298
Nectandra rigida 427
Neochlorogenic acid 444
Neocryptolepine 315
Neonauclea pallida 360
Nephropathy 113, 117
Nephroprotective 447, 452
Nephrosis 482
Nephrotoxic 114
Neriaside [3β-O-(D-Diginosyl)-8,14-seco-14α-hydroxy 22
Neritaloside [3β-O-(D-Digitalosyl)-16β-acetoxy-14-hydroxy 20
Nerium oleander 1
Nerol 227
Neuroblastoma cell lines 388
Neuropathic pain 386
Neurotoxic 382
Neurotoxins 382, 386
NF-*k*B 60, 84, 132, 136, 229
Niacin 443
Nitric oxide 216
N,N-diallyltoxiferine (alcuronium) 310
N,O-dimethylharnovine 424
Non-genotoxic 114
Non-insulin dependent diabetes mellitus (NIDDM) 80
Normalindine 296
Norpreocoteine 427
Norpurpureine 427
Nostoc 383
Novacine 294
Nuclear factor kappa B 216
Nuclear factor of activated T cells 216
Nuclear magnetic resonance spectroscopy (NMR) 345
Nuclear proteins DNA 480

O

O-methyl-cryptowoline 429
O-methyl-cassifoline 425
Obesity 128, 482
Ochrolifuanine A 312
Ocimum basilicum L. 227
Ocimum canum L. 227
Ocimum gratissimum L. 227
Ocimum sanctum L. 227, 360
Ocokriptine (N-methylhernandine) 424
Ocominarine 425
Ocopodine 425
Ocotea duckei 425
Ocotea minarum 428
Ocotea odorifera 414
Ocotea porosa 414
Ocotea pretiosa 262
Ocotea quixos 262
Ocotea vellosiana 425
Ocoteine 425
Ocotominarine 425
Odoroside H [3β-O-(D-Digitalosyl)-14-hydroxy-5β,14β-card 20
Oenanthe javanica 133, 183

Oldenlandia corymbosa 360
Oleandrin [3β-O-(L-oleandrosyl)-16β-aceoxy-14-hydroxy 20
Oleaside A [(8R)-3β-O-(D-Diginosyl)-14-oxo-15(14 →8)abeo-5β-card-20(22)-enolide] 22
Oleoresin 258
Olive leaf extract 147
Onobrychis armena 360
Ophiorrhiza nicobarica 339
Ophthalmic 438
Oral contraceptive 447
Orchidaceae 477
Orcinol glycoside 226
Orlistat 130
Oroxylum indicum 360
Ortho-azido aryl carbamate 298
Oscillatoria nigroviridis 383, 388
Osthol 141
Ovalbumin 216
Oxalis corniculata 360
Oxazole 382
Oxidation assay 406
Oxidative cell death assay 406
Oxidative stress 80, 130
Oxymatrine 132, 179
Oxytetracycline 333

P

P-cymen-8-ol 260
P-cymene 260
P-menth-3-ene 260
P38 MAPK signalling 90
Padina antillarum 405
Padina gymnospora 405
Padina tetrastomatica 405
Paeonia lactiflora 145
Palicoside 297
Palidine 414
Palmyrolide A 386
Panax ginseng 139
Panax notoginseng 145, 188
Panax notoginsenosides 139
Panganensines R 304
Panganensines S 304
Panganensines X 304
Panganensines Y 304
Papaver lateritium 360
Papaver somniferum 339
Parietaria diffusa 360
Passepartout 139
Passive cutaneous anaphylaxis 216
Pathogenesis 128
Pathogens 332
Pavine 413
Peganine 459
Pentoxifylline 132, 179
Peptides 396
Peracetyl-kinsenoside 489
Pergularia daemia 360
Perialdehyde 269
Peristrophe roxburghiana 151
Peristrophe tinctoria 360
Petitia domingensis 361
Phaganalon rupestre 361
Phagocytosis 117
Pharmacotherapy 130
Phaseolus trilobus 196
Phenolic compounds 79
Phenylpropanoids 256
Phoebe grandis 427
Phoebe molicella 427
Phoebe pittieri 427
Phormidium gracile 386
Phormidium tenue 383
Phosphoenolpyruvate carboxykinase

(PEPCK) 90
Phyllanthus acidus 361
Phyllanthus emblica 226, 361
Phyllanthus urinaria 152
Phytoalexins 335
Phytoanticipins 335
Phytochemicals 177, 277
Phytoconstituents 227
Phytomedicine 468
Picconioside I 287
Picea abies 361
Picrorhiza kurroa Royle. ex Benth. 152, 227
Pinus sylvestris 361
Piper aduncum 265
Piper bartlingianumm 266
Piper betel 195
Piper callosum 266
Piper guineense 361
Piper hispidinervium 265
Piper longum L. 226, 361
Piper nigrum L. 226, 361
Piper porphyrophyllum 361
Piper stylosum 361
Piperonal 266
Piperonil butoxide 266
Pistacia lentiscus 361
Pittosporum viridiflorum 361
PKC pathways 90
Plant kingdom 79
Plantago intermedia 361
Plasmodium falciparum 388
Platycodin 140
Platycodon grandiflorum 146
Plectonema 383
Pleurothyrium cinereum 427
Pleurotus serotinus 152
Plumbago indica 361
Polyalthia lateriflora 361
Polyalthia longijblia 361
Polydextrose 142
Polygonum cuspidatum 144
Polygonum multiflorum 145
Polygonum punctatum 361
Polyketides 396
Polyol pathway 83
Polypeptide chains 382
Polypeptides 339
Polyphenols 232
Polysaccharides 397
Polysiphonia urceolata 405
Posidonia oceanica 408
Potentilla chinensis 201
Pothomorphe umbellata 267
Pratensein 92
Preocoteine 427
Primula longipes 361
Proantohocyanidins 337
Prokaryotic 382
Propargylic silane 300
Prostaglandin 216
Prostaglandins E2 216
Protein kinase C 83
Proteus mirabilis 265, 270
Proteus vulgaris 265, 337
Protium hebetatum 260
Protium heptaphyllum 259
Protostrychnine 295
Prunus padus 362
Pruscaria celligrica 407
Pseudobrucine 294
Pseudocolubrine 293
Pseudomonas aeruginosa 333, 390, 451, 458, 465

Pseudostrychnine 293
Psoralea corylifolia 362
Psoriasis 216
Psychotria capensis 362
Psychotria nervosa 362
Pterosupin 92
Pueraria lobata 232
Puerarin 135
Pulicaria stephanocarpa 362
Pulmonary diseases 259
Punica granatum 362
Punica protopunica 362
Pureraira lobata 218
Purpureine 427
Pyridine 413

Q

QSAR 178
Quercetin 88, 136, 187, 239, 444, 459
Quercetine 467
Quercitrin 239
Quercus macranthera 362
Quercus pontica 362
Quinones 336

R

Rabdosiin 244
Radical scavenging 405
Radix ampelopsis 194
Radix polygoni multiflori 145
Rafflesia hasseltii 362
Randia spinosa 362
Raspberry ketone 136
Rat basophilic leukemic cells 216
Rat paw oedema 465
Rat peritoneal mast cells 216
Rauvolfia caffra 362
Ravensara anisata 430
Raw hawthorn 147
Reactive nitrogen species 82
Reactive oxygen species 82, 216, 404
Receptor tyrosine kinases (RTKs) 397
Red peony root 145
Reduced glutathione (GSH) 452
Reseda lutea 362
Resveratrol 136, 185
Reticuline 414
Retinol 137
Retoquinesine 461
Retuline 292
Rhamnetin 88
Rhaponitin 137
Rhaponticum carthamoides 362
Rhapontigenin 243
Rhein 135, 185
Rheum undulatum L. 232
Rhizophora apiculata 406
Rhizophora lamarkii 406
Rhizophora mangle 406
Rhizophora mucronata 406
Rhizophora stylosa 406
Rhococcus equi 267
Rhodamnia cinerea 362
Rhododendron ponticum 362
Rhoicissus digitata 362
Rhoicissus rhomboidea 363
Rhoicissus tomentosa 363
Rhoicissus tridentata 363
Rhubarb 144
Ribes nigrum 363
Riboflavin 443
Ricinus communis L. 228
Robinin 88
ROESY 385
Rosa canina 363
Rosa pisiformis 363

Rosemary leaf 147
Rosmarinic acid 187
Rosmarinus officinalis 363
Rubus chamaemorusa 363
Rubus idaeus 363
Rumex hastatus 363
Rungia parviflora 363
Ruscus aculeatus 363
Ruta chalepensis 363
Ruta graveolens 363
Ruvegacient 438

S

Safrole 264
Saikosaponin-d 188
Salacia microsperma 363
Salidroside 188
Salix caprea 364
Salix rizeensis 364
Salmonella sp. 265, 270
Salmonella typhi 333, 451
Salvia fruticosa 364
Salvia miltiorrhiza 193
Salvianolic acid B 186
Sanguinaria 469
Sanguisorba officinalis 364
Sansevieria hyacinthoides 364
Saponins 139, 232, 335
Sarcopoterium spinosum 364
Sargassum fusiforme 149
Sargassum marginatum 405
Sargassum wightii 405
Sassafras albidum 427
Saururus chinensis 199
Schefflera heterophylla 364
Schefflera oxyphylla 364
Schinus terebinthifolius 364
Schisandra chinensis 156
Schizandrin 188
Schotia brachypetala 364
Scindapsus officinals 364
Sclerocarya birrea 364
Scorzonoside 285
Scutellaria baicalensis 183
Scytonema 383
Seagrasses 407
Seal oil ω-3 polyunsaturated fatty acids 143
Sebastiania brasiliensis 364
Sebastiania klotszchiana 364
Secale cereale 364
Secondary metabolites 382, 396, 405
Sedum sarmentosum 152
Semen hoveniae 198
Senecio vulgaris 364
Sennapetersiana 364
Sesamine 461
Sesamoline 461
Sesquiterpenes 231, 256, 335
Sibutramine 130
Sida cordata 364
Sida shomibtia 364
Siddha 278
Silibinin 136
Silymarin 134, 186
Simpletoxine 461
Simplexoside 461
Sinapic acid 444
Sitophilus zeamais 266
Smila leucophylla 364
Solamargine 339
Solanum indicum L. 229
Solanum khasianum 339
Solanum nigrum L. 229
Solanum torvum 364
Solanum tuberosum 365

Sonerila begoniaefolia 365
Sonneratia apetala 406
Sophora tonkinensis 145
Soy protein concentrate 148
Soybean peptide 141
Spirostachys africana 365
Spirulina platensis 150
Spodoptera frugiperda 265
Spondias pinnata 365
Stachytarpheta indica 365
Staphylococcus aureus 265, 270, 333, 451
Staphylococcus sp. 337
Statins 130
Steatohepatitis 128
Steatonecrosis 128
Stellaria holostea 365
Stephania tetrandra 195
Stereochemistry 487
Steroids 396
Sterols 438
Stigmasterol 464
Stilbenes 232
Stilbenoids 336
Stimulants 259
Streptococcus mutans 337
Streptococcus pneumoniae 332
Streptococcus sobrinus 337
Streptozotocin 93
Strictosidine β-glucosidase 297
Strictosidinic acid 288
Stroke 386
Strychnine 278, 288
Strychnine N-oxide 301
Strychnobrasiline 298
Strychnogucine B 294
Strychnohexamine 295
Strychnopentamine 311
Strychnos 278
Strychnos axillaris 279
Strychnos bicirohssa 279
Strychnos diaboli 279
Strychnos diplotricha 279
Strychnos guianensis 280
Strychnos henningsii 281
Strychnos icaja 281
Strychnos innocua 316
Strychnos johnsonii 316
Strychnos lucida 316
Strychnos mellodora 317
Strychnos minfiensine 317
Strychnos moandaensis 317
Strychnos myrtoides 317
Strychnos nux-vomica 318
Strychnos panganensis 320
Strychnos potatorum 321
Strychnos pseudoquina 322
Strychnos spinosa 321
Strychnos trinervis 321
Strychnos usambarensis 321
Strychnos vanprukii 321
STZ diabetic rats 449
Suaeda monica 407
Sucrose 487
Sulphur glycosides 437
Sungucine 294
Superoxide anions ($\bullet O_2^-$) 82
Superoxide dismutase (SOD) 452
Suregada multiflora 231
Sweet potato vines 142
Sweroside 287
Symbiosis 438
Symploca sp. 383
Syphilis 438
Syringodium isoetifolium 407

T

Tachioside 283
Tachyphylaxis 447
Tachyspermum ammi 365
Tamarindus indica 365
Tanaecium nocturnum 270
Tannins 337
Tanshinone 183
Taraxerol 467
Taurine 140
TCM 128
Tecomaria capensis 365
Tenesmus 438
Tephrosia purpurea L. 229
Teratogenic 438
Terguide 314
Terminalia alata 365
Terminalia bellerica Roxb., 226, 365
Terminalia catappa 365, 406
Terminalia chebula Retz., 226, 365
Terminalia sericea 365
Terpene derivatives 137
Terpenoids 338, 396
Terpinen-4-ol 260
Tetracyclic-1,2,3,4,5,6-hexahydro-1,5-methanoazoci 307
Tetramethylpyrazine 191
Tetrandrine 180
Teucrium chamaedrys 156
Teuerium polium 156
Thalassia hemprichii 407
Thermogenic 438
Thespesia lampas 365
Thespesia populnea 365
Thiamine 443
Thiazole 382
Thottea siliquosa 365
Thymus vulgaris 365
Tilapia nilotica 461
Tinospora cordifolia 365
TLC-Bioautography 350
TNF-α 60, 132, 227, 403
TOCSY 385
Trachystemon orientalis 366
Traditional Ayurvedic medicines 227
Traditional Chinese medicine 130, 178
Traditional medicine 334, 438, 470
Traditional systems of medicine 278
Trevesia burckii 366
Trichocalyx obovatus 366
Trichomes 383
Trichopus zeylanicus 366
Tricyclic vinylidene ketone 300
Trigonella foenum graecum 148
Trimethoxyflavone 88
Triplostoside A 288
Tripterygium glycosides 139
Triterpeines 438
Triterpenoid α-amyrin 459
Trypanosoma cruzi 388
Trypanossoma brucei 420
Tryptothrine 315
Tubifolidine 300
Tubular cell hyperplasia 115
Tubulosine 311
Tumor necrosis factor-α 55, 216
Tumor necrosis factor receptor (TNFR) 398
Tumorigenesis 397
Turbinaria conoides 405
Turpentine 112
Tussilago farfara 366
Tylophora indica 231
Typha capensis 366

U

Ulva lactuca 398
Umbeliferone 466
Unani 278
Undaria pinnatifida 398, 405
Urena lobata 366
Uronic acid 399
Ursodeoxycholic acid 138
Ursodiol 130
Ursolic acid 191
Urticaria 226
Usambarensine 311
Usambrarane 307

V

Vaccinium ashei 156
Vaccinium myrtillus 366
Vaccinium oxycoccus 366
Vanilloloside 284
Vanprukoside 306
Vasicine 239
Vasicinol 226, 459
Vasicinone 226, 459
Vasicoline 226
Vasicolinone 226
Verbascum varians 366
Vernonia cinerea 366
Vero cells 388
Villalstonine 313
Viola diffusa 202
Vitex leucoxyhm 366
Vitex negundo 366
Vitis coignetiae 156
VLDL 484
Voacamine 314
Vomicine 294

W

Western Ghats 218
Withaferin A 240
Withananine 228
Withania adunensis 366
Withania riebeckii 366
Withania somnifera Dunal 228
Withanine 228
Withanolides A-Y 228
Woodfordia fruticosa 366

X

Xylocarpus granatum 407
Xylopia aethiopica 366
Xylopia emarginata 268

Z

Zedoary 145
Zhijuzi 148
Zingiber cassumunar Roxb. 228
Zingiber officinale Roscoe 226, 366
Zizyphus jujuba 367
Zizyphus spinachristi 198, 367
Zygophyllum quatarense 367